Workplace Health Surveillance

Workplace Health Surveillance

An Action-Oriented Approach

Edited by

Neil A. Maizlish

OXFORD
UNIVERSITY PRESS
2000

OXFORD
UNIVERSITY PRESS

Athens Auckland Bangkok Bogotá Buenos Aires Calcutta
Cape Town Chennai Dar es Salaam Delhi Florence Hong Kong Istanbul
Karachi Kuala Lumpur Madrid Melbourne Mexico City Mumbai
Nairobi Paris São Paulo Shanghai Singapore Taipei Tokyo Toronto Warsaw

and associated companies in
Berlin Ibadan

Published by Oxford University Press, Inc.,
198 Madison Avenue, New York, New York, 10016
http://www.oup-usa.org

Library of Congress Cataloging-in-Publication Data
Workplace health surveillance : an action-oriented approach /
edited by Neil A. Maizlish.
p. cm. Includes bibliographical references and index.
ISBN 0-19-512888-5 (acid-free paper)
1. Occupational health services.
2. Public health surveillance
I. Maizlish, Neil A.
RC968.W665 2000 616.6′803—dc21 00-022000

2 4 6 8 9 7 5 3 1
Printed in the United States of America
on acid-free paper

In memory of
my parents
and brother

Preface

Prevention of occupational injury, illness, and death is a daily concern of workers and their families, businesses, unions, government, workers' compensation insurers, health care professionals, occupational health and safety professionals, and lawmakers. With the goal of prevention, occupational health surveillance is the collection, analysis, interpretation, and feedback of information about workplace hazards and workers' health. The information describes the problem(s), the magnitude, the groups affected, and trends in time and location. It is information that guides prevention.

Over the last two decades, interest in occupational health surveillance has grown enormously. In part, the interest has been stimulated by government agencies concerned with modernizing and building capacity to meet national public health objectives. Escalating costs in workers' compensation and the emergence of managed care has also stimulated interest at the level of employers, workers' compensation insurers, and health care professionals. These and other factors have contributed to innovation and broadening of the knowledge of how to organize and carry out occupational health surveillance. Much of this knowledge and experience has been published in scientific journals. However, a wide audience of health and safety professionals has yet to be reached. This book is the first attempt to reach this wider audience.

At academic training centers, surveillance is usually a part of epidemiology instruction, but the practical aspects of establishing and maintaining a surveillance system are not usually taught. Surveillance is largely learned "on-the-job."

This book will explain how to design, implement, and maintain occupational health surveillance systems, and present case studies of actual surveillance systems. The material in the Principles chapters will explain how to:

- define goals, objectives, and scope of the surveillance system
- gain organizational support for surveillance
- organize the surveillance workgroup
- identify the information needed to carry out the objectives of the surveillance system
- construct reporting guidelines and case definitions
- make priorities for follow-up of cases
- establish mechanisms for case reporting and the screening of cases for follow-up
- carry out case management
- create and maintain databases for statistical reporting and case management
- analyze and interpret surveillance data
- use workplace epidemiologic surveillance data in cost-benefit and cost-effectiveness analysis of workplace interventions, and
- present and communicate findings and provide feedback to participants.

The case studies provide examples from industry, state health and labor agencies, and unions. Conditions covered include a wide array of acute and chronic health conditions, fatal injuries, and cancer mortality. Also included are the emerging areas of electronic commerce and electronic data interchange (EDI) in the design of workers' compensation information systems, disability surveillance, and the surveillance of quality and effectiveness of occupational health services. Several areas related to surveillance are beyond the scope of this book such as genetic screening or methods used in epidemiologic research or statistics. Nonetheless, a reader comfortable with high school algebra has the math skills to excel in surveillance.

This text book was written for professionals and students who wish to use surveillance as a tool to improve the effectiveness of health and safety programs. This includes corporate and plant level-medical officers, nurses, industrial hygienists, safety specialists, risk managers and other health and safety personnel. These individuals work in diverse settings: individual workplaces, state health and labor agencies, loss control departments of workers' compensation insurers, managed care organizations and medical groups, and universities.

This diverse audience poses a challenge in achieving the right balance in presenting general concepts and examples. The principles chapters apply to a wide audience and have sections that highlight employer- or government-oriented surveillance. The case studies and appendices are tailored to more specific interests and audiences.

This book was motivated by the desire to share the experience and knowledge that comes from public health practice. No book like this was available when I began my career in surveillance. Through surveillance, my colleagues and I have changed the lives of many workers and their employers for the better. Participating in prevention has been an immensely rewarding experience.

I thank Dr. Edward Baker, Dr. Lawrence Fine, Dr. William Halperin, Dr. Linda Rosenstock and other colleagues at the National Institute for Occupational Safety and Health who have promoted the development of the Sentinel Event Notification System for Occupational Risks (SENSOR) and other surveillance activities. I owe much thanks to my colleagues at the Center for the Study of Workers' Health, Maracay, Venezuela and the U.S. Fulbright Senior Scholar Program. They provided a supportive setting to develop the lecture series and training materials that evolved into the Principles chapters of this book. Dr. Maritza Tennasee and Dr. Gerry Eijkemans, Pan American Health Organization, are gratefully acknowledged for their collaboration in promoting occupational health surveillance throughout Latin America. This book reflects the insights gained through a decade-long collaboration with Linda Rudolph and Kathy Dervin. For this collaboration and enduring friendship, I am deeply grateful. The critique of early drafts of the Principles chapters by Linda Rudolph is also gratefully acknowledged. Lisa Maizlish is gratefully acknowledged for the cover design. I thank Aismara Borges for the companionship and understanding that sustained me through this project. My deepest gratitude goes to the co-authors who generously gave their time and energy to make this book possible.

December 1999 N.A.M.
Berkeley, California
Maracay, Venezuela

Contents

APPENDICES

Contributors

JIM BELLOWS, M.P.H., C.I.H.
Research Manager
California Division of Workers' Compensation
San Francisco, California

PAUL D. BLANC, M.D., M.S.P.H.
Associate Professor of Medicine
University of California
San Francisco, California

KATHY A. DERVIN, M.P.H.
Health Education Consultant
California Division of Workers' Compensation
San Francisco, California

E. LYNN JENKINS, M.A.
Chief, Analysis and Field Evaluations Branch
Division of Safety Research
National Institute for Occupational Safety and Health
Morgantown, West Virginia

ANTHONY D. LAMONTAGNE, SC.D., M.A., M.ED.
Instructor in Occupational Health
Dana-Farber Cancer Institute & Harvard School of Public Health
Boston, Massachusetts

NEIL A. MAIZLISH, PH.D., M.P.H.
Epidemiologist
Berkeley, California

FRANKLIN E. MIRER, PH.D.
Director, Health and Safety Department
United Automobile Workers Union
Detroit, Michigan

ROBERT M. PARK, MS.O.H.
Epidemiologist
National Institute for Occupational Safety and Health
Cincinnati, Ohio

MARY JO REILLY, M.S.
Epidemiologist
Michigan State University
East Lansing, Michigan

GORDON R. REEVE, PH.D.
Manager, Epidemiology
Ford Motor Company
Dearborn, Michigan

KENNETH D. ROSENMAN, M.D.
Professor of Medicine
Michigan State University
East Lansing, Michigan

LINDA A. RUDOLPH, M.D., M.P.H.
Medical Director
California Division of Workers' Compensation
San Francisco, California

A. JAMES RUTTENBER, PH.D., M.D.
University of Colorado Health Sciences Center
Boulder, Colorado

MICHAEL A. SILVERSTEIN, M.D., M.P.H.
Assistant Director
Washington State Occupational Safety and Health Administration
Olympia, Washington

MARTHA W. STANBURY, M.S.P.H.
Public Health Advisor
Division of Epidemiology, Environmental, and Occupational Health
New Jersey Department of Health and Senior Services
Trenton, New Jersey

DAVID H. WEGMAN, M.D., M.SC.
Professor and Chair
Department of Work Environment
University of Massachusetts, Lowell
Lowell, Massachusetts

I

PRINCIPLES

1

Introduction

NEIL A. MAIZLISH

The toll of work-related illness and injury is enormous. Each year in the United States, there are:

- 6500 fatal job injuries
- 60,000 deaths from work-related chronic diseases
- 14 million nonfatal job injuries and illnesses

The annual cost is at least $171 billion.[1] On a global scale, 120 million work injuries, 200,000 fatalities, and 68–157 million new cases of occupational disease are believed to occur annually.[2] In most regions of the world, work outranks tobacco, air pollution, illicit drugs, hypertension, and physical activity as a leading cause of premature death and disability.[3]

In theory, occupational injuries and illnesses are preventable because humans create and control the industrial process. Prevention can start at product design and carry through at each stage at which job exposures, illness, and disability might occur (Fig. 1.1).[4] Health and safety experts know that prevention requires an understanding of workplace exposures, action that anticipates potential harm, and an evaluation of individual incidents and their statistical patterns. At many workplaces the lessons that could be learned from prior experience are not used. Managers often run from one urgent problem to the next, and information vital for improving health and safety settles into filing cabinets and into computer hard drives. Where is the information control center that sizes up the problems, charts the patterns, alerts management to the possible solutions, and coordinates the response? In short, where is the surveillance system?

DEFINITION OF SURVEILLANCE

Surveillance is formally defined as:

> "continuous analysis, interpretation, and feedback of systematically collected data, generally using methods distinguished by their practicality, uniformity, and rapidity, rather than by accuracy or completeness."[5]
>
> "By observing trends in time, place, and persons, changes can be observed or anticipated and appropriate action, including investigative or control measures, can be taken."[6]

Applied to occupational health and safety, surveillance is the continuous analysis, interpretation, and feedback of data regarding the workplace and workers' health.

BACKGROUND

Surveillance is a basic problem-solving process used in many fields. In business, quality management involves a continuous cycle of measurement, analysis, interpretation, action, and feedback. For example, computer chip manufacturing is not perfect. A low level of defects is the norm. Perhaps 5 per 1000 chips made are defective. If the defect rate suddenly jumps to 10 per 1000 in any given lot, something is amiss. The specific type of defect may provide a clue to what the problem is. If the circuits are poorly formed, then perhaps the manufacturing process needs fine tuning. If dust particles settled on the chip, then air filters in the production area need to be evaluated. Sometimes the cause will be obvious, and immediate action can be taken with confidence. In other situations there may be sev-

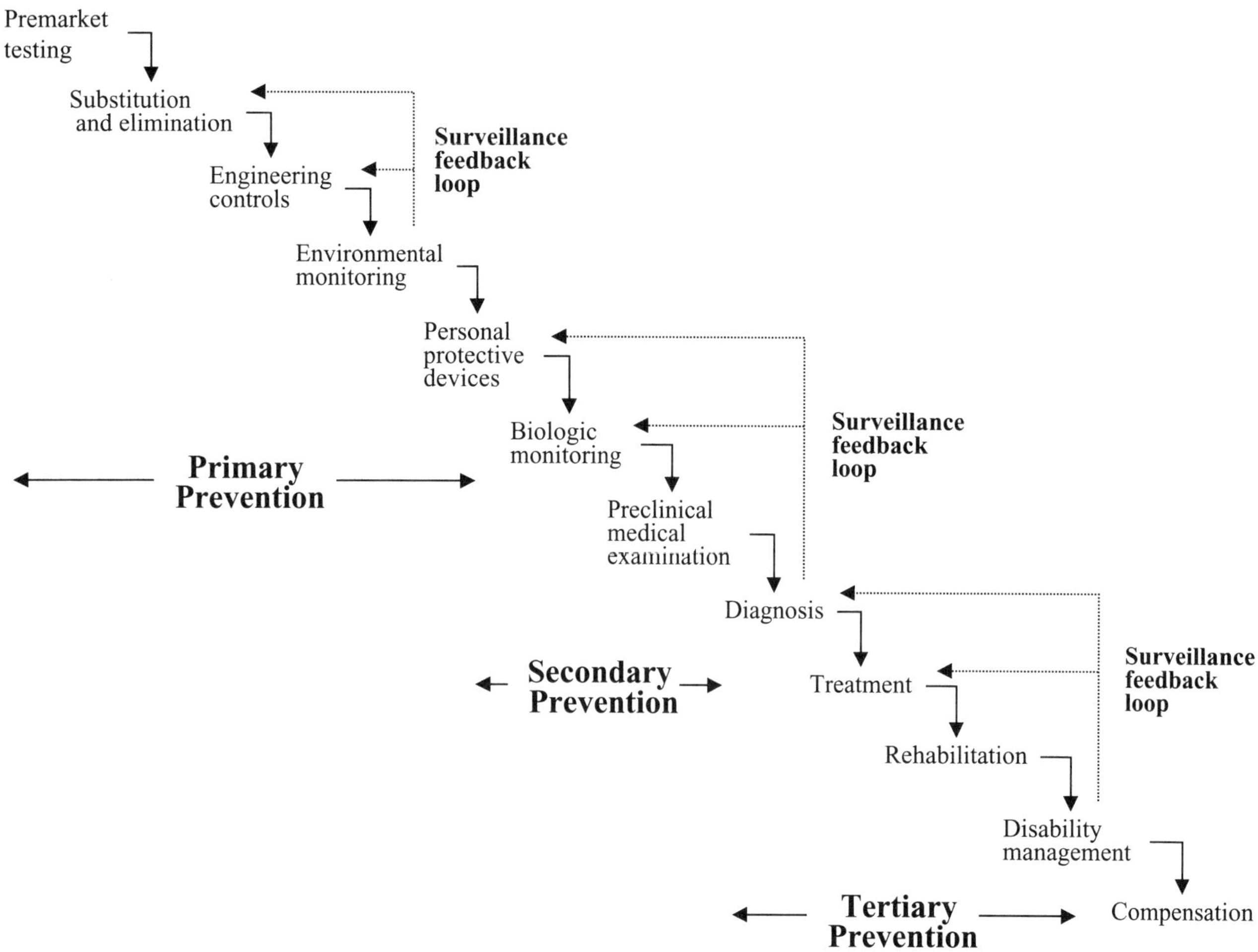

Figure 1.1 Eliminating exposures and hazards before they have an opportunity to do harm is called primary prevention. Examples are substituting safe materials and processes for hazardous ones, using engineering controls such as ventilation to reduce exposures, personal protective equipment if engineering controls are not feasible, administrative practices such as reducing the hours of contact with exposures, and education and training. Secondary prevention, such as medical examinations in workers exposed to hazards, is used to detect health effects at an early, reversible stage. If health has been damaged, several strategies are used to limit the consequences: medical care that reduces the clinical severity and promotes rapid healing, assistance in return-to-work, rehabilitation, and compensation for lost earning power. Surveillance can catch the lapses along the chain and provide feedback so prevention can be improved. (Adapted from Halperin.[4])

eral possibilities. After each is tested, the lots are sampled again to see if the rate goes back to the original level or is now lower. Some employers graph the number of defects by lot and day and the walls of their factories are filled with control charts.

Of course, the most relevant experience on surveillance comes from the field of public health, where surveillance is the link between health problems and prevention.[7–11] In public health surveillance, human populations are scanned for cases of ill health or the exposures that cause ill health. For up to 52 different infectious diseases, physicians, hospitals, and other health facilities are the eyes and ears of national surveillance systems.[12] Shortly after seeing a patient, they voluntarily report the basic facts to local and state health departments, and, in the United States, to the federal Centers for Disease Control and Prevention (CDC). They report by post card, fax, or electronically in a standard format that describes briefly the type of disease and date of diagnosis, as well as the age, gender, and residence of the patient. Each week, the health departments count the cases. The weekly tally is compared with averages from previous years. For example, if seven cases of mumps were expected, and 25 were reported, there may be an outbreak in the making.

Simple statistics are used to answer the journalistic questions of what, where, when, who, how, and why. *What* is the exposure or health event described by the signs, symptoms, physical examinations, and laboratory tests. *Where* is the physical or geographic location of the exposure, injury, or illness. *When* describes the occurrence of the health event by hour, day, month, year, or other cycle of time, and the time line of events between exposure and health effect. *Who* describes the personal characteristics of those being affected—men or women, young or old, African-American or white, rich or poor, and urban or rural. These characteristics are not necessarily a direct cause of illness. However, they may be linked in some way to illness, and provide clues as to where to start looking for the actual causes. They may suggest vulnerable populations that need to take special precautions. *How* details the chain of events that link exposures to the health effects. This can be the route of exposure of a chemical or the mode of transmission of an infectious disease. *Why* is not only the immediate cause, but also the chain of causes, which at each step may provide opportunities for prevention (Fig. 1.1).

To hone in on the causes, a response team goes into the field to gather more detailed information. They will review medical data, interview cases and their neighbors, and sample water, food, air, or other potential sources of contamination. Sometimes the immediate cause will be found quickly because a bacterium, virus, or contaminant (and their chemical fingerprints) shows up at high levels in both the environmental samples and medical tests. Sometimes there is no laboratory test, and educated guesses about the possible cause are made with the help of statistics. While the possible cause is being researched, educated guesses still help choose a course of action. There are many examples in public health when educated guesses saved lives.[13]

When surveillance is coupled to prevention programs the results are dramatic (Fig. 1.2). For example, after the development of a vaccine, efforts are made to get whole communities vaccinated. However, some residents miss their vaccinations, and sometimes the vaccine loses its potency because it is not handled properly. Cases will continue to occur in the groups not covered. New cases detected by the surveillance system help pinpoint which communities have not been reached. The process is repeated until there are no more cases.

Surveillance was a key component of the worldwide campaign to eradicate smallpox. In 1900, there were over 21,064 cases of smallpox reported in the United States. By 1949, zero cases were reported, and, by 1979, smallpox was eliminated from the rest of the world. For other infectious diseases like polio, measles, mumps, and influenza, vaccine programs linked to surveillance reduced the number of cases from tens of thousands of cases to just a few hundred by 2000.[14] After conquering infectious disease, other conditions have been added to the list of conditions for public health surveillance. These including chronic disease, injuries, violence, behavioral risk factors (such as smoking, lack of exercise, drinking alcoholic beverages, and not using seat belts), and occupational health. Risk factors are exposures, health hazards, personal characteristics, and behaviors that play either a direct or indirect role in causing disease or injury. The common classes of occupational risk factors are shown in Table 1.1.

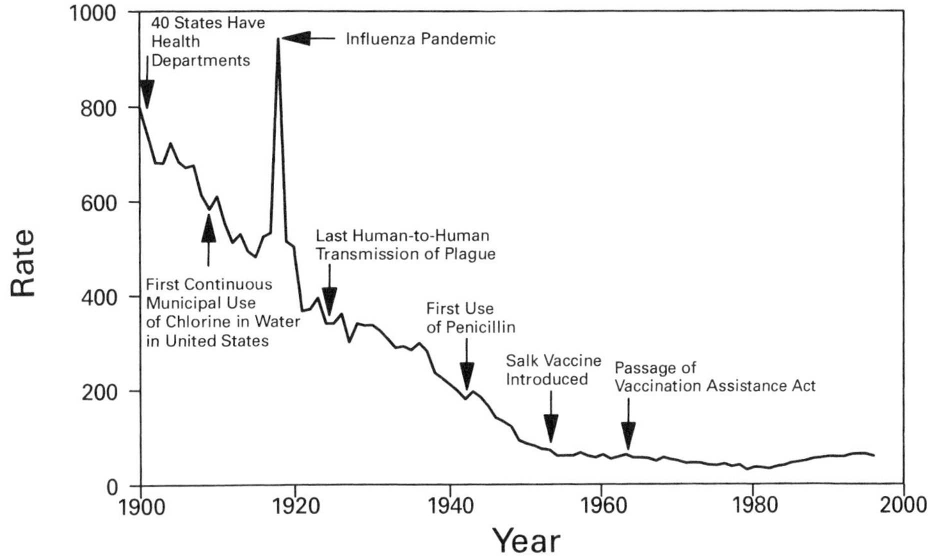

Figure 1.2 Crude death rate per 100,000 population for infectious diseases—United States, 1900–1996. Public health surveillance combined with improvements in sanitation, vaccination, antibiotics, and medical care played a significant role in conquering infectious diseases in the twentieth century. (Centers for Disease Control.[108–110])

Table 1.1 Categories of Occupational Risk Factors

Class of Risk Factor	*Examples*
Physical	Noise, vibration, heat, cold, radiation, electricity, extreme pressures
Mechanical	Moving objects, falls, unguarded machinery, cutting tools, conveyors, motor vehicles
Biomechanical	Movements that are forceful, repetitive, done with an awkward posture; prolonged static postures
Chemical	Strong acids and bases; organic solvents; dusts, aerosols, gases (asbestos, coal dust, cotton dust, hydrogen sulfide), lack of oxygen, pesticides
Biological	Blood-borne exposures (hepatitis B virus, HIV*), toxic plants, farm animals (brucellosis), shift work, fatigue
Psychologic	Level of autonomy, conflicts with supervisor, coworkers, and clients; stress, boredom, level of demands, skills and training, level of participation in decision-making
Work organization	Payment method (piece rate, hourly, salary), economic incentives, authority–responsibility, intensity and style of supervision, reward–punishment structure; organizational culture, style of leadership
General risk factors	
Person	Age, sex, race, medical conditions
Place/ environment	Occupation, department in a workplace, industry of employer, alcohol consumption, tobacco use, access to medical care and medications, hobbies, residence, education
Time	Date of hire, years of service, shift, duration of shift, overtime, cycles of production (daily, weekly, monthly, quarterly)

*HIV, human immunodeficiency virus.

PURPOSE AND USES OF SURVEILLANCE

The purpose of surveillance is to guide action. Managers in business and government need to assess problems, set priorities, and measure the effectiveness of their health and safety programs. Surveillance is a measurement tool and a decision tool for action. It is a distinct activity that helps organize the work of those who coordinate, deliver, and evaluate health and safety services. As Teustch and Churchill[8] point out, collection, analysis, and interpretation of health data without providing it to those who set policy or implement programs is better described as health information rather than surveillance. The main uses of surveillance are presented below and in Table 1.2.

Measure the Magnitude of Health Problems and Exposures

Putting a number or rank on the size of a problem is essential for setting priorities. Even though every workplace should regard health and safety as important as production, this is not always so. Health and safety competes with other programs for scarce resources. Within a health and safety program, there are also competing priorities. For planning, goals are expressed in terms of how much the problem can be reduced from the baseline—10%, 33%, 100% of cases, lost workdays, costs, etc. Thus, the magnitude can be used to establish a baseline. Knowing the magnitude also gives some idea of the amount of resources and time needed to solve the problem.

Identify High-Risk Groups

Whether the problem is evenly spread across the work force or concentrated in a few groups is critical for targeting an intervention. If the distribution is even, then a broad-based program may be most appropriate. But if the problem concentrates in a specific group, say maintenance welders, it makes sense to target that group. Knowing the age, sex, educational level, and ethnicity of those most likely affected also can be used to help design programs. Latino workers who have a hard time reading in English or Spanish are not going to get much out of materials written in English at a college reading level.

Monitor Time and Geographic Trends of the Health Problem or Exposure

Observing events over time is one of the most important uses of surveillance. Sudden changes in the number of cases may signal a new exposure, or an old one that is not being controlled. If monitoring is frequent, one can detect outbreaks in their early stages. If a prevention activity was recently put into place, a change in the number of cases may be a sign that its starting to work.

Table 1.2 Objectives and Uses of Epidemiologic Surveillance

OBJECTIVES

1. Identify and estimate the magnitude of a problem
2. Identify high- and low-risk groups
3. Monitor time and geographic trends
4. Identify cases, case clusters, coworkers, worksites, and industries for follow-up
5. Identify new diseases and syndromes
6. Identify new, hazardous exposures

USES

1. Prioritize health problems
2. Evaluate the progress, success, or failure of interventions and programs
3. Provide planning data for cost-effectiveness and benefit analyses
4. Generate hypotheses regarding disease–exposure relationships

Mapping cases or exposures onto the floor plan of a workplace or a geographic area also shows whether cases are distributed evenly or clustered. Injuries or illnesses that bunch together at the same location within a short time are a further clue that a job hazard may be present. One can use this information to target workplaces, departments, or work areas, and start an investigation into materials, work practices, safety procedures, and other plausible explanations.

Identify Possible Causes and Risk Factors of Health Problems

Many health hazards are well-known to health and safety experts but not recognized at individual workplaces. Surveillance plays an important role in identifying a well-established cause of illness and injury so that individual workplaces can launch prevention activities.

Over 65,000 new chemicals are introduced yearly into the industrial environment. Chemicals used in consumer products undergo far more toxicological testing than those destined for industry.[15] This puts workers at greater risk of exposures to new chemicals that may cause illness. Likewise, familiar chemicals may be used in new production techniques without adequately considering their health and safety impact. Surveillance can play a role in identifying these new exposures and diseases.

Mine Data to Find Previously Undocumented Cause–Effect Relationships

It is possible to track a health problem over time and with other variables that might be in a database. These include age, sex, department, occupation, year hired, chemicals used, etc. (Table 1.1). When variables are crossed with one another, some of the pairings will track together. When one variable, say age, is related to another, say high blood pressure, the variables have a correlation or an association—older people tend to have higher blood pressure.

Some associations show what others found before, and, if previously researched, these relationships may have accepted scientific explanations. Other associations may be statistical flukes: two variables that track together but do not have a cause–effect relationship. For example, asthma cases might track with the number of radios in a house. It is very unlikely that radios have anything to do with asthma, but they might occur together in a particular database. However, some associations are part of a real cause-and-effect relationship. For example, you might find that the number of cases of asthma are highest in the foam molding department of a plastics factory. Since toluene diisocyanate (TDI) is used at the plant and is an established cause of occupational asthma, the action should be clear—reduce the TDI exposures. However, in the same statistical analysis, breast cancer occurs unevenly throughout the plant and is mostly in female spray painters. This is interesting and has not been observed before (and is made up for this example). If this were found, one could say that there is a possible relationship between breast cancer and spray painting. This is a hypothesis. The statistical analysis would have to be repeated at other plants to see if this was a one-of-a-kind finding, or true in general. There are several possible interpretations for this type of finding (Chapter 7). Much more research will have to be done to show whether the spray paint operation is really related to breast cancer. In the meantime, one can still take precautions and reduce suspect exposures.

DIMENSIONS OF SURVEILLANCE

Surveillance systems are classified by their data source, health outcome, exposure, method of data collection or analysis, and other aspects of their design. A surveillance system can have several of these dimensions at the same time.

Sentinel Events

Certain health events call attention to lapses in prevention. The appearance of even a single case suggests a breakdown in medical care, environmental control, or organization.[16] In public health, a case of tuberculosis or the death of a woman in childbirth would be an example. In occupational health, cases of lead poisoning or asbestosis are examples.

In September 1990, the California state health department received a blood lead report of 84 μg/dl on a 31-year-old, male radiator repairer employed in Tulare County. The staff of the occupational health program interviewed the patient, his physician and employer, and followed up with information packets and referral to the consultation services of the California Occupational Safety and Health Administration (Cal/OSHA), who subsequently assisted the employer. The patient complained of symptoms consistent with lead poisoning, and reported that he performed his work without ventilation or a respirator, did not shower at work, or change out of contaminated work clothes before coming home, where he lived with his 11-month-old infant daughter, two other children aged 10 and 11, and wife. The state health department referred his infant daughter and other family members for blood lead tests at the local health department, which found that the infant's blood lead level was significantly elevated at 36 μg/dl. Household dust samples taken by the county health department, revealed excessive levels of 7646 part per million (ppm) for the worker's favorite chair and 5135 ppm for the carpet.—*This case illustrates that uncontrolled occupational exposures can cause toxic lead levels not only in workers, but also their family members, particularly children, who are most vulnerable to the effects of lead. The primary prevention of these take-home exposures starts in the workplace.*[17]

Sentinel health events/occupational (SHE/O) are health conditions that are caused by occupational exposures and occur at elevated frequencies in certain occupations and industries (Table 1.3).[18,19] Sentinel has been used to describe diagnoses in which occupation is always the cause, such as beryllium lung disease, or a rare liver cancer (angiosarcoma) from exposure to vinyl chloride monomer; or, when occupation accounts for a significant proportion of cases in the general population.[20]

Sentinel is also used to describe the sentries—health care and health and safety personnel—who alert the rest of the community to cases of occupational injury and illness. These are called sentinel health care providers, who, in some surveillance systems, are recruited into networks that report to a central agency. In the United States, the Sentinel Event Notification System for Occupational Risks (SENSOR)[21] is such a model (Fig. 1.3). This program is funded and coordinated by the National Institute for Occupational Safety and Health (NIOSH) and carried out by approximately 20 states. The model has many variations depending on the SHE/O and data source. The conditions include acute trauma and poisoning (pesticide illness, amputations); intermediate-term illnesses (carpal tunnel syn-

Table 1.3 Sentinel Health Events/Occupational

*ICD9**	*Diagnosis*	*ICD9*	*Diagnosis*
011	Pulmonary tuberculosis	283.1	Hemolytic anemia
011,502	Silicotuberculosis	284.3	Aplastic anemia
020	Plague	288.0	Agranulocytosis or neutropenia
021	Tularemia	289.7	Methemoglobinemia
022	Anthrax	323.7	Toxic encephalitis
023	Brucellosis	332.1	Parkinson's disease, secondary
31.1	Fish fancier's finger	334.3	Cerebellar ataxia
054.6	Herpetic whitlow	354	Mononeuritis of upper limb
037	Tetanus	354.0	Carpal tunnel syndrome
042	HIV†	354.2	Lesion of ulnar nerve
056	Rubella	354.3	Lesion of radial nerve
70.0,70.1	Hepatitis A	357.7	Inflammatory and toxic neuropathy
70.2,70.3	Hepatitis B	366.4	Cataract
70.4	Hepatitis, non-A, non-B	388.1	Noise effects on inner ear
071	Rabies	443.0	Reynaud's phenomenon
073	Ornithosis	493.0,507.8	Extrinsic asthma
082.0	Rocky Mountain spotted fever	495.4	Malt worker's lung
100.8	Leptospirosis	495.5	Mushroom worker's lung
115	Histoplasmosis	495.8	Grain hander's lung, sequoiosis
117.1	Sporotrichosis	495.9	Unspecific allergic alveolitis
147	Malignant neoplasm of nasopharynx	500	Coal workers' pneumoconiosis
155	Hemangiosarcoma of liver	501	Asbestosis
158,163	Mesothelioma, malignant neoplasm of peritoneum and pluera	502	Silicosis, talcosis
160.0	Malignant neoplasm of nasal cavities	503	Chronic beryllium disease of the lung
161	Malignant neoplasm of larynx	504	Byssinosis
162	Malignant neoplasm of lung, bronchus, trachea	506.0	Acute bronchitis
170	Malignant neoplasm of bone	506.1	Acute pneumonitis, pulmonary edema
187.7	Malignant neoplasm of scrotum	570, 570.3	Toxic hepatitis
188	Malignant neoplasm of bladder	584,585	Acute, chronic renal failure
189	Malignant neoplasm of kidney	606	Male infertility
204.0	Lymphoid leukemia, acute	692	Contact and allergic dermatitis
205.0	Myeloid leukemia, acute	733.9	Skeletal fluorosis
207.0	Erythroleukemia		

*International Classification of Diseases, 9th Revision.[54]
†HIV, human immunodeficiency virus.
Source: Mullan and Murthy.[19]

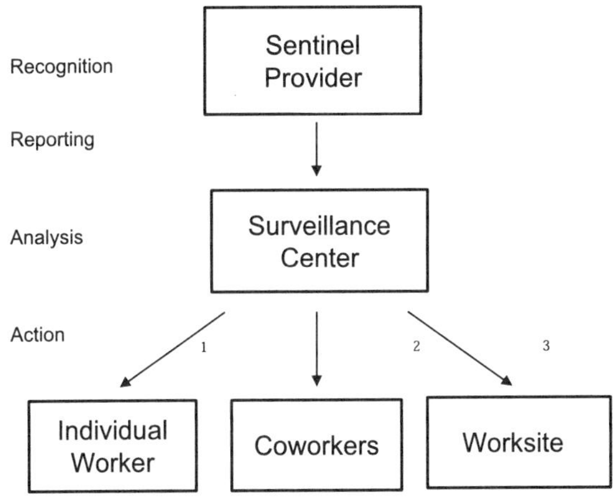

Figure 1.3 Schematic of the Sentinel Event Notification System for Occupational Risks (SENSOR) model. Cases of occupational health events are reported to a surveillance center, which screens, analyzes the case reports, set priorities, and coordinates the follow-up. Follow-up can include additional data gathering and case finding among coworkers, medical examinations, and worksite investigations, or industrywide prevention activities. (Baker.[21])

drome, lead poisoning, dermatitis), and chronic diseases (asthma, silicosis). These conditions were selected, in part, because they occur over a short to medium time frame. This allows case reports to be linked to a specific workplace, where follow-up can be carried out in real time. Different methods and data sources have been used, including workers' compensation, [22] hospital discharge data (Chapter 22), analytical laboratories for heavy metals (Chapter 11),[23] physician specialty offices (Chapter 14–16), and special networks of primary care doctors and nurses, specialists, and emergency rooms (Chapters 12, 13).[24,25]

Exposure and Health

Surveillance that focuses on exposure is called exposure surveillance or hazard surveillance (Chapter 21). Exposure surveillance allows prevention activities to be implemented *before* illness occurs. Surveillance that focuses on health is called health surveillance, health effects surveillance, health events surveillance, or health outcomes surveillance. Traditional measures of health include illness, injury, disability, or death. However, the definition of health can be considerably broadened to include quality of work life or satisfaction with occupational health care services. Exposure surveillance and health surveillance must be combined to minimize each other's shortcomings.

Active and Passive

Figure 1.3 shows two key stages of surveillance—the reporting of cases and follow-up. Recording of information is important. However, if it is not reported it cannot be acted upon. When little is done to promote the identification and reporting of cases, surveillance is passive. However, when the employer, government agency, or other surveillance organization takes positive steps to identify and report cases and exposures, the surveillance is active. The first step may be educating workers, supervisors, and health care providers about job hazards and the health problems they cause. This will increase the chance that health problems will be recognized. Afterward, regular contact can emphasize the importance of reporting cases, and be used to remind the participants of their responsibilities and the procedures to report cases. This interaction distinguishes active from passive reporting. The techniques for promoting reporting include written and telephone reminders, face-to-face meetings, newsletters, briefings on follow-up of cases, continuing education, dissemination of statistical summaries, public appreciation, professional recognition, and coauthorship on scientific publications. The heightened awareness frequently increases the number of reported cases as much as 2–5 times.[24,26,27]

It is also possible to make special efforts to find cases that the passive systems miss altogether.[28] A workplace health and safety committee or other group can use specially designed questionnaires and medical examinations. This often starts by using checklists of job hazards (exposure or risk factor surveillance) to identify jobs that have particular risks. Once the jobs are identified, all the workers with those jobs are given health questionnaires or brief medical examinations to see which among them are experiencing discomfort, symptoms, or medical evidence of a health problem. This approach has been effective in identifying musculoskeletal disorders, particularly in their early stages.[29]

Active and passive also describes the degree to which follow-up is pursued or linked to the surveillance system. Surveillance systems do not necessarily provide health or prevention services but may actively refer cases or provide information to others who have the responsibility for protecting workers' health. When surveillance systems do not provide services themselves, active follow-up often involves steps to educate, motivate, persuade, and pressure others to take action. After making referrals, active surveillance may also provide oversight to assure that prevention and control services are actually being delivered. In passive follow-up, few steps are taken to reach outside the surveillance organization. Even the dissemination of the results can be passive or active. The ability to carry out active or passive follow-up depends on the authority, responsibility, resources, and commitment of the surveillance organization.

Thus, the active and passive dimension can result in surveillance systems with passive reporting with active follow-up (Chapter 11), active reporting with passive follow-up, active reporting with active follow-up (Chapters 12–16), and passive reporting with passive follow-up.

Mortality and Morbidity

Mortality surveillance tends to be a specialized area of surveillance and depends on the collection and analysis of death certificates. For chronic diseases, there may not be immediate, practical follow-up because the business linked to the exposure has ceased to exist. There are notable exceptions (Chapter 14). Mortality surveillance of cancer and other chronic disease using general exposure information such as occupation, department, or industry may generate only the crudest of associations (Table 1.4). An appropriate response is more research. The advantage of mortality surveillance is that death is a definitive and serious outcome, and has a data source that counts a high percentage of cases.

Case-Based and Population-Based

The number of work injuries and illnesses are often expressed as a population rate: cases per 1000 workers per year, or per 100 full-time workers per year. This makes it easier to track trends over time when the population itself may be changing. For example, the population of workers at individual worksites goes up and down with cycles of layoffs and rehirings. By measuring injuries and illnesses with a common denominator it is possible to make comparisons across small, medium, and large plants or other groups. When population data are linked to injuries and illness, the sur-

Table 1.4 Occupations with the Highest Proportional Mortality Ratios for Cancer and Other Selected Chronic Diseases in Workers 20 Years Old and Older in 24 States in the United States 1984–1988[a]

Race and Sex	*Occupation (Census Code)*	*Cause of Death (ICD9[b])*	*Observed Deaths*	*PMR[c]*	*Excess Deaths[d]*
White men	Mining machine operator (616)	Coal workers' pneumoconiosis (500)	479	5146	470
	Electrical and electronic engineer (055)	Cancer of the brain and other parts of the nervous system (191–192)	57	224	32
	Insulation worker (593)	Cancer of the trachea, bronchus, and lung (162)	97	188	45
Black men	Mining machine operator (616)	Coal workers' pneumoconiosis (500)	24	7880	24
	Winding and twisting machine operator (738)	Acute myocardial infarction (410)	21	222	12
	Molding and casting machine operator (719)	Chronic obstructive pulmonary diseases (490–496)	26	196	13
	Painters, construction and maintenance worker (556, 579)	Cancer of the esophagus (150)	31	187	14
	Crane and tower operator (849)	Other ischemic heart disease (411–414)	66	164	26
	Farmer, except horticultural (473)	Cerebrovascular diseases (430–438)	1162	134	295
White women	Waitress	Cancer of the esophagus (150)	35	203	18
		Cancer of the lip, oral cavity, and pharynx (140–149)	49	191	23
		Chronic obstructive pulmonary diseases (490–496)	421	148	137
		Cancer of the trachea, bronchus, lung (162)	716	143	215
	Winding and twisting machine operator (738)	Diseases of the skin and subcutaneous tissue (680–709)	26	197	13
Black women	Teacher, except postsecondary (155–159)	Cancer of the breast (174, 175)	253	187	118
		Cancer of the ovary and uterine adnexa (183)	51	184	23
	Health aide, except nursing (446)	Other ischemic heart disease (411–414)	30	193	14
	Farmer, except horticultural (473)	Cerebrovascular diseases (430–438)	326	141	95

[a]Data includes deaths to residents of the 24-state reporting area occurring in the area. Criteria for inclusion in the table for white males was at least 50 deaths and a lower 95% confidence interval (not shown) of at least 150 for a cause of death–occupation combination. For white females and black males, at least 20 deaths and a lower 95% confidence interval (not shown) of at least 125 for a cause of death–occupation combination. For black females, at least 10 deaths and a lower 95% confidence interval (not shown) of at least 125 for a cause of death–occupation combination.

[b]International Classification of Diseases, 9th Revision[54]

[c]PMR (proportional mortality ratio) = observed deaths ÷ expected deaths × 100. (See Chapter 5 for details of PMR methods.)

[d]Excess deaths = observed deaths − expected deaths.

Source: National Institute for Occupational Safety and Health.[66]

veillance is rate-based. The population data can be calculated from personnel records, time keeping, or payroll that counts individual workers or their work hours. Sometimes these data are not available, or the population is difficult to track, such as migratory farm workers or construction workers. When this occurs, all that can be counted are cases. This is called case-based surveillance.

Mixed Modes

The dimensions can be combined creatively in the same surveillance system. Passively collected records in a rate-based surveillance system can be used to provide a statistical profile of the magnitude of the problems experienced by an employer or industry. As soon as cases with certain sentinel-event diagnoses are reported, there can be active follow-up at the worksite, an individual workstation, and with workers in the same occupation as the sentinel case.

DATA SOURCES FOR OCCUPATIONAL HEALTH SURVEILLANCE

Almost any health condition, exposure, or health service that can be measured can be included in surveillance. Data for surveillance ideally has information on exposures, health events, and how they vary by person, place, and time—the journalistic questions of who, what, when, where, how. The exact data needed will depend on the goals of specific surveillance systems (next chapter). Surveillance relies mainly on preexisting data from employment, medical care and insurance, industrial processes and materials, and health and safety activities. However, one is not restricted to preexisting data. Sometimes by making small changes, surveillance can piggyback onto data collected for a different purpose. Less often, surveillance systems can be designed from scratch with new data sources. The following reviews some of the existing data sources for surveillance. There are several more detailed reviews.[30,31] Most public data sources mentioned below are available on the internet as publications, interactive databases, or data products (Table 1.5).

Existing Data

Employment Data

The frequency of injuries, illnesses, or deaths is often measured on a population basis, such as injuries per *100 workers* employed. Employment data are used to identify the population of workers and provide information on potential exposures and high-risk groups. Within a company, personnel records summarize the important milestones of work life. They list the jobs and departments held, dates of hire, layoffs, retirement, and sick leave. For hourly workers, time keeping or payroll data often list individuals with the hours worked during the payroll period. Personnel files and payroll are becoming increasingly automated, which makes these sources a building block for rate-based surveillance.

In the United States, employees are covered by unemployment insurance and their employers must report summary data to state and federal employment agencies. In the ES202 program,[32] this includes a count of employees that worked during the mid-month payroll period. Government agencies code the employer's industry and tabulate the number of employees, wages, and employers. Summary tables are published by the state employment agencies, breaking down the counts by county, state, industry, and size of employer based on the number of employees.

The U.S. Bureau of Labor Statistics carries out detailed national surveys of employment on a sample of about 50,000 persons every month.[33] Questions are asked about occupations, wages, and type of employment, such as being self-employed or a government worker. Data on personal characteristics are also collected. Every 10 years, the Bureau of Census conducts a national census, and records occupation, industry, and demographic details of the U.S. population.[34] Special employment surveys target special groups, such as agricultural workers, children, and disabled persons.[35,36]

An important practical aspect of employment data is that they are almost always collected independently of illness and injury data. They are usually stored in a separate database and administered by a group within an organization that is different than those responsible for illness and injury data. How one gets access to the employment database and link it with the injury database requires both organizational and technical skills.

Employer Reports of Work Injury and Illness

Employers fill out forms on job injuries, illnesses, and deaths for their internal use and to satisfy requirements of their governments and insurers. In the United States, the OSHA form 200 (Appendix A) is the cornerstone of a national reporting system. Each job injury, illness, or death that meets the OSHA case definition has to be recorded on a separate line with the date of injury, onset of illness, and a notation for cases with lost workdays away from work, restricted activities at work, and the number of days involved. In addition, free-form text fields record usual job title, department, and a description of the injury with body parts affected. These logs are a building block of company-based surveillance

Table 1.5 Publications and Public Databases on the Internet

Topic	*Organization*	*Home Page*	*Additional Information*
Occupational hazards and health effects	National Institute for Occupational Safety and Health (NIOSH)	www.cdc.gov/niosh	*Industrial Environment: It's Evaluation and Control.* Publ No. 74-117. *Occupational Safety and Health Guidelines for Chemical Hazards.* Publ No. 95-121 Vendor list for *Registry of Toxic Substances (RTECS) NIOSH Analytical Methods*
	American Industrial Hygiene Association	www.aiha.org	Publisher of *The Occupational Environment—its Evaluation and Control.* Fairfax, Virginia: AIHA Press, 1997.
	National Library of Medicine	igm.nlm.nih.gov	MEDLINE, TOXLINE, and other bibliographic retrieval services for articles from scientific literature
Occupational health standards	Occupational Safety and Health Administration (OSHA)	www.osha.gov	Complete text of OSHA standards, PELs (www.osha-slc.gov/OshStd_toc/OSHA_Std_toc1910.html)
	American Conference of Governmental Industrial Hygienists	www.acgih.org	Publishers of *Threshold Limit Values ACGIH Ventilation Manual Occupational Health and Safety Management Systems*
Occupational surveillance publications, statistics, and data	Bureau of Labor Statistics	www.bls.gov	Census of Fatal Occupational Injuries Nonfatal occupational injuries and illnesses from the *Survey of Occupational Injuries and Illnesses* (stats.bls.gov/oshhome)
	National Institute for Occupational Safety and Health	www.cdc.gov/niosh	*National Traumatic Occupational Fatalities* (Publ. No. 93-108) Mortality by occupation, industry, and cause of death—24 reporting states (1984–1988). DHHS (NIOSH) Pub. No. 97-114. Gateway to occupational mortality data, FARS, SEER, and other data sets (wonder.cdc.gov)
	Occupational Safety and Health Administration	www.osha.gov	Database of OSHA citations from the Integrated Management Information System (IMIS) www.osha.gov/oshstats
	Mine Safety and Health Administration (MSHA)	www.msha.gov	MSHA Inspector Dust Sampling Results www.msha.gov/STATS/SAMPLING/MAINPGE.htm
	California Department of Pesticide Regulation	www.cdpr.ca.gov	Pesticide illness surveillance system of California
General health surveillance publications, statistics, and data	Centers for Disease Control	www.cdc.gov	*Morbidity Mortality Weekly Reporter (MMWR)*
	National Cancer Institute	www.seer.ims.nci.nih.gov	Cancer incidence rates
	National Center for Health Statistics	www.cdc.gov/wwwnchs	National Health Interview Survey Hospital discharge data
Employment data and industry/occupation coding	Bureau of Census	www.census.gov	1990 and 2000 Census data Census of Agriculture Occupation/Industry Codes (SIC, NAICS)
	Bureau of Labor Statistics	www.bls.census.gov	Current Population Survey (http://ferret.bls.census.gov) National Agricultural Workers Survey Standard Occupational Coding (SOC)
Additional health and safety organizations	Canadian Center for Occupational Health and Safety	www.ccohs.gov	Reports, statistics, educational materials Links to other health and safety sites
	World Health Organization	www.who.ch	Reports, statistics, educational materials Links to other health and safety sites
	Pan American Health Organization	www.paho.org	Materials in English and Spanish (www.cepis.org.pe) Links to other health and safety sites
	International Labor Organization	www.ilo.org	Publishers of ILO *Encyclopedia*
	National Safety Council	www.nsc.org	Publishers of *Fundamentals of Industrial Hygiene*
	Duke University, Occupational Environmental Medicine	occ-env-med.mc.duke.edu/oem/	Occupational health and safety list server and discussion group Links to other health and safety sites

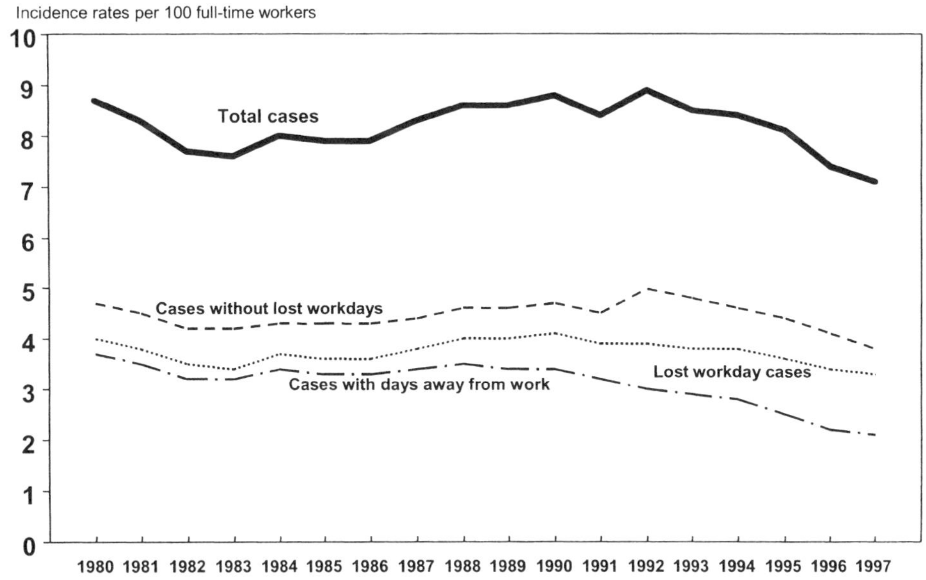

Figure 1.4 Incidence rates of nonfatal injury and illnesses by type of case—United States, 1980–1997. Each year a sample of employers' Occupational Safety and Health Administration (OSHA) logs is taken from about 164,000 private industry establishments. Excluded are about 20% of the work force who are self-employed, farms with fewer than 10 employees, private households, and local, state, and federal government agencies. About 30%–40% of cases lose workdays by being away from work or have work restrictions. (Bureau of Labor Statistics.[38])

systems[37] and are used by enforcement personnel during individual worksite inspections. A national sample of these forms are compiled by the Bureau of Labor Statistics in an annual statistical survey (Fig. 1.4).[38]

Most state agencies require employers to report new cases of injuries, illness, and death on special forms for use in their workers' compensation system. State agencies compile statistics from information recorded on the forms, and workers' compensation insurers use these forms to help establish individual claims. California's Employers First Report is typical (Appendix A) and devotes a full page to gather details on the employer's business, the worker, and the injury or illness.[39] Similar forms are used in other countries in the Americas (Canada, Mexico, Central, and South America) whose social security institutes are the major health care provider and insurer. They require workers, employers, and physicians to each fill out and sign different sections of the same form.

The diagnosis of some illnesses and extent of disability may not be apparent on the first report. Many occupational diseases are not recognized by employers, physicians, and workers, and are poorly captured from this source.

Physician Reports of Work Injury and Illness

At least 32 states have laws that require physicians to report occupational diseases.[10] Some states list specific conditions and others require reporting any suspected occupational disease. The report is usually filed once, usually a few days after the patient is first seen. In addition to the name and address of the business and the worker, the reports give details on the age, sex, occupation, industry, activity at the time of onset, diagnoses, treatment plan, and return to work. California's form is typical (Appendix A). As with employers first reports, for some cases the final diagnosis, complications, and full extent of disability unfold over time and are not known at the first office visit. About half the states in the United States require physicians and health facilities to report pesticide illnesses, a significant proportion of which are occupational.[40,41]

Workers' Compensation

All states in the United States and an increasing number of countries in Latin America require private employers to purchase insurance or self insure to cover the costs of work injuries and illness. Workers' compensation by its very nature captures data on reported job injuries and illnesses, medical care, disability, and payments. It is one of the few sources that collects cost data. Because the insurance coverage is for the lifetime of the claim, cases are followed over time, sometimes for decades. Chapter 24 explores this data source in detail. Private insurance companies do not release their data to the public at the individual claim level. Like other forms of insurance, state agencies regulate the rates insurance carriers can charge employers. Most states require the reporting of summary data for the purpose of establishing these rates.[42] A few states, however, underwrite the insurance themselves, or allow self-insurance, usually of large employers. For example, the State of Washington has been able to use their data for the surveillance of dermatitis,[43] burns,[44] cumulative trauma disorders of the upper extremities, [45] hearing loss,[46] injuries in adolescents,[47] and return-to-work.[48]

When doctors and hospitals get reimbursed for their services, the medical bills are sent to the insurance carrier or claim processor. Nowadays, insurance carriers or companies they contract with, review the bills and pay according to a contract or a fee schedule. In the United States, most bills are submitted on standardized forms for doctors' services and hospital services (Appendix A). These data contain the principal and secondary diagnoses, dates of treatment, treatment codes, information about the provider specialty, charged and paid amounts, and type of health care arrangement, such as a health maintenance organization, preferred provider network, etc. These medical bills are becoming increasingly automated[49,50] and are used in health services evaluation. However, because reimbursement often depends on coded diagnoses and treatments, there are concerns that the codes can be manipulated and are not reliable. Data not used for reimbursement are often missing.

Hospital Discharge

Approximately 20 states require their hospitals to summarize hospital stays in a standardized, electronic format called a hospital discharge abstract that follows the format of a hospital bill (Appendix A). The information includes codes for medical diagnoses such as asthma, low back pain, fracture, etc. For injuries, a separate code is used for the cause, such as a motor vehicle crash, suffocation, or a fall. These are called the external causes of injuries. Also included are admission and discharge dates, medical procedures, patient age, sex, race, and expected source of payment, including workers' compensation. These data have been particularly useful in sentinel health event surveillance.

Occupational Safety and Health Administration (OSHA) Medical Record Keeping

Medical care provided to injured workers is covered by workers' compensation. However, for workers with exposure to any of 21 specific hazards, OSHA requires periodic medical examinations and diagnostic tests to be carried out at the employer's expense.[51] These hazards include dusts that cause lung disease or cancer like asbestos, chemicals like lead that cause poisoning, or physical agents like noise that cause hearing loss. The medical tests detect the early health effects in individual workers so that appropriate action can be taken while the condition is still reversible. This is called medical screening of high-risk workers and is a type of surveillance. The records must be retained for 30 years by the employer.

Laboratories

Other health care facilities may collect and report data for surveillance. Laboratories that do specialized diagnostic tests for heavy metals, cholinesterase-inhibiting pesticides, hearing loss, and nerve conduction are examples. Commercial and public laboratories in 28 states that test for blood lead are required to report the results to a state health agency.[23] Most states use a standard form that identifies the doctor, patient, and employer, and give the results of the blood lead test, age, sex, and other important data (Chapter 11). Even though the patients include children and adults from the general population, most adult cases are occupational. States generally follow up reports with interviews and prevention activities.

Death Certificates and Other Vital Records

Death certificates are the most important source of data in most countries for fatal occupational injuries and deaths due to chronic disease.[52,53] The U.S. standard death certificate (Appendix A) records up to three causes of the death, other significant medical conditions, as well as age at death, sex, race, residence, and usual occupation and industry of employment. There is a box to indicate whether a fatal injury occurred at work. State health departments assign 4-digit codes for the causes of death from a standard list, the International Classification of Diseases.[54] Approximately 40 states code occupational and industry according to the Bureau of Census 3-digit classification.[55]

The statistical profile of fatal occupational injuries is part of an annual census carried out by the Bureau of Labor Statistics[56] (Fig. 1.5) and studies by the National Institute for Occupational Safety and Health[57, 58] (Figs. 1.6 and 1.7). In addition to death certificates, the annual census uses obituaries, OSHA notification, and workers' compensation records to identify deaths. In the NIOSH Fatality Assessment and Control Evaluation (FACE) program, individual cases of electrocution, falls, confined space, and other fatal injuries are followed up on site to identify the causes and recommend prevention activities that are typically broader than those made by enforcement agencies (Chapter 20).

Deaths due to cancer and other chronic diseases can also be studied with death certificates. For causes of death that are almost always due to occupational ex-

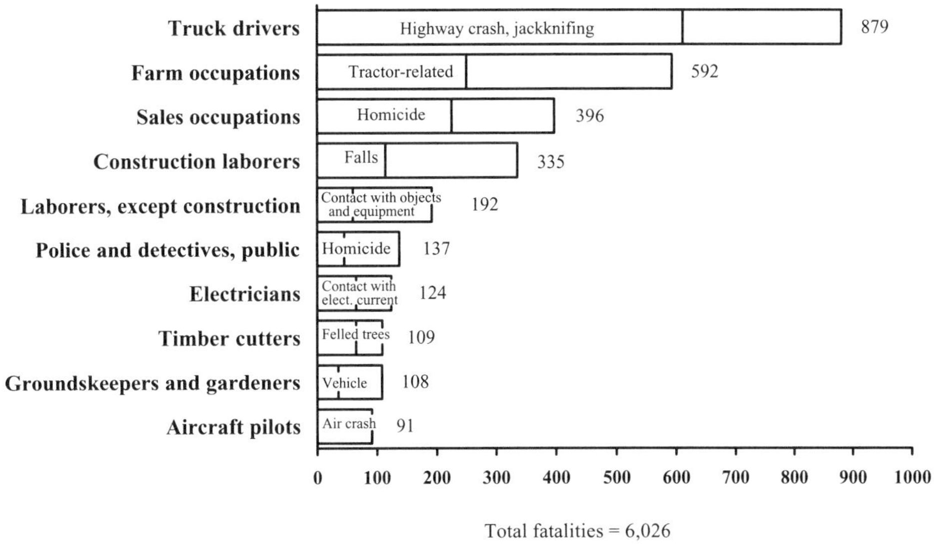

Figure 1.5 Occupations with large numbers of worker fatalities and the leading event—United States, 1998. (Bureau of Labor Statistics.[56])

posures, such as coal workers' lung (pneumoconiosis) or lung scarring caused by asbestos (asbestosis), it is possible to count the number of deaths (Fig. 1.8).[59] Cancer deaths at specific body sites (lung, liver, nasal cavity) that might be occupational can be studied by plotting cases on maps to see if they cluster near manufacturing facilities.[60]

It is possible to count the deaths of workers in a *particular* occupation or industry, and compare the tally with the average number of deaths in the *entire* workforce or general population. This can be done for an individual worksite [61] (Chapter 19), state,[62–65] or country (Table 1.4).[53,66]

Birth certificates have been used for the surveillance of miscarriages (spontaneous abortions), birth defects, and fertility of workers exposed to chemicals.[67,68]

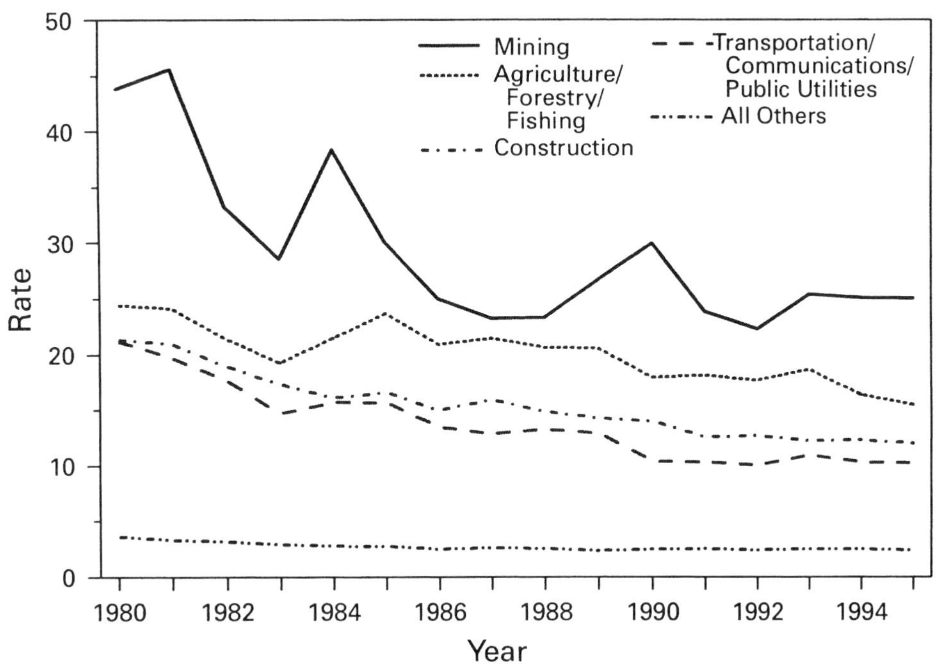

Figure 1.6 Occupational injury death rates per 100,000 workers by major industry division—United States, 1980–1995. (Centers for Disease Control.[102])

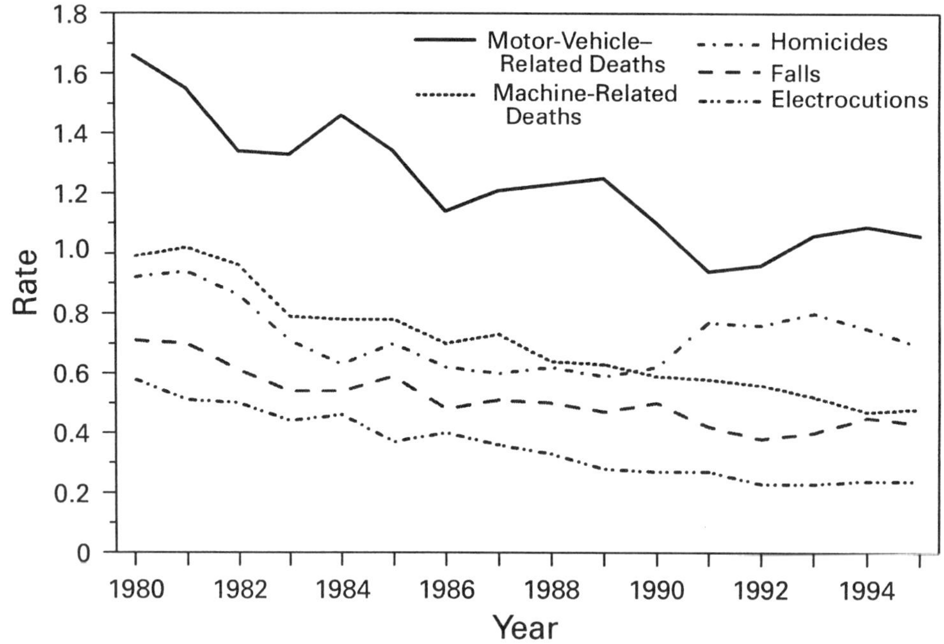

Figure 1.7 Rates per 100,000 workers for the leading causes of occupational injury deaths by cause—United States, 1980–1995. (Centers for Disease Control.[102])

Surveys

Much data are collected locally but not reported and centralized. Many organizations that have centralized databases are missing key pieces of information on an exposure or health condition. Periodic surveys are a potential solution to these problems. They use specially designed questionnaires, medical examinations, or physical measurements of the work environment. Sometimes it is impossible to survey every person or every workplace over a wide geographic area. Instead a representative sample is taken.[69]

Surveys require special skills and are usually undertaken by government, business, or research organizations. Large businesses routinely use surveys for customer satisfaction, market surveillance, and employees' satisfaction with their health care benefits.[70] Surveys of patient satisfaction are being used to assess the quality of medical care in workers' compensation.[71,72]

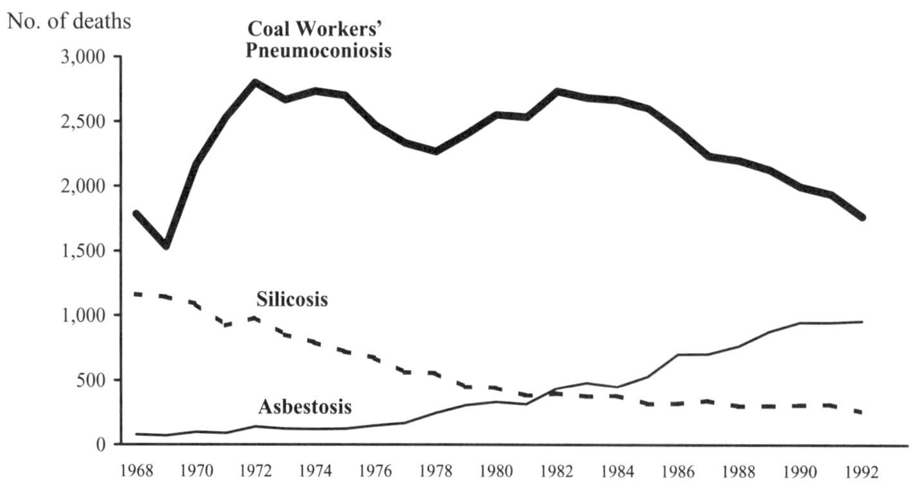

Figure 1.8 Deaths due to selected lung diseases listed on death certificates, residents 15 and over—United States, 1968–1992. Each is a chronic lung disease from occupational exposures to coal dust, asbestos fibers, or silica dust. The exposures for many of the decedents started in the decades prior to 1960. (Adapted from the Division of Respiratory Disease Studies, National Institute for Occupational Safety and Health (NIOSH).[59])

Exposure Surveys. The National Occupational Exposure Survey is the most extensive exposure survey in the United States.[73] It is a sample of 4490 worksites broken down by geographic area and employer size. The workplaces are visited by trained surveyors who directly observe the types of potential safety hazards and exposures to specific chemical, physical, and biological agents. Medical services and testing for occupational exposures is also recorded. It is possible to estimate the number of establishments and workers exposed to chemicals and physical hazards, a well as access to occupational health services and training programs.

Health Surveys. Occupational health has piggybacked onto routine health surveys carried out by the U.S. Public Health Service.[74] The Health Interview Survey interviews over 100,000 U.S. residents by telephone from about 43,000 households every year, and asks about the health problems they have experienced. In addition to the usual topics, the survey in 1988 added questions about work and low back pain, hand discomfort, and dermatitis.[75]

Company-Based Exposure Data

The sources of data for exposures include inventories of hazardous materials, production statistics, process flows, layout of work stations, invoices for materials, direct measurements, and the observations and experience of process engineers, supervisors, and workers. Although not ordinarily thought of as surveillance, the list of materials used by a company should be scanned to identify unsafe chemicals. In many countries, the hazards of chemicals must be disclosed by the manufacturer. Material Data Safety Sheets summarize this information; however, they may be incomplete, especially for chronic health effects. Electronic libraries of toxic chemicals and their health effects are now widely available in public and commercial databases.[76] Government enforcement agencies publish legal standards for safety and health.[77] Professional organizations [78,79] and research agencies[80] publish recommended exposure levels that are almost always more protective and based on more up-to-date information.

Sometimes it is not possible to find a safer substitute for hazardous materials or processes, and the hazard or exposure is part of production. Directly measuring the hazard or exposure is sometimes possible. This is done in the personal space of an individual worker, or over a broader area of several workers. The personal space can be the work area, breathing zone, work surface, or blood, urine, exhaled air, or skin washings. The method depends on the substance being measured. There are direct-reading meters for noise and illumination. Videotaping of workers is used for the analysis of lifting and repetitive motions that are forceful and awkward. For air-borne contaminants, there are air-draw tubes that change colors when contaminants react, exposure badges with chemical films, or air pumps that catch contaminants on filters that are later weighed or extracted with solvents in the laboratory. Textbooks and manuals are available to show how these measurements are made and analyzed.[81,82]

Government health and safety agencies and some employers that carry out safety inspections take samples and compile their observations in databases. OSHA's Integrated Management Information System [83,84] and the Mine Safety and Health Administration[85] are examples.

Potential Data Sources

The following data sources are not as widely used in occupational health surveillance. Each has at least one significant barrier. In several sources, occupational cases are not distinguished from nonoccupational cases. Others face the lack of standardization or use of text fields. However, these sources may gain importance with improvements in technology or changes in health care organization.

Medical Charts and Company Medical Services

Medical information is generally at the offices and hospitals where workers get medical care. The medical chart is a detailed source of information, but its use in occupational health surveillance has been limited. Medical records are sometimes confidential, or have restricted access. Even though important strides are being made to computerize medical records, much of the information is not standardized and is still written by hand. Nonetheless, statistical samples of medical charts may be used to assess the quality of health care.[70]

Companies that have on-site medical services are uniquely positioned to use their medical data. Many medical offices maintain a log that lists the patient and reason for the visit. Several large companies have automated some of the information they collect (See Chapter 17).[37,86]

Group Health Insurance

About 88% of the working U.S. population between the ages of 18 and 64 have some type of health insurance other than workers' compensation. This includes prepaid health maintenance organizations and other types of managed care.[87] Half of private sector employers offer health insurance, which covers about 58% of the employees.[88] Small employers are least likely to offer this benefit. Most persons over age 60 are enrolled in publicly administered health insurance (Medicare in the United States).

Even though these insurance systems specifically exclude work-related conditions from eligibility, a substantial amount of health care is provided for occupational diseases. This health care is recorded in the billing systems of insurance companies using the standard forms (Appendix A). Workers and their physicians may be truly unaware that the health problem is work-related. Some workers are discouraged by the adversarial nature of workers' compensation and seek treatment covered by other insurance. Chronic diseases caused by work may be first diagnosed in retirees enrolled in programs such as Medicare.

Even though cases are presumed to be nonoccupational, health insurance still may be used to identify cases of specific diagnoses for which occupation accounts for a high percentage of cases (sentinel events). At companies that offer private health insurance, this is a very valuable source of information for diseases that escape official reports of work injury and illness (Chapter 18).[89,90]

Disability Insurance

Disability insurance and sick leave are other benefits that are used for work injuries and illness. About 50% of the U.S. work force gets sick leave of a few days to a few weeks per year paid by their employer. Insurance programs for temporary disability lasting less than 6 months are administered by the states of California, New Jersey, New York, Hawaii, and Rhode Island.[91] Taken together with programs offered by private employers, about 44% of private sector workers are covered by some form of short-term disability insurance. Workers with serious long-term disabilities are covered by federal Social Security Disability Insurance (SSDI). The Social Security Administration has a computerized file of a sample of disabled workers who receive benefits under the disability insurance program. Data include age, sex, date of diagnosis, diagnoses, industry and occupation. This source has been used to investigate the links between occupation and disabling injuries and disease.[92,93] Data in private disability insurance, which paid out nearly $15 billion in 1994, are available at individual employers and can be a valuable resource for a company-based surveillance program (Chapter 18).

Disease and Exposure Registries

The U.S. National Cancer Institute and several states compile information on newly diagnosed cases of cancer at selected medical centers.[94] The information includes age, sex, race, residence, date of diagnosis, and clinical details such as cell type of cancer and stage of disease. Because occupation is sometimes coded, links between specific types of cancer and occupation can be established.[95] Similar types of registries exist for birth defects.[96]

Workers with exposures to specific chemicals are compiled into lists and followed up over time to determine if their health may be affected. Registries have been established for workers exposed to beryllium in arms manufacturing during World War II, [97,98] methylene bischloro aniline (MBOCA),[99] and dioxin.[100]

Other Data Sources

Several other data sources have been adapted for occupational health surveillance. Poison control centers record the patient's occupation and the details of the exposure (Chapter 23).[101] A national sample of approximately 60 emergency rooms electronically reports cases to the Consumer Product Safety Commission, which identifies consumer products that cause injuries. Occupation has been coded since 1982. Reports of coroners and medical examiners, highway transportation investigations for fatal motor vehicle injuries (FARS), and crime reports for violence are other examples of data sources.[31]

CHALLENGES IN OCCUPATIONAL HEALTH SURVEILLANCE

Occupational health and safety is also part of the public health tradition and has impressive accomplishments.[102] In 1913, in a work force of 38 million workers, approximately 23,000 U.S. workers died from work-related injuries. In 1997, the number of fatal work injuries was 6128 in a work force that had expanded to 131 million. Thus, the death rate was reduced over 90% from 61 deaths per 100,000 workers to 4.8 per 100,000.

National objectives for exposure and illness reduction for the year 2010 have been formulated for fatal injuries ($\leq$3.6 per 100,000), nonfatal injuries ($\leq$5.2 per 100 full-time workers) cumulative trauma disorders ($\leq$705,800 cases per year), skin disorders ($\leq$46 per 100,000), occupant protection systems, noise, blood lead greater than 25 μg/dL (0 cases), hepatitis B immunizations (100% of occupationally exposed), exposure standards for occupational lung disease, worksite back injury programs, and work-related homicides ($\leq$0.5 per 100,000). Several objectives have largely been met using baselines from the mid-1990s.[103]

The existing national surveillance system in the United States combines several different approaches based on employer reports, death certificates, surveys, and sentinel events notification systems. Without a doubt, surveillance has played an important role in reducing the burden of occupational disease and injury, and has helped formulate national occupational health objectives.[104] However, in the United States and many other countries, occupational health surveillance is "fragmented and 75 years behind" the rest of the public health community.[105] There are many reasons for this—technical, economic, political, and social. Difficulties are encountered at each stage of recognition, reporting, data collection, analysis, interpretation, and follow-up.

Recognition

Diagnosing a work-related illness is not as simple as diagnosing an infectious disease in the community. After the illness is diagnosed, the relationship to work has to be suspected or established. This means that workers, employers, and physicians have to be knowledgeable. Most physicians only get a few hours of training in occupational health in medical school. In the United States, nearly three-fourths of large employers (>500 employees) report having a regularly scheduled health and safety training program, but in small businesses (<100 employees), which employ about one-third of private-sector employees, only one in five say they provide regular safety training.[73,106] Recent immigrants face additional barriers of language, culture, and discrimination.

Many occupational diseases are not unique. Low back pain can be caused by lifting at work or lifting at home. It can start at home, but be made worse by work. Many are chronic conditions that develop over decades like cancer or chronic lung diseases. These time lags make it much harder for a worker or physician to link the illness to work. In addition, the employer where the exposure started may be out-of-business.

Reporting

There are incentives and disincentives for reporting cases. However, disincentives usually make underreporting the norm. Health care professionals say they are overwhelmed with paperwork, and that reporting takes time away from seeing patients. Some are unaware that they have to report or they do not know the procedures. There may be differences in the amounts physicians get reimbursed for the same medical care under workers' compensation and under general health insurance. If one pays more than the other, physicians may be more (or less) attentive to occupational health.

Some employers believe that they can avoid a rate hike on their workers' compensation insurance if they do not report injuries. This practice is illegal but it persists. Unfortunately, workers, health care professionals, and insurance companies can all get drawn into hiding cases. "Company" doctors may be biased in favor of the employer and not consider work as a cause of illness. They may unfairly suspect workers of faking illnesses to avoid work or to get benefits. Doctors who diagnose "too much" may be threatened with losing their contracts with employers.

Workers who report their health problems sometimes lose favor with their employer. Workers with a disability get labeled as *damaged goods*. Discrimination against the disabled is illegal in many countries, but it persists. Some workers hold out on reporting their injuries or illness as long as possible, fearing that they will lose their jobs. Waiting puts off early treatment and could hinder a full recovery.

Work injuries are sometimes linked directly to economic incentives for individual managers and workers. In some companies, workers' compensation costs come out of the company's overhead. But in others, costs are charged back to the departments where the injuries occurred. This might make a department manager more inclined to reduce costs by preventing injuries, or, with less effort, by hiding them. Policies on return-to-work also create incentives. If getting a replacement worker is out of the question, a supervisor may work more closely with the recovering worker and his or her physician to accommodate an early return-to-work. In other programs, if safety goals are met, managers, supervisors, or workers are rewarded with bonuses or prizes. There is always a danger that pressure from supervisors or peers will discourage workers from reporting their injuries.

Analysis, Interpretation, and Feedback

Surveillance data does not generally require sophisticated analysis to draw out meaning. But, many organizations face significant barriers, including automation of injury and employment databases, standardized coding, software for analysis, and skills for interpretation. Little research is available to shed light on the practice of occupational surveillance at private or public employers, insurers, health maintenance organizations (HMOs), or occupational health clinics. In the specialized area of occupational medical surveillance, about half of U.S. business establishments with more than 250 employees reported having a program in 1990. However, when establishments were visited to validate survey responses, very few were found to evaluate their program using even simple statistical techniques.[107] This suggests that surveillance skills are not put to use even by larger employers. A major challenge is to acquire the technical and organizational skills and to select appropriate surveillance models.

GENERAL READING

Industrial Hygiene and Safety

American Conference of Governmental Industrial Hygienists. *Industrial Ventilation: a Manual of Recommended Practice,* 20th edition. Cincinnati: ACGIH, 1989.

American Conference of Governmental Industrial Hygienists. *Threshold Limit Values and Biological Exposure Indices.* Cincinnati: ACGIH, 1999.

Burgess WA. Recognition of Health Hazards in Industry: *A Review of Materials and Processes.* New York: John Wiley, 1981.

Plog B. *Fundamentals of Industrial Hygiene,* Third Edition. Chicago: National Safety Council, 1988.

Proctor NH, Hughes JP, Fischman ML, eds. *Chemical Hazards of the Workplace,* Second Edition. Philadelphia: JA Lippincott, 1988.

Sax NI, Lewis RL. *Dangerous Properties of Industrial Materials,* 3 volumes. New York: Van Nostrand Reinhold, 1989.

Ergonomics

Eastman Kodak Ergonomics Group. *Ergonomic Design for People at Work,* Vol. 1 and 2. New York: Van Nostrand Reinhold, 1986.

Kuorinka I, Forcier L, eds. *Work Related Musculoskeletal Disorders (WMSDs): A Reference Book for Prevention.* London: Taylor & Francis, 1995.

National Institute for Occupational Safety and Health. *Revised Guide to Manual Lifting.* Cincinnati: National Institute for Occupational Safety and Health, 1991.

Putz-Anderson V, ed. *Cumulative Trauma Disorders: A Manual for Musculoskeletal Diseases of the Upper Limbs.* New York: Taylor & Francis, 1988.

Occupational Medicine and Diseases

Adams RM. *Occupational Skin Disease.* Philadelphia: WB Saunders, 1990.

Hayes WJ. *Pesticides Studied in Man.* Baltimore: Williams and Wilkins, 1983.

Levy BS, Wegman DH, eds. *Occupational Health: Recognition and Prevention of Work-Related Disease,* Second Edition. Boston: Little, Brown, and Co., 1988.

Morgan DP. *Recognition and Management of Pesticide Poisonings,* Fourth Edition. EPA 540/9-80-005, 1990.

Parkes WR. *Occupational Lung Disorders,* Second Edition. London: Butterworths, 1982.

Rom WN, ed. *Environmental and Occupational Medicine,* Second Edition. Boston: Little Brown & Co., 1992.

Weeks JL, Levy BS, Wagner GR, eds. *Preventing Occupational Disease and Injury.* Washington DC: American Public Health Association, 1991.

Epidemiology and Surveillance

Baker SP, O'Neill B, Ginsburg MJ, Li G. *The Injury Fact Book,* Second Edition. New York: Oxford University Press, 1992.

Monson R. *Occupational Epidemiology.* Boca Raton, FL: CRC Press, 1990.

Teusch SM, Churchill RE. *Principles and Practices of Public Health Surveillance.* New York: Oxford University Press, 1994.

Disability Management

Akabas SH, Gates LB, Galvin DE. *Disability Management: A Complete System to Reduce Costs, Increase Productivity, Meet Employee Needs, and Ensure Legal Compliance.* New York: AMACOM, American Management Association, 1992.

Economic Analysis in Occupational and Public Health

Haddix AC, Teusch SM, Shaffer PA, Duñet DO. *Prevention Effectiveness.* New York: Oxford University Press, 1996.

Oxenburgh M. *Increasing Productivity and Profit Through Health and Safety.* Chicago: Commerce Clearing House, 1991.

REFERENCES

1. Leigh JP, Markowitz SB, Fahs M, Chonggak S, Landrigan P. Occupational injury and illness in the United States. Estimates of costs, morbidity, and mortality. *Arch Intern Med* 1997; 157:1557–1568.
2. WHO Collaborating Centres in Occupational Health. *Global Strategy on Occupational Health for All.* Geneva: WHO, 1995.
3. Murray CJL, Lopez A. Global mortality, disability, and the contribution of risk factors: Global burden of disease study. *Lancet* 1997; 349:1436–1442.
4. Halperin W. The role of surveillance in prevention. *Am J Ind Med* 1996; 29:321–323.
5. Eylenbosch WJ, Noah N. *Surveillance in Health and Disease.* Oxford, England: Oxford University Press, 1988.
6. Last J. *A Dictionary of Epidemiology.* New York: Oxford University Press, 1995.
7. Langmuir A. William Farr: Founder of modern concepts of surveillance. *Int J Epidemiol* 1976; 5:13–18.
8. Teutsch SM, Churchill R. *Principles and Practice of Public Health Surveillance.* New York: Oxford University Press, 1994.
9. Centers for Disease Control. National notifiable disease reporting—United States, 1994. *MMWR* 1994; 43:800–801.
10. Centers for Disease Control. Mandatory reporting of infectious disease by clinicians and mandatory reporting of occupational diseases by clinicians. *MMWR* 1990; 39 (RR-9).
11. Centers for Disease Control. Summary of notifiable diseases, United States, 1997. *MMWR* 1997; 46 (54).
12. Pan American Health Organization. Health conditions in the Americas. Washington, DC: Pan American Health Organization, 1994.
13. Centers for Disease Control. Reduced incidence of menstrual toxic-shock syndrome—United States, 1980–1990. *MMWR* 1990; 39:421–423.
14. Centers for Disease Control. Ten great public health achievements—United States, 1900–1999. *MMWR* 1999; 48:241–243.
15. National Research Council. Toxicity Testing. Washington, DC: National Academy of Sciences, 1984.
16. Rutstein DD, Berenberg W, Chalmers TC, Child CG, Fishman AP, Perrin E. Measuring the quality of medical care. *N Engl J Med* 1976; 294:582–588.
17. California Occupational Health Program. Elevated blood lead in California adults, 1987–1990. Berkeley, CA: California Department of Health Services, 1991.
18. Rutstein DD, Mullan RJ, Frazier TM, Halperin WE, Melius JM, Sestito JP. Sentinel events (occupational) for physician recognition and public health surveillance. *Am J Public Health* 1983; 73:1054–1062.
19. Mullan RJ, Murthy L. Occupational sentinel health events: an updated list for physician recognition and public health surveillance. *Am J Ind Med* 1991; 19:775–799.
20. Matte TD, Baker EL, Honchar P. The selection and definition of targeted work-related conditions for surveillance under SENSOR. *Am J Public Health* 1989; Suppl 79:21–25.

21. Baker E. Sentinel event notification system for occupational risks (SENSOR): The concept. *Am J Public Health* 1989; Suppl 79:18–20.
22. Hanrahan LP, Higgins D, Anderson H, Haskins L, Tai S. Project SENSOR: Wisconsin surveillance of occupational carpal tunnel syndrome. *Wisconsin Med J* 1991; 90:80–83.
23. Centers for Disease Control. Adult lead epidemiology and surveillance—United States, Second and third quarters 1998, and annual 1994–1997. *MMWR* 1999; 48:213–223.
24. Maizlish NA, Rudolph LA, Dervin K. Surveillance of work-related pesticide illness: an application of the Sentinel Event Notification System for Occupational Risks (SENSOR). *Am J Public Health* 1995; 85:806–811.
25. Maizlish NA, Rudolph LA, Dervin KA, Sankaranarayan M. Surveillance and prevention of work-related carpal tunnel syndrome: an application of the Sentinel Event Notification System for Occupational Risks (SENSOR). *Am J Ind Med* 1995; 27:715–729.
26. Hinds MW, Skaggs JW, Bergeisen G. Benefit-cost analysis of active surveillance of primary care physicians for Hepatitis A. *Am J Public Health* 1985; 75:176–177.
27. Vogt RL, LaRue D, Klauke DN, Jillson D. Comparison of active and passive surveillance systems of primary care providers for hepatitis, measles, rubella, and salmonellosis in Vermont. *Am J Public Health* 1983; 73:795–797.
28. Silverstein BA, Stetson DS, Keyserling WM, Fine L. Work-related musculoskeletal disorders: comparison of data sources for surveillance. *Am J Ind Med* 1997; 31:600–608.
29. Silverstein B. Health and risk factor surveillance for work related musculoskeletal disorders. In: Kuorinka I, Forcier L, eds. *Work Related Musculoskeletal Disorders (WMSDs): A Reference Book for Prevention.* London: Taylor & Francis, 1995:213–245.
30. Melius J, Sestito JP, Seligman P. Occupational disease surveillance with existing data sources. *Am J Public Health* 1989; Suppl 79:46–52.
31. Stroup NE, Zack MM, Wharton M. Sources of routinely collected data for surveillance. In: Teutsch SM, Churchill R, eds. *Principles and Practice of Public Health Surveillance.* New York: Oxford University Press, 1994:31–85.
32. Department of Labor. Employment and wages covered by unemployment insurance. *BLS Handbook of Methods.* Washington, DC: US Department of Labor, 1982:Bulletin 2134-1.
33. *Current Population Census. The Employment Situation: July 1999.* Washington, DC: Bureau of Labor Statistics, USDL 99–221, 1999.
34. Bureau of Census. *Characteristics of the Population. 1990 Census.* Washington, DC: U.S. Government Printing Office, 1992.
35. Mines R. *Findings from the National Agricultural Workers Survey (NAWS) 1990.* Washington, DC: U.S. Department of Labor, 1992.
36. National Agricultural Statistics Service. *Census of Agriculture, 1997.* Washington, DC: U.S. Department of Agriculture, Volume 1, Geographic Area Series, 1999.
37. Sorock GS, Smith GS, Reeve GR, Dement J, Stout N, Layne L, Pastula S. Three perspectives on work-related injury surveillance systems. *Am J Ind Med* 1997; 32:116–128.
38. Bureau of Labor Statistics. *Survey of Occupational Injuries and Illnesses, 1997.* Washington, DC: U.S. Department of Labor, USDL 98-494, 1998.
39. Division of Labor Statistics and Research. *Occupational Injuries and Illness in California, 1991.* San Francisco: California Department of Industrial Relations, 1993.
40. Research Triangle Institute. *Statistical Support of Survey and Reporting Activities of Pesticide Exposure Incidents.* Research Triangle Park, NC: Research Triangle Institute, EPA Contract No. 68-01-6826, 1986.
41. Worker Health and Safety Branch. *California Pesticide Illness Surveillance Program Report—1996.* Sacramento: California Department of Pesticide Regulation, HS-1776, 1999.
42. National Council on Compensation Insurance. *Classification Codes and Statistical Codes for Workers Compensation and Employers Liability Insurance.* Boca Raton, FL: National Council on Compensation Insurance, 1995.
43. Kaufman JD, Cohen MA, Sama SR, Shields JW, Kalatt J. Occupational skin diseases in Washington State, 1989 through 1993: using workers' compensation data to identify cutaneous hazards. *Am J Public Health* 1998; 88:1047–1051.
44. McCullough JE, Henderson AK, Kaufman J. Occupational burns in Washington State, 1989–1993. *J Occup Environ Med* 1998; 40:1083–1089.
45. Silverstein B, Welp E, Nelson N, Kalat J. Claims incidence of work-related disorders of the upper extremities: Washington State, 1987 through 1995. *Am J Public Health* 1998; 88:1827–1833.
46. Daniell WE, Fulton-Kehoe D, Smith-Weller T, Franklin G. Occupational hearing loss in Washington State, 1984–1991: II. Morbidity and associated costs. *Am J Ind Med* 1998; 33:529–536.
47. Miller ME, Kaufman J. Occupational injuries among adolescents in Washington State, 1988–1991. *Am J Ind Med* 1998; 34:121–132.
48. Cheadle A, Franklin G, Wolfhagen C, Savarino J, Liu PY, Salley C, Weaver M. Factors influencing the duration of work-related disability: a population-based study of Washington State workers' compensation. *Am J Public Health* 1994; 84:190–196.
49. IAIABC EDI Development Project. *Medical Bill Payment Report.* Release 1. Kansas City: International Association of Industrial Accidents Boards and Commissions, 1996.
50. American National Standards Institute. Accredited Subcommittee X12. *Electronic Data Interchange Standards. Transaction Sets 148 (First Report of Injury), 837 (Health Care Claim).* Alexandria, VA: Data Interchange Standards Association, 1995.
51. Silverstein M. Analysis of medical screening and surveillance in 21 Occupational Safety and Health Administration standards: support for a generic medical surveillance standard. *Am J Ind Med* 1994; 26:283–295.
52. Dubrow R, Sestito JP, Lalich NR, Burnett CA, Salg J. Death certificate-based occupational mortality surveillance in the United States. *Am J Ind Med* 1987; 11:329–342.
53. Registrar General for England and Wales. *Occupational Mortality. Decennial Supplement for Great Britain, 1979–1980, 1982–1983.* London: Her Majesty's Stationary Office, Series DS No. 1, 1986.
54. World Health Organization. *International Classification of Diseases.* 9th Revision. Geneva: WHO, 1978.
55. Bureau of the Census. *Classified Index of Industries and Occupations. The 1990 Census of the Population.* Washington, DC: U.S. Government Printing Office, 1992.
56. Bureau of Labor Statistics. *National Census of Fatal Occupational Injuries, 1997.* Washington, D.C.: U.S. Department of Labor, USDL 98-336, 1998.
57. Division of Safety Research. *Fatal Injuries to Workers in the U.S., 1980–1989: A Decade of Surveillance.* Cincinnati, OH: National Institute for Occupational Safety and Health, DHHS (NIOSH) Publ. No. 93-108, 1993.
58. Centers for Disease Control. Fatal occupational injuries—United States, 1980–1994. *MMWR* 1998; 47:297–302.
59. Division of Respiratory Disease Studies. *Work-Related Lung*

Disease Surveillance Report, 1996. Morgantown: National Institute for Occupational Safety and Health, DHHS(NIOSH) Publ. No. 96-134, 1996.

60. Frazier TM, Lalich NR, Pedersen D. Uses of computer-generated maps in occupational hazard and mortality surveillance. *MMWR* 1984; 33:27–31.
61. Silverstein MA, Maizlish NA, Park R, Mirer F. Mortality among workers exposed to coal tar pitch volatiles and welding fumes at a stamping plant. *Am J Public Health* 1985; 75:1283–1287.
62. Milham S. *Occupational Mortality in Washington State, 1950–1979.* Springfield VA: National Technical Information Center, NIOSH Publ. No. 83-116 (No. PB-84-199-769/E09), 1989.
63. California Department of Health Services. *California Occupational Mortality, 1979–1981.* Sacramento: California Department of Health Services, 1987.
64. New York Department of Health. *Mortality in New York State, 1980–1982: A Report by Industry and Occupation.* Albany: New York State Department of Health, 1986.
65. Dubrow R, Wegman D. *Occupational Characteristics of White Male Cancer Victims in Massachusetts, 1971–1973.* Springfield VA: National Technical Information Center, NIOSH Publ. No. 84-109 (PB-85-218-683/E09), 1984.
66. National Institute for Occupational Safety and Health. *Mortality by Occupation, Industry, and Cause of Death—24 Reporting States (1984–1988).* Washington DC: Government Printing Office, DHHS (NIOSH) Publ. No. 97-114, 1997.
67. Vaughn TL, Daling JR, Starzyk P. Fetal death and maternal occupation: an analysis of birth records in the state of Washington. *J Occup Med* 1984; 26:676–678.
68. Starr TB, Levine R. Assessing effects of occupational exposure on fertility with indirect standardization. *Am J Epidemiol* 1983; 118:897–904.
69. Levy PS, Lemeshow S. *Sampling for Health Professionals.* Belmont, CA: Lifetime Learning Publications, 1980.
70. National Committee for Quality Assurance. *HEDIS 1999 (Health plan employer data and information set).* Washington, DC: National Committee for Quality Assurance, Technical Specifications. Volume 2, 1998.
71. Kyes KB, Franklin G, Weaver M. Reliability and validity of medical outcome and patient satisfaction measures among injured workers in Washington State: a pretest. *Am J Ind Med* 1997; 31:427–434.
72. Rudolph L, Wiley J, Dervin K, Garrett K, Maizlish N, Chang Y. *What Do Injured Workers Think of Their Medical Care?* San Francisco: Division of Workers' Compensation, 1998.
73. National Institute for Occupational Safety and Health. *National Occupational Exposure Survey.* Cincinnati: National Institute for Occupational Safety and Health, DHHS (NIOSH) Publ. Nos. 88-106, 89-102, 89-103, 1989.
74. National Institute for Occupational Safety and Health. *Occupational Health Supplement. 1988 National Health Interview Survey (NHIS).* Washington, DC: National Center for Health Statistics, 1992.
75. Behrens BJ, Seligman PJ, Cameron LL, Mathias CGT, Fine L. The prevalence of back pain, hand discomfort, and dermatitis in the US working population. *Am J Public Health* 1994; 84:1780–1785.
76. National Institute for Occupational Safety and Health. *Registry of Toxic Effects of Chemical Substances (RTECS).* Cincinnati, OH: National Institute for Occupational Safety and Health.
77. Code of Federal Regulations. *Occupational Safety and Health Administration.* Washington DC: US Government Printing Office, Parts 1900 to 1910, 1988.
78. American Conference of Governmental Industrial Hygienists. *Documentation of the Threshold Limit Values and Biological Exposure Indices.* Cincinnati, OH: American Conference of Governmental Industrial Hygienists, Publ. No. 206, 1999.
79. American Conference of Governmental Industrial Hygienists. *1999 TLVs® and BEIs®.* Cincinnati, OH: American Conference of Governmental Industrial Hygienists, Inc., Publication 0099, 1999.
80. National Institute for Occupational Safety and Health. *Occupational Safety and Health Guidelines for Chemical Hazards.* Cincinnati, OH: National Institute for Occupational Safety and Health, DHHS(NIOSH) Publ. Nos. 81-123, 88-118, 89-104, 92-110, 95-121, 1995.
81. American Industrial Hygiene Association. *The Occupational Environment—Its Evaluation and Control.* Fairfax, VA: AIHA Press, 1997.
82. National Institute for Occupational Safety and Health. *NIOSH Manual of Analytical Methods (NMAM®).* Cincinnati, OH: National Institute for Occupational Safety and Health, DHHS (NIOSH) Publ. No. 94-113, 1994.
83. Occupational Safety and Health Administration. *Integrated Management Information System.* Washington, DC: U.S. Department of Labor, http://www.osha.gov/oshstats/, 1999.
84. Froines JR, Baron S, Wegman DH, O'Rouke S. Characterization of the airborne concentration of lead in U.S. Industry. *Am J Ind Med* 1990; 18:1–17.
85. Mine Safety and Health Administration. *MSHA Inspector Dust Sampling Results (Metal and Nonmetal Mines).* Washington, DC: U.S. Department of Labor, http://www.msha.gov/STATS/SAMPLING/MAINPGE.htm, 1998.
86. Gowers DS, Carpenter AV, Ellis HM, Best AM, Nash D, Holzner CL, Keith JB, Sherrard H. Health surveillance using an occupational medical database. *J Occup Environ Med* 1998; 40:685–696.
87. Centers for Disease Control. State-specific prevalence estimates of uninsured and underinsured persons—Behavioral risk factor surveillance system, 1995. *MMWR* 1998; 47:51–55.
88. National Center for Health Statistics. *Employer-Sponsored Health Insurance: State and National Estimates.* Hyattsville, MD: Centers for Disease Control and Prevention, 1997.
89. Park R, Nelson NA, Silverstein MA, Mirer F. Use of medical insurance claims for surveillance of occupational disease. An analysis of cumulative trauma in the auto industry. *J Occup Med* 1992; 34:731–737.
90. Park RM, Krebs JM, Mirer F. Occupational disease surveillance using disability insurance at an automotive stamping and assembly complex. *J Occup Environ Med* 1996; 38:1111–1123.
91. Kerns W. Cash benefits for short-term sickness, 1970–1994. *Soc Sec Bulletin* 1997; 60:49–53.
92. Fischbach TJ, Dacey EW, Sestito J, Green J. *Occupational Characteristics of Disabled Workers, 1975–1976.* Cincinnati OH: National Institute for Occupational Safety and Health, Publ. No. 86-106, 1986.
93. Brackbill R, Maizlish NA, Fischbach T. Risk of neuropsychiatric disability among painters in the United States. *Scand J Work Environ Health* 1990; 16:182–188.
94. Ries LAG, Kosary CL, Hankey BF, Miller BA, Clegg L, Edwards B. *SEER Cancer Statistics Review, 1973–1996.* Bethesda, MD: National Cancer Institute, 1999.
95. Peters JM, Garabrant DH, Wright WE, Bernstein L, Mack T. Uses of a cancer registry in the assessment of occupational cancer risks. *Natl Cancer Inst Monogr* 1985; 69:157–161.
96. Katz EA, Shaw GM, Schaffer D. Exposure assessment in epidemiologic studies of birth defects by industrial hygiene review of maternal interviews. *Am J Ind Med* 1994; 26:1–11.
97. Williams W. United Kingdom Beryllium Registry: Mortality and

autopsy study. *Environ Health Perspect* 1996; 104S:949–951.
98. Sprince NL, Kazemi H. U.S. beryllium case registry through 1977. *Environ Res* 1980; 21:44–47.
99. Ward E, Halperin W, Thun M, Grossman HB, Fink B, Koss L, Osorio AM, Schulte P. Bladder tumors in two young males occupationally exposed to MBOCA. *Am J Ind Med* 1988; 14: 267–272.
100. Messerer P, Zober A, Becher H. Blood lipid concentrations of dioxins and furans in a sample of BASF employees included in the IARC registry of workers exposed to phenoxy acid herbicides and/or chlorophenols. *Environ Health Perspect* 1998; 106:733–735.
101. Blanc PD, Rempel D, Maizlish N, Hiatt P, Olson K. Occupational illness: case detection by poison control surveillance. *Ann Intern Med* 1989; 111:238–244.
102. Centers for Disease Control. Improvements in workplace safety—United States, 1900–1999. *MMWR* 1999; 48:461–469.
103. Centers for Disease Control. *Healthy People 2010 Objectives. Occupational Safety and Health (draft for public comment).* Hyattsville, MD: U.S. Department of Health and Human Services, 1999.
104. National Institute for Occupational Safety and Health. *National Occupational Research Agenda.* Cincinnati, OH: National Institute for Occupational Safety and Health, 1996.
105. Millar D. *OSHA Injury and Illness Information System: Testimony Before a Subcommittee of the Committee on Governmental Operations.* U.S. House of Representatives, 98th Congr. Second Session, 1984.
106. National Institute for Occupational Safety and Health. *Identifying High-Risk Small Business Industries.* Cincinnati, OH: National Institute for Occupational Safety and Health, DHHS-(NIOSH) Publ. No. 99-107, 1999.
107. Conway H, Simmons J, Talbert T. Effects of occupational surveillance programs as perceived by respondents to the Occupational Safety and Health Administrations 1990–1991 survey. *J Occup Med* 1993; 35:687–697.
108. Centers for Disease Control. Control of infectious diseases. *MMWR* 1999; 48:621–629.
109. Armstrong GL, Conn LA, Pinner R. Trends in infectious disease mortality surveillance in the United States during the 20th century. *JAMA* 1999;281:61–66.
110. American Water Works Association. *Water Chlorination Principles and Practices: AWWA manual M20.* Denver, CO: American Water Works Association, 1973.

2

Getting Organized

NEIL A. MAIZLISH

STEPS FOR SURVEILLANCE SYSTEMS

Workplace epidemiologic surveillance is difficult because it challenges our skills to stay focused on a problem-solving process that has numerous steps and details. Each step generates information that is both input to future steps and feedback to earlier steps. Table 2.1 shows the basic sequence of steps for surveillance systems, including active reporting and active case follow-up. The steps are applicable to surveillance done by an employer at a single worksite; a medical group, health maintenance organization, or insurance company that has multiple clients; or, a governmental agency at the local, state, or national level.

Naturally, there are important differences whether surveillance is being done by the employer or by another organization. Many job hazards, exposures, injuries, and short-term illnesses are readily observed at work. Employers have the authority and responsibility for working conditions at their worksites, and can make changes accordingly.

In contrast, government agencies and other organizations are farther removed from the sources of job hazards. They have a broader mission that includes oversight of occupational safety and health or provision of workers' compensation services. They have a special role in occupational disease surveillance because of the difficulties in recognizing occupational disease. They can combine data over many different worksites and small employers, and observe risk factors common to an industry, occupation, or geographic area that may not be apparent to an individual employer. Nonemployer organizations also initiate follow-up of injured workers and worksites because they provide a contracted service such as workers' compensation medical care or loss control. For government agencies, labor and public health laws provide a basis for enforcement, investigations, or other actions.

Because employers are required to record injuries, report cases to their workers' compensation carrier, tabulate their Occupational Safety and Health Administration (OSHA) logs, and post the summaries annually, some of the elements of data collection, analysis, and feedback are already in place at most U.S. workplaces. Employers, trade association, workers' compensation carriers, managed care organizations, and government agencies can build surveillance systems that meet specific goals, based on the foundation of existing data and established surveillance methods.

STEP 1. DEFINE GOALS, OBJECTIVES, AND SCOPE

The most important discussion that should take place before creating a surveillance system is defining the goals, objectives, and scope. This will determine the range of possible outcomes and risk factors that might be part of the surveillance system, the data needed and potential data sources, the appropriate surveillance methods, and the amount of resources and the number of personnel. All other aspects of surveillance will in some way be determined by this initial decision. The most important goals in occupational health and safety are to:

- prevent workplace injuries and illness (Goal 1)
- minimize disability once it occurs (Goal 2)
- improve the quality and effectiveness of occupational health and safety services (Goal 3)

Table 2.1 Steps in Planning and Implementing a Surveillance System

1. Define the goals and scope
2. Gain management support and that of all participants
3. Assemble a multidisciplinary team
4. Make case definitions, reporting guidelines, and define the minimum data set
5. Make an inventory of information and analyze the flow of information
6. Establish mechanisms for case reporting and its promotion
7. Select, recruit, and train the reporters
8. Establish protocols to prioritize cases for follow-up*
9. Activate case reporting, collect and code data into a database, follow-up,* and manage individual cases*
10. Analyze and interpret the data, identify groups at high risk, possible interventions, cost-benefit, and prepare standardized reports
11. Provide feedback to participants and disseminate the results
12. Evaluate the surveillance system

*Frequently a component of active and sentinel event surveillance systems.

Surveillance systems can be oriented to one or more of these goals. This book focuses almost entirely on Goal 1, the prevention of worksite injuries and illnesses. Disability surveillance and the surveillance of the quality and effectiveness of health services are emerging topics in occupational health and are discussed in Chapter 26.

Once goals have been established, surveillance systems should be organized around specific objectives derived from the general objectives and uses of surveillance (Chapter 1, Table 1.2). Examples of specific objectives are:

- track compensable injuries in order to reduce workers' compensation costs
- identify priority areas for a health and safety department of an employer, or areas of emphasis for enforcement and prevention by government agencies
- monitor the year-to-year changes in the number and rate of lost-time back injuries
- identify industries and occupations at risk for specific types of injury or illness
- identify individual workers and workplaces to target prevention services
- link case reporting to individual case follow-up

It is important to ask, "What objectives are possible given the available data sources and other limitations?" Many factors influence the degree to which objectives can be met. They are summarized in Table 2.2 and discussed in the following sections.

Table 2.2 Factors that Influence Objectives and Design of Surveillance Systems

Objective	*Factors that Influence Meeting Objective*	*Questions and Issues for Surveillance Methods and Data Sources*
Link case reporting to active follow-up	Timely reporting	Is the time lag between diagnosis and reporting to the surveillance system short enough to allow preventive actions to be relevant? Can active reporting shorten the time lag?
	Nature of injuries and illnesses	Is there a long time interval (latency) between exposure and onset of injury and illness? Diseases that are diagnosed years after the exposure may not be appropriate for active follow-up. Active follow-up may be appropriate for disability management or medical screening of coworkers.
	Nature of the exposure	Is the exposure likely to be present when diagnosis is made? Is the employer still in business? Has the industrial process changed so much over time that the exposure has ceased to exist?
	Availability of interventions	What can be done to lessen severity among those already affected and to prevent additional cases? Are there interventions for exposure reduction, medical treatment, and medical screening?
	Personal identifiers	For government agencies, do existing data sources provide a practical way to obtain names, addresses of cases, employers, and health care providers?
Estimate magnitude of a problem	Nature of injury or illness	Is the primary interest injuries or diseases? Passive systems are most likely to capture injuries and illnesses of short duration and miss diseases with long latencies.
	Availability of employment data	Is the magnitude of the problem expressed as case counts or as rates? Is employment data available to calculate rates?
Identify high-risk groups	Availability of employment data subgrouped in the same categories as the cases database	Does the employment database list individuals or aggregate employment data (hours worked, number of workers) using the same categories (occupation, department, industry, county) as the injury or illness database? If they vary in detail, can the categories be combined or aggregated to make the definitions of occupation, exposure, or industry alike for the cases and employment data?
Monitor trends in time and geography	Representativeness of cases	Passive systems may be suitable even if there is underreporting, as long as the cases that are reported have similar characteristics (such as industry, occupation, type of injury or illness, etc.) as the cases not reported.

Active Case Follow-up

Several questions can help determine whether active follow-up can be an important part of a surveillance system.

- Is there anything the surveillance system can offer to improve the health of specific individuals and their employers?

For a state agency interested in cancer surveillance, if all the cases died years ago and their employers are now out of business, the answer is probably no. Research may be appropriate, but not active surveillance.

- Has the disease or injury already run its full course, can follow-up alter the severity in the case or in coworkers, and can follow-up help identify still uncontrolled exposures?

Most injuries and short-term illnesses lend themselves to active follow-up. In contrast, health conditions like cancer or chronic occupational lung diseases develop slowly and appear decades after the first exposures.

- Are medical screening tests available and feasible for exposed coworkers who do not yet show signs of illness?

While it may be too late to alter events for the case, it may be possible to lessen the severity of illness in the coworkers through early detection and medical treatment.

- Is it likely that uncontrolled exposures can be identified, and acted upon?

Sentinel event surveillance is geared toward individual case follow-up because a high proportion of cases are related to known exposures that can be readily identified.

- Are identifiers (name, address, telephone number) available to contact the case, his or her employer and health care provider?

Active follow-up may be difficult for government agencies who are not in direct contact with the case or employer, but receive case reports from physicians or laboratories. The name, address, and telephone numbers may not be completely reported. Even when personal identifiers are available, it may not be feasible to routinely trace individuals.

Magnitude of the Problem, High-Risk Groups, and Trends

Estimating the magnitude of the problem, identifying high-risk groups, and monitoring trends can be achieved with counting cases in passive surveillance systems (Table 2.2). Even with undercounting, if the number of cases is significant, the estimate can still be useful for setting priorities.

These objectives can be more completely met when employment data are used to construct rates. Expressing the number of injuries and illnesses as a rate per 100 workers provides a common denominator for comparisons. (Employment data are also called population data or denominator data.) For example, if the shipping and receiving department at a company has 50 back injuries per year and the production department has 50 injuries also, we might think that the problem in both departments has the same magnitude. However, if shipping and receiving has only 100 employees and production has 1000 employees, the employees in shipping are 10 times more likely to have a back injury during the year: 50 per 100 in shipping versus 5 per 100 (50 per 1000) in production. Perhaps we should reconsider which department is the priority for follow-up. This reasoning is true whether surveillance is carried out by the employer, government agencies, or others. An important limitation is that rates may not be reliable for any group with few workers (e.g., a workplace with fewer than 10 persons, a small department in large factory, or uncommon occupations with few workers for an entire state).

One must ask whether employment data are available and accessible, whether they cover the same time period as the injury and illness data, and whether they can be subgrouped into the same categories that apply to injuries and illness. For example, if the number of injuries per year has not changed over time, the injury rate in the most current year will be overestimated by using 5-year-old employment data in a company that has continuously expanded employment over the past 5 years.

Some employment data are not automated or are counted at an aggregate level using preset categories. For example, a company may have a routine data run for the number of employees in each department. If you are interested in injury rates broken down by job title (occupation), the data run by department will not answer your question. It is very likely that the information for job title exists in the company database, but is not tabulated or circulated to all staff. If the database lists each person individually, a new data run can count employees in each job title. If no such database exists, an alternative is to manually count employees by job title. Obviously, lack of automation and poor database design are serious barriers to surveillance.

Sometimes the categories for subgrouping are defined more broadly or narrowly than one would like. For example, if one wishes to calculate the annual rate of injuries among carpenters, all carpenters and all of the injury cases among carpenters must be counted. If a company- or statewide employment database does not have carpenter as a unique category but lumps carpenters with skilled trades, the purpose will be thwarted. One is then faced with underestimating the injury incidence rate among carpenters, or broaden the detail to include cases among other skilled trades workers. This change may fit in with the original purpose or may be unacceptable.

Making the Scope More Manageable

Most surveillance systems make strategic decisions to bring resources into alignment with objectives. This is part of the trade-off between the quantity and the quality of any endeavor: to do more in less detail, or to do less with greater detail. Scope can be limited by selecting fewer outcomes, restricting the coverage of the surveillance system to specific geographic areas or employment groups, or using statistical samples.

One Outcome or Many

Restricting surveillance to a few health outcomes can make the surveillance system more manageable. It may be more feasible to collect data on cases with lost workdays than all cases that saw a doctor or that received first aid. Thus, how one defines the cases (Chapter 3) has an impact on the scope. If certain sentinel health events/occupational (SHE/Os) are a concern, focusing on one or a few may be a reasonable way of limiting the scope.

Even with a general outcome such as a reported case of illness or injury, it may be possible to collect data on diagnoses of each case. Surveillance systems such as the Bureau of Labor Statistics (BLS) or workers' compensation routinely collect, code, and analyze cases by diagnosis (nature and type), body part, and agent or exposure.

In passive systems, the scope is usually limited by the number of variables in the database, their level of detail, and the number of statistical analyses that can be carried out, interpreted, and written up. In contrast, systems with active reporting and active follow-up usually cannot manage more than a few specific health conditions or exposures at the same time because case reporting and follow-up are labor intensive.

Geographic and Population Coverage

Geographic targeting is usually an option of government agencies or large companies. It may also be used to pilot surveillance programs. At individual workplaces, targeting often involves deciding which departments, operations, and employee types (production as opposed to administrative) to include.

The scope can be changed by defining the cases or population under surveillance as those covered by workers' compensation or OSHA, or those reported from any potential data source. For employers, this latter option may require assessing first-aid cases, pension records, or group health and disability insurance (Chapter 18). State agencies may seek data from hospital discharge data, emergency rooms, poison control centers, or other publicly available data sources. These alternative sources include occupational cases that were not diagnosed as such, and work-related cases in self-employed workers not covered by workers' compensation.

Samples or the Entire Population

Sometimes data are so voluminous or geographically dispersed that it is not feasible to collect information on every injury and worker. Passive systems of government agencies and workers' compensation insurers can use samples to achieve surveillance objectives. The BLS surveillance system for nonfatal injuries and illnesses draws a statistical sample of OSHA logs and is a model for such an approach.

Active surveillance performed by government health agencies often cannot be maintained because resources are diluted below their effective level. The frequency, intensity, and quality of contact with health care providers reporting cases just cannot be maintained over a wide geographic area. Active surveillance can be made manageable by recruiting a sample of health care providers for reporting.

Samples of workers are also appropriate for special surveys, especially when the outcome of interest is not in any existing data source. Surveys of patient satisfaction or prevalence of pain are examples (Appendix B).

STEP 2. GAIN SUPPORT

Employer-Based Programs

The elements of successful employer-based health and safety programs have been known for decades:

- Commitment from the participants: workers, supervisors, managers, unions, health professionals
- Structure and process such as health and safety committee with real participation and clear lines of authority and responsibility
- Resources for personnel, equipment, supplies, communication
- Training and expertise in hazard recognition and control
- Methods for identifying problems (e.g., surveillance system for exposures and health events)
- Standards and guidelines for priorities and taking action
- Evaluation and goals for continuous improvement

These success factors apply to surveillance systems as well. Strong management commitment, and frequent close contacts between workers, supervisors, and management on health and safety issues are perhaps the most important. However, commitment must translate into resources for trained personnel, equipment, and methods for recognizing and anticipating problems. Without standards or guidelines for taking action, priorities and decision-making will be guided by anecdote and whim; action will be improvised or misguided. Ideally, surveillance should be a tool for measurement, evaluation, and coordination of other health and safety activities, rather than operating apart from an existing heath and safety program.

Support directly benefits the design and functioning of surveillance systems. Support improves the participation of workers, health professionals, employers, labor unions, government agencies, and professional groups. It lowers barriers so that participants will (*1*) share information that improves case reporting and follow-up and (*2*) be receptive to recommendations of the surveillance system.

Gaining and maintaining this support from the participants and stakeholders should be an explicit part of the development and maintenance of the surveillance system. It should start early and be ongoing. Support is rarely automatic or unconditional, but must be negotiated, taking into account benefits and risks. The benefits of surveillance include information that can:

- reduce injuries and illness
- reduce or avoid costs
- improve productivity
- improve the quality of goods and services
- increase morale and quality of work life

Surveillance can:

- increase the number of reported injuries and illness, and, as a consequence, their costs
- identify problems for which there are no easy solutions

Because benefits and risks vary among the participants and have the potential to conflict, considerable skill is needed in presenting an honest case for each benefit, cost, and risk. There are legitimate issues of who receives the benefits and takes the risks. Surveillance is most acceptable when all the stake holders benefit, the risks are minimal, and the tradeoffs are fair. Often the promise of improved health is not a sufficient incentive. If surveillance and follow-up contribute to savings, increased productivity, and profits, workers will be more willing to participate if they share in the benefits. Likewise, if a problem identified by surveillance has a solution that eliminates jobs through automation, many workers will prefer jobs with pain to losing their incomes altogether.

Meetings among members of a surveillance work group, workers, and managers during the planning stage can identify barriers and issues that drive concerns in health and safety, production, and quality of work life. Before appealing to upper management for support, one must be well-prepared. A brief presentation may be all that one gets to make a case and to seek approval. In that brief time, one must educate the management on the issues, outline the plan of action, and provide a rundown of the costs and the benefits, all in a style that transmits confidence, trust, and competence. Talking points for a 5–10-minute presentation geared to upper management in a company is outlined in Table 2.3. Because some of those involved might be

Table 2.3 Points of Discussion for a Brief Presentation to Upper Management at an Employer

- Our workers' compensation costs are rising. We have too many job injuries and illnesses.
- We can't afford this and we have do something. We cannot control the problem without a better understanding.
- We don't know whether it is a:
  - widespread problem or localized to a few areas
  - the result of ____ (name of specific medical problem) or
  - a wide range of injury and illness types, and whether it is getting worse over time
- We cannot identify their causes because we do not have a tracking (surveillance) system.
- A tracking system will tell us whether the problem is primarily in the ____ occupations in the ____ departments (where the problem is most severe)
- There appears to be a range of solutions, each with its own effectiveness and cost-benefit
- We might expect to get the following benefits:
  1. reduce productivity losses
  2. avoid costs and generating cost savings
  3. increase productivity
  4. improve product quality
- We have to act because
  1. there are OSHA* or other legal compliance issues
  2. workers are dissatisfied and we are losing good employees
  3. workers' compensation costs will go up
  4. it is the right thing to do
- We want your approval to move to the next step, which is:
  1. design and implement the surveillance system
  2. your visible commitment so that others will see that it is a priority. We will need resources for planning, establishing the system, and its maintenance. We will need to cross organizational lines to collect some of the data, so we need your support so that we will be taken seriously as we move about the plant.

*OSHA, Occupational Safety and Health Administration.

located outside of the organizational unit responsible for occupational health and safety, it is particularly important to emphasize the need for cooperation across organizational lines.

Government Agencies and Other Organizations

Gaining support for surveillance in government health agencies and other organizations involves similar issues inside the bureaucracy and with organized political constituencies. Even though occupational health and safety is part of the mission of most public health agencies, it competes for priority with other health concerns. At a societal level, the costs and benefits can be quantified,[1,2] but the potential benefits and costs usually affect different organized political constituencies in different ways. Managed care organizations and insurance companies may believe that surveillance is not a core business function, unless it can be developed into a product line or service, or unless customers demand such services. Nonetheless, the benefits and barriers need to be identified, and interest groups need to be consulted for their ideas, concerns, and possible solutions to real or perceived barriers.

Local health departments may view state officials as saviors in situations in which local expertise or resources are lacking, or as a threat by providing data that fuel controversies. The results of surveillance may generate a demand for health services that exceed local resources or clash with local priorities. Employers, unions, health care providers, and insurers excluded from the process may challenge the findings and be less receptive to implementing recommendations. Political considerations can affect the financing and design of surveillance systems and cannot be ignored.

Government agencies often find it advantageous to create an advisory board or select community advisors as a way of gaining and maintaining support. This sometimes is structured as a group that meets regularly and that includes members of labor and business organizations, health and safety professionals, civic groups, and representatives of other important community organizations.

Gaining support also has symbolic elements that require involving and even paying homage to influential individuals. These individuals may be beyond the outer most ring of your work unit or organization, or may be opinion leaders in the community. Aside from the symbolism, one should use this opportunity to gather information regarding their interests, concerns, and fears. One should also ask who else they recommend contacting so that the relevant social and professional networks are adequately explored.

Gaining support is an ongoing activity that needs periodic booster shots. The routine dissemination of surveillance data plays an important role in maintaining support.

STEP 3. FORM A SURVEILANCE TEAM

Active surveillance systems span five activities: data collection, analysis, interpretation, follow-up, and feedback. The skills and knowledge to implement them come from several different fields: epidemiology (health statistics), database management and administration, occupational medicine, industrial hygiene, ergonomics, safety engineering, health education, and communications. To put the results of surveillance into action, employer-based programs need input from plant engineers and product designers, supervisors, workers, professionals in strategic planning, business operations, procurement, and others who play some role in providing information to the surveillance system or are consumers of the information (Fig. 2.1).

For employers, the issues in building surveillance capacity are:

- coordinating existing staff and resources
- providing additional training (rather than getting new staff or contracting for consultants)
- demanding additional value from those who already provide contracted services for loss control or medical care
- any combination of the above

Some employers may find that their workers' compensation carrier has pertinent data that require more detailed analysis. Surveillance capacity can be phased in,

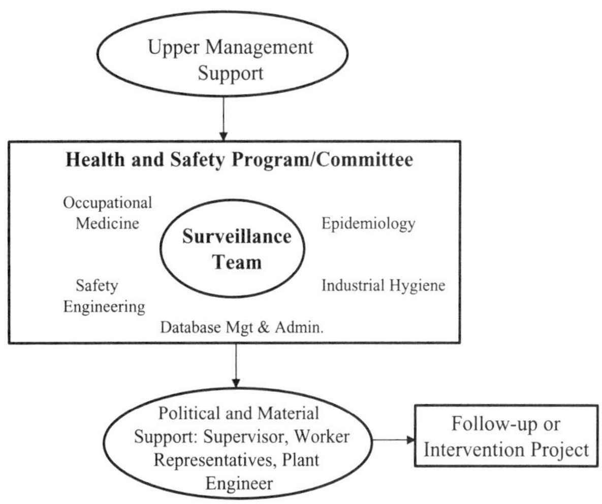

Figure 2.1 A company-based surveillance work group should have the support of upper management and be linked to the health and safety program. Ideally, some members of the work group should be involved in follow-up and intervention to help evaluate their impact.

starting with improvements in an existing passive data collection system, and later adding active case reporting and follow-up.

Passive systems generally require less staff than active systems. The skills of the staff are focused on data processing, statistical analysis, interpretation, and dissemination of information. If data are not automated, key entry and coding of text fields are labor-intensive steps.

Table 2.4 lists some of the functions and ideal job descriptions for a employer-based work group for active surveillance. Ideally, these functions are carried out by existing health and safety staff who work on surveillance tasks only part time. Staffing must be adequate to define objectives, identify the data to meet the objectives (Chapter 3), design or use a database (Chapter 10), analyze and interpret data (Chapter 7), and link cases to prevention activities (Chapter 6).

Government agencies and nonemployer organizations face similar issues in creating a surveillance work group. Compared to passive systems, surveillance that links case reporting by health care providers to work-site follow-up is labor intensive and requires staff with skills broad enough to handle or refer cases. Among the skills are occupational medicine, industrial hygiene

Table 2.4 Tasks and Functions of Personnel Carrying Out Surveillance

Position	*Education*	*Responsibilities*
Coordinator	Bachelors, master's, nursing or medical degree in health, industrial hygiene, safety, risk management, actuarial, or related science; or, an appropriate level of skill gained from experience.	Coordinate and provide overall guidance for the surveillance system; establish the administrative arrangements between departments (or government agencies), medical personnel, supervisors, health and safety committees, production, quality control committees, and community contacts. Develops and implements policies and protocols for case reporting, priorities for case follow-up, and carry out case follow-up. Document actions taken and not taken, assure data quality, carry out and interpret statistical analyses, help develop intervention strategies with in-house or external consultants on safety engineering, ergonomics, industrial hygiene; participate in cost-benefit analysis of interventions, prepare statistical summaries and reports for management and participants of the surveillance system; develop and carry out a dissemination plan appropriate to multiple audiences (management, technical, supervisors, workers, etc.). Provide functional supervision of the surveillance workgroup including technical assistants and analysts and information services. Identify and correct administrative problems, and when necessary, bring them to the attention of management.
Analyst or technician	Associate bachelor's degree or greater in accounting, biology, computer science, economics, engineering, psychology, or other fields that involve data collection or management; or, an appropriate level of skill gained from experience.	Carry out the protocols of the surveillance system under the supervision of the surveillance coordinator. Participate in the reporting of cases, collecting data, filling out of data collection forms, follow up when the information is incomplete, maintain routine contact with reporters and participants, collect information regarding the costs of cases and participate in data quality assurance and control.
Information technician	Associate bachelor's or greater in information systems, database management, computer programming, accounting, statistics, or other field related to information technology and data management; or, an appropriate level of skill gained from experience.	Enter data or oversee data entry including injury and illness reports and employment information (manual entry or relational linkage), establish and administer a database, and create or adapt the report generators to the needs of the surveillance system. Capable of carrying out simple statistical analysis using Structured Query Language (SQL) to identify subgroups of interest. Participates in data quality assurance, data maintenance, and the export of data to analysis packages.
Technical advisors and consultants* 1. Physician and occupational nurse	Postgraduate training or degree in occupational health; or, an appropriate level of skill gained from experience.	Apply clinical knowledge to assist in case confirmation; adapt or develop guidelines and protocols for medical treatment, disability, and return-to-work management.
2. Engineer, hygienist, ergonomist	Postgraduate (BS, MS, etc.) training or degree in occupational health; or an appropriate level of skill gained from experience.	Apply knowledge to assist with case confirmation, exposure classifications in statistical analyses, and develop protocols for follow-up interventions. Work with product-, process-, and production-engineers to develop modifications of workstations, processes, tools, and work practices.
3. Strategic and financial planner	College degree or appropriate skills gained from experience.	Apply knowledge of economic analysis to assess the cost-effectiveness of proposed interventions based on inputs from the surveillance system.

*In-house or external.

and safety, health education, communications, epidemiology or statistics, and database management.

In any organization, strong communications skills are necessary to present and market the surveillance findings. Government agencies sometimes carry out surveillance in culturally diverse populations. Multilingual and multicultural staff should be part of the team to increase access and acceptance by participants. Because government often works in coalitions with business, labor, health care, and professional groups, strong communications and organizational skills are needed to obtain effective results.

Organizational Issues

Surveillance functions do not necessarily follow the official organization chart. It is almost always necessary to cross organizational lines and involve staff from different work units. For company-based programs, this requires that managers and a surveillance coordinator or work group clearly lay out the lines of authority and responsibility to guarantee access to staff and information. A problem of organizing surveillance activities in some company-based programs is a confusion of the roles and responsibilities between the operational team and the expanded group of players who play largely supporting roles.

There are two distinct levels of support: (*1*) upper management who authorize the surveillance activity in general, and (*2*) middle management, department heads, supervisors, and the workers directly involved in case reporting, follow-up, and interventions (Fig. 2.1). Under ideal circumstances, surveillance is integrated into follow-up and interventions to help with their evaluations. A surveillance coordinator or work group can help identify whether data to evaluate an intervention are already part of the exiting surveillance system, or whether additional data are needed.

For government agencies, interagency agreements may be required to share data and protect the confidentiality of health and employment data.

REFERENCES

1. Leigh JP, Markowitz SB, Fahs M, Chonggak S, Landrigan P. Occupational injury and illness in the United States. Estimates of costs, morbidity, and mortality. *Arch Intern Med* 1997; 157: 1557–1568.
2. Murray CJL, Lopez A. Global mortality, disability, and the contribution of risk factors: Global burden of disease study. *Lancet* 1997; 349:1436–1442.

3

Collecting Data

NEIL A. MAIZLISH

STEP 4. MAKE CASE DEFINITIONS AND REPORTING GUIDELINES

To count health events or exposures, one must first carefully define them (Table 3.1). The definition can be based on:

- an authoritative source such as medical diagnosis made by a health professional or an exposure classification made by an industrial hygienist or safety professional
- an administrative definition that is used to fill in an OSHA log or to report an injury or illness to a workers' compensation insurance carrier or state agency
- an operational definition created by the surveillance system

In passive surveillance systems, cases are usually defined by administrative rules. These rules have thresholds of severity to trigger case reporting. In OSHA recordkeeping and workers' compensation these triggers are treatment beyond first aid and causing lost time from work. This favors more severe cases that have medical testing, treatment, and data available to show objective evidence of an injury or illness.

Active systems build on this information, but often collect additional data to meet a specific surveillance objective. Additional data may be available from first medical visits, questionnaires filled in by workers, industrial hygiene reports, and searches of other databases. For example, musculoskeletal disorders (MSDs) in their early stages often generate complaints of aches and pains that affect productivity but may not be serious enough to generate workers' compensation claims. To estimate the magnitude of this particular problem and identify high-risk groups at a company, case definitions can be based on first medical visits or symptoms reported on questionnaires filled in by workers. Some active surveillance systems make a concerted effort to find cases below the severity thresholds of passive systems and cases of occupational disease not reported on OSHA logs or workers' compensation. Appendix B illustrates questionnaires used for active risk factor surveillance and active case finding of MSDs in employer-based surveillance programs.[1,2] Thus, the way a health event is defined and whether the surveillance system is active or passive influences the number of cases counted.

Case Definitions Used in Public Health Surveillance Systems

The next sections are oriented to case definitions used by governmental public health agencies particularly for the surveillance and follow-up of occupational diseases reported by health care professionals. Employers and other organizations may create operational case definitions for their own purposes.

These definitions often combine data from several data sources. Data collection involves contact with health care providers, patients, or employers to gather details after a simple case report is filed. In addition to clinically confirmed cases, health care professionals are instructed to inform public health authorities of suspected cases and those that are waiting confirmation. Thus, the data available for each case may be variable in quality and quantity, and may change over time.

Data provided on report forms and other sources,

Table 3.1 Ways of Defining a Case

Type	*Criteria*	*Examples*
Authoritative	Professional judgement	Medical diagnosis
		Industrial hygiene, safety, or ergonomic assessment
Administrative	Threshold of more than first aid (OSHA*)	Beyond one-time treatment and subsequent observation—even when administered by a doctor or nurse—for minor scratches, cuts, burns, or splinters that do not ordinarily require medical treatment
	Threshold of disability for workers' compensation	Illness and injury that results in lost time beyond the date of illness or injury, or requires medical treatment beyond first aid. Occupational illness is any abnormal condition or disorder caused by exposure to environmental factors associated with employment, including acute and chronic illnesses or diseases or diseases that may be caused by inhalation, absorption, ingestions, or direct contact
		Lost work time injury or illness of at least 3 or more days beyond the shift of occurrence
		Insurance claim in which a payment was made to a worker or physician
Surveillance or epidemiologic research	Signs, symptoms, and physical findings	A classification system that takes symptoms, signs, and physical findings into account and sometimes gives levels of certainty such as definite, probable, suspect or possible.
	Laboratory confirmation	Worker with a breathing zone sample exceeding 10% of the recommended exposure level
		Blood lead levels > 25 μg Pb/dL
		Red blood cell cholinesterase inhibition > 30% of baseline
		Forced expiratory volume at 1 sec (FEV_1) < 70% than predicted
		Hearing loss with a displacement of 25 dB or greater at 4000 KHz

*OSHA, Occupational Safety and Health Administration.

when available, are compared against criteria to determine whether a reported case meets the definition for public health purposes. The general format follows rules of logic and has the sequence:

A. Symptoms and signs present
   and (or)
B. Objective findings present
   1. Physical findings
      and (or)
   2. Laboratory confirmation

and

C. Evidence of Work Exposure
   1. A history of occupational exposure
      and (or)
   2. Physical findings

Parts A and B are criteria for the health problem, and part C are criteria for the degree to which the problem is work-related. One can make the definition more restrictive by requiring parts A *and* B to simultaneously be in effect, or less restrictive by using *or*, which requires only one of the two criteria to be met. Thus, how the logic is applied influences the number of cases. This is discussed in more detail in this chapter under the topic of sensitivity and specificity of Scientific Classification Systems. Some disease control programs begin case follow-up even if the relation to work (part C) is not initially established. When more information is available the case may be reclassified.

Case definitions also have specific criteria that exclude certain cases that are not eligible because they are caused by other medical conditions or exposures not related to work. Likewise, certain criteria may help include cases, based on the existence of mini-outbreaks or symptomatic coworkers with similar exposures at the same worksite. Table 3.2 applies this type of logic to work-related carpal tunnel syndrome.[3]

Certainty Levels

The case definition in Table 3.2 places workers into two categories: case and not a case. Case definitions for surveillance also use multipoint scales to indicate the level of certainty. For example, cases can be categorized on a three-point scale: confirmed case, suspected case, and not a case. Five-point scales are common: definite, probable, possible or suspect, not a case, and not classifiable. Confirmation is often associated with a laboratory test or other hard evidence. Multipoint scales are particularly useful when laboratory results are not available or applicable, exclusion or inclusion criteria are missing on many cases, or when other aspects of data quality vary from case to case. In these situations, it is difficult to generate rapid and reproducible classifications unless there are explicit rules.

A multipoint scale is shown in Table 3.3, and uses a matrix method for assigning probability to suspected cases of work-related carpal tunnel syndrome in an ac-

Table 3.2 Surveillance Case Definition for Work-Related Carpal Tunnel Syndrome

A. One or more of the following symptoms suggestive of carpal tunnel syndrome (CTS) is present:[a] parethesias, hypothesia, pain, or numbness affecting at least part of the median nerve distribution[b] of the hand(s).

AND

B. Objective findings consistent with CTS are present in the affected hand(s) and wrist(s):

EITHER

1. Physical examination findings—Tinel's sign[c] present or positive Phalen's test[d] or diminished or absent sensation to pin prick in the median nerve distribution of the hand.

OR

2. Electrodiagnostic findings indicative of the median nerve dysfunction across the carpal tunnel.[e]

AND

C. Evidence of work-relatedness—a history of a job involving *one or more* of the following activities before the development of symptoms[f]:

1. Frequent, repetitive use of the same or similar movements of the hand or wrist on the affected side(s)
2. Regular tasks requiring the generation of high force by the hand on the affected side(s).
3. Regular or sustained tasks requiring awkward hand positions on the affected side(s).[g]
4. Regular use of vibrating hand tools.
5. Frequent or prolonged pressure over the wrist or base of the palm on the affected side(s).

[a]Symptoms should have lasted at least 1 week or, if intermittent, have occurred on multiple occasions. Other causes of hand numbness or paresthesias, such as cervical radiculopathy, thoracic outlet syndrome, and pronator teres syndrome, should be excluded by appropriate clinical evaluation.

[b]Generally includes palmar side of thumb, index finger, middle finger, and radial half of ring finger; dorsal (back) side of the same digits distal to PIP joint; and radial half of palm. Pain and paresthesias may radiate proximally into the arm.

[c]Parethesias are elicited or accentuated by gentle percussion over the carpal tunnel.

[d]Parethesias are elicited or accentuated by maximal passive flexion of the wrist for 1 minute.

[e]Criteria for abnormal electrodiagnostic findings are generally determined by the individual laboratories.

[f]A temporal relationship of symptoms to work or an association with cases of CTS in coworkers performing similar tasks is also evidence of work-relatedness.

[g]Awkward hand positions predisposing to CTS include the use of pinch grip (as when holding a pencil), extreme flexion, extension, or ulnar deviation of the wrist, and use of the fingers with the wrist flexed.

Source: Cummings et al.[3]

tive surveillance system (Chapter 13). The sources of information available to the surveillance team included a standardized report form for symptoms, signs, and physical findings completed by the physician, data abstracted from medical charts, and telephone interviews with the worker and the employer. Upon entering the matrix the reports were evaluated for whether they met the criteria for a possible or suspected case. If the case met *all* the criteria at the next higher certainty level, the case moved up the matrix. Some reported cases were so sketchy that they had to be placed in the category for unclassifiable or uncertain. Unlikely cases were those in which the time sequence between stated exposures and the disease seemed improbable, or information on job risks also made it unlikely that work was a cause.

There is a difference between the lack of data and a report of a negative finding. In Table 3.3, possible and probable cases differ because some physicians reported exclusion criteria (probable) and some did not (possible).

Public Health Versus Clinical Definitions

Public health case definitions are similar to clinical definitions and incorporate the same type of scientific information. Ideally, they would be the same. However, public health authorities often use case definitions that are broader than those used by doctors to treat individual patients, or by administrative systems. There are several reasons for this. First, the purpose of the definitions is different. The purpose or goal of the clinical case definition (or diagnosis) is to assure appropriate medical treatment of an individual patient. Administrative systems such as workers' compensation define cases for the purpose of determining eligibility for benefits. For occupational health surveillance, the goal is to treat the workplace, in the sense of identifying and preventing the exposures that cause injury or illness.

Second, for many occupational diseases, such as soft tissue injuries, there is considerable uncertainty of the clinical diagnosis and no diagnostic test is a gold standard. Only the most severe cases may generate enough medical data to make a firm diagnosis. Thus, if surveillance is limited to only severe cases, important objectives such as estimating the full magnitude of the problem may go unmet. There may be many lost opportunities for prevention as mild cases progress to full blown cases that are not reversible. Thus, surveillance definitions sometimes include cases that might be considered mild by clinicians as long as they meet other scientific criteria. The relation to occupation may also be uncertain, which reflects a physician's lack of information or knowledge about workplace risks, the availability or access to exposure data, and the knowledge of workers and employers.

Table 3.3 Surveillance Case Definition for Work-Related Carpal Tunnel Syndrome: Minimum Requirements for Classification

	Medical Information						*Temporal Sequence*		*Work*
Case Probability	*NCV*[a]	*Signs*[b]	*Symptoms*[c]	*Mimicking Conditions*[d]	*Associated Conditions*[e]	*Acute Trauma*[f]	*Symptom Onset*[g]	*Exacerbation*[h]	*Job Risk*[i]
Definitive	[(+ and	(≥ 1 or	≥ 1) and	– and	– and	–] and	[(+ or	+)]	and [+]
Probable		[(≥ 1 and	≥ 1) and	– and	– and	–] and	[(+ or	+)]	and [+]
Possible or suspect		[(≥ 1 or	≥ 1)]						and [+]
Improbable or no							– and	–	and [–]
Uncertain									

Cases enter the confirmation matrix at the "possible or suspect" level and move upward or downward according to the available information. The minimum information on any case is the physician report form (see Chapter 13).

[a]+ = Nerve conduction velocity (NCV) for the distal median nerve, which is abnormal according to normal laboratory range. The data source is the physician report form. Cases reported without a normal laboratory range uses: NCV < 38 m/s as abnormal; latencies for motor nerve > 3.5 ms are abnormal and latencies for sensory nerve > 4.4 ms are abnormal.

[b]+ = Tinel's sign present or positive Phalen's test or decreased or absent pin prick sensation in the median nerve distribution of the hand. Source: Physician's report form.

[c]+ = 1 or more of the following: pain, tingling, or numbness affecting at least part of the distribution of the median nerve with symptoms lasting more than one week or occurred on two or more occasions (>1 episode). Sources: physician report form and patient questionnaire.

[d]– = No history of cervical root compression, generalized peripheral neuropathy, thoracic outlet syndrome, or pronator teres syndrome. For definite source is medical record; for probable the source is the patient questionnaire.

[e]– = No history rheumatoid arthritis, insulin dependent diabetes, hypothyroidism, gout pregnancy, or bilateral oophorectomy. Source is patient questionnaire.

[f]+ = Reported symptoms started as the result of a sudden wrist or arm injury such as fracture, or injury due to automobile or sports activity.

[g]+ = Symptoms started after starting job. Source: patient questionnaire.

[h]+ = Symptoms have become worse after starting job. Source: patient questionnaire.

[i]+ = Presence of one or more job risks. Source: case questionnaire or report form.

There are potential consequences of using surveillance rather than clinical definitions. Even if surveillance definitions are admittedly more tolerant of false positives, it does not mean that employers are more tolerant. Minimizing both false positive and false negative cases is highly desirable for case definitions. For employers, this raises a concern that their legal liability will increase if broad definitions are used, or if separate books are maintained for OSHA, workers' compensation, and a more proactive surveillance system. Some employers have already solved this by creating a single computerized database for injuries and illness in which a standardized logic program categorizes cases reported for any reason as (*1*) cases reportable to their insurance carrier, (*2*) cases recordable on OSHA logs, and (*3*) cases for internal company follow-up (Chapter 17).

Scientific Classification Systems

The following characteristics should be considered in any scientifically based method to classify health conditions and exposures:

- natural
- mutually exclusive categories
- exhaustive
- standardized
- rapid
- reproducible
- manageable
- accurate
- valid

The data and criteria used to classify cases should be natural to the classifier. Personnel should be appropriate and be familiar with what is scientifically known about the health condition and the exposure of interest.

Mutually exclusive means the same health event or exposure belongs to only one category at a time. For example, one is either a case, or not a case; or a person is male or female.

Exhaustive means that each case has been classified. Missing data should be discouraged, but sometimes the quality of the data is so poor that some cases are labeled unclassifiable.

Standardized means that the decision process follows set rules, definitions, inputs, procedures, and outputs.

Rapid means that each case can be classified in a relatively short period of time. Once all the source documents (e.g., report forms, laboratory results, interviews, follow-up investigations, etc.) are collected, this is usually on the order of minutes. If all the criteria and data are computerized, this process may be automated.[4] A classification system is not practical if much time is spent debating each case.

Reproducible means that the decision is the same each time a list of potential cases is classified. This operates at the line item level rather than in the aggregate. Even if a list of 10 candidates is judged to have 5 cases by 2 different raters, the process is not reproducible if Rater A says the 5 cases occur in persons 1, 3, 5, 7, and 9 and Rater B says the 5 cases occur in persons 2, 4, 6, 8, and 10. This is true for the same rater who classifies the same list on different occasions, or for different raters using the same list.

Manageable means that a reasonable number of categories are created by the classification. For employers, a practical problem arises in classifying exposure groups using a department or job title. Large workplaces have dozens of administrative departments or job classifications that have just a few persons. To work around this problem, it is necessary to group together small departments into a single group that has similar exposures.

Accurate means the degree to which true cases are always classified as cases (sensitivity) and true noncases are classified as noncases (specificity) (Fig. 3.1).

Valid means that classification criteria and results are consistent with professional judgement and scientific knowledge.

In addition to expert opinion, accuracy and validity are assessed by comparing the results of the classification system against a gold standard, such as an accepted laboratory test. For example, it might be possible to classify cases of acute, organophosphate pesticide poisoning from a questionnaire of symptoms and signs. The validity of this classification will be enhanced if it can be shown that all the questionnaire cases have an abnormal laboratory result (30% or greater cholinesterase inhibition from a baseline measure), and all the questionnaire normals have less than 30% inhibition, which is considered a normal laboratory result. The questionnaire cases that are true normals (<30% inhibition) are called false positives, and the questionnaire normals that are true cases (≥30% inhibition) are called false negatives (Fig. 3.1).

Questionnaire:	**True Case** ≥ 30% Inhibition	**True Normal** < 30% Inhibition
Positive	(a) True positive	(b) False positive
Negative	(c) False negative	(d) True negative

$$\text{Sensitivity} = \frac{\text{True positive}}{\text{All true cases}} = \frac{a}{a+c}$$

$$\text{Specificity} = \frac{\text{True negative cases}}{\text{All true normal cases}} = \frac{d}{b+d}$$

$$\text{Positive Predicitive Value} = \frac{\text{True positive cases}}{\text{All positive cases on questionnaire}} = \frac{a}{a+b}$$

$$\text{Proportion of Agreement} = \frac{\text{True positive cases and true negative cases}}{\text{All cases}} = \frac{a+d}{a+b+c+d}$$

Questionnaire:	**True Case** ≥ 30% Inhibition	**True Normal** < 30% Inhibition
Positive	40	10
Negative	5	45

$$\text{Sensitivity} = \frac{40}{45} = 89\%$$

$$\text{Specificity} = \frac{45}{55} = 82\%$$

$$\text{Positive Predicitive Value} = \frac{40}{50} = 80\%$$

$$\text{Proportion of Agreement} = \frac{40+45}{100} = 85\%$$

Figure 3.1 A method for evaluating the accuracy of classification systems or individual raters. In this example, the pattern of symptoms reported by patients on a questionnaire is being compared against their own laboratory tests. Before making the comparison with the laboratory tests, the designers of the questionnaire determine which items on the questionnaire must be positive in order to classify the person as a case of pesticide illness. This follows a set of fixed decision rules, such as 3 or more symptoms checked off on a list of 10. The laboratory test is considered to be a gold standard and reflects the true state of health.

Guidelines for Reporting

Reporting a case and determining whether a case meets a surveillance case definition are two distinct but related functions. Case definitions are for the internal use of the surveillance system, and reporting guidelines are for the case reporters. Guidelines for reporting act as a primary filter that orients the surveillance system toward greater or lesser sensitivity and specificity. The surveillance case definition acts as a secondary filter that attempts to apply uniform criteria to carry out the goals of the surveillance system.

Guidelines parallel the case definition in content and serve an educational purpose. An example guideline for work-related carpal tunnel syndrome is shown in Table 3.4. Most administrative systems do not have active outreach to educate or remind case reporters (workers, supervisors, health care professionals) of the details of what they are required to do. To help improve the reporting, guidelines can be provided by the surveillance system. The guidelines should state:

- the type of case(s) that should be reported and examples of those cases

Table 3.4 Guidelines for Reporting Carpal Tunnel Syndrome Cases for Epidemiologic Surveillance

Health Care Providers. You are being asked to report all suspected cases of carpal tunnel syndrome that are related to work, nonwork activities, or are of unknown etiology to the California Department of Health Services. To assist our surveillance program, we are requesting reports of severe, moderate, and mild cases.

Reported cases should meet the criteria below:

A. Symptoms compatible with carpal tunnel syndrome including cases of unknown etiology (Table 3.4A)

—OR—

B. Objective findings compatible with carpal tunnel syndrome (Table 3.4B)

Job characteristics with risks for carpal tunnel syndrome (Table 3.4C) and occupations associated with cumulative trauma disorders (Table 3.4D) are presented in the following tables.

Table 3.4A Symptoms Compatible with Carpal Tunnel Syndrome

Symptoms suggestive of carpal tunnel syndrome include any combination of the following symptoms affecting at least part of the median nerve distribution of the hand(s):

Pain

Paresthsia

Numbness

Weakness

Table 3.4B Objective Findings Suggestive of Carpal Tunnel Syndrome

1. A tingling sensation in the nerve distribution with percussion over the median nerve in the affected wrist(s) (Tinel's sign).
2. Pain or tingling with sustained hyperflexion of the wrist (Phalen's sign).
3. Decreased sensation in the sensory distribution of the median nerve in the affected hand(s) (pin prick).
4. Thenar atrophy.
5. Electrodiagnostic findings of sensory or motor nerve dysfunction (as a conduction velocity reported in meters per second or latency in milliseconds).

Table 3.4C Job Characteristics with Risks for Carpal Tunnel Syndrome

1. Regular use of the hand(s) on the affected side(s) in tasks involving repetitive or forceful movements.
2. Regular use of the hand(s) on the affected side(s) in tasks involving awkward hand postures. Is the wrist used in position other than neutral? i.e. lateral deviation, flexion, rotation or wringing motions?
3. Frequent or prolonged pressure over the wrist(s) or base of the palm(s) on the affected side(s).
4. Prolonged constrained postures. Is one posture held for long, uninterrupted periods throughout the workshift?
5. Regular use of vibrating hand tools or work surfaces.
6. Finger tips and thumb opposed for frequent or prolonged periods in a pinch grip.

Table 3.4D Occupations and Jobs at Risk for Cumulative Trauma Disorders (Partial List)

• Buffing and grinding	• Letter carriers
• Punch press operators	• Carpenters
• Overhead assemblers	• Material handlers
• Key entry	• Construction workers
• Sewers and cutters	• Butchers and meat packers
• Assembler (small parts)	• Core makers
• Musicians	• Cooks
• Operating room personnel	• Secretaries
• Dental hygienists	• Welders
• Truck drivers	• Packers

- the type of case(s) that should not be reported and examples of those cases
- the deadline for reporting after the case has been detected or diagnosed
- where the case report form should be sent and by what mechanism (mail, fax, electronic, etc.)
- the thresholds of severity and how to handle mild cases
- how to handle suspect cases due to uncertain diagnosis or an uncertain relationship to work
- how to handle cases pending further diagnostic testing

STEP 5. MAKE A DATA INVENTORY

Defining the Data Needed

The specific objectives of the surveillance system will determine the data needed. To meet the basic objectives of defining the problem(s), estimating the magnitude of the problem(s), identifying high-risk groups, and monitoring trends, most of the following items should be considered in a minimum or core data set (Table 3.5), whether surveillance is company- or government-based:

- a case definition or diagnosis
- the date of the injury or onset of the illness
- industry
- occupation
- date of hire
- age (date of birth)
- sex
- race or ethnicity
- location (department for employers) and geographic area (county, state, region).

Some systems for classifying the diagnosis of injuries give additional information on body part(s) affected and the external cause or agent (e.g., motor vehicle, hand tools, struck by object).

Table 3.5 Data to Be Considered in Selecting a Minimum Data Set for Surveillance Systems

Category	*Data Element*
CASES	
Person and injury/illness	Identifier and name
	Diagnosis* or other case definition
	External cause of injury
	Date of birth
	Gender
	Race or ethnicity
Place/environment	Department (industry), geographic or location code
	Occupation or job
	Hire date, dates of transfers to new jobs*
Time	Date of injury, onset of illness
	Date of return to work*
EMPLOYMENT (POPULATION)	Hours worked, full-time equivalents, persons a. individually listed, or b. grouped by person-place-time data elements
CASE MANAGEMENT	Proposed action*
	Deadline for proposed action*
	Person responsible for taking action*
COSTS	Cost per case or cost per hour of production (direct and indirect)
HEALTH SERVICES	Diagnoses*
	Type and date of treatments* (linked to diagnoses)
	Cost of treatment
	Provider credential, provider specialty
	Treatment setting (hospital, physician office)
	Health system characteristic (e.g., managed care)

* Can have multiple per case.

When surveillance is rate-based, it is necessary to collect:

- employment data for each worker or subgroup in appropriate categories for at least occupation and industry, and, for employers, job title and department

To meet the objective of linking case reporting to worksite follow-up:

- personal identifiers (names of workers, employers or supervisors, health care providers, telephone numbers and addresses) are necessary

Data to meet the broad goals of disability management and evaluation of the quality and effectiveness of health services are also presented in Table 3.5 and discussed in Chapter 26.

Evaluating Data Sources

Most surveillance systems build on existing injury and illness reporting and data collection systems. Each potential data source has strengths and weaknesses. Scope, population coverage, accuracy, timeliness of data collection, accessibility, standardization, and linkability to other databases are criteria to help evaluate potential data sources.

In active reporting systems, there are practical limits on what data providers may be reasonably expected to report. Those with high workloads will be reluctant to do little more than what their current practice allows. However, small, but important changes to forms for reporting and to procedures may be possible. Data providers generally ignore requests to report a long list of data elements. This results in incomplete reports with low data quality.

Appropriate Scope

The scope of the data is the breadth of the information on health, exposure, risk factors, costs, and their relevance to the objectives of the surveillance system. One tests the scope by asking which health outcomes, exposures, and characteristics of the work force such as age, sex, race, education, and residence are part of the data source. Are occupational cases distinguished from nonoccupational cases? Does the data source have information on just illness and injuries or does it is also have data on the population and employment?

Coding and the Level of Detail. Coding of information determines the level of detail available to answer key questions. Diagnosis, industry, and occupation are challenges for coding. In the United States, employers, insurance companies, and government agencies have their own coding systems. Because the categories do not match, an injury or illness rate calculated by an individual employer cannot be easily compared to publicly available data.

The two main public coding systems for diagnosis are the International Classification of Diseases (ICD), 9th or 10th Revision,[5] and the American National Standards Institute (ANSI Z16) nature-type-body part-agent.[6] Both coding systems have strengths and weaknesses. The ICD provides more medical detail, whereas the ANSI Z16 has more detail on the external cause of the injury. (The external cause describes what in the environment came into contact or caused an injury, such as a fall, a motor vehicle crash, an electrocution, or being struck by an object.) Until the 10th Revision of the ICD, the level of detail for body part was greater in the ANSI classification. Workers' compensation insurers use a variant of the ANSI system, which codes nature, body part, and external cause.

There are also several major industry and occupation (I/O) coding systems. Some have as few as three digits and others as many as nine. Nearly all are hierarchical with increasing detail as digits are added. Nearly all reflect economic activity rather than job risks or actual exposures. Increased precision comes with combining industry and occupation into unique categories, such as the Job Exposure Matrix.[7]

United States government agencies use four principal I/O classification schemes. The Bureau of the Census (BOC)[8] classification has over 200 three-digit industries and 505 three-digit occupations. The Standard Industrial Classification (SIC)[9] is used by many state labor departments and economic planning agencies. The Dictionary of Occupational Titles (DOT) with nine-digit codes is used by the Social Security Administration, and rehabilitation and job placement professionals. The Standard Occupational Classification (SOC) used by the Bureau of Census has five-digit detail.[8] Many U.S. government agencies will be moving to the six-digit North American Industrial Classification (NAIC)[10] over the next decade.

In the insurance industry, the National Council of Compensation Insurers (NCCI) uses four-digit codes that often combine industry and occupation into insurance risk groupings.[11]

There are several international lists for industry and occupation in use. The United Nations has developed the International Standard Industrial Classification (ISIC)[12] and the International Labor Organization uses the International Uniform Classification for Occupations.[13]

Cross-walks that translate codes between some of these lists have been developed, but the results at detailed levels are often unsatisfactory.

The choice of the coding system will depend on many factors besides the desired level of detail: the skill level, training, and supervision necessary to maintain the system; available software; the need to maintain comparability with historical data or other coding systems; and, legal mandates.

Appropriate Population Coverage

Some data sources capture only part of the work force. Self-employed and government workers are typically left out of state employment agencies' data on wage employment, but are included in national census data. Cases of occupational disease that are not reported to workers' compensation enter other insurance systems, or are paid out-of-pocket by the worker. Thus, the actual coverage may be less than officially stated.

Accurate

Using data that are riddled with errors may lead to flawed interpretations and ineffective action. Many large databases have some variables that are mostly missing because the data collection forms were not filled in or key entered. By looking at a paper form, database design, or record layout one cannot know whether fields have actually been filled in with data. The surest way to find out is to request a count and percent of missing data (null fields) for each key data element.

Data Quality. The basic integrity of the data collected must also be assessed and promoted through a program of data quality control. The inventory of data should examine whether the basic elements of a data quality program have been in place. These include:

- standardized procedures for data collection
- training of staff in those procedures
- supervision
- explicit written data quality standards for accuracy of individual fields and completeness (missing data, missing records)
- an ongoing monitoring system that takes measurements and compares the results to the standards
- feedback to the participants
- corrective action taken when performance falls short of the standards

If the accuracy of files are checked with automated edits, the frequency of errors should be calculated and fed back to those responsible. Edits can be performed at the point of data entry, or with computer programs after data entry. Typical edits at the level of a data element include:

- missing data
- nonlegal codes or values outside of ranges (outliers)
- illogical date sequences (e.g., discharged from hospital before admitted)
- illogical age-diagnosis combinations (e.g., suicide in a 6-month old)
- illogical gender-diagnosis combinations (e.g., men with ovarian cancer)

At the level of entire records, edits include:

- duplicate records
- blank records
- orphans or dangling records that are left over after relational linking. For example, a record of a medical bill for a worker whose work injury was not reported

Several national organizations have issued guidelines on data quality standards,[14] including edits on specific fields and error tolerances.[15,16]

Standardized
Data that are not standardized are difficult to use for statistical counting or subgrouping. Free-form text generally cannot be used until it is coded, which is a labor-intensive process. For example, we can code occupations using the letters SR for shipping and receiving and MM for material handlers. However, the code must be fixed, or standardized. For computer processing, even small spelling errors, such as S instead of SR will inadvertently create a new category that will be considered a separate department. Recent improvements in computerized databases have made it possible to read text descriptions, such as occupation, and assign a code,[17] or help users select a code from pull-down menus that present a pick list.

Timely
Data that are not available in a timely fashion may not be relevant if exposures or the population have already changed, or if cases have left the workplace. If an objective of surveillance is to identify individual cases in real time, timeliness is very important.

Accessible
Some data are not accessible because they are confidential, and require permission from patients, employers, or government agencies. Data on paper forms are not nearly as useable as computerized databases or scannable forms for optical character recognition. Some records are physically archived in remote locations and literally buried under boxes.

Linkable
Linkable refers to personal identifying information used to link information on the same individual from two different electronic data sources. For example, social security number is reported on the standard death certificate (Appendix A), which in many states is computerized. It may be possible to find out whether workers at a specific workplace died from cancer by linking personnel records that list each worker's social security number to computerized death certificates. This is called record linkage (Chapter 19).

Employer-Based Surveillance

Figure 3.2 shows business processes that occur in every workplace. Information flows when a worker fills out an employment application, is counted present at the start of his or her work shift, gets injured on the job, and seeks medical treatment. The details are captured on official and unofficial forms and in the memory of the participants.

It is worthwhile to construct a map of information flows like Figure 3.2 and compile all the forms and database documentation. The database documentation should include the name of files, data elements, their definitions, widths, data types (numeric, character, date), code lists, and the edits that are performed. If the database is relational, the primary keys that link tables together should also be identified.

One should compare the data elements in case definition and minimum data set in STEP 4 with the data map. This will show whether the data element is collected at all, the physical location of the data (filing cabinet or server), and the organizational unit that is responsible. Some of the desired data elements will be listed in several sources, others may not be collected at all, and some may be available outside your organization. Redundancy and gaps will highlight the need for better designed business processes and computerized information systems (Chapter 10).

Figure 3.2 illustrates that the key information for surveillance is usually in several different locations throughout the workplace. This reinforces the need for the surveillance team to have access. Because the health care system and insurers have key data, it may also be necessary to have a formal agreement to share data between employers and insurers if these data are needed to meet a specific surveillance objective.

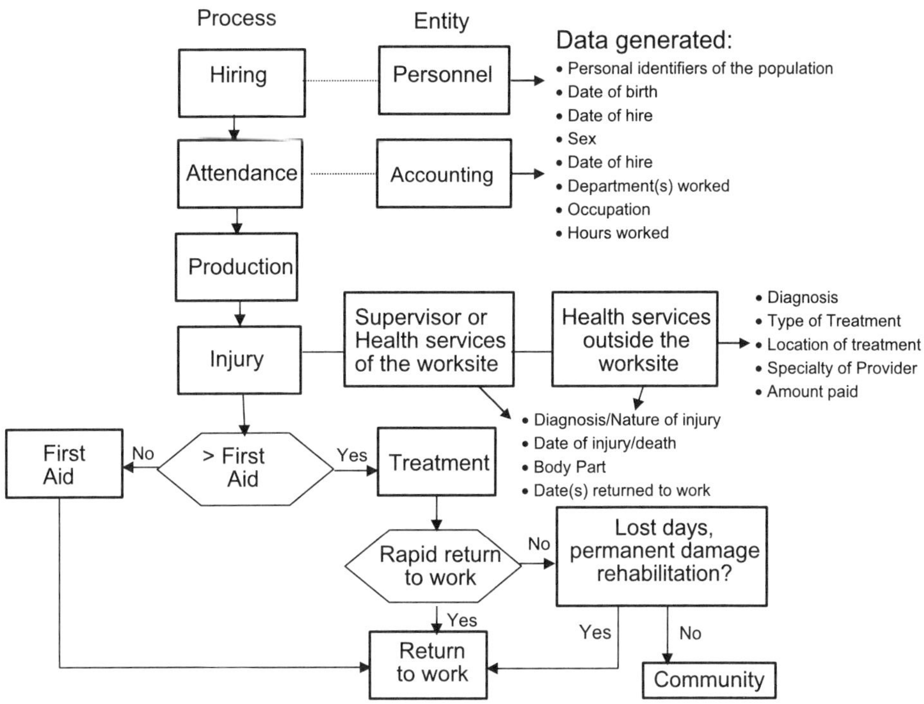

Figure 3.2 The flow diagram illustrates where data elements for surveillance are likely to be encountered in routine business processes at a company.

Government Agencies

Publicly available data sources in the United States were reviewed in Chapter 1. Several data collection forms are shown in Appendix A and Chapters 11–25. Readers should consult the Internet addresses listed in Chapter 1 (Table 1.5) to obtain additional details.

STEP 6. ESTABLISH MECHANISMS FOR CASE REPORTING AND DATA COLLECTION

There are numerous mechanisms for data collection and case reporting. Each involves a different level of technology and contact between data providers and the surveillance system:

- surface mail (e.g., U.S. Postal Service), interoffice mail, and electronic mail (E-mail)
- telephone
- facsimile (fax) with and without optical character recognition of printed forms
- electronic data interchange (EDI)
- manual record abstraction

The trade-offs between methods include costs, timeliness, training of personnel and case reporters, and the degree of sharing of workload between the case reporters and the surveillance organization.

Mail

Many passive surveillance systems use mail as the mechanism for data collection. Mail involves the lowest level of technology and the least amount of interaction. While it is relatively cheap, it may not be sufficiently timely for active follow-up. Reporting is usually done on a post card or standardized report form that is filled out by the reporter on a scheduled time interval such as weekly or monthly, or within a fixed time after contact with the case such as 24 hours, or 5 days. Employer's First Reports of Injury (Appendix A) used in many state's workers' compensation systems are an example of mail data collection, although automated methods are being introduced (see Electronic Data Interchange below). Active surveillance systems improve the response by supplying the reporter with preprinted forms and prepaid, self-addressed return envelopes or postcards.

Telephone

Active surveillance systems often report cases by telephone. Telephone reporting can be initiated by either the case reporter or the surveillance organization. The conversation follows the sequence of items on a standardized form or computerized data intake screen. Telephone reporting can improve data quality by prompting the caller to complete all items. When the intake is done by trained personnel, such as a nurse using a computer, receiving reports can be coupled to the beginning of individual case follow-up. Toll-free numbers also make reporting easier by removing cost barriers. Pager technology may be used to report cases after normal business hours. Interactive voice response systems that prompt and record responses on telephone push buttons are also possible reporting mechanisms, but are probably too cumbersome to gain wide acceptance.

Facsimile

Facsimile (fax) combines some of the advantages of telephonic and written communication. It can increase timeliness and reduce the work of transcribing reports by hand. It does not, however, produce information that can be loaded into a database. Optical character recognition has been used in combination with fax technology to complete key entry, but this is not widespread.

Electronic Mail

E-mail has become a popular way to communicate. In employer-based surveillance, it can be a rapid way of notifying a supervisor or others that a case has occurred before an official case report form is filled out. However, messages that are free-form cannot be loaded into databases without rekeying. E-mail attachments that follow a structured format (e.g., spreadsheet) can be loaded into databases.

Electronic Data Interchange

Electronic data interchange, or EDI, allows information to flow between data providers and the surveillance system using standardized electronic data elements. It is ideal for passive surveillance systems using administrative data in workers' compensation or health insurance. In EDI, data are already key entered by the data provider into an electronic database using commercial spreadsheets and databases or custom products. The data are sent as ASCII flat files, or other standardized format via an electronic network between a computer in the data provider's organization and a computer (or electronic mailbox) in the data receiver's organization. Specially designed computer programs facilitate the transfer, encrypt data for security purposes, and check for missing or erroneous data. A variant of EDI is sending database records or flat files on magnetic media (e.g., flexible diskettes, magnetic tape) via mail or courier service.

Standards organizations have already begun to create standards for electronic commerce, including workers' compensation (Chapter 24).

Electronic data interchange requires a higher level of technological sophistication and the appropriate computer hardware and software. Large amounts of data can be transferred rapidly and relatively inexpensively. With decreasing costs and increasing power of microprocessors, EDI will overtake other methods in the near future.

Manual Data Abstraction

Lastly, when data providers are unable to report cases, manual abstraction of records may be the only option. It is the most labor intensive mechanism for collecting data. Manual abstraction requires the surveillance organization to periodically visit a workplace, medical office, or hospital. The U.S. Bureau of Labor Statistics uses this data collection method when it visits a sample of employers selected into its annual survey of workplaces.[18]

Physical and administrative access may be barriers. Data may not be captured on standardized forms, difficult to locate within files, or illegible. For medical records, the personnel doing the extracting may require specific training in medical terminology. Supervision and periodic tests of data quality control are important. Manual abstraction involves a low level of technology, but productivity can be increased by abstracting data directly into a database on a portable computer.

REFERENCES

1. Silverstein B. Health and risk factor surveillance for work related musculoskeletal disorders. In: Kuorinka I, Forcier L, eds. *Work Related Musculoskeletal Disorders (WMSDs): A Reference Book for Prevention.* London: Taylor & Francis, 1995; 213–245.
2. Silverstein BA, Stetson DS, Keyserling WM, Fine L. Work-related musculoskeletal disorders: comparison of data sources for surveillance. *Am J Ind Med* 1997; 31:600–608.
3. Cummings KC, Maizlish NA, Rudolph LA, Dervin KA, Ervin A. Occupational disease surveillance: carpal tunnel syndrome. *MMWR* 1989; 38:485–489.
4. National Center for Health Statistics. *Proceedings of the International Collaborative Effort on Automating Mortality Statistics,* Volume I (7/99). Hyattsville, MD: Centers for Disease Control and Prevention, 1999.
5. World Health Organization. *International Classification of Diseases.* 9th Revision. Geneva: World Health Organization, 1978.
6. Z16.2 Subcommittee. *Method of Recording Basic Facts Relating to the Nature and Occurrence of Work Injuries,* ANSI Z16.2-1962 (R1969). Alexandria, VA: American National Standards Institute, 1995.
7. Sieber WK, Sundin DS, Frazier TM, Robinson C. Development, use, and availability of a job exposure matrix based on national occupational hazard survey data. *Am J Ind Med* 1991; 20:163–174.
8. Bureau of the Census. *Classified Index of Industries and Occu-*

pations. The 1990 Census of the Population. Washington, DC: US Govt Printing Office, 1992.

9. Office of Management and Budget. *Standard Industrial Classification Manual, 1987.* Washington, DC: US Govt Printing Office., 1989.
10. Office of Management and Budget. *North American Industry Classification System—United States, 1997.* Washington, DC: US Government Printing Office, 1998.
11. National Council on Compensation Insurance. *Classification Codes and Statistical Codes for Workers Compensation and Employers Liability Insurance.* Boca Raton, FL: National Council on Compensation Insurance, 1995.
12. United Nations. *International Standard Industrial Classification of Economic Activity.* New York: United Nations, 1990.
13. International Labor Office. *International Standard Classification of Occupations (CIUO-88).* Geneva: International Labor Office, 1998.
14. Insurance Data Management Association. *Data Quality Certification Model for Insurance Data Management.* New York: Insurance Data Management Association, 1995 (www.ins-data-mgmt.org).
15. IAIABC EDI Development Project. *First Report of Injury. Release 1.* Kansas City: International Association of Industrial Accidents Boards and Commissions, 1996 (www.iaiabc.org).
16. Health Information Division. *Patient Discharge Data Manual for California Hospitals.* Sacramento, CA: Office of Statewide Health Planning and Development, 1999.
17. Division of Safety Research. *The SOIC System User's Manual, Version 1.3.* Morgantown, WV: National Institute for Occupational Safety and Health, 1998.
18. Bureau of Labor Statistics. *Survey of Occupational Injuries and Illnesses, 1997.* Washington, DC: US Department of Labor, USDL 98-494, 1998.

4

Measuring Injury and Disease Frequency

NEIL A. MAIZLISH

Several surveillance objectives are met when the health or exposure outcome is expressed as a rate. This chapter is oriented to surveillance systems that are capable of combining case counts with employment data to construct rates for injury, illness, or death.

Methods for analyzing case counts and rates come from the field of epidemiology. Epidemiology is the study of the patterns of diseases and their causes in human populations. Measuring the health of a whole population is what sets epidemiology apart from related fields such as clinical medicine whose focus is the individual who seeks medical care.

Occupational epidemiology attempts to answer how workplace hazards alter the frequency and pattern of injuries, illness, and deaths in groups of workers. These questions are the journalistic who, what, how, when, where, and why, expressed at both the individual and population level. For an individual, the answers to "who was exposed or made ill to what, how, when, where, and why did it happen at all?" may be in an incident report like this:

> Susan hit her hand on a roller bar and bruised her thumb on July 18th while she was unloading parts off a jammed conveyor belt in the Finishing Department.

For the population of workers at the entire plant:

> During 1998, there were 50 injuries among the 500 hourly employees, or 10 injuries per 100 employees. Women, who are 200 of the 500 employees, had a higher injury rate than did men: 16 per 100 women versus 6 per 100 men. Twenty-five percent of all injuries were contusions, 25% were sprains and strains, 30% were cuts and abrasions, and 10% were eye irritation. The department with the most injuries (30 of 50, 60%) was the Shipping and Receiving Department for a rate of 30 per 150 workers. However, the department with the highest rate was Finishing (10 injuries in 25 workers) for a rate of 40 per 100. After reviewing all the incident reports in the Finishing Department by the plant health and safety committee, the main cause of injuries appeared to be conveyor line breakdowns (33% of injuries), which increased the manual handling of parts.

In the above example, working in the Finishing Department alters the frequency of injuries by fourfold: 40 per 100 versus the plant average of 10 per 100. The plantwide frequency is also influenced by gender with women being more than twice as likely to be injured than men (16 versus 6 injuries per 100 workers). By reviewing the individual incident report, it is not apparent that Susan in the Finishing Department is a member of two groups at increased risk for an injury. Only by including employment data was this revealed.

PERSON–PLACE–TIME

In epidemiology, the journalistic questions that help describe the variation in injury and illness rates are usually put in three major categories: person, place, and time. Personal characteristics that influence rates are biological and cannot be altered. These include age, gender, race, height, and preexisting medical conditions. Other characteristics, acquired through the envi-

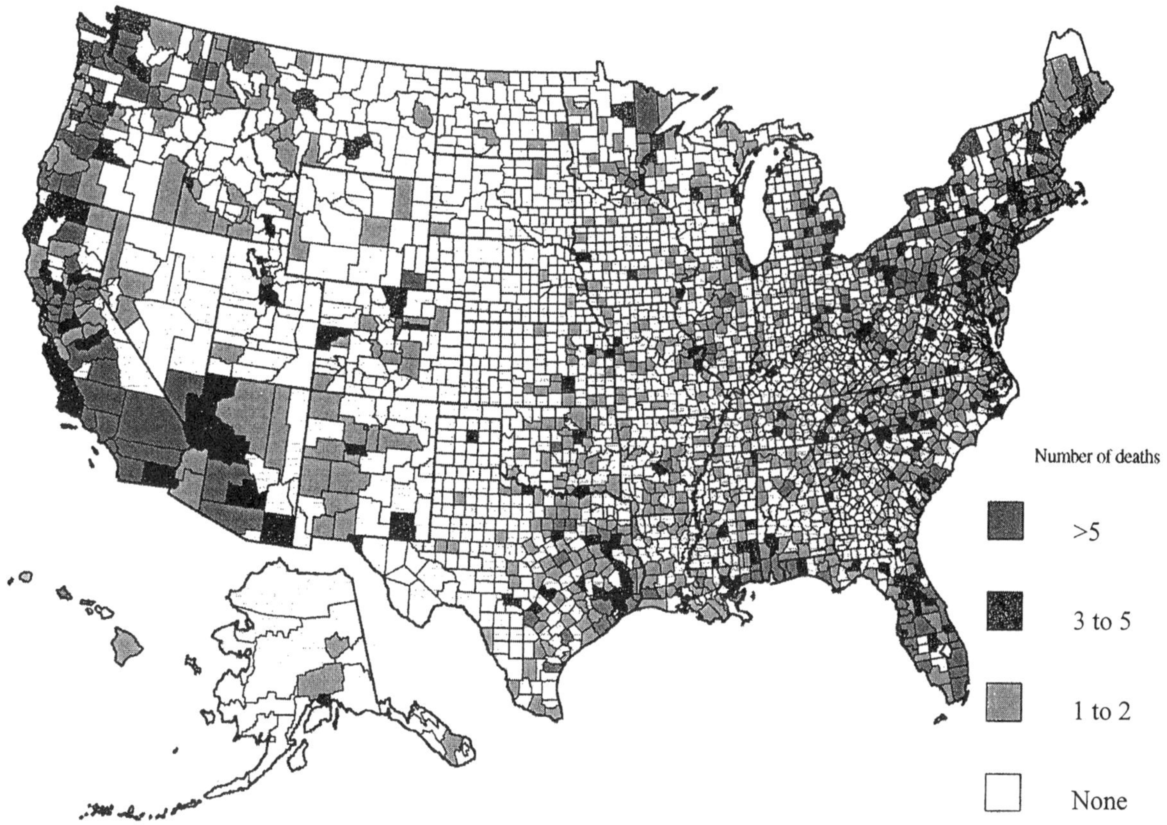

Figure 4.1 Asbestosis: total number of deaths by county, U.S. residents aged 15 and over, 1983–1992. (Division of Respiratory Disease Studies.[6])

ronment (place) may be altered. These include work-related items such as work practices, job training, safety training, supervision, management style, and organizational culture. Environmental characteristics also include literacy, languages spoken, income, access to health care, socioeconomic status, alcohol intake, and cigarette smoking. Place, whether it is the specific work station, county, state, or country of residence, exerts a strong influence on the frequency of health events. Geographic maps (Fig. 4.1) and spot maps (Fig. 4.2), which plot exposures or injuries and illnesses at the work location where they occurred, are powerful tools to observe the variation in frequency of health events. By using different symbols one can plot several characteristics of person, place, and time on the same map. For example, burn injuries can be displayed with dot symbols and fractures with triangles. Likewise, different symbols can be used for injuries that occur on the first, second, and third shift.

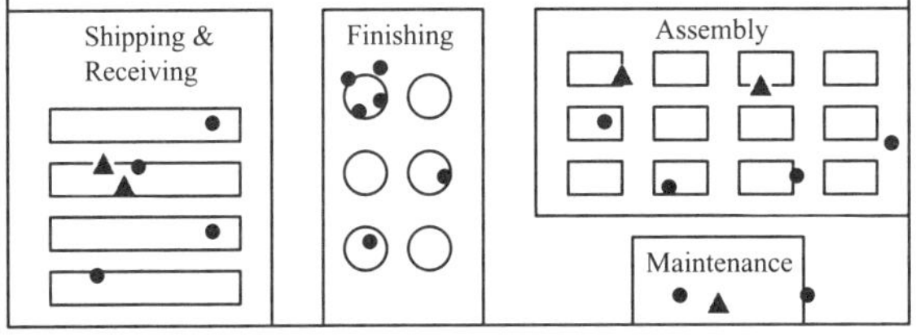

Figure 4.2 Spot map of a hypothetical factory showing the spatial distribution of injuries and illnesses. There appears to be a clustering of cases on Line 3 in Fabrication and in one of the 6 work areas in Finishing. Cases on the first shift are circles (●) and cases on the second shift are triangles (▲).

The frequency of health events is strongly influenced by time. The pace of work and changes in exposures often track with production cycles that vary daily, weekly, monthly, quarterly, or yearly. Even within a day of production, there can be large variations in the injury and illness rate between the first, second, and third shifts. Over a span of years, injury and illness rates can change markedly as old processes and their hazards are phased out and new ones are introduced.

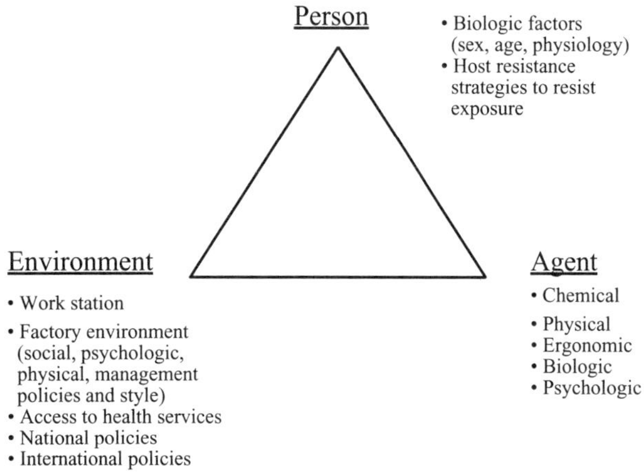

Figure 4.3 The epidemiologic model of health and disease says there is a dynamic (time) interplay between persons (person), their environment (place), and the agents that harm or promote health.

DISTRIBUTION OF INJURY AND DISEASE

Distribution is another basic concept and is reviewed in Appendix C. A model that explains why injury and illness rates vary says that health (or illness) results from the interplay between agents that harm or promote health, characteristics of the workers, and the environment (Fig. 4.3). The interaction between the person, agent, and environment affects the dose that ultimately is delivered to and absorbed into the body. The interaction also affects the body's ability to counteract damage to the cells, tissues, and organs that are targeted by the exposure. This is like a tug-of-war in which each worker is pushed or pulled closer or farther away from ill health.

Workplace hazards also fall along a distribution (top of Fig. 4.4). They are rarely the same for each worker because intensity and duration of exposures depend on the production process, individual tasks, distance from the source of exposure, and the ability of workers to avoid the exposure. During the tug-of-war, each individual's health will also fall along a distribution in the population (bottom of Fig. 4.4). Unless there are two extremes of exposure—totally absent or overwhelming—one may not always see an exact one-to-one relationship between level of exposure and health effect. Also, an exposure may not always produce an observable health effect for all exposed individuals in the population. This helps explain what often seems inex-

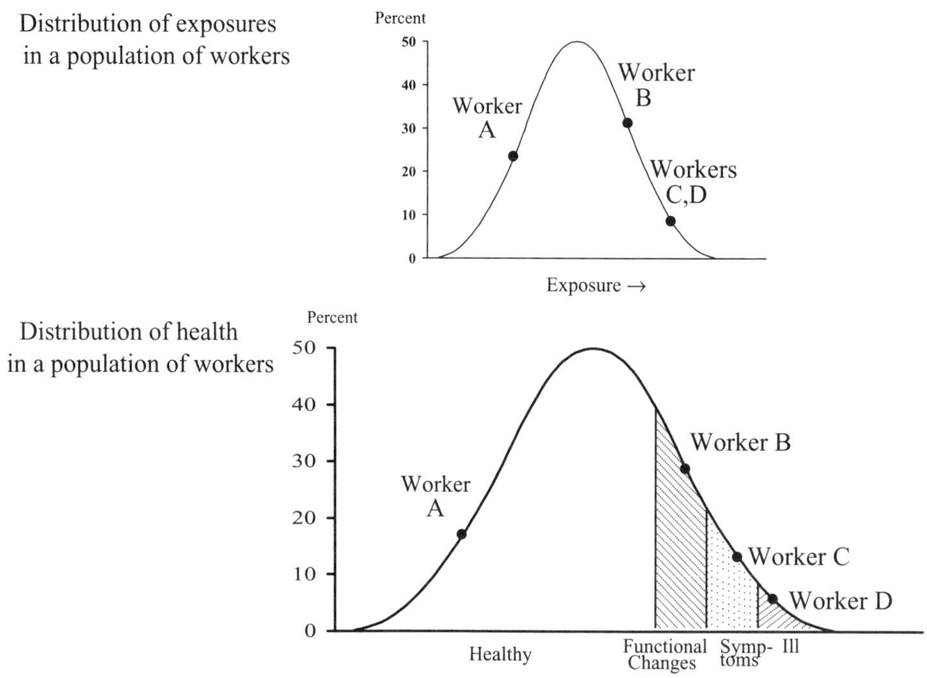

Figure 4.4 In this hypothetical example, workers A, B, C, and D work at different workstations in the same department of a factory. Even though they work in the same department, the exposures each experiences can be quite different because of differences in productive process, individual tasks, work practices, health and safety training, availability and use of protective equipment, and other factors. Workers A and B are outwardly normal. Worker B has functional changes that can be an early sign of ill health unless the exposure is lowered. (Functional changes are normal responses of the body subjected to a physical or mental stress, and include changes in physiologic measures such as pulse, body temperature, respiration, fatigue, etc.). Workers C and D have the same level of exposure (*upper distribution*), but D is outwardly ill and C shows symptoms (*lower distribution*). Workers C and D may vary in age or other ways that makes Worker D more vulnerable to the same level of exposure.

plicable to many employers and workers: why some workers become ill and some do not when work exposures seem equal. The other explanation is that the exposures are only outwardly the same because two workers can have the same workstation and are supposedly doing the same tasks, but closer examination can reveal important differences.

MEASURING POPULATIONS AND EMPLOYMENT

The denominator of injury and illness rates is based on employment data or population counts. Measuring working populations is difficult because populations change in time, and the task of identifying hundreds, thousands, or even millions of persons is daunting. Worker populations are unique because production and business cycles create fluctuations in employment, layoffs, and rehiring (Fig. 4.5). The net result is a complex pattern.

Not all workers have the same employment relationship at a given company. Collective bargaining agreements and employment practices create different categories of workers. These include management, permanent salaried workers, hourly workers, contract workers, and independent contractors. Separate payroll and accounting systems often exist for these different categories, making it difficult to count all the workers. Employment status may be complicated: full-time, part-time, vacation leave, short-term absences due to work or nonwork injuries or illness, long-term absence due to disability-,

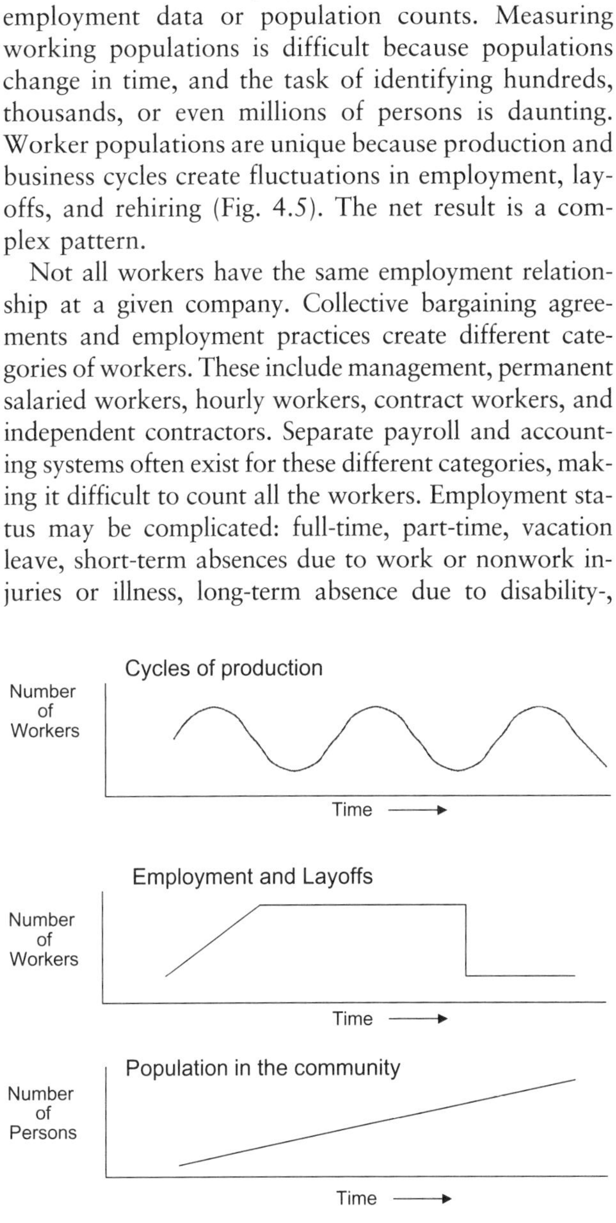

Figure 4.5 Working populations are dynamic, and experience fluctuations that are related to cycles of production, employment, and layoffs. The population in the community tends to increase in a steady manner.

study-, military-, or family-leave, unexcused absence, suspended without pay, laid off, retired, quit, or even died while employed. Given this complexity, what are the methods available to count workers? In each method there are several considerations: what to count and how often the population will be counted.

Persons, Positions, Hours Worked

Counts of workers can be based on persons, positions, or hours worked. Counting persons is perhaps the simplest way of measuring a population. Each person is counted once whether he or she is full- or part-time, and the population is the total number of persons working. Another method tallies the number of positions—full- and part-time—and expresses the total in terms of full-time equivalent (FTE) positions. Two persons each working half-time are counted as one FTE worker. Lastly, a more precise count is based on the hours a person actually works, or person-hours. These hours are added up and expressed as work hours of a fictitious full-time worker putting in 40 hours a week for 50 weeks per year, or 2000 hours per year. Thus, another way of expressing the number of FTE workers is the total hours divided by 2000 hours per FTE. For example, 386,290 work hours is 193.15 FTEs. Counts based on person-hours and positions are the most accurate, and a method usually available to employers. Counts of persons is usually done when data on person-hours are not available.

Typical sources of data for population counts are governmental census data or company-based payroll lists, seniority lists, or daily attendance records. Payroll lists are usually issued on a given date after the end of a payroll period lasting 1 week, 2 weeks, or 1 month.

Hours actually worked, hours of service credit, and hours paid may in fact be different. Paid hours can include sick days, vacation days, personal leave, and other days when one is not actually working. Similarly, seniority lists may include furloughed workers and those on long-term disability. Some collective bargaining agreements pay a premium or give extra service credit to night shifts, overtime, or hazardous work. If one compares two plants that have the same number of injuries and employment, the plant that counts hours actually worked instead of hours paid will appear to have a higher injury rate.

Of note, in many workers' compensation systems, denominator data is based on dollars of payroll or premium paid. This may not be accurate for surveillance purposes. For example, two workplaces with an identical number of injuries and employment could have different injury rates per 100 payroll dollars. The workplace that pays higher wages will appear to have a lower rate.

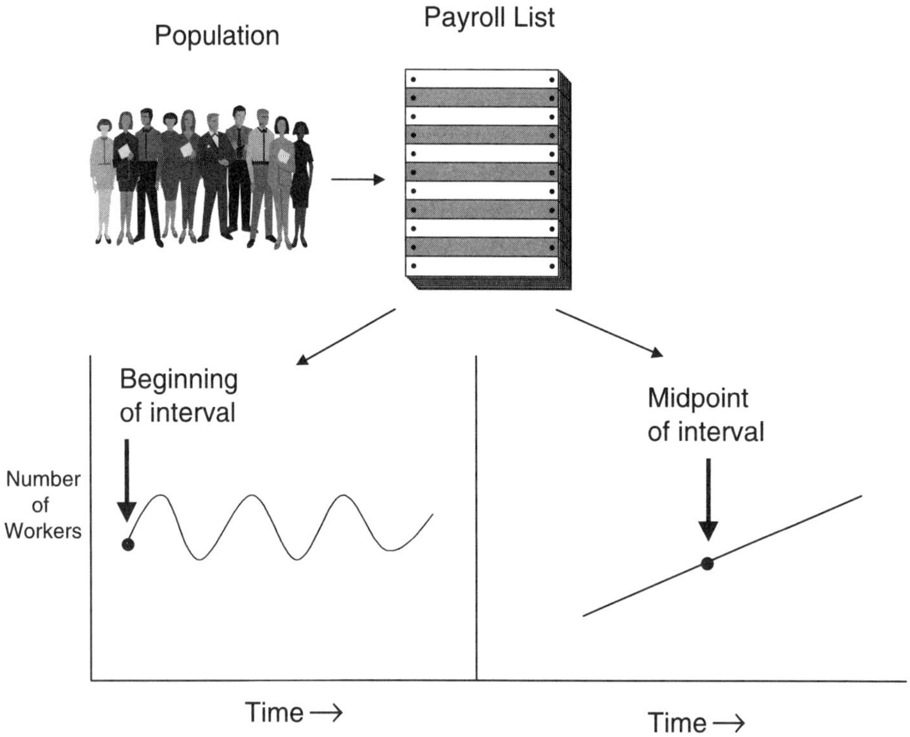

Figure 4.6 Single point estimates of the population are taken at the beginning or midpoint of the time interval of observation.

Estimation at a Single Point in Time

The simplest way to count a population is a single measurement or census of persons or positions at a single point in time. This is a snapshot, or a cross section in time. A single moment can be a day, week, month, or year. The measurement can be taken at the beginning of a time interval and will be accurate if the number of persons or positions is not changing or expected to change. If the population is experiencing steady growth it may be more accurate to take a single measurement in the middle of the time period (Fig. 4.6). This is done for annual population counts in the United States, where the population present on July 1 of a given year is used to estimate the population for the entire year, January to December.

Average Employment

When a population fluctuates, a single point in time will not be accurate. The next option is to take a census at two or more points in time and compute an average (Fig. 4.7). It does not matter whether the same worker or a replacement is counted at each census. For employment statistics, many states tabulate employment based on monthly employer reports of the number of workers they paid wages to during the week that includes the 12th day of the month. By averaging 12 monthly censuses, a single number represents the average population of workers and is referred to as average annual employment.

Person-Time

Another option, usually available to employers, involves tracking each worker over time and counting the number of hours, days, months, or years each works, and then adding each worker's total to the population total. This method of counting is called person-time. It follows up a group of individuals, or cohort, over time. The population is measured by the contribution of hours of everyone who worked without regard to the number of specific individuals. One full-time worker putting in 40 hours a week for a year will contribute the same number of hours as two half-time workers putting in 20 hours each. If a worker's attendance is recorded by time- and date-stamping of a time card, hours worked are tabulated daily.

MEASURES OF INJURY AND DISEASE FREQUENCY

The general format for calculating a rate is:[1]

$$\text{Rate} = \frac{\text{What and How Much Happened}}{\text{To Whom}} \times \text{Within What Time Period}$$

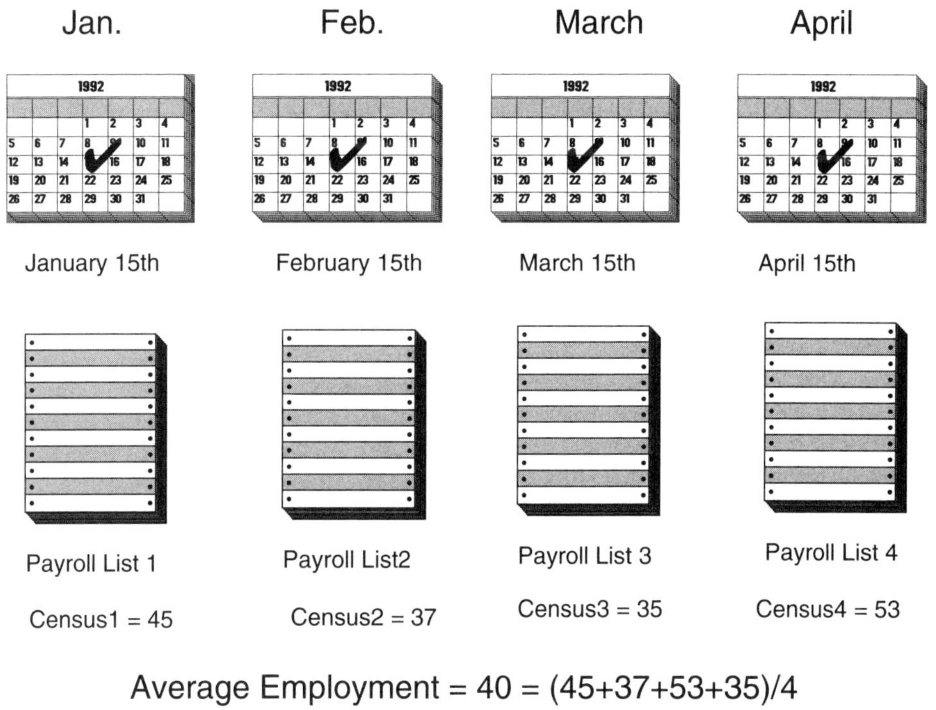

Figure 4.7 A series of censuses taken once a month can be averaged. This is called the average employment.

What and how much happened is the number of health events that meet the case definition. *To whom* is the population or individuals that are eligible to experience the health event. *Within what time period* is the measure of time over which the cases and population are observed. We have several options to express *To whom* using single, average, and person-time population counts.

It is important to point out that when we count the number of cases per population unit, the injuries and illnesses arise in the same population that we have specified. For example, if we limit the population of interest to production employees, the injuries should be among production employees, and management employees and their injuries should not be included. This concept is sometimes called the population at-risk, or eligible population.

Likewise, the time period for case counting must match the period for the population count. For example, if the period for counting cases starts on January 1 and ends August 31, the population must also be counted from January through August. If monthly censuses were taken, the average will have eight points in time. Even if no cases occurred in January, as long as workers were working, January's population count should be included. Likewise, if the population count stops in August, one should not include September's cases.

Prevalence

Suppose each worker in a population is evaluated on the same day to determine if they are ill, injured, or meet the criteria for being a case. The number of cases of injury or illness that exist at that time is a measure of frequency called prevalence.

$$\text{Prevalence} = \text{Cases Counted at a Single Point in Time}$$

Some text books call this point prevalence. For example, Figure 4.8 shows 10 days in the lives of five workers. A day when the worker is ill is shaded. The prevalence of illness is:

- 2 on day 6
- 1 on days 2, 5, and 7
- 0 on days 1, 3, 4, 8, 9, and 10

The number of cases can also be expressed as a proportion of the entire population. This measure of frequency is called the prevalence rate in many text books. The population is counted at the same point in time as the cases. The way the population is counted is usually by a census of persons.

$$\text{Prevalence Rate} = \frac{\text{Cases Counted at a Single Point in Time}}{\text{Population Counted at a Single Point in Time}}$$

The prevalence rate is a proportion that ranges from 0 to 1, or 0% to 100%. Sometimes it is expressed per 100 workers. In Figure 4.8, the prevalence rate on day 6 is 2/5, 40%, or 40 cases per 100 workers. The preva-

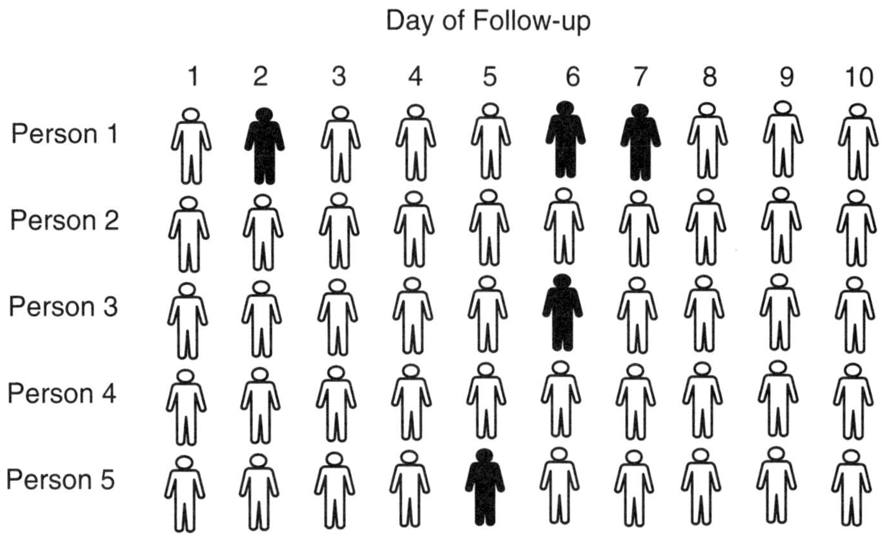

- Prevalence, day 6 = 2/5 = .4 = 40% = 40 per 100 workers
- Cumulative Incidence (days 1-10) = 4/5 = .8 = 80% = 80 per 100
- Person-Day Incidence = 4/45 person-days = 9 per 100 person-days

Figure 4.8 Measures of frequency of injury and illness: prevalence and incidence.

lence rate is 1/5 (20%) on day 2 and 7, and 0/5 (0%) on days 1, 3, 4, 8, 9, and 10.

Prevalence rates are particularly useful to estimate the magnitude of exposures and longer-term health problems such dermatitis, back pain or musculoskeletal disorders.[2] Data are usually collected with health or exposure questionnaires. In active surveillance, prevalence surveys may be part of active case finding[3] (Appendix B) and investigations of high-risk groups to identify exposures.

Incidence

Incidence is the frequency of new health events or cases counted within a specified time period. The specified time period is usually defined as a specific beginning date and a specific ending date. A group of workers without illness or injury at the start of a time period is followed up and new cases are counted until the end of the interval.

$$\text{Incidence} = \text{New Cases Occurring in a Specified Time Period}$$

Returning to Figure 4.8, we may ask "How many new cases are there?" There are three workers with an illness, but worker 1 is sick on day 2, goes back to work on days 3–5, and gets sick again on days 6–7. Is this a single case with two episodes, or just a single case? This depends on the definition of a case. If on day 2 worker 1 had a sprained ankle that recovered quickly, and if on days 6–7 worker 1 burned his forearm, we may conclude that the two injuries were different and worker 1 had two different cases within the 10-day follow-up period.

However, if worker 1's case was low back pain, which first started on day 2, went away on days 3–5, but flared up again on days 6–7, we may conclude that this is a single case with two episodes. Both measures of incidence (3 or 4 cases) are correct in the context of their definition.

Incidence rates are usually expressed in terms of a standard population size (per 100 workers, per 1000 workers) and unit of time, such as per year. Because there are three options for measuring the population (single point in time, multiple times to calculate an average, and the sum of person-hours), there are three ways to express an incidence rate.

Cumulative Incidence Rate

When the worker population is stable, the population count can be the number of disease-free persons at the beginning of the follow-up period. The single point in time is the beginning of the time interval. The cumulative incidence rate is the number of new cases expressed as a proportion of the initial population.

$$\text{Cumulative Incidence Rate} = \frac{\text{New Cases Within a Specified Time Period}}{\text{Number of Workers Without Illness at the Beginning of the Time Period}}$$

In Figure 4.8, assuming there are two distinct cases in worker 1—day 2 is one case and days 6–7 a separate case—there are four cases overall. The cumulative incidence rate is four cases per five workers, 0.8, 80%, or 80 per 100 workers.

Cumulative incidence rates are not frequently encountered in surveillance but are in epidemiologic research. However, a type of cumulative incidence rate for return-to-work is used in disability surveillance (Chapter 26).

Incidence Rate Using Average Employment

When the population count is the average of repeated censuses, or a single midpoint count, the incidence rate is:

$$\text{Incidence Rate} = \frac{\text{New Cases Within a Specified Time Period}}{\text{Average Number of Workers or FTEs Within the Specified Time Period}}$$

In Figure 4.8, there are five persons in the population whether we average 10 daily censuses or take a single census on day 5. It is customary to include persons on the active payroll who are not present on the day of the census due to vacation, sick leave, or other absence. Assuming there are four cases in Figure 4.8, the incidence rate is four cases per 5 workers, 0.8, 80%, or 80 per 100 workers.

Incidence rates based on average employment are commonly calculated in passive surveillance systems of government agencies.[4]

Person-Time Incidence Rate

When the population is measured as the sum of person-time, the measure of incidence is called the person-time incidence rate:

$$\text{Person-Time Incidence Rate} = \frac{\text{New Cases Within a Specified Time Period}}{\text{Sum of Person-Time Within the Specified Time Period}}$$

In some text books, person-time incidence rate is called incidence density or incidence density rate. This is the rate most employers would use for an injury and illness surveillance system based on OSHA record keeping.

In Figure 4.8, the five persons who start off disease-free on day 1 have the potential of contributing 50 person-days (5 persons × 10 days), if no one gets sick by day 10. However, workers 1, 3, 5 each get sick, worker 1 for 3 days and workers 3 and 5 for 1 day each. The three workers miss 5 work days due to their illnesses. Thus, the five workers put in 45 person-days at work (50 − 5), and 45 person-days is the denominator of the person-time incidence rate. During the sick days when the workers are away from work, they are not contributing work hours to the population total. Assuming there are just four new cases, the incidence rate is four per 45 workdays, or 9 per 100 workdays.

Person-time incidence rates are expressed in a common denominator of 100 full-time equivalent workers in the United States and 1 million work-hours in other countries. Because 1 full-time worker contributes 2000 work hours per year (40 hours per week for 50 weeks), 100 full-time workers will contribute 100 × 2000 or 200,000 hours per year. The proper way to calculate an incidence rate per 100 FTEs using hours worked is shown in Table 4.1. One multiplies the number of injuries by the conversion factor of 200,000, and then divides by the number of hours worked.

Lost Time Incidence

To describe the severity of injuries and illness, the case definition is sometimes limited to cases with lost workdays, or days with restricted activity. As a rate, lost-time case incidence is:

$$\text{Lost Time Case Incidence Rate} = \frac{\text{Number of New Cases with Lost Workdays Within a Specified Time Period}}{\text{Sum of Person-Time Within a Specified Time Period}}$$

Table 4.1 Calculation of Annual Incidence Rates: Case Incidence Rate and Lost Time Incidence Rate Using Lost Workdays

Health Event	*Number of Health Events*	*Hours Worked in Calendar Year*	*Conversion Factor*	*Formula*	*Rate per 100 FTES**
	(*A*)	(*B*)	(*C*)	$\frac{A \times C}{B}$	
Cases	102	386,861	200,000	$\frac{102 \times 200{,}000}{386{,}861}$	52.7
Lost workdays	180	386,861	200,000	$\frac{180 \times 200{,}000}{386{,}861}$	93.1

*FTE, full-time equivalent.

Cases that have not lost workdays do not meet the case definition and are not counted. There are several common thresholds of 1, 3, and 7 lost workdays used to define lost time cases. This reflects different laws regarding workers' compensation benefits in different states and countries.

Another common way to measure severity of injuries and illness is counting lost workdays as the health event and expressing the number of lost workdays per population and time unit.

$$\text{Lost Workday Incidence Rate} = \frac{\text{Sum of Lost Workdays of Cases Within a Specified Time Period}}{\text{Sum of Person-Time Within the Specified Time Period}}$$

In Figure 4.8, there are five lost workdays with 45 person days of follow-up giving a lost workday incidence rate of 11.1 per 100 person-days. Table 4.1 shows how to calculate the lost workday incidence rate per 100 FTEs using hours worked.

While this measure seems straightforward, in practice, it is difficult to carry out. Some injuries are so severe that their lost workdays will continue weeks or months after the date of injury. Lost workdays may also extend beyond the date specified for case incidence. For example, an annual person-time measurement of a population begins on January 1 and ends December 31. Some of the incident cases (January to December) will continue to lose workdays into the next calendar year. If we stop counting lost workdays on December 31, the lost time incidence rate will be underestimated. The lost workdays occurring in the new calendar year should be counted. In one study, employers estimated rather than counted lost workdays after December 31. When researchers counted the actual days lost after December 31, the lost time incidence rate was eight times greater than the employer's estimate.[5]

Period Prevalence

What happens if one combines prevalence and incidence? For incidence we begin with a disease-free population and observe new cases. If we include the cases existing at the beginning of the time interval as well as new cases, we have another measure of disease frequency called period prevalence. The 12-month period prevalence of several common occupational illnesses is listed in Table 4.2.[2]

Diagnosis-Specific Incidence Rates and Proportional Morbidity

In addition to combining all injuries and illnesses into a single category, it is important to examine specific diagnoses. This is important because a few diagnoses with many cases will contribute most heavily to the overall injury rate, and potentially overwhelm smaller categories that may also be important. Sometimes nature of accident, or cause of illness or injury is used instead of diagnosis.

When calculating cause-specific rates, one uses the same population in the denominator even though the numerator changes for each specific cause. Because the specific causes add up to the all-causes total, the sum of the cause-specific rates will add up to the incidence rate of all injuries and illnesses.

Another way to express the distribution of causes is to calculate the proportion of cases that are due to

Table 4.2 12-Month Prevalence of Selected Occupational Health Conditions in the United States Working Population, 1988

Health Condition	*Occupation*	*Prevalence (Number of Cases)*	*Prevalence (%)*
Back pain from repeated activities at work	U.S. Working Population	4.75 million	4.5
	Mechanics and repairers of vehicles, engines, and heavy equipment		10.5
	Operators of extractive, mining, and material moving equipment		10.4
	Construction trades and other construction occupations		10.1
Hand discomfort	U.S. Working Population	11.6 million	10.7
	Operators of machines that process metal, plastic, stone, and glass		23.5
	Assemblers and people in hand-working occupations		21.9
	Operators of machines that process wood, paper, textiles and leather		17.8
Carpal tunnel syndrome	U.S. Working Population	2,645,300	1.55
Dermatitis from substances at work	U.S. Working Population	1.87 million	2.8
	Physicians, dentists, nurses, pharmacists, and dieticians		5.6
	People in personal service occupations		4.9
	Health care therapists, technologists, technicians, and assistants		3.5

Source: Behrens et al.[2]

Table 4.3 Lost Time Incidence Rates and Proportional Morbidity by Cause of Injury and Illness, California, 1990

Cause of Injury or Illness	*Cases** *(A)*	*Incidence Rate per 1000 Workers†* $\frac{\text{Specific Cause (A)}}{\text{Population (12,969,200)}} \times 1000$	*Proportional Morbidity (%)* $\frac{\text{Specific Cause (A)}}{\text{All Causes (444,886)}} \times 100$
All causes	444,886	34.3	100.0
Injury	376,866	29.1	84.7
Illness	36,378	2.8	8.2
Not stated	31,642	—	7.1
Strains, sprains, dislocations, hernias	218,212	16.8	49.0
Cuts, lacerations, punctures	57,296	4.4	12.9
Contusions and crushing injuries	44,048	3.4	9.9
Fractures	25,738	2.0	5.8
Scratches, abrasions	16,268	1.3	3.7
Anxiety reactions and other mental disorders	10,444	0.8	2.3
Burns and scalds	9160	0.7	2.1
Systemic poisoning	4278	0.3	1.0
Dermatitis	3810	0.3	0.9
Musculoskeletal disorders, excluding CTS‡	2690	0.2	0.6
Infective and parasitic diseases	2298	0.2	0.5
Conditions of the circulatory system	2196	0.2	0.5
Concussion	1748	0.1	0.4
CTS	1244	0.1	0.3
Radiation effects	1184	0.1	0.3
Amputation or enucleations	614	<0.1	0.1
Stomach ulcers, other stomach conditions related to stress	588	<0.1	0.1
Other occupational illnesses	7646	0.6	1.7
Other occupational injuries	3782	0.3	0.9

*Cases are defined as illnesses or injuries with 1 or more lost workdays. (In 1990, there were approximately 1 million other reported injuries that involved less than 1 day of lost work time.)

†The estimated worker population (12,969,200) is based on the arithmetic average of 12 monthly employment censuses counting workers receiving wages during the week of the 12th day of the month in 1990.

‡CTS, carpal tunnel syndrome.

Source: Division of Labor Statistics and Research.[4]

specific diagnoses. This is called proportional morbidity. The denominator of these calculations is not the population, but rather the total number of cases. These proportions are expressed as percentages that add up to 100%. Rates however, do not have to add up to 100%.

Table 4.3 shows the difference between incidence and proportional morbidity using First Reports of Injury by California employers in 1990.[4] The population unit chosen for incidence is 1000 workers rather than per 100. This was chosen to improve the appearance of the presentation by avoiding many categories whose rates only have decimal digits.

Other Measures of Injury and Illness

As mentioned in the previous chapter, broad goals in occupational health and safety include prevention of workplace injuries, limiting disability once health is impaired, and improving the quality and effectiveness of occupational health services. Several objectives aimed at disability surveillance use return-to-work rate as a key outcome. These and other measures of frequency are discussed in Chapter 26.

MEASURES OF FREQUENCY AND QUESTIONNAIRES

Questionnaires can be an important component of active surveillance systems to help identify cases and gather information during field investigations. The way one asks the question about injury or illness determines the measure of frequency. There are key words that set the time frame and others that place the onset before or during the time frame of interest. Table 4.4 illustrates how easy it is to change a question from prevalence to incidence or period prevalence

Table 4.4 Epidemiologic Measures of Frequency and the Phrasing of Questions

Frequency	*Sample Question*	*Key Words*
Prevalence	Do you have bronchitis today?	*Today* is the key word for single point in time
Incidence	In the last 12 months, have you had bronchitis diagnosed for the very first time? Or, Have you ever had a case of bronchitis? If yes, when was the diagnosis made?	*Last 12 months* is specified time period; *for the first time* indicates a new case. If the first question is true, the diagnosis has to occur in last 12 months to be incident case in the last 12 months. Cases that occurred before are incident in a different reference period
Period prevalence (12-month)	In the last 12 months, have you had bronchitis?	Cases that started before but continued during the 12-month period are counted
Period prevalence (lifetime)	Have you ever had bronchitis?	The time period for each person will be different depending on his or her age

with a slight variation in wording. Many discrepancies in published articles about the frequency of health events can be explained in part by the differences in the measure of frequency, and the time period used in period prevalence measures such as 1 week, 1 month, or 1 year.

GENERAL READING ON OCCUPATIONAL EPIDEMIOLOGY AND STATISTICS

Checkoway H, Pearce NE, Crawford-Brown, DJ. *Research Methods in Occupational Epidemiology. Monographs in Epidemiology and Statistics. Vol. 13.* New York: Oxford University Press, 1989.

Kleinbaum DG, Kupper LL, Morgenstern, H. *Epidemiologic Research: Principles and Quantitative Methods.* Belmont, CA: Lifetime Learning Publications, 1982.

Monson RR. *Occupational Epidemiology.* 2nd Edition. Boca Raton: CRC Press, 1990.

Selvin S. *Statistical Analysis of Epidemiologic Data. Monographs in Epidemiology and Statistics. Vol. 17.* New York: Oxford University Press, 1995.

REFERENCES

1. Kazandjian V. Indicators of performance or the search for the best pointer dog. In: Kazandjian V, ed. *The Epidemiology of Quality.* Gaithersburg, MD: Aspen Publishers, Inc., 1995.
2. Behrens BJ, Seligman PJ, Cameron LL, Mathias CGT, Fine L. The prevalence of back pain, hand discomfort, and dermatitis in the US working population. *Am J Public Health* 1994; 84:1780–1785.
3. Silverstein B. Health and risk factor surveillance for work related musculoskeletal disorders. In: Kuorinka I, Forcier L, ed. *Work Related Musculoskeletal Disorders (WMSDs): A Reference Book for Prevention.* London: Taylor & Francis, 1995:213–245.
4. Division of Labor Statistics and Research. *California Work Injuries and Illnesses, 1990.* San Francisco: Department of Industrial Relations, 1991.
5. Oleinick A, Guire KE, Hawthorne VM, Schork MA, Gluck JV, Lee B, La S. Current methods of estimating severity for occupational injuries and illnesses: data from the 1986 Michigan comprehensive compensable injury and illness database. *Am J Ind Med* 1993; 23:231-252.
6. Division of Respiratory Disease Studies. *Work-Related Lung Disease Surveillance Report, 1996.* Morgantown: National Institute for Occupational Safety and Health, DHHS(NIOSH) Publ. No. 96-134, 1996.

5

Comparing Rates of Injury and Disease

NEIL A. MAIZLISH

It is natural to ask whether the frequency of health events is changing over time or whether one particular group of workers has a higher or lower frequency compared to other workplaces, industries, or the general population. Typical questions are:

- "How do the number and rate of injuries at our workplace (our state, our country) compare to last year's figures?"
- "How does the injury rate at this plant compare to other plants in the same industry?"
- "Are we having an epidemic of back injuries at work?"
- "Which industries and occupations have the highest rates of injury and illness?"
- "What blood lead distribution is normal for this group of workers?"

Epidemiology provides several methods for comparing the frequency of health events in groups. This chapter explains these methods, which apply to both surveillance and research. Surveillance and research are often linked. When high-risk groups are identified by surveillance, the specific causes may still not be known. Research is often the follow-up activity.

MEASURES OF ASSOCIATION

Let's carry out a survey during one day in an automobile factory to investigate the prevalence of reported symptoms of asthma in two departments. In Department A, a plastic resin is used to make steering wheels. In Department B, this resin is not used. We ask each worker in both departments whether he or she is experiencing cough, pressure in the chest, or difficulty breathing, and afterward, we classify each worker in a 2 by 2 table (Table 5.1).

Rate Ratio or Relative Risk

We can compare prevalence in the group exposed to resin with the prevalence in the group not exposed to resin. We can make a ratio of the two prevalence rates or calculate their difference.

The ratio of two measures of frequency is called the rate ratio (RR), or relative risk,

$$\text{Rate Ratio} = \frac{\text{Rate in the Exposed Group}}{\text{Rate in the Nonexposed Group}}$$

In the example,

$$\text{Rate Ratio} = \frac{a/(a+b)}{c/(c+d)} = \frac{0.4}{0.04} = 10$$

The rate ratio has no units, and ranges from 0 to infinity. In the above example we say:

- The exposed group has a rate of asthma symptoms 10 times higher than the nonexposed group.
- The prevalence of asthma symptoms is increased by 1000% in the exposed group.
- Exposure appears to increase the rate of asthma symptoms 10 times (1000%).

Table 5.1 Classification Table* for Disease and Exposure Categories

	Asthma Symptoms? Yes	No	
Department A **Exposed**	10 (a)	15 (b)	25
Department B **Not Exposed**	3 (c)	72 (d)	75
	13	87	100 (N)

N = Total in the population, 100
a = Number of exposed cases, 10
c = Number of nonexposed cases, 3
b = Number of exposed without symptoms, 15
d = Number of nonexposed without symptoms, 72
$(a + c)$ = Number with symptoms, prevalence, 13
$(a + b)$ = Number with exposure, exposure prevalence, 25

$\frac{a+c}{N}$ = Prevalence rate of symptoms in the population, $\frac{13}{100} = 0.13$, or 13%

$\frac{a+b}{N}$ = Prevalence rate of exposure in the population, $\frac{25}{100} = 0.25$, or 25%

$\frac{a}{a+b}$ = Prevalence rate of symptoms in the exposed group, $\frac{10}{25} = 0.4$, or 40%

$\frac{c}{c+d}$ = Prevalence rate of symptoms in the nonexposed group, $\frac{3}{75} = 0.04$, or 4%

*When setting up the 2 by 2 classification table, the disease is usually put on top with cases in the left column and the noncases (normals, non-ill) in the right column. Likewise, exposure is put on the left side of the table with the exposed group in the upper row and nonexposed in the lower row. Many statistical packages list the column headings of categories in alphabetical or numeric order (No before Yes). This makes the output harder to interpret. Appropriate codes (e.g., 1 = Yes, 2 = No) make the output easier to understand.

- There is a positive association between exposure to resin and asthma symptoms.

These expressions convey the idea that there is a statistical link between exposure and illness. There may be a true cause-and-effect relationship or there may be other plausible explanations. Chapter 7 gives details on the interpretation of surveillance data and explores some alternative explanations.

The above statements are not equivalent in emotional charge or impact. Using large numbers such as 1000% will make the risk seem larger than 10-fold. When the RR is less than 1 the rate in the exposed group is lower than the nonexposed group. We say the exposure is protective. For example, pregnant women on a diet enriched with folic acid (exposure) reduces the rate of certain kinds of birth defects compared to women with an ordinary diet (nonexposed).

If we had measured incidence rates, rather than prevalence, we would describe the rate ratio as an incidence rate ratio. When using person-time rates, the rate ratio is sometimes called the incidence density ratio. Rate ratios can also be calculated using lost work time incidence rates (Chapter 4).

Attributable Risk and Excess Cases

The prevalence or incidence rate in the exposed group minus the rate in the nonexposed group is called attributable risk (ARE) or the risk difference. It provides the frequency of illness and injury attributable to the exposure after subtracting out the background frequency.

Attributable Risk = Rate in the Exposed Group − Rate in the Nonexposed Group

In the example,

Attributable Risk $= a/(a + b) - c/(c + d) = 0.4 - 0.04 = 0.36$

The attributable risk has the units of attributable cases per exposed population and time period, where the population unit can be per exposed worker, per 100 exposed workers, or per person-time. In the above example, the attributable risk is 0.36 cases per worker in the exposed population, or 36 cases per 100 exposed workers.

If exposure could be eliminated, how many cases in the exposed group could be prevented? The cases theoretically eliminated are called attributable cases. Other terms are excess, preventable, or avoidable cases. Excess cases are cases in excess of that expected if the exposed group had the lower injury and illness rate of the comparison group. Excess or attributable cases are calculated by multiplying the attributable risk times the *population* at risk or with exposure:

$$\text{Excess Cases} = \text{Attributable Risk} \times \text{Population at Risk}$$

In the example, the population at risk to exposure is the 25 workers in Department A.

$$\text{Excess Cases} = 0.36 \text{ per Exposed worker} \times 25 \text{ Exposed workers} = 9 \text{ Cases}$$

Alternatively, the number of excess cases can be calculated from the difference between the observed number in the exposed group and the expected number of cases in the exposed group.

$$\text{Excess Cases} = \text{Observed} - \text{Expected}$$

If the exposed group had the prevalence of asthma symptoms that exists in the nonexposed group, the expected cases are:

$$\text{Expected Cases} = \text{Rate in the nonexposed group} \times \text{Population in the exposed group}$$

In the example,

$$\text{Expected Cases} = 0.04 \text{ Cases Per Worker} \times 25 \text{ Exposed Workers} = 1$$

Ten cases occurred or were observed in the exposed group.

$$\text{Excess Cases} = 10 - 1 = 9$$

Thus, 9 of the 10 (90%) exposed cases in Department A are excess. Attributable risk is sometimes expressed as a percent of exposed cases. It can be calculated as the (Observed − Expected)/Observed, or

$$\text{Attributable Risk \%} = \frac{\text{RR} - 1}{\text{RR}} \times 100 = \frac{10 - 1}{10} \times 100 = 90\%$$

It should be pointed out that even if the attributable risk or rate ratio is small, say less than 2, when multiplied by a large population at risk, the number of excess cases can be large.

Attributable risk can be calculated for lost time incidence rates. Instead of excess cases, the result is excess lost workdays or work hours.

Rate ratios, excess cases, and excess lost workdays have important implications for setting priorities, prevention, and analysis of cost-effectiveness/benefit. Whereas all cases should be considered excess or preventable, a reasonable first step is to take corrective and preventive action in departments, jobs, and industries with the highest rates and numbers of excess cases.

The potential economic impact of work injuries and illnesses can be estimated by multiplying the number of cases by the average cost per case, or by multiplying the number of lost work hours (or days) by the average cost of a worker-hour (day) of production. Appendix F explores the use of surveillance data in economic analysis of occupational safety and health problems.

Odds Ratio

Another way of comparing groups with exposure and health problems is based on ratios of exposed to nonexposed, which is called the odds. In Table 5.1 exposure is defined as working in Department A. In the group of asthma cases, the odds of exposure is:

$$\text{Odds of Exposure in Asthma Cases} = \frac{\text{Cases with Exposure}}{\text{Cases without Exposure}} = \frac{a}{c} = \frac{10}{3} = 3.33{:}1$$

Likewise, in the group without asthma, the odds of exposure is:

$$\text{Odds of Exposure in Non-ill} = \frac{\text{Non-ill with Exposure}}{\text{Non-ill without Exposure}} = \frac{b}{d} = \frac{15}{72} = 1{:}4.8$$

The odds of exposure in the asthma cases is far from even, or 1:1. There are over 3 times as many exposed as nonexposed. The odds of exposure in the group without asthma symptoms is also far from 1:1. But this time, the number of nonexposed is over 4 times greater than exposed. Interpreting these ratios together, one would conclude that it is far more likely to work in Department A than B if you had asthma. Or, if you worked in Department A it is more likely you would have asthma than if you worked in Department B. The odds of the two groups (asthma cases and non-ill) can be made into a ratio called the odds ratio (OR).

$$\text{Odds Ratio} = \frac{\text{Odds of Exposure in the Cases}}{\text{Odds of Exposure in the Non-ill}}$$

The calculation can be made simple by rearranging the terms:

$$\text{Odds Ratio} = \frac{a/c}{b/d} = \frac{a \times d}{b \times c} = \frac{10 \times 72}{15 \times 3} = \frac{720}{45} = 16$$

Odds ratios are suited to surveillance and research in which it is not possible to identify or count the individuals in the population. Census data may not be available or up to date. Personnel records of an employer may be not be computerized, and it is not feasible to manually tabulate data for each worker. However, data are often available to identify a group of cases ($a + c$ in Table 5.1). Data may also be available to select a sample of workers ($b + d$) from the same population who are healthy, or at least do not have the same health problem as the cases. This second group without the illness or injury of interest is called controls. It is possible to calculate the odds of exposure in the cases (a/c) and controls (b/d). Chapters 18 and 19 provide examples of the use of ORs in surveillance.

What is the relationship between the odds ratio and the rate ratio? They have similar interpretation. If the OR is greater than 1, the disease occurs more frequently in the exposed group than in the nonexposed group. For the same data, it can be shown that when the odds ratio is 1, the rate ratio is also 1. However, the OR will be higher than the RR for RRs greater than 1, and the OR will be lower than the RR for RRs less than 1. When the overall rate of disease is less than 5% (5 cases per 100 population) the difference between the OR and RR is small. In Table 5.1, there is a marked difference (RR = 10 versus OR = 16). This is because the prevalence rate of asthma is 13% (13 cases per 100 population), much higher than 5%.

Examining Trends and Risk Factors: Rates for Comparisons

So far, the examples have compared just two groups where the exposure was known in advance. This is most appropriate for a researcher who designs a study that tests a hypothesis of whether a known exposure might be a cause of a health problem. However, in surveillance, one of the objectives is to identify possible exposures. By examining how rates of injury, illness, and death vary by characteristics of workers, their work, and time, we may get clues based on risk factors to which exposures might explain high and low rates. Rather than specific exposures, we compare groups with and without risk factors:

$$\text{Rate Ratio} = \frac{\text{Rate in the Group with the Risk Factor}}{\text{Rate in the Group without the Risk Factor}}$$

Reference Rates for Company-Based Surveillance. There are several options for the reference rate that is the denominator of the rate ratio and for the rate subtracted in attributable risk. At individual workplaces, the department, occupation, or the work area with the lowest rate can be the reference rate. A second option is to use the rate of the entire workplace. This is the average of the workplace. Third, if the actual exposures such as noise, solvents, dusts, heavy lifting, etc. have been measured throughout the workplace, one can make exposure categories and assign each worker to his or her category. The rate in the category with the lowest exposure level may be an appropriate reference rate.

The reference rate can also be a previous time period. For example, plantwide and department-specific rates for the most recent full year can be compared to those of the previous year. Likewise, rates for the most current quarter can be compared to the corresponding quarter from last year. Sometimes the comparison rate is an administrative goal such as a 10% improvement (decrease) compared to last year's rate based on improvements in health and safety.

The work area or occupation with the lowest rate and the plantwide rate are examples of internal comparisons because they are based on data from the same workplace. Data collected at the same workplace is generally more uniform than that collected from different workplaces. Another reference rate can be external to the specific workplace under surveillance. This is usually the industry-specific rate given by the three or four-digit SIC code published by the Bureau of Labor Statistics.[1]

Reference Rates Used in Surveillance by Governmental Agencies. There are similar options for reference rates used in surveillance done by governmental agencies. Within an industry grouping, it is common to compare injury and illness rates of specific industries to that of the broad group. For example, injury rates in meat packing can be compared to all manufacturing or all private employers. In the United States this is usually done using industry or occupation codes published by the Bureau of Labor Statistics[1] or by the Bureau of Census.[2]

Strengths and Weaknesses of Different Comparison Rates. It is desirable to calculate RRs using several different reference rates. Each reference rate has strengths and weaknesses that are countered by others. For example, the advantage of rates based on large populations (whole plant, state, nation) is that the rate is less susceptible to statistical fluctuations due to small numbers. Rate ratios that use reference rates from the same data source, data collection methods, and case definitions will be more comparable. Reference rates based on populations from the same geographic area have the advantage of minimizing the effects of social class, race, or ethnicity. These factors influence injury and illness rates and vary by geographic area.

With several reference rates, the results can be interpreted in different contexts. For example, the production department with the lowest rate may still have a rate that is twice as high as the external industry-specific rate. This suggests even the "safest" work area could need improvement to catch up to the industry average.

Calculating Rate Ratios in Multiple Categories

The rate ratio, attributable risk, excess cases, and odds ratio apply to situations with more than two work areas, job classifications, or any other characteristic that has multiple categories. Let's now assume, the automobile plant in the earlier example has four departments—A, B, X, and Y—and that we do not know beforehand about exposure levels in each department. Table 5.2 shows the results of classifying the workers in the various departments by the presence or absence of asthma symptoms. The departments have been put in descending order of prevalence rate and RR of asthma (RRs = 10, 6 2, 1). Twenty of the 27 cases (74%) are excess if each department had the lowest prevalence rate of asthma. About half the excess cases occur in Department A and half in Department X.

Rate ratios greater than 1 raise concerns that exposures might be increasing the rates, and the causes of the increase need to be investigated. In the example above, a review of materials at this plant might show that toluene diisocyanate (TDI)—a known allergen in the production of foam-molded plastic—is used in Department A, but in no other department. This may be enough information to start taking precautions such as examining the work practices and ventilation system to identify the sources of exposure and to control them.

By comparing the differences in production processes and physical locations we might be able to see other patterns that point to Department A. For example, if no walls separate the departments, and Department B

Table 5.2 Classification Table for Disease and Multiple Categories of Exposure and Risk Factors*

	Disease or Injury?							
Department	Yes	No	*N*	Department	Rate per 100 workers	Rate Ratio	Attributable Risk	Excess Cases
A	10 (a)	15 (b)	25	A	40	10	0.36	9
X	12 (c)	38 (d)	50	X	24	6	0.20	10
Y	2 (e)	23 (f)	25	Y	8	2	0.04	1
B	3 (g)	72 (h)	75	B	4	1	0	0
	27	148	175	Total				20

Disease or Injury

Rate Formula	*Rate Data*	*Rate per 100 workers*	*Rate Ratio Formula*	*Rate Ratio*	*Attributable Risk Formula*	*Attributable Risk*	*Excess Cases*
$\frac{a}{a+b}$	$\frac{10}{25}$	40	$\frac{a/(a+b)}{g/(g+h)}$	10	$a/(a+b) - g/(g+h)$	0.36	$9 = 0.36 \times 25$
$\frac{c}{c+d}$	$\frac{12}{50}$	24	$\frac{c/(c+d)}{g/(g+h)}$	6	$c/(c+d) - g/(g+h)$	0.20	$10 = 0.20 \times 50$
$\frac{e}{e+f}$	$\frac{2}{25}$	8	$\frac{e/(e+f)}{g/(g+h)}$	2	$e/(e+f) - g/(g+h)$	0.04	$1 = 0.04 \times 25$
$\frac{g}{g+h}$	$\frac{3}{75}$	4	$\frac{g/(g+h)}{g/(g+h)}$	1	$g/(g+h) - g/(g+h)$	0	$0 = 0 \times 75$
							20

* The reference rate will be the denominator for the Rate Ratio for each different category being compared. The Rate Ratio for the reference category will always be 1 because it will have the same rate in the numerator and denominator. This reference category will not have any excess cases because observed minus expected will always be zero.

is physically the farthest, and Departments X and Y are adjacent to Department A, one plausible explanation is: an airborne exposure has a gradient with a maximum in Department A and a minimum in Department B. The RRs are consistent with a dose-response relationship, and point to a possible cause located in Department A. Industrial hygiene measurements of airborne TDI in area samples of Departments A, X, Y, and B might be taken to confirm high levels or to show an exposure gradient. These industrial hygiene measurements can also serve as a baseline for a comparison before and after steps are taken to control the exposures.

In this example, the exposure level to resin was not determined for each worker. It was assumed that just by working in Department A each worker had a uniform level of exposure. Department is not the exposure per se but is a group label (risk factor) that substitutes for the actual exposure. A more accurate way of classifying the exposure is to measure the resin levels in the breathing zone of each worker and then create categories such as high, medium, and low (instead of Departments A, X, Y, and B). There may be workers in Department X or Y whose actual exposures to resin are greater than some workers in Department A.

Even though this example illustrates health surveillance using epidemiologic methods, it should be evident that if the TDI exposure was already known, periodic monitoring of airborne TDI in Department A could have been used to identify unhealthy levels before asthma cases developed. Chapter 21 describes such an exposure surveillance system.

Standardized Incidence and Mortality Ratios

What happens when *all* the workers are exposed and there is no appropriate comparison group within a workplace? How can one make comparisons when workplaces are so small that prevalence or incidence is based on just a few cases? One solution is to use injury, illness, or death rates based on state or national censuses and vital statistics.

In most industrialized countries, health statistics are collected for deaths and newly diagnosed cancer cases for all or key segments of the population. In the United States, states and counties issue death certificates (Appendix A), and a federal agency, the National Center for Health Statistics, compiles this information along with age at death, gender, race, cause of death, year of death, and state and county of residence.[3] Periodically, industry and occupation are also compiled.[4] Death rates are calculated using all the deaths that occur in a calendar year as the numerator, and the mid-year population estimate as the denominator.

$$\text{Mortality Rate} = \frac{\text{Number of Deaths in U. S. Residents from January 1 to December 31}}{\text{U. S. Resident Population July 1}}$$

Incidence rates for newly diagnosed cases of cancer in several major U.S. cities and regions are tabulated by the organ site affected. The data are collected from a network of hospitals whose laboratories and pathologists confirm the type of cancer.[5]

Although incidence and mortality rates of the general population could be used directly as the denominator of a rate ratio, the usual approach is a variation of the observed versus the expected calculations. The general population rate is substituted for the reference rate. The expected number is this reference rate multiplied by the number of workers at risk.

$$\text{Expected} = \text{Mortality Rate in the Standard Population} \times \text{Population of Workers at Risk}$$

This is similar to asking how many cases would we expect if the workers at risk had the same incidence or mortality rate as the general population. At a company, the number of workers at risk are those who work at a specific workplace or work area. In government surveillance systems, the number of workers at risk is based on data of the U.S. Bureau of Census, which counts workers in standard categories of industry and occupation.

The observed number of cases are those that actually occurred. The ratio of observed to expected is called a mortality ratio.

$$\text{Mortality Ratio} = \frac{\text{Observed Deaths}}{\text{Expected Deaths}}$$

This ratio can be calculated for each specific cause of death. It is common to review 50 to 100 specific causes of death, including infectious diseases related to work; cancers at up to 20 different sites; heart disease; respiratory diseases such as asthma, emphysema, pneumoconioses; and, traumatic injuries. Public domain software is available to carry out these calculations.[6,7]

Likewise, the expected number of cancer cases can be calculated from cancer incidence rates of the standard population.

$$\text{Expected} = \text{Cancer Incidence Rate in the Standard Population} \times \text{Population of Workers at Risk}$$

The ratio of observed new cancer cases to expected new cancer cases is called the cancer incidence ratio.

Cancer Incidence Ratio

$$= \frac{\text{Observed New Cancer Cases}}{\text{Expected New Cancer Cases}}$$

Age, Sex, Race, Calendar Year Adjustment

Age, sex, race, and year of diagnosis are factors that influence injury, illness, and death rates in both the general and the working population. However, the working population differs in its demographic profile from the general population. For example, heavy industry has a work force with a much higher percentage of men in middle age groups than the general population. Inaccurate mortality or cancer incidence ratios can result from using the general population rates without taking into account age, gender, race, and other potential differences. This is a type of systematic error in comparing rates called confounding and is discussed in more detail in Chapter 7.

These differences are taken into account by breaking up the general population and the particular group of workers into distinct categories of age, sex, race, and then calculating the observed versus the expected in each category. These distinct categories are also called strata. The expecteds are summed up over all the strata for a grand total. Likewise, the observed cases are summed up over all the strata for a grand total. The observed total is then divided by the expected total to make up the mortality or incidence ratio.

This is shown in Table 5.3 for a hypothetical group of 4366 workers—1676 males and 2690 females—12 of whom died of cancer in 1995. Twelve cancer deaths is indeed a small number, but over twice as many as the 5.17 expected based on the U.S. population, adjusting for strata of age, sex, and year of death. Fractional expected (e.g., 5.17) is not an error, and expecteds should be accurate to several decimal digits. These fractions do contribute to the overall sum, even if the idea of a fractional case exists only in statistics. When the mortality ratio reflects age, sex, race, and year of death of a standard population, the ratio is called a Standardized Mortality Ratio (SMR). When the rate is based on incidence rather than mortality, the ratio is called the Standardized Incidence Ratio (SIR). Rate ratios adjusted for a single risk factor such as age are called age-adjusted rate ratios.

Proportional Mortality Ratio

A variation of the above approach is used for specific causes of death based on the proportion of deaths due to a specific cause instead of the mortality rate. This technique is particularly useful when the population of workers at risk cannot be identified at a workplace or in census data, but all deaths are recorded. This mortality ratio is called the Proportional Mortality Ratio (PMR). The observed number of deaths is the same as before—those actually occurring—but the expected is

Table 5.3 Standardized Mortality Ratio for Cancer Deaths by Age and Sex, 1995

	U.S. Population			*Specific Workplace*			*Standardized Mortality Ratio*
	A	B	C = A/B	D	$E = \frac{C \times D}{100{,}000}$	O	O/E
Age Group	*Cancer Deaths**	*U.S. Population**	*Cancer Mortality Rate × 100,000*	*Worker Population*	*Expected Cancer Deaths*	*Observed Cancer Deaths*	*Observed / Expected*
Men							
15–24	1009	18,352,070	5.5	440	0.02	0	
25–44	10,069	41,493,598	24.3	875	0.21	0	
45–64	70,077	25,225,709	277.8	336	0.93	3	
65+	199,536	13,688,675	1457.7	25	0.36	1	
Total	280,691	98,760,052		1676	1.50	4	$2.7 = \frac{4}{1.5}$
Women							
15–24	633	17,594,565	3.6	544	0.02	1	
25–44	11,916	41,847,260	28.5	1220	0.35	0	
45–64	62,007	26,984,135	229.8	759	1.77	4	
65+	181,606	19,843,622	915.2	167	1.53	3	
Total	256,162	106,269,582		2690	3.67	8	$2.18 = \frac{8}{3.67}$
Men and Women					5.17	12	$2.32 = \frac{12}{5.17}$

*Source: National Center for Health Statistics.[9]

based on the proportion of deaths due to a specific cause in the standard population.

$$\text{Expected} = \frac{\text{Deaths Due to a Specific Cause in the Standard Population}}{\text{All Deaths in the Standard Population}} \times \text{Deaths in Workers}$$

In a company, *deaths in workers* are those that occurred in all employees or those who worked in a specific production area or job title. In government surveillance systems, *deaths in workers* are the number of deaths of workers who worked in specific occupations or industry. These data are obtained from the death certificate itself (Appendix A), which lists usual occupation and employer, and are coded into standard categories. Table 1.4 is an example of this approach to mortality surveillance using data on death certificates from 24 states.[4] Chapter 19 is a detailed example of surveillance of cancer mortality using PMRs.

Table 5.4 shows age-standardized proportional mortality ratios of motor vehicle fatalities that occurred among men in 1995 at a hypothetical workplace. The workplace had 775 total deaths, of which 58 were motor vehicle deaths (about 7.5% of all deaths). Based on the distribution of age-at-death for all deaths at this workplace and the age-specific proportions of motor vehicle fatalities in U.S. men, only 28.7 deaths were expected to occur at the workplace. Fifty-eight actually occurred. The PMR is 2.02 (58/28.7). If we just had ignored the age categories and used the crude proportion of motor vehicle fatalities in U.S. men, we would have expected 19.5 deaths, based on 775 total deaths at the workplace and a proportion of 0.0251 (29,038/1,156,006) in U.S. men. This would have led us to overestimate the mortality ratio at 2.98 instead of 2.02.

Pros and Cons of Standardization

The advantage of using vital statistics for deaths and cancer is that the data sets are large, collected in a uniform manner with data quality control, and have information on subgroups of age at death or diagnosis, sex, geographic area of residence, year of diagnosis or death, and specific cause of death or site of cancer.

There are disadvantages, too. Certain causes of death are not reported accurately on death certificates. Moreover, it may be inappropriate to compare the working population with the general population because working populations are usually healthier than the general population. Individuals who are born with or acquire severe medical conditions may not be able to work or hold jobs with high physical or mental demands. Also, depending on the country, the employed population has increased access to health insurance or health services. These health benefits, along with regular wages that pay for food, clothing, shelter, education, and medicines, help maintain health. Thus, one expects the incidence rates for most health conditions to be lower in workers compared to the general population in the absence of harmful work-related exposures. This systematic difference in incidence rates is a type of bias that is called the *healthy worker effect.* This suggests that when workers and the general population have a similar incidence, workers may already be experiencing ill effects of occupational exposures that do not occur in the general population.[8] Even with these drawbacks, health data from large populations can be used as one type of comparison.

Table 5.4 Standardized Proportional Mortality Ratio for Motor Vehicle Fatalities in Males, 1995

	U.S. Population†			*Specific Workplace*			*Proportional Mortality Ratio*
	A	B	C = A/B	D	E = C × D	O	O/E
Age Group	*MV* Deaths*	*All Deaths*	*MV Mortality*	*All Deaths*	*Expected MV Deaths*	*Observed MV Deaths*	*Observed / Expected*
Men							
1–4	454	3609	0.1258	0	0.0	0	—
5–14	1255	5219	0.2405	0	0.0	0	—
15–24	7594	25,777	0.2946	28	8.2	15	1.89
25–44	10,547	111,957	0.0942	137	12.9	27	2.09
45–64	4974	233,212	0.0213	266	5.7	12	2.11
65+	4214	776,232	0.0054	344	1.9	4	2.11
Total	29,038	1,156,006		775	28.7	58	2.02 = 58/28.7

*MV, motor vehicle.
†Source: National Center for Health Statistics.[9]

REFERENCES

1. Bureau of Labor Statistics. *Survey of Occupational Injuries and Illnesses, 1997.* Washington, DC: US Department of Labor, USDL 98-494, 1998.
2. Bureau of the Census. Classified index of industries and occupations. *The 1990 Census of the Population.* Washington, DC: US Government Printing Office, 1992.
3. Anderson RN, Kochanek KD, Murphy S. *Report of Final Mortality Statistics, 1995.* Atlanta: National Center for Health Statistics, 1997.
4. National Institute for Occupational Safety and Health. *Mortality by Occupation, Industry, and Cause of Death—24 Reporting States (1984–1988).* Washington, DC: Government Printing Office, DHHS (NIOSH) Pub. No. 97-114, 1997.
5. Ries LAG, Kosary CL, Hankey BF, Miller BA, Clegg L, Edwards B. *SEER Cancer Statistics Review, 1973–1996.* Bethesda, MD, 1999.
6. Steenland K, Beaumont J, Spaeth S, Brown D, Okun A, Jurcenko L, Ryan B, Phillips S, Royce R, Stayner L, Morris J. New developments in the NIOSH Life Table Analysis System. *J Occup Med* 1990; 32:1091–1098.
7. Steenland K, Spaeth S, Cassinelli R, Laber P, Chang L, Koch K. NIOSH life table program for personal computers. *Am J Ind Med* 1998; 34:517–518. (Available at www.cdc.gov/niosh.)
8. Park RM, Maizlish NA, Punnett L, Moure-Eraso R, Silverstein M. A comparison of PMRs and SMRs as estimators of occupational mortality. *Epidemiology* 1991; 2:49–59.
9. National Center for Health Statistics. *Health, United States, 1995.* Hyattsville, MD: Centers for Disease Control and Prevention, 1997.

6

Protocols for Case Reporting and Follow-Up

NEIL A. MAIZLISH

STEP 7. SELECTING, RECRUITING, AND TRAINING REPORTERS

This step is oriented to surveillance systems with active case reporting by health care professionals and active case follow-up. Sentinel event surveillance systems created over the last decade by state public health agencies provide many examples (See Chapters 11–16).

Selecting Reporters

There are several considerations in selecting case reporters for active case reporting. These include available resources, the objectives of the surveillance system, the nature of the condition under surveillance, and the worker population.

Managing Resources

To balance resources and the demands for active case reporting and follow-up, surveillance systems must estimate how many case reporters and institutions they can handle to maintain a desired level of contact. The surveillance system must also estimate the total number of cases expected to be reported, and the number in any subgroup that will be given special priority. When there are too few cases, additional providers must be recruited or the geographic area must be expanded. Having too many cases can be solved, in part, by setting priorities so that fewer cases get active follow-up (see later under Step 8. ESTABLISH PRIORITIES AND PROTOCOLS FOR FOLLOW-UP).

Probability Sample. A key decision in managing resources is whether the case reporters or data providers will be a statistical sample. When the probability of being selected into the sample is known, one can accurately estimate the magnitude of the problem—a key surveillance objective. Probability samples draw from complete lists of: patients, workplaces, health care providers, or health care facilities. Most states maintain lists of employers and licensed health facilities. Professional licensing boards and professional associations may make lists of their members available. Even the yellow pages of telephone directories have been used to identify health facilities and providers.

To improve representativeness, the sample can be broken down by geographic area, type of treatment facility (hospital, medical office), and other characteristics of providers, employers, or patients. There are several sampling techniques such as stratified random sampling and cluster samples that can increase precision of the estimate. Readers should consult experts before undertaking complex sample designs.[1]

Purposive Sample. The choice of reporters in a sample can be guided by a specific objective of the surveillance system. If the objective is identifying cases for follow-up at specific worksites, selecting a small number of providers that report a large number of cases may be appropriate. This approach may skew the representativeness, favoring more severe cases, patients who can afford specialty care, particular geographic areas, or particular industries.

Other criteria have been used in selecting provider networks for reporting. Selecting a diverse group of specialties or practice settings allows the surveillance organization to experiment and assess the pros and cons of working with each type of provider, including alternative health care providers. This is useful during the development phase of sentinel reporting networks (Chapter 13).

Nature of the Health Condition

The health condition under surveillance, its severity, and stage will determine the likely treatment settings and medical specialties of providers. Serious traumatic injuries will be found in emergency departments of hospitals. A wide variety of occupational illnesses, particularly those in their early stages, will be treated by primary care physicians in the community, industrial clinics, or on-site medical services. The occupational case load of community physicians is generally small, unless they serve a particular population such as farm workers. Severer cases will often be referred to specialists.

For sentinel health conditions, certain types of specialists are ideal for reporting. Audiologists will have a patient load of individuals exposed to noise (Chapter 15). Chronic lung diseases such as silicosis or asthma will be referred to pulmonary specialists (Chapters 14 and 16). Neurologists and hand surgeons are likely to see severe cases of carpal tunnel syndrome (Chapter 13). Orthopedists will see joint and back disorders. Rehabilitation medicine specialists are likely to see cases at a later stage. Besides being a rich source of potential cases, severer cases seen by specialists may generate more definitive medical data that will make it easier to confirm cases.

Some health services are highly centralized and may be ideal for reporting. For example, reporting by a few dozen centralized analytic laboratories for elevated blood lead covers 28 different states.[2] Other laboratories that perform cholinesterase testing or electrodiagnostic tests may also be ideal, especially if occupation and employment data are captured on laboratory report forms. Regional centers for trauma, burns, and poison control also funnel cases to a central location.

Nonphysician specialists play an important role and should not be overlooked as case reporters. These include occupational health nurses, chiropractors, vocational rehabilitation professionals, physical therapists, occupational therapists, and unions.

Health Beliefs of the Population and Health Access

Recent immigrants and certain resident ethnic groups often have health beliefs that differ from the mainstream. This affects their choice of health care providers. These groups and undocumented workers also have less access to the health care system because they lack the awareness of workers' compensation, health insurance, or actively avoid contact with mainstream institutions. These groups may place greater emphasis on physical medicine, including chiropractors, and alternative providers such as acupuncturists and folk healers (e.g., curanderos).

Lack of cases in surveillance systems may reflect a lack of access to health care, or that patients are using alternative health care. Accessing these groups requires a special understanding of their needs and of surveillance personnel that are multilingual and multicultural.

Recruitment

After geographic areas, the types of facilities, and medical specialties are identified, individual institutions and individuals within the institutions must be approached and recruited. In active systems this is often done in face-to-face meetings in which the goals of the surveillance system are explained and details of participation are described. Voluntary participation and patient confidentiality are questions of health professionals that frequently come up during recruitment. The existence of a passive surveillance system (in which reporting is already legally required) and laws that allow confidential medical information to be shared with public health authorities lower barriers to participation. Active systems build on this foundation, but extra data reporting is usually voluntary.

Training

There are two training needs. First, reporters must be trained to recognize occupational injuries and illnesses. In active surveillance, the surveillance system can provide targeted education to improve case recognition.

Second, reporters must be trained to report cases using the specific procedures of the surveillance system. These procedures include the reporting guidelines: the details of who must report to whom, the content of the report, the method of transmitting the report, and the time interval between the incident and the reporting of the case. Providers' preferences should be taken into account when making these decisions so that reporting will not interfere with their work flow and workload. Several reporting mechanisms may need to be offered. This will simplify the surveillance system from the viewpoint of the provider, but increase the complexity for the surveillance system. Training must include the administrative staff and paraprofessionals who are often the actual link between the reporter and the surveillance organization.

Written instructions in the form of a guide may be developed with provider input and disseminated to providers. This will facilitate both general education and the specifics of case reporting.

Promotion of Reporting

Active surveillance promotes reporting by reminders, incentives, and building personal relationships. To enhance participation, the surveillance organization should consider what it can offer reporters to make their participation worthwhile and sustainable. There are many kinds of incentives, including opportunities for professional education and development organized by the surveillance organization, clinical consultation, receiving scientific publications relevant to cases actually reported, participating in the writing of peer-reviewed scientific publications, or receiving certificates, awards, and public recognition.

In employer-based programs, the policy and practices regarding case reporting has an impact on the number and types of cases reported. Supervisors may neither actively encourage nor discourage workers from reporting work-related health concerns; however, when this occurs, the full magnitude of cases may not be attained. In some cases, workers who report an illness or file a workers' compensation claim may be met with hostility, threats to continued employment, or other reprisals. Fear of retaliation can drive reporting underground, and keep many mild and moderate cases from view. Threats for not reporting or hiding a job-related illness or injury are less common.

A sincere and active policy of prompt reporting without reprisals is most desirable. For many mild cases, this creates an opportunity to intervene when the problem is still reversible. When this policy is adopted after any of the previous ones, the number of reported cases temporarily increases and then subsides as the pent up milder cases finally come to attention. While the case incidence rates go up, the lost time incidence rates generally do not increase as steeply. Management should expect these changes, which have been likened to riding a roller coaster. The surveillance program is working (not failing) because there is an initial, short-lived increase in the number of reported cases.

As mentioned in Chapter 1, economic incentives influence reporting of cases. Linking incentives to production goals, assigning the costs of workers' compensation, and safety prizes may discourage case reporting.

STEP 8. ESTABLISH PRIORITIES AND PROTOCOLS FOR FOLLOW-UP

This step is applicable to company-based health and safety programs and governmental surveillance that link data collection and case reporting to active workplace follow-up.

Protocols for Case Reporting

The surveillance system should have written protocols with a flow diagram that shows the steps for case reporting and follow-up. A generic flow diagram for employer-based reporting is shown in Figure 6.1. Several of the case studies (see Chapters 11–25) have similar diagrams.

Protocols for Case and Worksite Follow-up: Epidemiologic Triage

During case reporting or analysis, there may be situations in which the nature of a case report or pattern of injuries, illness, or exposure triggers a response by the surveillance organization. This may be to disseminate the information rapidly, gather more information, or recommend or take immediate prevention measures.

On an operational level, the objectives of active follow-up are:

- confirm reported cases
- identify other cases not yet reported
- collect information on uncontrolled exposures at the worksite of cases
- manage cases and workplaces through the coordination of prevention, medical, and disability services. This includes medical screening of exposed coworkers and workplace health and safety investigations.

Not all cases, work areas, or worksites may merit individual follow-up, and, among the cases that do, there may be a range of action that follows in a priority sequence. Surveillance data can be used to help set priorities. Protocols help decide what to do in specific cases.

Emergency rooms sort cases into three categories: those that will get better with little or no follow-up, those that will not get better no matter how much follow-up is provided, and those that will survive only with vigorous follow-up. This is called triage and is applied to individual patients. A similar triage applies to workplaces using epidemiologic criteria. Chapter 19 is an example of epidemiologic triage of cancer mortality at specific workplaces. Criteria for prioritizing follow-up generally consider characteristics of individual cases, case clusters, total number of cases, and rates.

Individual Case Characteristics

Severity of individual cases is a well-recognized method of establishing priorities (Table 6.1). Severity may be defined by the clinical presentation of the case (signs, symptoms, physical findings), the nature and extent of organ or tissue damage (e.g., fatality, amputation), level of exposure (blood lead level, percent cholinesterase depression), the delivery of emergency or in-patient care

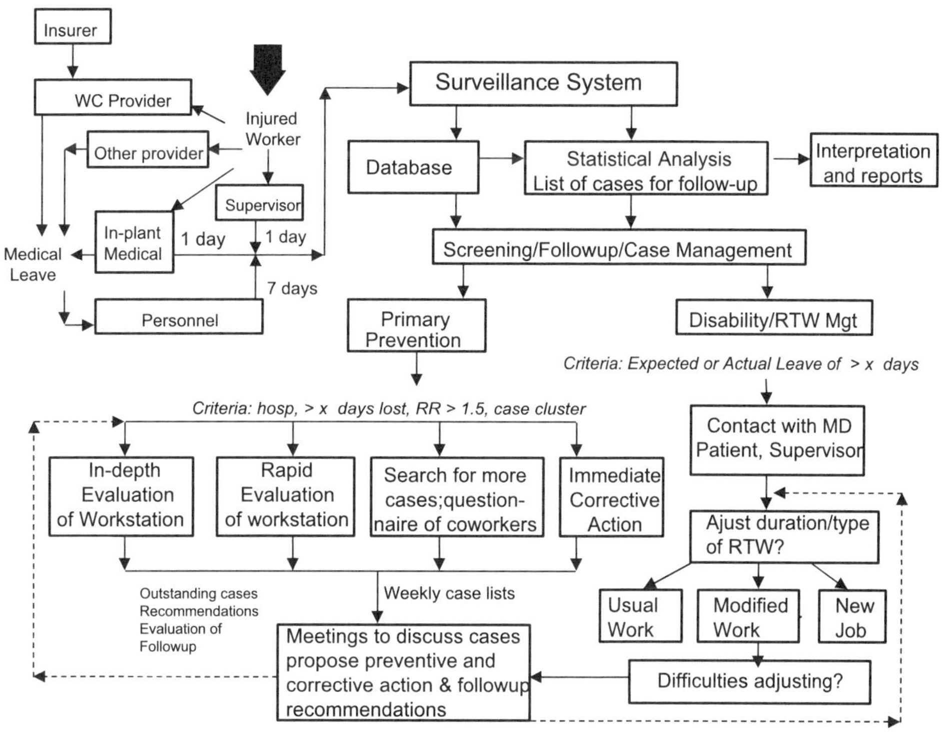

Figure 6.1 Flow chart of case reporting and follow-up in a generic workplace. Cases can flow into the surveillance center via any one of three paths: reports made by supervisors, in-plant medical personnel, and workers notifying their personnel department that either their personal physician or a worker's compensation provider has given them a medical leave of absence. (In many worksites this involves injuries and illnesses of three or more days.) Supervisors and in-plant medical services have 1 day to report the injury to the surveillance center and the personnel department compiles lists on a weekly basis, which are retrieved by the surveillance team. The case reports are key entered into a database that generates lists of workers and carries out statistical analyses. Cases are screened against criteria to guide prevention and disability management. Those meeting the criteria are followed up through a system of epidemiologic triage—graduated actions depending on the individual case characteristics and epidemiologic presentation as clusters, elevated rates, relative risks or incidence ratios.

(e.g., emergency room or hospital admission), or the type and amount of disability. Administrative indicators, such as the filing of a workers' compensation claim or attorney involvement, have been used as a severity measure.

Statistical Characteristics

The total number of cases in a subgroup, such cases per worksite or department, is the simplest way of prioritizing follow-up (Table 6.2). This tends to favor large worksites or departments that may have low incidence rates.

Cases reported in a brief time interval and originating from the same location are called time-space clusters, or case clusters. Some clusters are public health emergencies such as explosions and fires at manufacturing facilities, spills or releases of toxic materials, and group poisonings.

Incidence and prevalence rates, rate ratios, attributable risk, and excess cases are another way of estab-

Table 6.1 Examples of Triggers for Individual Case Follow-up

Treatment Setting	*Disability*	*Lost Workdays*	*Diagnostic or Clinical Criteria*	*Public Health*
Hospital (stay > 24 hours)	Death	30+ plateau of rapid RTW†	Amputation	Sentinel Event*
Emergency room	Permanent and total	8–30	Crushing injuries, fracture,	
Specialist care	Permanent and partial	1–7	Blood lead > 25 μg/dl	
Primary care (2 or more visits)	Temporary and total	No lost work	Cholinesterase decrease ≥ 30% from baseline	
First aid or 1 medical visit with no follow-up	Temporary and partial			
Self-treatment				

*See list in Chapter 1 (Table 1.3).
†RTW, return-to-work

Table 6.2 Examples of Priority Setting Criteria and Graduated Actions*

Individual Case Characteristics†	*Epidemiologic Indicators*†
• Death	• Elevated rate ratio (RR)
• Hospitalization	• Excess cases based on attributable risk‡
• Sentinel Health Event/Occupational (SHE/O)	• High rate
• Lost work days	• Large number of cases
• Clinical severity	• Mini-outbreak (e.g., 3 or more cases within a few weeks or months)

POTENTIAL ACTIONS

A. If causes are known, immediate preventive and corrective actions: stop dangerous operations, yellow tag dangerous machinery and equipment; medical removal, halt dangerous work practices, medical screening of exposed coworkers

B. Investigation of possible causes
   1. Quick investigation of workstation of case(s) to identify problems, and, if possible causes are found, use the information for immediate prevention at workstations of all exposed workers (quick fixes, short-term or interim prevention strategy)
   2. In-depth investigation to identify causes, if unknown, and examination of long-term prevention strategies based on engineering controls, process change, or redesign

C. Reassurance to workers that work-related health problems have not been demonstrated (e.g., low rate or RR = 1 for cancer, heart disease, respiratory disease, or other chronic health problem that is not a sentinel event), and are unlikely to have occurred and that little additional action is needed

*Quantitative data based on case characteristics and epidemiologic measures can help choosing among alternative courses of action (A, B, C) at a given workplace and in determining priorities among different workplaces according to relative urgency.

†Not listed in a particular order.

‡When the incidence rate is small, but the population at risk is large, the number of attributable (or excess) cases may be large.

lishing priorities. If the workplace has a few hundred workers it may be possible to:

- directly compare the departments or jobs with high and low rates within the same facility
- compare each department with the plant-wide rate

When the worksite or a particular department is small, it is possible to predict the expected number of cases if one knows:

- the number of workers at risk
- a published incidence rate from a comparable industry or from the community

The observed number of cases divided by the expected number of cases is called an incidence ratio (See Chapter 5). When the incidence ratio is greater than 1 based on at least a few observed cases, it is well advised to investigate the possible causes of the increased rate, or take preventive action if the cause is easily identified (e.g., sentinel event).

Epidemiologists are familiar with the idea that the size of the rate ratio helps identify cause-and-effect relationships. In Monson's classification,[3] rate ratios of 1.2–1.5 are considered weak, 1.5–3.0 moderate, 3.0–10 strong, and >10 as infinite. This type of information is useful and can be part of setting priorities when several workplaces or several areas within a single workplace have high incidence rates. Table 6.2 illustrates the linking of epidemiologic criteria to a graduated sequence of actions. These suggestions are not meant to be mechanically applied; these criteria should be relaxed or tightened depending on available resources and the seriousness of the consequences.

Protocols for Confidentiality and Ethical Issues

Government agencies need to consider the confidentiality of information and ethical treatment of individuals involved in public health surveillance and research. These issues are discussed in detail by Hahn.[4] In many states, government agencies have the legal authority to collect surveillance data and enter individual workplaces to carry out investigations. There is an ethical dimension how this is done.

An ethical checklist[4] for public health surveillance adapted to occupational health asks:

- Can the surveillance system be justified in terms of maximizing potential public health benefits while minimizing potential harm to the public and to individuals?
- Can the use of identifiers and maintaining records with identifiers be justified?
- Have the surveillance protocols been reviewed by colleagues?
- What procedures are used for informed consent when personal contact or records are being used?
- What steps have been taken to assure the confidentiality of information from workers, health care providers, and employers?
- Have health care providers been informed of conditions of their patients identified through surveillance?
- What steps have been taken to share data with colleagues and findings with the workers, unions, employers, and the public?

Absolute confidentiality can rarely be guaranteed because laws covering workers' compensation and Americans with Disabilities Act (ADA) may allow personal information to be divulged in legal proceedings. Insurance companies have access to personal medical information during claims processing. Nonetheless, steps should be taken to protect confidentiality and not permit the release of personal information without the permission of the affected party.

Some governmental surveillance systems collect data on medical testing that may not be part of employer-sponsored surveillance programs. An example is blood lead tests requested by a family physician, performed by a clinical laboratory, and reported to a state health agency. If the test result is urgent, the state agency may contact the patient before the physician. Government agencies should be sensitive to being the first to notify the worker of an abnormal result. Some workers may not want their employer to be contacted by the government health agency. In situations that immediately imperil life and limb, public health agencies do not hesitate to contact employers and recommend appropriate action. However, there may be situations that raise concerns about uncontrolled exposures, but are not emergencies. The risks of reprisals to an individual have to be balanced with the rights of coworkers to information that may affect their health. In the case of take-home exposures to lead, pesticides, and other substances, families of the patient and of coworkers may also be affected. At large workplaces, a government health agency might be able to contact the employer in a way that keeps the affected worker anonymous. At small workplaces, this approach may not work. However, some workers may not object to having their names acknowledged, and will give permission to contact their employers, if asked.

STEP 9. COMMENCE CASE REPORTING, DATA COLLECTION, AND FOLLOW-UP

This step is also oriented to company-based surveillance and governmental surveillance systems with active reporting and active case follow-up. As cases are reported, they need to be screened for completeness, coded, key entered into a computerized database (if they have not already been downloaded into one), and compared against the protocols to give direction to follow-up activities.

Unless the intake is done by a skilled surveillance technician, this will require the coordination of the secretarial, database, and technical staff of the surveillance team. In an unautomated environment, the mechanical steps are to physically check the mail, fax, or e-mail; take a report over the telephone; screen for completeness of the report; and, then deliver it to the person who actually reviews the report for triage. Case reports often contain less than the minimum amount of information to start the follow-up. These cases require re-contact with the reporter so that complete information can be obtained, if possible.

Managing Individual Case Follow-up

Some case reports will be coded and key entered into a statistical database and that is the extent of the follow-up. Cases requiring active follow-up usually have a file folder made up and are assigned to a case manager according to the protocols of the surveillance system. Depending on the number of individuals involved in case follow-up, case file routing or copying needs to be arranged. Otherwise, the paper file will have to be broken into different physical parts, each of which may be updated at different rates. With network computing and software, it is possible to design a central case file in which each case manager has an assigned authority to read, modify, create, and delete information in case files.

There is a generic process (Fig. 6.2) and a minimum data set to manage cases. The data are:

- a proposed action
- a deadline for taking the proposed action
- assignment of a staff person (case manager, line

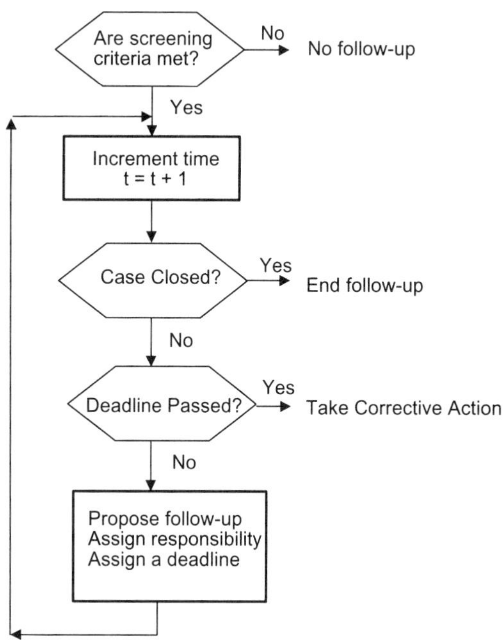

Figure 6.2 Algorithm for case management. One needs criteria for deciding which cases to follow-up. Once a case is opened it needs to be fed into a regular review cycle with other open cases. Explicit criteria are needed to decide that a case is closed so that cases do not fall through the cracks of the surveillance system. Deciding what actions to take, a deadline for completing the action, and staff person responsible for the follow-up are the other basic ingredients of case follow-up.

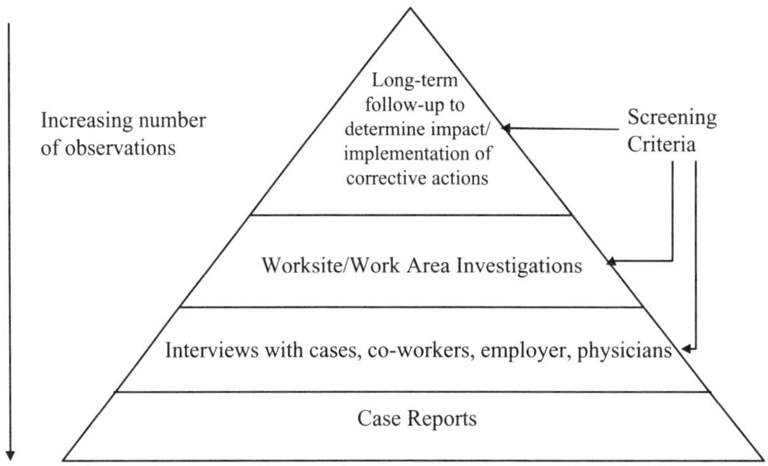

Figure 6.3 Active follow-up using increasingly strict priorities generates more detailed information for fewer cases. Initial case reports with the minimum data for all cases can be followed with interviews with the case, coworkers, physician, employer; worksite investigations, and long-term follow-up of recommendations and evaluation of corrective actions.

supervisor) who is responsible for carrying out the proposed follow-up

Criteria to trigger case opening are suggested in Table 6.1. Case closing criteria are also needed so that case managers will know when to stop follow-up. Closing criteria may include a completed injury investigation report, the implementation of recommendations, or a return-to-work within a specified time period. Ideally, management information should be entered into a database. Open cases with a due date for action that has lapsed need to be identified and listed.

Meetings of case managers to discuss cases should be planned on a regular basis depending on the urgency and the case load (e.g., daily, weekly, monthly, etc.). Unanticipated situations, gaps in the protocols, and other problems will inevitably be identified during case follow-up. Case management meetings play a crucial role in refining the protocols and assuring the protocols are consistently applied by all case managers. These meetings can be used to open new cases, formally close old cases, adjust workload, assign priorities, and help identify case studies that can be used for educational purposes. An example of individual case management is described in Chapter 11 on surveillance of elevated blood lead.

Data collected in surveillance systems with active follow-up typically have several layers of detail and breadth (Fig. 6.3). Case reports and other data collected during follow-up are among the input to statistical analysis, which is described in the next chapter.

REFERENCES

1. Levy PS, Lemeshow S. *Sampling for Health Professionals.* Belmont, CA: Lifetime Learning Publications, 1980.
2. Centers for Disease Control. Adult lead epidemiology and surveillance—United States, second and third quarters 1998, and annual 1994–1997. *MMWR* 1999; 48:213–223.
3. Monson R. *Occupational Epidemiology.* 2nd Edition. Boca Raton: CRC Press, 1990.
4. Hahn R. Ethical issues. In: Teutsch SM, Churchill R, ed. *Principles and Practice of Public Health Surveillance.* New York: Oxford University Press, 1994:175–189.

7

Analysis and Interpretation

NEIL A. MAIZLISH

STEP 10. ANALYZE AND INTERPRET DATA

Analysis and interpretation are essential steps in all surveillance systems. They transform raw data into meaningful information so decision-making is rational rather than improvised. The complexity of the analysis will depend on whether the surveillance system is case-based or population-based, and whether the surveillance system is linked to follow-up activities. There are several levels of analysis:

- case narrative or case report
- case series (case-based data)
- rate-based comparisons

Case Narrative

A case narrative is a concise description of an injury, an illness or an exposure affecting one or more individuals. Case narratives highlight emerging problems, sentinel events, or widely recognized problems with the intent to raise awareness and educate the reader. Case narratives, also called case reports, are often the first warning of a more wide spread problem, and capture interest because of their severity or novelty. Chapter 1 gives an example of a lead-poisoned radiator repair worker and there are hundreds of examples in occupational health and safety.[1–3]

The narrative describes the details of person-place-time such as age, sex, race, residence, occupation, industry and other demographic features of the case. Clinical details include the nature and timing of symptoms, signs, and physical evidence that support the diagnosis, a description of the medical treatment, and the response of the case. The known or presumed exposures are described by job activity or exposure using biologic and environmental samples when available. Case narratives are often accompanied by an editorial comment that links the current observation with previous reports, describes the limitations of the findings, and emphasizes established control measures.

General Considerations in Statistical Analyses

Timing of Events and the Analysis

There are several options for analyzing case incidence depending on when cases actually occurred or when they were reported. Additionally, in analyses of rates, the time period of case incidence must match employment data.

The surveillance system usually specifies the time period for analysis such as year, quarter, month, week, or other duration defined by two dates. How often data are analyzed reflects the urgency of the information, the rate of data collection, and the workload of the surveillance organization.

Date of Occurrence. Date of injury, date of onset of illness, and date of diagnosis are common ways to define actual occurrence. Analyses based on occurrence are easier to interpret and are generally preferred. For example, analyses can be based on "all cases diagnosed between January 1 and December 31, 2000," rather than "all cases received (reported) between January 1 and December 31, 2000." Some reported cases may have occurred in 1999 or earlier, and some cases that occurred in 2000 will not have been reported until 2001.

Analyses based on date of occurrence may have to be repeated when a few reports are received after the analysis is done. This may require revising the previous final report and notifying those with an old version of changes. Some organizations issue preliminary or provisional reports followed later by a final report.

Date Reported. There can be lags of weeks or months between the date of actual occurrence and the date the report was received. Waiting for every last case may cause substantial delays in analysis and in reporting the results. Analyses based on the date the report was received may be more timely and relevant.

If the time lag between date of occurrence and date reported is reasonably constant and the underlying employment (the population) is not changing over time or by subgroups, the results will be similar.

Matching Time Periods for Injury and Illness and Employment and Population Data. For rate-based analyses, employment data may be collected on a different time schedule than case data. For example, cases reported last month may be available today for analysis, but the most recent employment census or hours worked may be over a year old. The options include waiting until the population and employment data are available, making employment projections,[4] or using the available data.

Lost workdays, costs, and return-to-work can occur beyond the time period of case incidence (Chapter 26). This requires that the analysis is done after a meaningful length of time after the cut-off date of the case incidence period. It is possible to estimate the number of lost workdays after this date. However, underestimates often occur.[5] Analyses of costs and disability are commonly repeated and updated annually over a period of 2–5 years so that all the lost work time, disability, and costs are recorded.

Time Lags Between Exposures and Disease: Latency Effects. Chronic work-related diseases such as occupational cancer or asbestosis are usually diagnosed decades after exposures initiate the disease process. During this time lag, workers may have changed jobs either at the same employer, at different employers, or have changed occupations. The job he or she held at the time of diagnosis may not reflect the circumstances of exposure that led to his or her illness. If *current* occupation or industry is examined as a possible risk factor, the results may not be accurate. This type of error is called misclassification and is discussed later in this chapter in the section on validity and precision.

Analyses that examine the effects of latency may limit potential exposures or risk factors to a specified time interval in the latency period. For example, occupation can be defined as:

- occupation at the time period of first exposure
- "usual" occupation—longest duration (from date of first exposure to diagnosis)
- occupation on a specific date or decade

The analysis of silicosis cases in Chapter 14 illustrates these points.

Type of Frequency Measure of Injury and Illness

The analysis should take into account whether the cases are incident, prevalent, or period prevalent (Chapter 4). Some databases record data on the initial diagnosis and additional episodes in a continuous history that spans several years. A decision must be made to include or exclude cases that are not incident in the time period of analysis but carry over due to additional medical care or disability.

Sometimes it is important to analyze both prevalent and incidence cases. Case managers in active surveillance systems are keenly aware of their current workload—How many cases do I have now? This is a measure of prevalence. In contrast, monitoring trends or evaluation of prevention activities focuses on whether the rate of new cases (incidence) is going down.

Unit of Observation

Important aspects of clustering of health events can be revealed in statistical analyses in which outcomes and their characteristics naturally group together:

- episodes
- cases
- persons
- incidents
- workplaces
- industries
- occupations

A case can be made up of several episodes or repeated laboratory tests. Each person may have several different cases per year. Cases can occur alone or in incidents that affect many persons at the same time such as a burns from a fire or an explosion.

When examining trends or high-risk groups, analyses by different units of observation may indicate important changes in the pattern of risk factors. For example, when comparing case incidence in two time periods, it may be noted that the case incidence may not have changed, but that the number of episodes per case decreased or were of shorter duration. Likewise, if many cases occur in the same incident, the change in the number of multiple case incidents per year may be of interest as well as the total number of cases.

When data are available, these different groupings should be described. For example, the distribution of blood lead reports received annually by a statewide blood lead registry might be described as: 38 laboratories reported 1000 blood lead tests taken on 700 workers employed by 200 employers in 45 four-digit Standard Industrial Classification codes.

Data that include a large number of cases from a few workplaces or exposure incidents require a separate analysis to better understand their impact on the combined analysis. This is particularly true for catastrophic events such as explosions, fires, chemical releases, and mass poisonings. For example, 45 physicians reported 250 cases of occupational pesticide illness, of which 100 cases (40%) occurred in a single mass poisoning of citrus harvesting workers exposed to parathion.

These types of descriptive analyses are facilitated by good relational database design (Chapter 10). For example, laboratory reports of blood lead levels are placed in a database table linked to an episode table, which is linked to a case table, which is linked to a worker table, which, in turn is linked to an employer table, which, in turn, is linked to an industry table.

Case Series and Case-Based Analysis

A statistical analysis of case information is appropriate for sentinel event surveillance and for passive surveillance systems in which employment data are not available. A case series is a statistical summary of cases. Sometimes this summary accompanies individual case narratives.

The analysis should be driven by the objectives of the surveillance system, which include describing the problem and its magnitude, identifying high-risk groups, monitoring trends, and linking cases to follow-up activities. Each objective involves the analysis of health outcomes with specific variables that are known or possible risk factors. The statistics that are generated are frequency counts and percentages for categorical variables such as sex and race; and, means, medians, standard deviations, and range for continuous variables such as age, years of service, etc. Appendix C discusses distributions and descriptive statistics.

Description of Cases and Univariate and Bivariate Analysis

The typical analysis begins with a statistical profile—one variable at a time—starting with the outcome of interest, demographics, and occupational characteristics of the cases. Table 7.1 illustrates this approach and gives the distribution for blood lead (outcome), age, sex, Hispanic surname, selected industries, geographic area, and time period for adults with a laboratory-reported blood lead test. The goal is to describe cases noting the subgroups with the greatest and fewest number of cases or percentage of a particular characteristic, such as teenage workers or very severe cases.

When the health outcome is not restricted to a single diagnosis, it is important to describe the diagnoses that make up the cases. Table 7.2 shows the number and percent of cases specified by diagnosis.

After describing the outcome and risk factors separately, the next step examines how the outcome varies with other variables, one variable at a time. This is called univariate analysis. The variable crossed with the outcome is usually one of several possible risk factors based on person-place-time. For example, Table 7.3 (upper part) compares the blood lead distribution by sex, a possible risk factor for elevated blood lead. This example shows that men have a slightly higher percentage (6%) of cases with blood lead levels of 60 μg/dL or greater than do females (4%). Additional tables could be made for blood lead by age, blood lead by Hispanic surname, blood lead by industry, blood lead by year of report, etc.

Bivariate analyses examine how the outcome varies with combinations of two variables. Table 7.3 (lower part) illustrates how blood lead varies by age and sex. In this example, the younger men and younger women have a very similar blood lead distribution (percent columns for <40 years). For men, the percentage of cases with blood lead levels of 60–80+ μg/dL increases from 4% at ages younger than 40 to 9% for cases 40 and older—a 5% increase. Likewise, for women, the percentage of cases with blood lead levels of 60–80+ μg/dL increases from 3% at ages younger than 40 to 5% for cases 40 and older—a 2% increase. Age appears to increase the percentage of higher blood lead levels for both men and women. However, the increase with older age is more pronounced in men than in women—5% versus 2%.

In employer and government databases that code occupation, industry or department, body part and nature of injury and illness, there are many possible two-variable combinations with the same outcome. Three-way and even four-way combinations of nature, body part, occupation, industry, agent or external cause may be possible. Some combinations may have too few events (or none). But, if there are sufficient data, two-, three-, and four-way combinations of risk factors should be attempted.

Analysis of Magnitude of Problem and High-Risk Groups

A common analysis strategy attempts to identify the largest number or percentage of outcomes in the fewest number of categories. The more cases aggregate in specific subgroups, the easier it may be to identify high-risk groups, possible causes, and preventive action.

Table 7.1 Blood Lead Distribution and Demographic Characteristics of California Adults with a Blood Lead Report 25 μg/dL or Greater, 1987–1990

Item	*Number*	*Percent*	
Total adults	4069	100	
Blood lead level (μg/dL)			
25–39	2566	63	
40–59	1271	31	Health
60–79	170	4	Outcome
80+	62	2	
Age[a] (years)			
16–19	44	2	
20–29	574	25	
30–39	700	30	
40–49	547	23	
50–59	311	13	
60+	165	7	
Sex[b]			Person
Male	3730	95	
Female	199	5	
Surname[c]			
Non-Hispanic	2009	49	
Hispanic	1958	50	
Asian	22	1	
Top 10 Industries[d]			
Lead battery manufacture	1089	39	
Secondary lead smelting	473	17	
Brass/copper foundry	251	9	
Radiator repair	124	5	
Firing ranges—sport	78	3	
Brass pipe/valve manufacturing	65	2	
Pottery manufacturing	58	2	
Nonferrous foundries	51	2	Environment/
Firing ranges—police	51	2	Place
Porcelain electrical supplies	35	1	
County of Employer[e,f]			
Los Angeles	9053	67	
Orange	2164	16	
San Bernardino	679	5	
San Diego	370	3	
Year Test Reported[e]			
1987	3025	13	
1988	5874	26	Time
1989	7622	33	
1990	6539	28	
Total	20060	100	

[a]Excludes 1728 individuals with reports not stating age.
[b]Excludes 140 individuals for whom gender was not stated or determined.
[c]Excludes 80 individuals for whom surname was not classified.
[d]Excludes 1292 individuals for whom industry was not classified.
[e]Number of blood lead tests rather than persons.
[f]Excludes missing data.

Table 7.2 Number and Percent of Injuries and Illnesses by Diagnosis, 01/01/1999–12/31/1999

*ICD 9**	*Nature of Injury or Illness*	*Number*	*Percent*	*Cumulative Percent*	
710-739	Musculoskeletal diseases	98	26	26	
840-848	Sprains and strains	90	24	50	
870-904	Open wounds	36	10	60	
320-389	Diseases of the nervous system	22	6	66	← Cut-Point (67%)
960-989	Poisoning	19	5	71	
800-829	Fractures	19	5	76	
910-924	Superficial wounds	18	5	81	
950-959	Injuries to the spinal cord and nerves	13	3	84	
860-869	Internal organ injuries	11	3	87	
001-139	Infectious diseases	8	2	89	
830-839	Dislocations	7	2	91	
940-949	Burns	6	2	93	
390-459	Diseases of the circulatory system	6	2	95	
140-239	Cancer	5	1	95	
460-519	Respiratory diseases	4	1	96	
850-854	Intracranial injury and concussion	4	1	97	
520-579	Digestive organ diseases	4	1	98	
680-709	Skin diseases	3	1	98	
780-799	Symptoms and ill-defined conditions	2	1	99	
580-589	Diseases of the genito-urinary system	2	1	99	
999-999	Other illness and injury, nec	1	<1	100	
001-999	Total	378	100	100	

*International Classification of Diseases, 9th Revision

Table 7.3 Univariate Analysis of Blood Lead with Sex and Bivariate Analysis of Blood Lead with Sex and Age

UNIVARIATE ANALYSIS: SEX

Blood Lead Level (μg/dL)	*Male* N	*Male* %	*Female* N	*Female* %
25–39.9	2336	63	139	70
40–59.9	1166	31	52	26
60–79.9	151	4	6	3
80+	77	2	2	1
Total	3730	100	199	100

BIVARIATE ANALYSIS: SEX AND AGE

Blood Lead Level (μg/dL)	*Male*				*Female*			
	Age < 40		*Age ≥ 40*		*Age < 40*		*Age ≥ 40*	
	N	%	N	%	N	%	N	%
25–39.9	1342	63	994	62	72	64	67	78
40–59.9	701	33	465	29	37	33	15	17
60–79.9	55	3	96	6	3	2	3	4
80+	28	1	49	3	1	1	1	1
Total	2126	100	1604	100	113	100	86	100

For example, we may start with the observation that the diagnosis or body part with the largest number of cases is back injuries, which are typically 20%–30% of the disabling injuries in workers' compensation databases. We then may ask what is the leading cause or agent of back injuries? The number of cases under *lifting objects* may be the largest. We may then ask what are the leading occupations among back injuries because of lifting? The occupation with the largest number of cases may be packagers.

This process can be extremely repetitive and generate numerous categories with small numbers of cases. To set priorities and make the groupings more manageable, a threshold is sometimes used to limit the output (e.g., subgroups with 10 or more cases). Likewise, a cutoff based on a specific cumulative percent may be applied to a list sorted in descending order of number of cases. For example, in Table 7.2, two-thirds of cases occurred in only 4 of the 21 (~20%) diagnoses.

Analysis of Trends

To observe trends, the number of cases can be plotted on a time axis using bar charts or line charts. Figure 1.8 illustrates this approach with the number of deaths due to several chronic occupational lung diseases. To examine geographic trends, maps can be used to display the number of deaths (or rates) that occur in a specific geographic area. There are several common techniques to indicate the number or rate of events. Each geographic unit that makes up the map (e.g., county, state) can have a label for the number of deaths, shading or a pattern that corresponds to a category of events (e.g., 0, 1–9, 10–49, 50+), or dots, each of which represents a set number of cases. Figure 4.1 illustrates asbestos deaths in the United States by county. Counties with darker gray shades have more deaths than those with lighter shades.

Linking Case Reporting to Follow-up

In sentinel event surveillance systems with active follow-up, the statistical analysis is oriented to producing lists of cases or worksites that meet the criteria for follow-up (Step 8). Tables 6.1 and 6.2 give examples of criteria based on case severity, case clustering, and high rates. Data may include information in the initial case report form, laboratory tests, and interviews of cases, their physicians, and their employers. The analysis can be done by manually comparing logical criteria to each case or by applying Structured Query Language (SQL) of database software. Table-driven edits and menu-driven sort functions and filters are widely available in commercial spreadsheets and database programs to generate lists.

For example, a state blood lead registry that receives thousands of laboratory reports each year may decide to contact a case and his or her employer when one employee has a single blood lead test greater than 60 μg/dL or the worksite has three or more cases between 40 and 59.9 μg/dL within a 6-month period. Workers' compensation carriers have long practiced this type of analysis using cost criteria. Loss runs for an individual employer lists cases that have incurred more than a threshold amount of medical or indemnity payments or both.

The production of active surveillance systems is the number and the quality of statistical reports issued, cases followed up or referred, interviews conducted, field investigations carried out, and recommendations made and implemented. Counting these activities is facilitated by administrative databases. This is part of an efficiency evaluation. An evaluation of effectiveness examines whether surveillance is contributing to lowering injury and illness incidence. Chapter 8 discusses evaluation in more detail.

Limitations of Case-Based Analyses

The interpretation of a case series depends generally on whether the health condition is a sentinel event/occupational (SHE/O) or not. The cause-effect relationship between the occupational exposure and illness has already been proven. The evidence comes not only from epidemiologic research but also from other fields such as clinical medicine or toxicology. A control group is not usually necessary: a high percentage of those who have been exposed have the illness, and a high percentage of those who have not been exposed do not.

Case series of diseases that are not SHE/Os are generally harder to interpret without a comparison group. If a high percentage of the case series has an exposure to a specific substance that is present in very few workplaces in a specific industry, suspicions are raised even if the exposure has not been previously identified as a cause of occupational health problems. This is one of the uses of surveillance: to identify new occupational diseases and exposures.

However, finding that a high proportion of cases has an apparent exposure to a fairly widespread industrial exposure (e.g., a common industrial solvent) may reflect that a high proportion of the industrial population has that exposure (Fig. 7.1). Case series do not collect data on the distribution of exposure in the population. Until these data are collected (rate-based analyses or case-control studies), it is an open question, or untested hypothesis whether a new exposure causes the illness in the case series. One of the uses of case-based surveillance is to generate hypotheses to be followed-up by research.

Time trends in case-based data are also difficult to interpret unless there is reasonable certainty that the

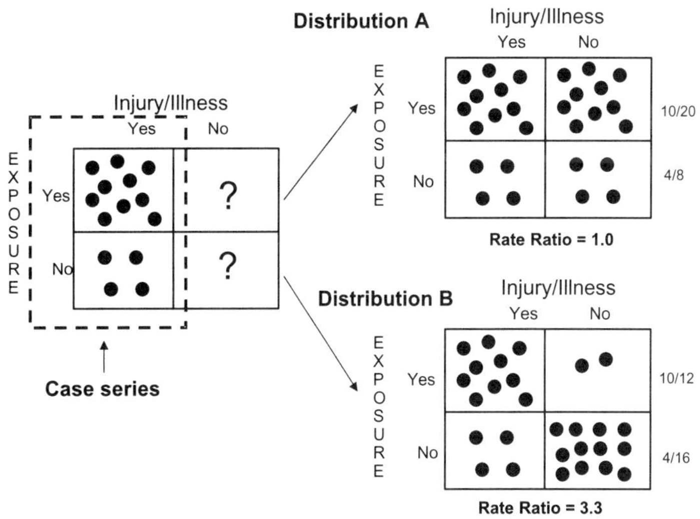

Figure 7.1 Case series collect data only on the distribution of exposures in the cases and not in the healthy population. This is illustrated by the half of the 2 × 2 table set off with dashed lines. In *A*, the distribution of exposure is the same in the cases as in the healthy population, and the exposure is not associated with the illness (RR = 1). In *B*, the distribution of exposure in the healthy population is different than that in the cases. Exposure and disease appear to occur together more in the cases than in the healthy population (RR = 3.3).

population and employment are not changing over time. An increase in the number of cases may occur when the population increases and the rate stays the same over two time periods.

Rate-Based Analyses

When data on cases and employment are available, employer and governmental programs can carry out surveillance using rates as the outcome. Data analysis in the rate-based approach is similar to that of case-based, with the exception that the outcome is a rate. The typical rate-based analysis also begins with a statistical profile in which the cases are described using frequency counts, percentages, and rates—one variable at a time. When data are available, the rates should be broken down by diagnosis, external cause of injury, body part, and agent. Appendix D (Table D.1 through D.4) illustrates rates for specific diagnoses.

The next step is univariate analysis of the outcome. When a rate is calculated for a particular subgroup, the rate is called subgroup-specific. For example, rates calculated individually for men and women are sex-specific rates. Univariate analyses are shown for department (Table 7.4) and job title (Table 7.5) at a hypothetical employer. The rates are department-specific and occupation-specific. Each table shows that rates vary considerably by department and occupation.

Selected bivariate analyses should also be examined. In governmental and workers' compensation surveillance programs, data are sufficient to examine rates by two-, three-, and four-way combinations of risk factors.

Table 7.4 Case Incidence Rate per 100 Full-Time Equivalents by Department, Employer A, 1999

Department	*Cases*	*Hours Worked*	*Rate**	*Rate* $Ratio_{S\&R}$†	*Rate* $Ratio_{plant}$‡	*Rate* $Ratio_{ind.}$§
Line 1	99	900,000	22.0	3.4	1.7	
Line 2	109	1,300,000	16.8	2.6	1.3	
Inspection	69	1,200,000	11.5	1.8	0.9	
Maintenance	65	1,500,000	8.7	1.3	0.7	
Shipping and receiving (S&R)	36	1,100,000	6.5	1.0	0.5	
Total Plant	378	6,000,000	12.6	—	1.0	1.3

*Rate per 100 full-time equivalent (FTE)s = $\frac{\text{Cases} \times 200{,}000}{\text{Hours Worked}}$.
†Shipping and Receiving rate used as reference, 6.5 per 100 FTE.
‡Plantwide rate used as reference, 12.6 per 100 FTEs.
§Industrywide rate from published data used as reference rate, 9.8 per 100 FTEs.

Table 7.5 Case Incidence Rate per 100 Full-Time Equivalents by Occupation, Employer A, 1999

Occupation	*Cases*	*Hours Worked*	*Rate*
Mechanics	71	2,000,000	7.1
Inspectors	66	1,500,000	8.8
Material handlers	75	1,000,000	15.0
Machine operators	166	1,500,000	22.1
Total	378	6,000,000	12.6

Table 7.6 displays the rates for combinations of department and job title at a hypothetical employer. Many combinations have too few cases (or none) to analyze. But, there are enough machine operators to analyze their rates separately for production Lines 1 and 2. Likewise, there are enough material handlers in Line 1 and Shipping & Receiving to analyze their rates separately. This bivariate analysis shows that the overall high rate in machine operators in the univariate analysis (22.1 cases per 100) is largely accounted for by the very high rate of machine operators in Line 1 (42.9 per 100). This is a high risk group that would merit follow-up.

Appendix D illustrates a univariate analysis at a hypothetical employer whose 3000 employees work in five departments and have four occupations. It examines both case incidence and lost workday incidence rates broken down by diagnosis, external cause, body part (for musculoskeletal disorders), department, and occupation.[6] The results are interpreted and presented in a brief technical summary. Appendix E is an additional example that shows step-by-step how to carry out an analysis of rates, rate ratios, and excess cases using data from a log of first medical visits and an operational case definition. Chapter 10 illustrates the computer logic and SQL to automate this process.

Magnitude of Problem, High-Risk Groups, and Trends

The emphasis in rate-based analyses is to identify specific subgroups with high rates and low rates. Follow-up can be directed to identify the possible causes of the high rates. Chapter 5 discusses different options to compare rates and calculate rate ratios. In government databases, the state-wide rate or the rate of all private sector workplaces is sometimes used. The major industrial group (2 digit SIC) is sometimes compared to a more specific 4-digit grouping. Attributable risk and excess cases can be calculated, but these data are not customarily presented in government reports of health and safety statistics.

Rates can be plotted on a time axis to observe trends and on maps to show geographic trends. Figure 1.4 illustrates time trends of injury and illness rates and Figure 1.6 illustrates the trend in death rates over time. In some surveillance systems it is possible to group industries and occupations into categories (e.g., high, medium, low) that reflect possible exposures to chemical substances or other hazards.[7] This type of classification of exposure allows us to examine whether there is a trend for dose-response: rates that increase with increasing levels of a risk factor.

An important advantage of rate-based analysis is that changes in the number of cases between two time periods can be explained by changes in employment and changes in rates. An increase in the number of cases from year 1 to year 2 may occur if the rate is steady but there are more hours worked. Alternatively, if employment stays constant over time, an increase in the number of cases reflects an increase in the rate. Plotting rates over time allows us to determine if the rates are changing.

Relationship Between Case Incidence Rate and Lost Workday Incidence Rate

Many employers calculate both case incidence rates and lost workday incidence rates from data in workers' compensation or OSHA record keeping. How these rates track together from year to year may shed light on potential workplace hazards, medical care issues, disability management, and other factors. For example, if the case incidence does not change from year 1 to

Table 7.6 Case Incidence Rate per 100 Full-Time Equivalents by Department and Occupation, Employer A, 1999

	Machine Operators			*Material Handlers**			*Mechanics**		*Inspectors**	
Department	*Cases*	*Hours*	*Rate*	*Cases*	*Hours*	*Rate*	*Cases*	*Rate*	*Cases*	*Rate*
Line 1	60	280,000	42.9	39	480,000	16.2	—†	—	—	—
Line 2	106	1,220,000	17.4	—	—	—	—	—	—	—
Shipping and receiving	—	—	—	36	520,000	13.8	—	—	—	—
Inspection	—	—	—	—	—	—	—	—	—	—
Maintenance	—	—	—	—	—	—	—	—	—	—
Total	166	1,500,000	22.1	75	1,000,000	15.0	71	7.1	66	8.8

*Nearly all inspectors are assigned to the Inspection Department and Mechanics to the Maintenance Department.
†— indicates a cell with no or too few cases to analyze.

year 2, but the lost workday incidence increases in the second year, among the possible explanations are:

- increase in intensity of exposures
- a few catastrophic cases
- increase in the proportion of diagnoses that require more medical treatment (change in case-mix)
- diminished access to medical treatment
- less demanding return-to-work program (e.g., a change in policy or personnel, new physicians, supervisor, case manager)
- less effective medical treatment

Likewise, if the lost-time incidence rate stays the same from year 1 to year 2, but the case incidence rate increases, possible explanations include:

- more sensitive case definition
- earlier recognition and reporting of milder cases

Several other general considerations should be taken into account when interpreting surveillance data.

INTERPRETATION OF SURVEILLANCE DATA

Validity and Precision

The interpretation of epidemiologic data is guided by the concepts of validity and precision. This applies to surveillance data as well. It is a judgement of whether what one intended to measure about illness and exposure was actually measured. This refers to the definitions of disease, exposure, and other variables; the integrity of the data; and the methods used to collect and analyze the data. Validity often comes down to the standards held by the community of occupational health and safety professionals. These standards reflect the appropriate use of established methods and scientific processes. Databases that are riddled with errors or missing a substantial amount of data are not considered valid no matter how sophisticated the analysis.

Precision is related to error. Some error is random and reflects a natural variation in populations. This is likened to shots that cluster around a bull's-eye. The cluster can be very loose (much variation) or very tight (little variation). However, the average of the shots falls right on the center of the bull's-eye. Random error is discussed in the section below on variation in populations and samples.

Other types of error are systematic and may be introduced by the surveillance team or those providing data to the surveillance system. In this case, the cluster of shots is off the mark, because the center of the cluster is high, low, left, or right of the bull's eye. The average calculated from data with a systematic error is more or less than it really should be. This is called bias, or a biased estimate. Averages, proportions, rates, and rate ratios can have biases.

Some types of systematic error are under the control of the surveillance system or the researcher. For example, before taking measurements, we calibrate the instruments and train interviewers.

Reporting Bias

Most surveillance systems are susceptible to a systematic error introduced by reporting practices. Before one accepts that an increase or decrease in incidence is due to a change in a workplace exposure, it is prudent to ask whether reporting has changed. Reporting depends on the knowledge and skills to detect a case, the motivation to report it, and the case definition. Increases in reporting often follow training programs or reminders. These increases are temporary, partly because they need to be reinforced and partly because the personnel originally trained transferred or left the workplace and have been replaced with individuals without specific training. Because of new scientific knowledge, the case definition itself can change, as has happened several times with the reporting of those infected with the human immunodeficiency virus (HIV) or acquired immune deficiency syndrome (AIDS).[8]

Sometimes the explanation for a sudden decrease in reporting is exasperatingly simple or bureaucratic, e.g., the clerk who gathers and mails reports to the surveillance center goes on vacation and has no back-up. A new, zealous (or lackadaisical) supervisor, a change in the employer's medical group or workers' compensation carrier are other examples. In the start-up phase of surveillance projects, an increase in cases may merely reflect that more data reporters are being brought on board or the geographic area is being expanded. Sudden decreases can also occur when a single employer that accounts for a large percentage of cases, goes out of business or eliminates a product line that generated many cases.

Some lapses in reporting should be tolerated by the surveillance team rather than demand a level of perfection that alienates reporters. However, in other situations, the surveillance system exercises good judgment by contacting a reporter to find out whether an administrative bottleneck has occurred. For example, laboratory reports of blood lead levels over 80 μg/dL should not just sit on a clerk's desk while he or she is on vacation.

Reporting bias can affect the total number of cases and the representativeness of the cases that are reported. It has been mentioned previously that severe cases are more likely to be reported (severity bias). But other characteristics of the case can be skewed, including age, sex, race, industry, occupation, or geographic area. For example, a low proportion of cases in rural areas may reflect the lack of case reporters or lack of access to health services compared to urban areas.

Confounding

Another type of systematic error called confounding is related to the population rather than to the reporters. For example, smokers as a group have a much higher incidence of respiratory diseases than do nonsmokers. In a workplace, we might observe a high incidence of respiratory disease in a department where workers are exposed to resins that are respiratory irritants. We also observe that some of the workers in that department smoke. How can we tell whether smoking, exposure to resin, or both are the cause of the high incidence rates?

The simplest way to untangle the effects of smoking from those of working with resin is to calculate the respiratory illness incidence rates in four different subgroups:

- smokers with resin exposure
- nonsmokers with resin exposure
- smokers without resin exposure
- nonsmokers without resin exposure

This is an example of a particular type of bivariate analysis used to control the effects of confounding. That is, two variables (e.g., smoking and resin) influence the same outcome (e.g., respiratory disease) and occur together (e.g., smoking and resin). By breaking the population into subgroups, we can examine the effect of resin apart from the effect of smoking. Using the rate of respiratory illness in nonsmokers without resin exposure as a reference rate, we can make comparisons with the other groups. The comparison with the rate in nonsmokers with resin exposure provides information on the independent effect of resins on respiratory disease. The comparison with the subgroup with both resin exposure and smoking provides clues on the combined effects of resin and smoking (Fig. 7.2).

This technique of breaking the population into subgroups is called stratification and can be used when there are sufficient numbers of workers with the exposure and risk factor in each subgroup. This technique is often used in passive surveillance systems with large databases. Readers should consult the text books listed at the end of Chapter 4 for additional details on confounding and interaction between variables.

Misclassification

Occupational surveillance often relies on occupation, department, or industry for classifying exposures rather than on precise measurements of contaminants in the air or on physical hazards. As mentioned in Chapter 3,

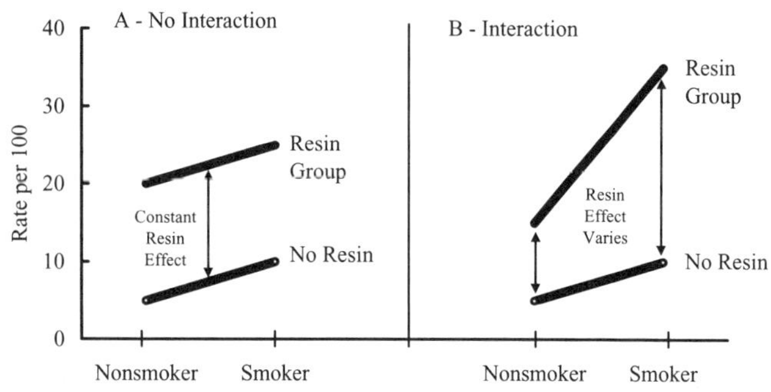

Figure 7.2 Using stratification to untangle the effects of smoking and resin exposures on the rate of respiratory disease. In *A*, both smoking and resin exposure each increase the rate of respiratory disease. The amount of increase because of resin exposure is the same (15 per 100) for smokers and for nonsmokers. The slopes of the two lines are parallel. When the effect is constant across the levels there is no interaction. In *B*, the amount of increase in the rate because of resin exposure depends on whether one is a nonsmoker or a smoker. The lines are not parallel and there is interaction between smoking and resin exposure. The graph of the interaction may appear as lines that funnel out as in *B* above, funnel in, or cross.

classifying cases or exposures is not foolproof, and there will be false negatives and false positives in almost every data set. The errors in classification can be systematic or random also. When the errors are systematic, the true rate ratio can be higher or lower than that actually measured. When classification errors are random, the association between the illness or injury and the risk factor will be weaker, and the rate ratio in the surveillance data will be closer to 1 than to the true value. Random, rather than systematic misclassification is often assumed to occur in surveillance data.

Other Biases

Other biases occur in surveillance data. The healthy worker effect is mentioned in Chapter 5. The reader is referred to introductory texts in epidemiology in Chapter 4 for a discussion of other kinds of biases.

Variation in Populations and Samples

As mentioned earlier, some error is random and can be caused by the natural variation in populations. Variation between individuals in age, sex, height, weight, blood pressure, etc. is an essential part of populations and is not created by surveillance or by a researcher. Measurements of disease and exposure in populations of workers have variation also. We rarely get to measure the entire working population, but can only take a sample of workers such as those present in a single workplace. The variation in the entire population will be present in a sample also. Averages based on a large number of observations vary less than those based on just a few observations. This variation often appears in a set fashion, such as the bell-shaped curve of the normal distribution (Fig. 4.4).

Every once in a while due to the luck of the draw, we might take two samples and observe that the two averages are so different, that, if we did not already know that the samples came from the same original population, we might think that they came from two different populations. Comparing rates in two groups with supposedly different levels of exposure or different levels of a risk factor is much like comparing two samples. Is it the natural variation reflected in the samples, or is exposure the reason why the rates are different? This is like inspecting a cluster of shots on a blank background and guessing whether there was one target or two targets set closely side by side.

When the difference in rates between groups appears to be very unlikely because of natural variation, scientists declare the difference "statistically significant." This indicates that the observed difference is not likely to have occurred by chance alone. It does not mean that the difference is important. A statistician asks, What is the chance of seeing a difference in rates of that size or bigger when comparing two samples taken from the same population? The *p* value used in the tables in several of the case study chapters of this book describes this probability. *P* values less than 5% are usually considered unlikely by health researchers.

Thus, a random variation in illness or injury rates can make two groups (samples) that are not really different appear different. However, when the difference between rates or an elevated rate ratio meets criteria for follow-up, a false-positive result occurs. Random variation in incidence rates can also make two groups that are really different appear the same. In this case our criteria for follow-up are not met, and we do not respond to the true situation.

Assessing random variation in rates is only one aspect of interpreting surveillance data. Certain situations such as SHE/Os merit follow-up whether statistical differences can be demonstrated or not. Small workplaces are at a statistical disadvantage. The lack of statistically significant results alone should not justify inaction. Several text books mentioned in Chapter 4 give more detailed discussions of concepts, such as statistical power, which apply to epidemiologic and surveillance data.

Management of Data Analysis

The analysis of surveillance data should follow a formal written plan or protocol. The analysis plan is a technical document for internal use of the surveillance organization. It should include an introduction or background; a statement of purpose and objectives; the method of data collection; data quality assurance and control program; case definition and a definition of variables from report forms and variables created in analysis; a prioritized list of proposed analyses; statistical tests, if applicable; and limitations of the data and analysis, and potential biases.

Because surveillance reports are issued in a standard format on a regular schedule, computer commands that execute the analysis should be written into batch files or standard queries. Batch files and saved queries provide written documentation. Interactive analysis can not always be documented and therefore not easily reproduced.

The overall time and resource budget for the analysis step should be in the range of 10%–25%. Most resources of surveillance should be spent on data collection, data quality, and follow-up. Unplanned and endlessly repeated statistical analyses that produce at least one statistically significant finding are called data dredging. It is a waste of resources and can be questioned on the grounds of intellectual honesty. One of the uses of surveillance is to generate hypothesis. This often arises as an unanticipated result during a formal, structured analysis rather than one that is improvised or contrived.

What one chooses to collect, analyze, and present reflects not only what data are available, but also what kind of story or message one wants to communicate. A mix of analyses that appeals to different audiences should be considered. A case vignette that tells the story of a real person carries greater emotional impact than columns of numbers that bespeak the same serious problem. Presentation and dissemination of surveillance data are explored in more detail in the next chapter.

REFERENCES

1. Centers for Disease Control. Fatalities attributed to entering manure waste pits—MN, 1992. *MMWR* 1993; 42:325–329.
2. Centers for Disease Control. Silicosis Deaths Among Young Adults—United States, 1968–1994. *MMWR* 1998; 47:331–335.
3. Centers for Disease Control. Carbon monoxide poisoning from use of gasoline-fueled power washers. *MMWR* 1995; 44:363–364.
4. Stroup D. Special analytic issues. In: Teutsch S, Churchill E, ed. *Principles and Practice of Public Health Surveillance*. New York: Oxford University Press, 1994:136–149.
5. Oleinick A, Guire KE, Hawthorne VM, Schork MA, Gluck JV, Lee B, La S. Current methods of estimating severity for occupational injuries and illnesses: data from the 1986 Michigan comprehensive compensable injury and illness database. *Am J Ind Med* 1993; 23:231–252.
6. Maizlish N. Designing prevention-oriented software for workplace health and safety. *Am J Ind Med* 1997; 31:64–74.
7. Sieber WK, Sundin DS, Frazier TM, Robinson C. Development, use, and availability of a job exposure matrix based on national occupational hazard survey data. *Am J Ind Med* 1991; 20:163–174.
8. Centers for Disease Control. Case definitions for infectious conditions under public health surveillance. *MMWR* 1997; 46 (RR10).

8

Feedback

NEIL A. MAIZLISH

STEP 11. GIVE FEEDBACK

The product of surveillance is information for action. Those who need the information include the individuals directly involved—workers, their health care providers and their employers—and organizations with an interest in surveillance findings. The actions themselves may be part of the responsibilities of the surveillance organization or of a different organization. The actions may be introduced at many points in the prevention pathway (Fig. 1.1) and are based on education, engineering, research, and enforcement. Occasionally, there are gaps in responsibilities and surveillance may bring this to the attention of policy makers. Depending on the design of the surveillance system, the feedback can be based on individual case reports or statistical analyses of cases and population data. The type of feedback is influenced by the type of health outcome (e.g., sentinel event) and whether active case follow-up is part of the surveillance system. In this chapter feedback is discussed broadly and includes not only dissemination of information, but also other possible actions.

One-On-One Feedback

Sentinel Event Surveillance

For state health agencies, sentinel event surveillance with active case follow-up provides opportunities for feedback with individual workers, their physicians, and their employers. These individuals are contacted by the surveillance organization after the case is diagnosed and reported, and the illness and exposures may still be in progress.

One of the objectives of individual case follow-up is to collect additional data and this can be combined with individual education. An illness that involves a group of individuals who know each other and work together can represent a *teachable moment*. People are naturally concerned and may be more receptive to educational messages and taking action.

The general health effects of exposure and the means for prevention can be discussed with sentinel cases and their employers if follow-up includes telephone or in-person interviews. Physicians who lack expertise in occupational medicine can benefit from telephone consultation or a referral to occupational medicine experts. Following telephone or in-person interviews, written educational materials can be provided to workers, employers, and physicians. This material should include a list of referrals to other organizations for additional information and services. Injured and ill workers may need information on how to contact the state workers' compensation agency, legal aid, rehabilitation consultants, the local OSHA office, and other service organizations. Attending physicians may need referrals to clinical consultation from experts located at university occupational health programs. In addition to their own workers' compensation carrier, some employers may need to contact an OSHA consultant or private consultants.

Data Providers

Feedback to data providers is an essential element in active reporting to surveillance systems. Feedback is facilitated when the data reporters are a well-defined group such as analytic laboratories reporting blood lead, or a sentinel network of medical specialists. These groups react positively to statistical summaries of their own cases, to those of the entire system, to reports of field investigations, press clippings, and other follow-up activities. Seeing that the information was used is an important ego-boost to reporters and helps maintain the flow and quality of reports.

Feedback should also be given to data reporters on their timeliness, coverage (e.g., each case diagnosed was reported), completeness and accuracy of information, and adherence to reporting guidelines. Reminders, retraining, and changes in reporting procedures may be necessary. If compliance is a problem, it is important to understand and document why providers do not report their cases.

Worker and Employer Notification

Government agencies that conduct active case follow-up, field investigations, and research have a responsibility to notify the affected worker and his or her employer.[1] Before workers and employers are notified, the surveillance system has to carefully consider:

- which workers will be notified
- how they benefit from medical referrals or screening
- who will perform the medical screening if it is recommended
- who will pay
- what kind of support services workers and their families may need (e.g., psychologic counseling)
- how workers will be protected from potential job discrimination due to their illnesses

Some occupational exposures like lead and pesticides can be brought home by the worker and expose family members. Therefore, some of the referrals may also include nonemployees. These concerns need to be taken into account before case follow-up is initiated and when protocols for follow-up are developed (Chapter 6, STEP 8). It takes great skill to carry out notification, which is often met with anger, frustration, depression, and denial.[2] These responses may be appropriate, overreactions, or underreactions.

Field Investigations

Field investigations are another type of feedback, but aimed at the worksite, rather than at individual cases. They are used to identify the specific operation, process, work practice, material, and deficient safety measure that led to the illness in a reported case. When the role of work in the illness has not yet been identified, a field investigation is appropriate, and may be structured like a research project. Hundreds of examples of health hazard investigations have been published by the National Institute for Occupational Health in the Health Hazard Evaluation (HHE) and Technical Assistance program[3] and by state health and labor departments.

Field investigations may be voluntary or compulsory. This depends on whether an enforcement agency is involved and whether a nonenforcement agency has access to the worksite. Some state and federal health agencies have the legal authority to carry out health investigations at individual worksites. Workers' compensation carriers may conduct investigations as part of their loss control services.

The structure of investigations are similar whether they are conducted by enforcement or other type of agency. Appropriate personnel and equipment need to be assembled prior to the investigation. Depending on the nature of the illness and potential exposure, the team of the investigators can include an industrial hygienist, ergonomist, safety engineer, physician or nurse, health educator, or industrial engineer or other specialist who may play a role in prevention. In work forces with a large percentage of non-English speaking employees, bilingual personnel or an interpreter may be necessary. Having coworkers or supervisors translate for the investigators may make some workers uncomfortable. If personal, medical, or potentially embarrassing information is being collected, it should be obtained in a private, confidential manner by the investigators. Chapter 6 discusses informed consent and other ethical issues faced by surveillance organizations.

The on-site part of the investigation usually begins with an opening conference with the investigators, management, worker representatives. Sometimes employers' health care professionals or workers' compensation representatives attend. The investigators explain the purpose and the events leading up to the investigation and describe the procedures used by the investigators (review of records, interviews of workers and management employees, medical tests, air measurements, etc.). This is followed by directly observing and taking measurements in the workplace.

In sentinel event surveillance, the observations usually start at the workstation of the sentinel case. Depending on the scope of the investigation, other work areas with similar hazards or ill coworkers may be included. When the causes of the illness are not readily identifiable, medical tests, health surveys, exposure measurements might be taken of the entire plant to identify high-risk groups.

At the conclusion of the worksite visit, a closing conference is held with management and worker representatives. The closing conference gives feedback on items that require immediate attention or can be solved with relatively little effort (quick fixes), confirms issues that management was already aware of, and identifies new or unresolved concerns. Some field investigations require an analysis of data by the investigators, which may take several days or weeks. The product of the field investigation is a written report with recommendations. Sometimes, a draft report is presented to management and worker representatives for comment before a final report is issued.

The focus of the field investigations will differ depending on whether the investigation is done by an enforcement agency, private consultants, workers' compensation carrier, a public health agency, university, or the employers' own health and safety staff, if present. Each has a different mission, which will change the emphasis of the investigation. Enforcement agencies will pay more attention to potential violations of existing standards. Public health agencies may include health and safety conditions that are not addressed by laws, but may be important elements of prevention. Appendix H is an example of a public-health oriented field investigation carried out by a state health department in response to sentinel cases of carpal tunnel syndrome at an individual workplace.

Research

An objective of surveillance is to identify high-risk groups and potential causes of workplace injury and illness. When the causes of the health problem cannot be easily identified in the high-risk groups, epidemiologic research is one of the responses. Research projects are specifically designed to collect data of greater detail than that available through surveillance. Data of greater detail may shed light on the specific agents responsible for the health outcome. For example, mortality surveillance in several states has found that certain construction industry trades have higher risks of lung cancer than other trades do.[4,5] One hypothesis is that construction materials that contain asbestosis are responsible. Research may then examine lung cancer and asbestos exposures in specific occupations such as insulation workers, pipe trades workers, or demolition workers.

Research projects also can overcome some of the limitations in surveillance. Research can examine health effects and exposures that fall below the thresholds for reporting to surveillance systems. This includes the warning signs of occupational disease based on symptoms or other early effects. In research, the definition of the health outcome and exposures can be more precise, thus reducing misclassification bias. Researchers can make a systematic effort to identify all the cases, thus reducing bias due to underreporting. By selecting comparison groups, research may be able to minimize the effects of confounding. The methods used in occupational epidemiologic research are reviewed in text books listed at the end of Chapter 4.

Communication of Information

Getting information to those with a need to know is an essential function of surveillance. The traditional approach of many governmental surveillance organizations has been based on dissemination of information, in which there is a one-way flow from surveillance organization to a target audience. Many public health experts consider true communication of surveillance information to be a two-way exchange that should follow the accepted practices in the field of communications:

- establish the message
- define the audience
- select the channel and time slot
- market the information
- evaluate the impact[6]

Establishing the message answers the question "What should be said?" The messages should reflect the objectives and purposes of the surveillance system. Changes in the magnitude of the problem, high-risk groups, time and geographic trends, and the detection of new illnesses or exposures will be among the possible messages. The analysis and interpretation of surveillance data will provide the specific content for establishing the message and the target audience. For example, a finding that teenage workers in fast-food restaurants have a high incidence of burns, identifies the problem, a high-risk group, and the industry to where the message should be directed.

Define the audience addresses "To whom should it be said?" There are usually several different audiences with an interest in surveillance findings. Within a workplace there are workers, supervisors, management, unions, health care providers, and a workers' compensation carrier. In government surveillance programs, the target audience includes several different government agencies, employer organizations and trade associations, unions, health professionals, industrial hygiene and safety organizations, academic research and training centers, workers' compensation insurers, managed care organizations, lawmakers, government agencies, and the public or press. Many organizations operate at the local, state, and federal level; therefore, the scope of feedback may be narrow or broad.

Some government surveillance systems consider feedback in their design by seeking out advisors or establishing an advisory board made up of members of the target audience (see Chapter 2, STEP 2. Gaining Support). This is useful in building long-term relationships with groups who also play a role in implementing recommendations.

Select the channel answers "Through what communication medium?" Once the audience and message are chosen, it is easier to select an appropriate channel.

Most employers will use print (memos) and in-person meetings. Government surveillance organizations will also use electronic and mass media. Print communication is most familiar and includes memos, newsletters, special alerts or bulletins, reports, and scientific publications. Electronic communication includes the Internet, fax, and telephone or video conferences. Mass media include news releases and news conferences. In-person meetings can be small group briefings, news conferences, legislative hearings, or regularly scheduled meetings of professional associations. The demographic characteristics of cases may provide insight into how to frame the message and what media to deliver it. For example, providing written materials at a high school reading level may not be effective if most of the intended audience stopped formal education at the fifth grade. However, radio programs may be extremely effective if the target audience listens to the radio while working.

Marketing the information addresses "How should the message be stated?" Marketing of information is more than dissemination. Much thought is necessary to tailor the message to each targeted audience. Successful marketing requires focusing the overriding message rather that presenting detail that might be overwhelming. Marketing anticipates what is likely to capture the interest of the audience. Graphical presentations are more appealing than tables. For some audiences, the information needs to be personalized rather than statistical. Information in a case narrative may help focus the message. The timing and method of release of surveillance information may be crucial.

Evaluating the impact answers "What effect did the message create?" Two key aspects of evaluation are whether the message was communicated to those with a need to know and whether the information had a positive effect on the problem.

A written plan for communicating surveillance findings may help organize feedback and be part of the overall description of the surveillance system.

Broadening the Impact of Surveillance

To be effective, surveillance systems should examine ways to maximize their impact.

Sentinel Event Notification

As a part of sentinel event surveillance, findings at one workplace can be extended to others with similar exposures by notifying individual establishments, their trade association, and their unions. This approach can be highly successful when the there are a limited number of easily identifiable establishments, the health condition is serious, the exposure is specific, and control measures are readily available. For example, local and state health departments in collaboration with the National Institute for Occupational Safety and Health received several reports of carbon monoxide exposures in operators of gas-powered machines used to resurface the ice of indoor ice rinks.[7] The Colorado Health Department contacted ice rink owners and the manufactures of this specialized type of equipment. The owners, manufacturers, and government worked together to educate individual ice rink operators on how to control this type of exposure.

Program Planning and Economic Analysis

Surveillance data can be an important input to program planning (next chapter) and the economic analysis of alternative strategies for controlling exposures. At the employer level, some problems raised by surveillance data are not solved by a quick fix and require a formal analysis. Appendix F discusses surveillance data and economic analysis in occupational safety and health. It also gives an example of how an individual employer can measure the costs and benefits of an intervention using rate-based surveillance data.

Intervention Programs

Surveillance data on high risk groups are used by government agencies to target prevention and enforcement, and to identify areas that need additional research funding, policy development, and legislation. Several states have special emphasis programs to reduce injury and illness in high-risk industries such as construction, manufacturing, agriculture, mining, forestry, meatpacking, small establishments, and other groups such as working adolescents and immigrant workers.

Some sentinel event surveillance systems increase workers' access to clinical and preventive services through individual case follow-up. This one-on-one approach is overwhelmed by problems that are widespread. It is also reactive and may miss many cases because of underreporting. Broader-based interventions that emphasize primary prevention—controlling exposures at their source—are the long-term solution. Surveillance can be used to target such intervention programs. In addition to controlling exposures, some intervention programs can channel previously unreported cases back into the surveillance system. The intervention program benefits by having a mechanism for its evaluation. The surveillance system improves because previously unreported cases are captured. This helps meet surveillance objectives by providing a more accurate estimate of the magnitude of the problem, trends, and high-risk groups. This linkage between surveillance and intervention—closing the loop—is highlighted in Chapter 25.

REFERENCES

1. Schulte PA, Boal WL, Friedland JM, Walker JT, Connally LB, Mazzuckelli LF, Fine LJ. Methodologic issues in risk communications to workers. *Am J Ind Med* 1993; 23:3–9.
2. Boal WL, Friedland J, Schulte PA. Workers' response to risk notification. *Am J Ind Med* 1995; 27:471–483.
3. National Institute for Occupational Safety and Health. *Health Hazard Evaluations, Final Reports, 1990–1996*. Cincinnati, OH: National Institute for Occupational Safety and Health, DHHS (NIOSH) Publ. No. 97-144 (CD ROM), 1997.
4. Dubrow R, Sestito JP, Lalich NR, Burnett CA, Salg J. Death certificate-based occupational mortality surveillance in the United States. *Am J Ind Med* 1987; 11:329–342.
5. Dubrow R, Wegman D. *Occupational Characteristics of White Male Cancer Victims in Massachusetts, 1971–1973*. Springfield VA: National Technical Information Center, NIOSH Publ. No. 84-109 (PB-85-218-683/E09), 1984.
6. Goodman RA, Remington PL, Howard R. Communicating information for action. In: Teutsch SM, Churchill R, ed. *Principles and Practice of Public Health Surveillance*. New York: Oxford University Press, 1994:150–157.
7. Centers for Disease Control. Carbon monoxide exposures at an ice skating rink–Colorado. *MMWR* 1986;35:435–436.

9

Evaluation and Planning

NEIL A. MAIZLISH

STEP 12. EVALUATE THE IMPACT AND FUNCTIONING OF THE SURVEILLANCE SYSTEM

Surveillance must be evaluated to identify strengths, weaknesses, and areas for improvement. Much has been written about program evaluation. The purpose of this chapter is not to review the extensive literature, but to offer a few practical tools.

Evaluation is sometimes left until the end of a project, when participants are completing deadlines and are exhausted. This reflects the notion that planning, implementation, and evaluation are three separate sequential stages, rather than a continuous process repeated many times over the life of a project. The evaluation of any project has roots in the planning process. Data for evaluation may be lost forever if it is not anticipated at the planning stage and saved the moment it is generated.

There are two basic types of evaluation. The first is impact or effectiveness evaluation. This addresses the question "Is the program having the impact it is supposed to?" The second type of evaluation is process or efficiency evaluation. This addresses a narrower but important question of "Are the processes internal to the program appropriate and using resources efficiently?" A bird that flaps its wings at the prescribed beats per minute (efficiency), may never get off the ground (effectiveness). Likewise, an occupational health and safety program may not decrease the incidence and severity of workplace injuries and illness (effectiveness) despite the fact that 100% of workers viewed a safety video (efficiency).

To avoid a disconnect between impacts and processes it is very important to define the problem and analyze its causes. The problem may be defined in terms of objectives of a surveillance system such as "because occupational pesticide poisoning is underreported, we cannot estimate the magnitude of the problem." Or, the problem may be defined in terms of the goals of a prevention program (e.g., to reduce the incidence of pesticide illness) in which a surveillance system or surveillance data plays a role.

The first part of this chapter highlights planning and evaluation in this broader sense and is oriented to injuries and diseases with causes that are well established (SHE/Os and workplace injuries). The presentation points out links to surveillance. The second part is aimed at the evaluation of surveillance systems. The evaluation techniques described below can be conducted by many different types of organizations from an individual employer to a national government agency.

THE ROLE OF SURVEILLANCE IN PLANNING AND EVALUATION

Figure 9.1 shows a multistep model for planning and evaluation of public health programs.[1] Planning and evaluation start with goals (Step 1.0, Fig. 9.1), which are usually expressed in general terms: to control or eliminate the exposures that cause occupational health and safety problems. Planning and evaluation begin with straightforward questions:

- Where am I?
- Where do I want to be in the future?
- How do I get there?
- Am I doing things right?
- Am I doing the right things?
- How do I know I'm getting there?

Surveillance plays a critical role in answering the question "Where am I?" Surveillance data reveal the mag-

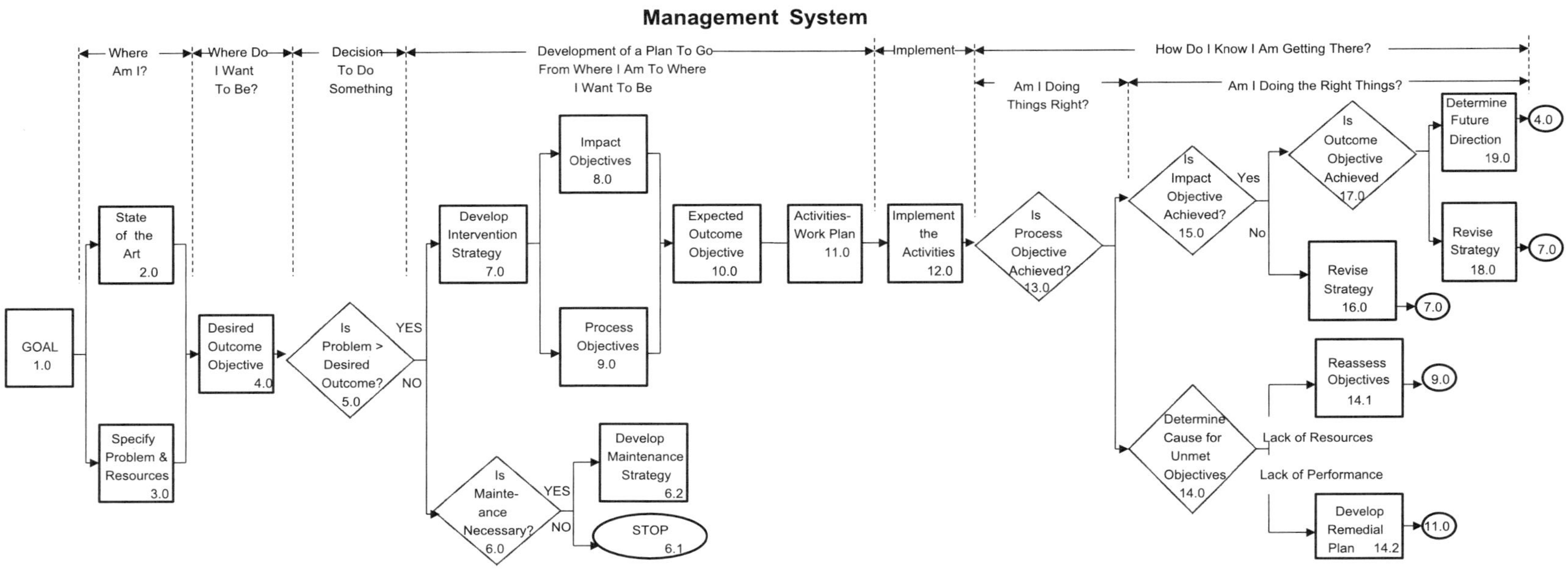

Figure 9.1 Management system for program planning and evaluation. (Centers for Disease Control.[1])

nitude of pressing health problems (Step 3.0, Fig. 9.1), in terms of their incidence, prevalence, or severity, and the population groups that are bearing the greatest burden. "Where am I?" also requires knowledge about the established causes of the problem and the solutions. This includes the state of the art (Step 2.0, Fig. 9.1) for exposure control strategies, medical treatment, and disability management. To identify the most feasible solution, one evaluates the stage of technical development of possible solutions, their effectiveness, and their costs. Lastly, to answer "Where am I?" one must make an inventory of the resources available within the program, such as personnel, equipment, travel, supplies, consultants, and resources that might be shared or available from others (Step 3.0, Fig. 9.1).

"Where do I want to be?" restates the problem as a desired outcome objective (Step 4.0, Fig. 9.1) such as a diminished level of injury, illness, or exposure in the population. "Where am I now?" may be 15 injuries per 100 full-time workers. "Where do I want to be?" in 3 years may be 7.5 injuries per 100. The outcome objective is the problem envisioned at a future point in time after an intervention. Unless the problem has already been solved (Step 5.0, Fig. 9.1), and needs maintenance (Step 6.0), a decision must be made to develop an intervention strategy (Step 7.0). A coherent intervention strategy develops specific objectives from a thorough analysis of the problem, its determinants, and its contributing factors (Fig. 9.2).

CAUSAL WEBS FOR PLANNING AND EVALUATION

Causal webs are a useful way to understand how workers interact with the work environment. While it is sometimes useful to focus on the last item in a chain of events, most injuries and illnesses at work are the result of a chain of events or multiple factors. By repeatedly asking "Why did this happen?" or "What are the contributing factors?" one can create a detailed model to explain what happened and possible modes of prevention. As one threads backwards, ignorance and inadequate training, supervision, lack of availability of safer tools, materials, processes, work practices, product designs, policies and procedures, work organization, organizational culture, societal attitudes, presence or absence of positive or negative economic incentives, lack of standards, laws and regulations, national and international economic policies all play some role. If the organizational environment permits, it is recommended highly that the surveillance team or health and safety committee construct such models in a group exercise in which everyone expresses their views of the problem.

Figure 9.3 shows a very simple cause and effect model of lead poisoning at a hypothetical battery plant. The problem should be stated as specifically as possible, and ideally as a measurable quantity. For example, there is a high prevalence—15 cases per 100 FTEs—of elevated blood lead, defined as workers with blood lead levels over 40 μg/dL. The primary determinants are:

- environmental lead exposures are too high
- medical care is not aimed at prevention and treatment is inadequate, perhaps because physicians do not recognize the diagnosis

Two (among the many) contributing factors are:

- established risk factors are not being recognized by supervisors and workers
- available control technology is not being used

The lack of training contributes to not recognizing the established risk factors. Lack of awareness contributes

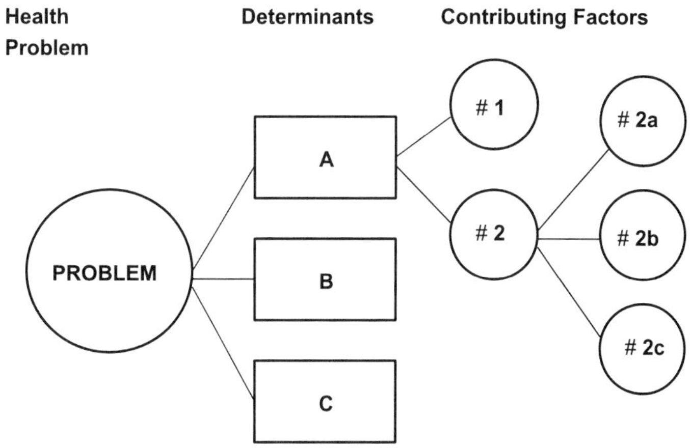

Figure 9.2 Generic causal web made up of the problem, determinants of the problem, and contributing factors. (Centers for Disease Control.[1])

to employers not using existing control technology. This process can be repeated for the contributing factors themselves, creating detailed causal webs.

The branches of the causal web must be examined carefully to identify determinants and contributing factors that:

- are strong and prevalent in the population of interest
- you have direct control over
- are shared responsibilities with others within your organization so that you can involve them in planning
- are responsibilities of others outside your organization so that you can explore possibilities working with them
- require policy development, legislative action, technical knowledge and expertise, or basic research

Ideally, planning should be organized around activities that change contributing factors that: one controls directly, are linked to strong determinants of the health problem, and have readily available solutions.

A balanced strategy will also identify tasks and participants beyond the usual work group. These are potential target audiences to whom surveillance findings must be marketed. It may be necessary to develop allies within and outside of your organization to promote prevention goals. If the model is valid, altering the contributing factors alters the determinants, which in turn, diminishes the health problem.

The objectives used in planning and evaluation are rephrased from the contributing factors and determinants themselves. Impact objectives (Step 8.0, Fig. 9.1) state the future level of a determinant, such as 30% reduction in lead exposure (Fig. 9.3). One generally cannot alter the level of determinants directly, but must create a process that acts on the contributing factors by selecting appropriate activities in a work plan (11.0). Process objectives (Step 9.0, Fig. 9.1) state the future level of a contributing factor (Fig. 9.4). If the contributing factor is lack of recognition of risk factors of lead poisoning, a process objective is for 100% of workers and supervisors in lead-using departments to recognize these risk factors. Training is an activity that uses program resources to meet this objective. Evaluation that merely counts the number of workers attending a training is not a measure of this objective. The knowledge of risk factors needs to be measured pre- and posttraining. Although this may not be easy, this is the appropriate objective to measure. Given limited resources one may need to scope up or down the activities and objectives to determine whether the desired outcome objective is really possible, and whether the expected outcome (Step 10.0, Fig. 9.1) is still worthwhile. Perhaps, 7.5 cases per 100 FTEs, a 50% reduction from baseline, is not realistic, but 10 cases per 100 (a 33% reduction) is a reasonable projection.

If the process objective is not being met (Step 13.0, Fig. 9.1), one must ask "Am I doing things right?" Is the objective not being met because there is a lack of effort, poor quality of work, inappropriate methods, or insufficient resources? For example, if workers still do not recognize hazards after training sessions, one must ask whether the training program was done correctly. Was the trainer qualified? Was the basic design useful? For a manager, the corrective actions for "not doing things right" are motivate, hire, train, supervise, discipline, get more resources, and select appropriate work methods.

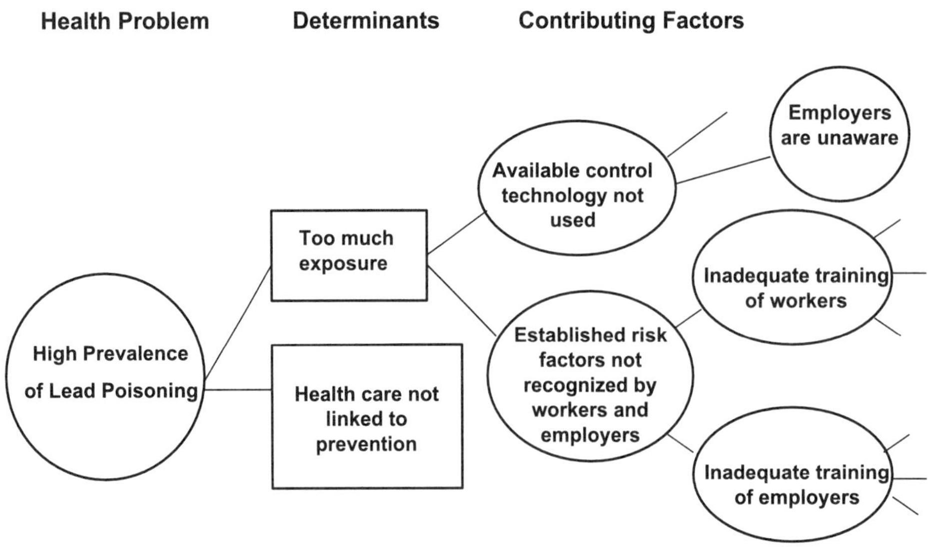

Figure 9.3 The problem of occupational lead poisoning using causal webs to analyze the problem. (Adapted from Centers for Disease Control.[1])

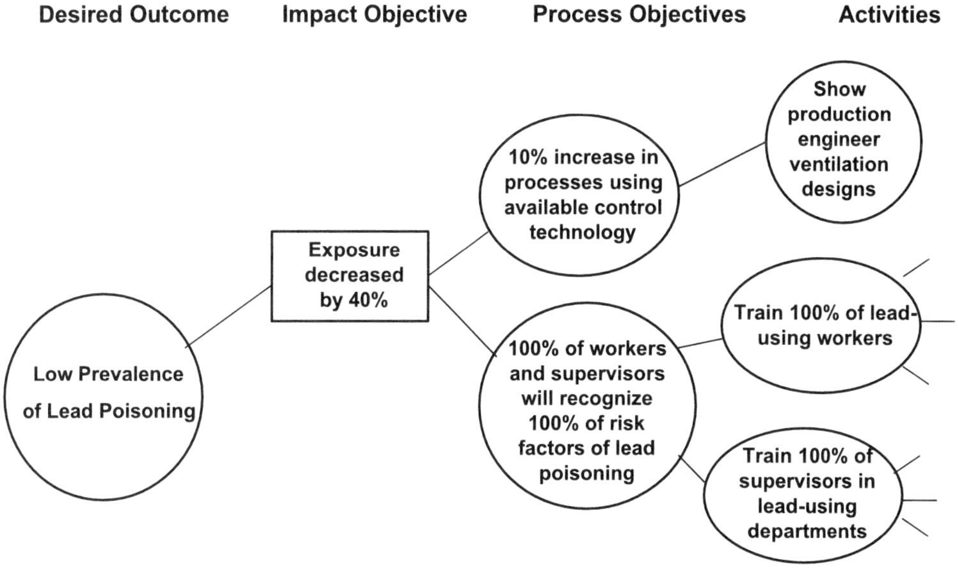

Figure 9.4 Objectives for planning and evaluation are based on changing determinants and contributing factors. The desired outcome is lowering the level of a problem. Impact objectives are a future level of a determinant. Process objectives are a future level of a contributing factor. The model assumes that a cascade of changes in contributing factors and determinants lowers the problem. (Adapted from Centers for Disease Control.[1])

If process objectives are met, but impact objectives are not, the organization may not be "doing the right things." No amount of praising or exhorting workers to do their job, or getting more resources is likely to change this situation, because the cause-effect model is incomplete or incorrect. It is a manager's job to distinguish between "doing things right" and "doing the right things." This requires reevaluation of the model to see where determinants or contributing factors may have been left out, or misstated. For example, if supervisors encourage workers to take shortcuts that increase production, but are unsafe, recognizing the risk factors may not change the determinant (too much exposure). If this was not taken into account in the original model, then production incentives of supervisors and their contributing factors need to be included in the model.

The causes of injury and illness must be changed before the impact is felt, and, one usually observes changes in the process objectives before the impact objectives or the outcome objective. In large-scale public health programs, the expected time frame to evaluate process objectives is usually several months to 1 year; impact objectives, 1–3 years, and the outcome objective even longer. Along this time frame, evaluation should be carried out by comparing the objectives put forth in the planning stage with the real situation. Data collection to measure these objectives should be planned in advance and may come from surveillance.

Causal models, such as Figure 9.5, can be developed that provide detail and insight. The lack of a surveillance system itself is a determinant of many occupational health problems because injuries and illness occur and there is no feedback to those responsible for taking corrective action and additional workers are harmed. Ignorance, apathy, and the lack of priority are also contributing factors. This impacts workers, supervisors, management, unions, business associations, insurers, suppliers, product designers, enforcement personnel, and legislators.

EVALUATION OF SURVEILLANCE SYSTEMS

The traditional framework for evaluating surveillance systems was advanced by Klauke and coworkers at the Centers for Disease Control.[2] This framework can be applied to occupational health surveillance systems, though few have been formally evaluated.[3,4] The first question is "Should a particular health event be under surveillance?" Second, if so, "How useful and efficient is a surveillance system in absolute terms and compared to alternate designs?"

The first question is external to the surveillance system and applies to starting up a new surveillance system or the continuation of an existing one. The question is usually answered by ranking the health event under surveillance among priorities. The criteria used to set priorities include the magnitude of the problem (expressed as incidence or prevalence of the injury, illness, or exposure), severity, economic costs, and feasibility of prevention. Sometimes the estimates of the magnitude of the problem are drawn from poorly func-

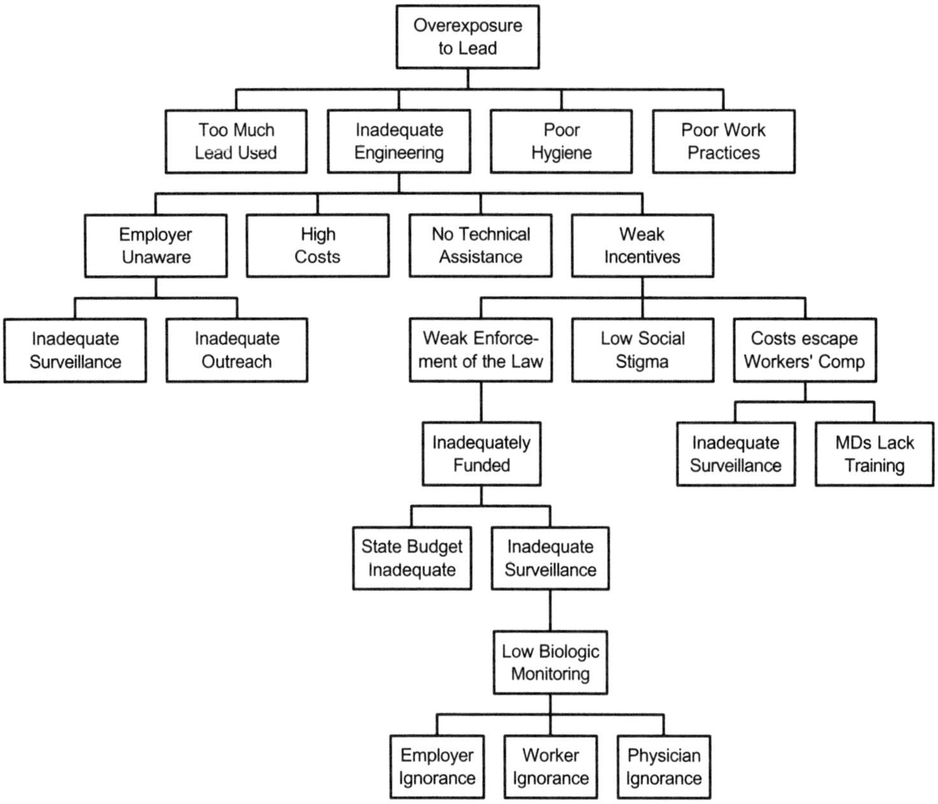

Figure 9.5 Part of a causal web that analyzes the determinants and contributing factors to occupational lead poisoning. The lack of surveillance and the lack of dissemination of surveillance data are contributing factors.

tioning surveillance systems. The decision not to develop a surveillance system then feeds a circular argument: occupational health conditions are not a priority because so few cases are apparent. Legal requirements also influence the health conditions potentially under surveillance. At individual workplaces, employers are legally required to control recognized hazards and collect certain kinds of health data. As pointed out in Chapter 1, surveillance systems for employers can be based on a foundation of existing data.

To answer the second question of usefulness and efficiency, the operation of the system must be evaluated against its goals and objectives. A good written description of the operation of the system is essential to evaluation. Moreover, evaluation will be significantly streamlined if all the relevant materials are compiled in a written system manual that addresses the points in the following section.

Objectives

Goals and Scope

- Are the goals and objectives clearly stated?
- Are the outcomes clearly stated? (e.g., exposure, cases, disability, health services, mortality, etc.)
- Is the objective to:
  - measure the magnitude of the problem?
  - detect trends in cases or rates in time, pre-postintervention, geographic area?
  - identify high-risk groups?
  - link cases to specific worksites or work areas in real time?
- Is the approach case-based or population-based or both? Are employment and population data available?
- Are there multiple outcomes, or is a single condition or sentinel event under surveillance?
- Is the condition geographically or otherwise targeted?
- Will the surveillance organization play an active or passive role in promoting reporting and follow-up?

System Operation

Support

- Does the surveillance activity have organizational support from
  - upper management?
  - middle management, health and safety committee, department heads, unions, and workers?

- What support was sought?
  - permission to carry out surveillance as an official activity?
  - access to information in various organizational units?
  - access to individual workers, supervisors, and records?
  - material support and resources?
- Was the support periodically renewed, and what were the methods to maintain support?
- What do the participants in the workplace or community say they know and feel about the project?

Multidisciplinary Team

- What are the skills needed to carry out the surveillance project? Are they consistent with the objectives?
- Does the surveillance team have these skills?
- How is the surveillance team organized? How do the surveillance functions fit within the structure of the organization?
- Who on the surveillance team carries out data collection, analysis, interpretation, and feedback?
- Are the responsibilities and authority of each team member clear?

Case Definition and Minimum Data Set

- What is the written definition of a case?
- What are the data elements and their sources that are needed to define or confirm a case?
- Who will define the case: the case reporter or the surveillance team?
- How long does it take to classify a case? Is it reproducible?
- What percentage of reports do not meet the case definition (positive predictive value, or false positive rate)?
- How are reporting guidelines defined?
- How are the guidelines for reporting communicated to the reporters?

Flow of Information

- What is the flow of information in the surveillance system? From whom to whom?
- Are the time steps between reporters stated clearly? Is the actual performance measured? Is there feedback to reporters on their performances?
- What does the system flow diagram look like?

Mechanism of Reporting

- What are the mechanisms for reporting? Telephone, fax, written forms, mail, electronic?
- Do the reporters think the mechanisms are acceptable, or too time consuming or complex?
- What steps are made to facilitate and promote reporting?
- What are the policies of the workplace that put barriers on the reporting of cases?

Selecting, Recruiting, and Training reporters

- How were the case reporters selected? Self-selected, probability sample, other?
- What training do case reporters have to recognize occupational injury and illness?
- What training do case reporters have in the procedures of the surveillance system?

Protocols for Follow-up

- What are the follow-up activities and are they consistent with the objectives?
- How are priorities for follow-up established?
  - Characteristics of individual cases: clinical severity, days lost or disability, treatment setting?
  - Case clustering, mini-epidemics?
  - Epidemiologic measures of rates such as rate ratios or attributable cases?
- What is the flow diagram for follow-up?

Data Collection and Coding

- Is the case report easily key entered? Are there tools for searching for preexisting entries or duplicates, coding by pick lists? Can rekeying be eliminated by electronic data interchange?
- Are there data collected that are never used or key entered?
- What text fields require coding? Who will do the coding? What level of detail is needed? For hierarchical classifications (ICD, SIC, SOC, etc.) what is the appropriate level of aggregation? What is the skill level needed for coders?
- What is the structure of the database? Is the database relational?
- Is there a data quality control program? Are there standards, training, supervision, a method to sample and compare source documents to the database for accuracy and validity?
- Is there a data security program to prevent unauthorized access to confidential information. Is there appropriate archiving, storage, and back-up?

Manage Cases

- What is the scope of case follow-up—medical care, primary prevention, disability management?
- Are take-home exposures considered?
- Who is responsible for notification of the worker, health care provider, others within the company, health officials, OSHA, or NIOSH?

Analysis

- Is there a written data analysis protocol that describes the types of analyses, the time period of analyses, outcomes, and stratification variables?
- Are the analyses documented and reproducible?
- Do the analyses reflect the objectives and show magnitude, severity, high-risk groups, clusters, or trends?
- Are the results of analyses used in setting priorities?
- Are the results of analyses written up and presented in useful ways?

Feedback

- Did those who were asked to support the surveillance system receive updates, results, recommendations, and other information?
- What is the message or content of the dissemination? Does it reflect the key findings of the analysis?
- Who is the target audience and have the messages been tailored to their organizational needs, educational background, and time constraints?
- What are the channels for communicating the message?
- How is the message marketed?
- Is the information available in a timely way for decision-making?
- Are the recommendations made by the surveillance system followed up? If not, why?
- What are the actions taken by those who receive or use surveillance data (investigations, research, interventions)?
- Does the surveillance system contribute to taking and evaluating interventions? If not, why?
- Are surveillance data used in program planning and evaluation and economic analyses of potential interventions?
- Are surveillance activities contributing to lowering the number or rate of injuries, illness, or deaths?

In addition to these points, Klauke et al.[4] also point out several issues that relate to the validity and biases in surveillance data. First is whether the surveillance system captures all the true cases. This is the sensitivity (Chapter 3). If the only goal is to estimate the magnitude of the problem and most cases escape the surveillance system, one needs to question whether the surveillance system should exist or identify ways it can be improved. Perhaps a periodic prevalence survey is more suited to answer the question. Nonetheless, if the percentage of cases that are captured remains reasonably constant over time, one can still observe trends even if the absolute magnitude is underestimated.

Second is whether the characteristics of the reported cases differ from those of the cases not reported. This is called representativeness. For example, compared to the cases not in the surveillance system, how do the reported cases differ by case severity, age, sex, race, ethnicity, education, occupation, or industry? Unless these are measured in the population eligible for surveillance, it may not be possible to assess representativeness.

Costs and Cost-Benefit of Surveillance Systems

Cost is another important element in the evaluation of surveillance systems. Traditional accounting models are useful for describing costs in the categories of personnel, equipment, travel, supplies, consulting, and administration. The fixed or one-time costs are related to establishing and maintaining the infrastructure: defining the scope and purpose and developing protocols (case reporting, prioritizing case follow-up, statistical analysis, dissemination), supervision of data collection, and data quality. Certain aspects of statistical analysis, report writing, dissemination and communication of results can reuse templates. Most statistical analyses can be performed using batch commands or saved queries. Some fixed costs are not limiting. For example, with a single desktop computer and public domain statistical software, simple descriptive statistical analyses of hundreds of thousands of cases can be accomplished within minutes.[5,6] The variable costs associated with surveillance are related to the number of outcomes under surveillance, whether case follow-up is an objective, and whether the relevant data are already collected and automated.

Costs of surveillance systems can vary significantly during the development and maintenance phases. Many significant costs will be borne primarily in the first years such as development of protocols, design of databases, analysis programs, and report templates. During the development phase, output may be relatively low, but this preparation avoids costly errors and additional costs in subsequent years. Costs will also vary depending on the scope and the objectives. Passive reporting systems that process large numbers of cases with few data elements may not provide much insight on prevention activities, even if their cost per case is low. Case follow-up is a labor intensive task. However, the specificity of the information may allow very accurate and timely targeting of interventions that may diminish the severity of existing cases and prevent additional cases. While the cost of the intervention may not be part of the surveillance system, the benefits (less severe and averted cases) may be ascribed fairly to the surveillance system.

Within a given surveillance system, cost may also be

evaluated from the standpoint of how resources are internally allocated. What percentage of the budget is spent on seeking and maintaining support, case reporting, gathering data for case confirmation, database maintenance, case follow-up and management, analysis, report writing, dissemination, etc.? This information may help prioritize areas within the surveillance system. The cost implications of expanding or narrowing the objectives also should be included in the evaluation.

ACKNOWLEDGMENTS

Dr. Edward Baker and Mr. Joseph Webb, Public Health Prevention Practice Office, Centers for Disease Control and Prevention, are gratefully acknowledged for providing technical assistance in planning and evaluation techniques.

REFERENCES

1. Centers for Disease Control. *Program Management: A Guide for Improving Program Decisions.* Atlanta, GA: US Department of Health and Human Services, 1987.
2. Klauke DN, Buehler JW, Thacker SB, Parrish RG, Trowbridge FL, Berkelman RL. Guidelines for the evaluation of surveillance systems. Centers for Disease Control. *MMWR* 1988; 37 (Suppl. No. S-5).
3. Geidenberger C, Nestel G, Soce EM, Gromen K. Evaluation of a public health program: Silicosis surveillance and prevention in Ohio, 1989–1995. *Am J Epidemiol* 1998; S28.
4. Rosenman DK. What is the most cost-effective way to identify silica problem worksites? *Am J Ind Med* 1999; 35:434–435.
5. Dean AG, Dean JA, Coulombier D, et al. *Epi Info, Version 6: A Word Processing, Database, and Statistics Program for Epidemiology on Microcomputers.* Atlanta, GA: Centers for Disease Control and Prevention, 1994.
6. Maizlish N. Designing prevention-oriented software for workplace health and safety. *Am J Ind Med* 1997; 31:64–74.

10

Surveillance and the Design of Occupational Health Information Systems

NEIL A. MAIZLISH

Occupational health and safety stands at a crossroads of the information highway. Decision-making based on data is becoming more commonplace due to several recent developments in information technology and health services organization.

Electronic commerce and the Internet are becoming a routine part of business practice. The American National Standards Institute has produced drafts for an electronic health insurance claim form,[1,2] which is likely to evolve into the national standard for U.S. government payors.[3] Motivated by the year 2000 transition, large businesses reengineered their business processes and updated their information systems. They are now in a better position to integrate health and safety, loss control, health benefits, workers' compensation, short-term and long-term disability, compliance with the Americans with Disabilities Act (ADA), and employee assistance programs.

Unfettered growth of computer and communications technologies is increasing processing power and mass storage at lower unit costs. Multiuser, networked, relational databases for microcomputers and midrange computers are capable of tasks that could be achieved with mainframes only a few years ago. Open architecture now enables different databases, formerly incompatible by virtue of different operating systems and hardware, to communicate seamlessly.

Managed care is gaining momentum in the delivery of workers' compensation medical care.[4] Many of its processes are data intensive: enrollment, utilization management, network selection based on provider profiling, the setting of capitation or case rates, evaluating health outcome measures of quality or performance, patient satisfaction, and the synthesis of several of these measures into consumer report cards.

This information revolution offers many potential benefits. Reducing costs and increasing efficiency of bill payment and claims management have been the primary focus. This chapter presents issues that users and information specialists should consider to enhance their information systems for surveillance and prevention. The term information system is used in this chapter for data collection that a business or government does on its work injuries and illness, rather than information retrieval from electronic libraries or databases such as Medline or the Registry of Toxic Effects of Chemical Substances (RTECS).

CONCEPTUAL FOUNDATION

Information systems are not just the hardware and software for networked relational databases of daily business transactions. Information systems should be viewed broadly as all of the data collection strategies and the knowledge they impart to an organization.

Surveillance and information systems overlap greatly in function, but information systems often deal with a broader range of questions and often have nonroutine components such as research.

Until recently, government agencies and businesses that collected a vast amount of business transactions did not have integrated platforms, affordable mass storage, and analytical capacity to examine statistical patterns in their data. These patterns guide management decisions for priority setting, planning, and evaluation. Decision support is becoming an integral component of business software applications. There are commercial off-the-shelf (COTS) products as well as in-house custom applications. Health and safety managers need to have a basic understanding of these tools, and to assure that they are applied for decision-support in occupational health and safety. The principles of epidemiologic surveillance are the basis for decision-support (Chapters 4 and 5).

Information systems are useful decision-support tools to the extent they answer key questions. From the many possible questions, there is a routine subset that should be anticipated for surveillance purposes. The following are broadly applicable to most workplaces and workers' compensation systems.

- What are the problems? Who has the problem?
- What is the magnitude of each problem?
- What is the severity?
- What are the costs?
- How effective are the persons (or organization) responsible at solving the problem(s)?
- How long does it take to solve the problem(s)?
- How efficient is the management of resources?

Many managers and policy makers assume that the data they need to answer these questions is a byproduct of routine business transactions; and, that they need only tweak a database to get the answer. Rarely is it so simple.

USER INVOLVEMENT AND THE KEY QUESTIONS

Many information systems do not meet user's expectations and some fail outright. Sometimes the failure is because the design is focused narrowly on one particular requirement. Several distinct, but similar requirements spawn different forms, computer systems, and management structures. This is common in many businesses. In occupational health and safety one sees OSHA reporting done by one department, workers' compensation by another, and group health and disability by yet a third. Tremendous redundancy arises because data cannot be shared by different departments. Sometimes contractual arrangements do not consider sharing data with outside organizations such as a workers' compensation carrier or health insurer.

Rather than conceiving the problem as not having computers or automating an existing form, one needs to step back and analyze the basic problem (Chapter 9). Sometimes users themselves do not know or agree as to what information they need to meet process or impact objectives (Chapter 9). Before coming to the design table, users must know what they want and why.

The lack of meaningful user involvement in the design process is another common problem. Communication between information technology (IT) specialists and users is often difficult because of differences in vocabulary and culture. Information technology staff may not fully understand the business needs, and users generally do not fully understand the technical requirements. This gap can be irreconcilable if some of the participants do not have a boundary spanning role; that is, capable of doing the simultaneous translation of business needs and technical detail. It is ideal to have a multidisciplinary development team that includes health and safety staff and some participants with boundary spanning roles.

IDENTIFYING INFORMATION NEEDS

The following steps are an overview of a methodology to help users identify their information needs and express the results in a way that is accessible to those who design decision-support systems:

- ask key questions from users' point of view and vocabulary
- refine the questions and express them as measurable outcomes
- identify additional variables (data elements) used to stratify or subgroup the outcomes by their chief attributes such as person-place-time
- make an inventory of existing data sources with an emphasis on the data elements needed to answer the key questions and data quality
- sort the outcomes and their data elements into those that can be collected from existing data sources and those that require new data collection methods
- develop a model(s) of an information system that considers several strategies for data collection based on route business transactions, samples, surveys, and record linkage

In larger organizations, the models may be subject to formal feasibility studies, in which technical details, timelines, cost-benefit analysis of alternative designs are examined using accounting models and technology risk assessments.

Ask the Key Questions in Plain Language

Asking questions one wants to answer is the starting point for information system design (See Chapter 24 for an example). When done in a mixed group of users and IT staff, these questions often validate organizational concerns and build consensus among participants. If questions are phrased in a way that an informed layperson will understand, the process will be more inclusive. The questions are also the anchor to the following steps that involve operational detail. Without this anchor, some participants will lose sight of why certain data elements are requested and will not be able to defend their collection.

Express Each Question as a Measurable Outcome

The key questions describe an outcome. The principal outcomes in occupational health surveillance include injury and illness incidence, severity, costs, return-to-work, and satisfaction with services. Outcomes are also called performance indicators, benchmark statistics, and dependent variables. National benchmarks for selected occupational health conditions have been developed by the National Institute for Occupational Safety and Health and are published in Healthy People 2010.[5] Many important outcomes are expressed as a statistic that has a numerator that describes a health or exposure event, a denominator that describes the population to whom the event is applicable, and boundaries of time. Thus, many performance indicators are similar to epidemiologic incidence rates or prevalence.

$$\frac{\text{Health Event}}{\text{Population of Workers}} \times \text{Time Period}$$

For example, the following performance indicator could be a way of defining "What is the injury and illness rate based on reported injuries and illnesses from any of our different databases?"

$$\frac{\text{Entry on OSHA Log or Employers' First Report to Comp Carrier or Comp Filing}}{\text{Hours Worked by Hourly and Salaried Workers}} \times \text{Jan 1, 1999 to Dec 31, 1999}$$

For illustration purposes, this definition says that unique instances of an injury during calendar year 1999 that is OSHA recordable, workers' compensation reportable, or arose from a workers' compensation filing (accepted or not) meets the case definition for an injury.

Software engineers will immediately recognize the implications for database structures and formulas for calculation. A simplified relational database model is shown in Figure 10.1. The Structured Query Language

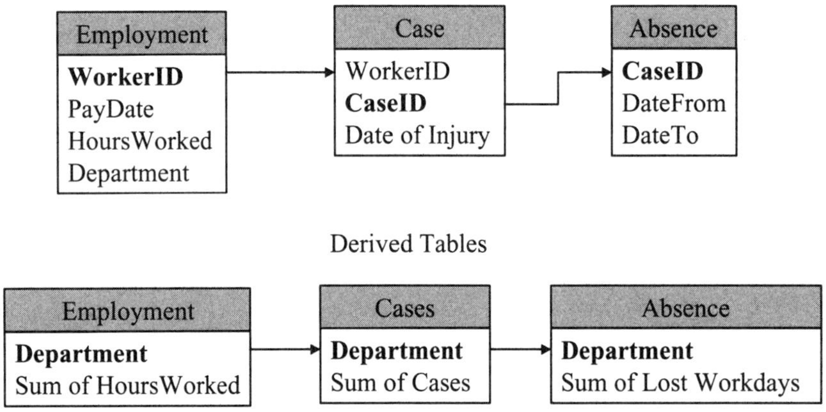

Case Incidence Rate Calculation - Database View

Department	Cases(A)	Hours Worked (B)	Rate (A/B)	Rate Ratio
Shipping	7	93,333	15.0	3.1
Fabrication	12	233,010	10.3	2.1
Assembly	15	612,225	4.9	1.0

Figure 10.1 Database skeleton for the calculation of case and lost time incidence rates. There are three main tables that are linked through worker and injury identifiers. The tables are (*1*) employment hours of individual workers in a specified pay period, (*2*) cases, and (*3*) episodes of absence. To calculate incidence rates by department, each main table has a derived table that sums hours, cases, or lost work days by department. This model can be expanded by additional tables in which a case links to diagnoses and diagnoses link to episodes. If work hours are not available, a monthly census of workers may be used to calculate average employment, as is done in many state-based injury surveillance systems.

Table 10.1 Structured Query Language that Implements an Epidemiologic Rate

Component of Rate	*Structured Query Language Commands*
A. Incidence rate by department	
1. Sum of hours by department (denominator)	SELECT DISTINCTROW Employment.Department, Sum(Employment.Hours) AS [Sum Of Hours] INTO Hours_sum FROM Employment WHERE (((Employment.PayDate)>= #1/1/99# And (Employment.PayDate)<= #12/31/99#)) GROUP BY Employment.Department;
2. Count of injuries by department (numerator)	SELECT DISTINCTROW Employment.Department, Count(*) AS [Count Of Injury] INTO Inj_sum FROM Employment INNER JOIN Injury ON Employment.WorkerID = Injury.WorkerID WHERE (((Injury.[Date of Injury])>=#1/1/99# And (Injury.[Date of Injury])<= #12/31/99#)) GROUP BY Employment.Department;
3. Incidence rate calculation	SELECT Hours_sum.Department, Hours_sum.[Sum Of Hours], Inj_sum.[Count Of Injury], (([Inj_sum].[Count Of Injury])/([Hours_sum].[Sum Of Hours]))*200,000 AS Rate FROM Hours_sum INNER JOIN Inj_sum ON Hours_sum.Department = Inj_sum.Department;
B. Lost workday incidence rate by department	
1. Sum of hours by department (denominator)	SELECT DISTINCTROW Employment.Department, Sum(Employment.Hours) AS [Sum Of Hours] INTO Hours_sum FROM Employment WHERE (((Employment.PayDate)>[t=] #1/1/99# And (Employment.PayDate)<= #12/31/99#)) GROUP BY Employment.Department;
2. Sum days lost (numerator)	SELECT Employment.Department, Sum(Days_absense.Days) AS SumOfDays INTO Sum_days FROM Employment INNER JOIN (Days_absense INNER JOIN Injury ON Days_absense.InjuryID = Injury.InjuryID) ON Employment.WorkerID = Injury.WorkerID WHERE (((Injury.[Date of Injury])>= #1/1/99# And (Injury.[Date of Injury])<= #12/31/99#)) GROUP BY Employment.Department;
3. Lost workday incidence rate*	SELECT Hours_sum.Department, Hours_sum.[Sum Of Hours], Sum_days.SumOfDays, ([SumOfDays]/[Sum Of Hours])*200,000 AS Rate FROM Sum_days INNER JOIN Hours_sum ON Sum_days.Department = Hours_sum.Department;

*Lost workday rate should have an explicit date for end of follow-up. Workdays lost may accumulate beyond the year of case incidence. If the case has not returned to work as of the date of the end of follow-up, lost workdays days must be added between the date last worked and the end of follow-up.

(SQL) or equivalent table-driven queries that generates performance indicators will have a logic sequence as shown in Table 10.1. Hours worked is an aggregate function of hours of individual workers stored in one database table.

Employment Table

Worker ID	*Payroll Date*	*Hours Worked*
001	1/29/99	160
002	1/29/99	158
003	1/29/99	166
001	2/28/99	145
002	2/28/99	160
003	2/28/99	154
. . .	. . .	. . .
001	12/29/99	160
002	12/29/99	158
003	12/29/99	166

Injury is a different entity with three attributes (columns) called OSHA (Yes or No), Employer's First Report (Yes or No) and Workers' Compensation (Yes or No).

Injury Table

Worker ID	*Injury ID*	*Injury Date*	*OSHA*	*Employer's First Report*	*Workers' Compensation Claim*
001	A	1/14/99	Y	Y	N
003	B	6/22/99	N	N	Y

The data elements for the population (Employment Table) include worker ID, hours worked, date of payroll, and hours worked during the payroll period. For the injury table, data elements include worker ID, injury ID, and Injury Date. Because the same worker can have more than one injury during the year, the injury ID is necessary. Injured workers who are not listed in the population (employment table) may indicate data quality problems.

Identify the Significant Variables to Stratify or Subgroup the Outcomes

Outcomes vary by person, place, and time. Each outcome may have a different set of subgrouping variables. However, diagnosis (nature of injury, body part, external cause), age, gender, department, and occupation are frequently needed by employers. In addition, industry, income, education, race or ethnicity, and residence may be important stratification variables for government agencies.

Some stratification variables apply to both the numerator and denominator of rate. For example, to calculate the injury incidence rate for a group of 30- to 34-year-olds requires that only this age group be counted in the denominator and that cases 30 to 34 years old at the time of the injury be included in the numerator.

Employment Table

Worker ID	*Payroll Date*	*Hours Worked*	*Age*
001	1/29/99	160	31
002	1/29/99	158	34
003	1/29/99	166	18
001	2/28/99	145	31
002	2/28/99	160	34
003	2/28/99	154	18
. . .	. . .	. . .	. . .
001	12/29/99	160	31
002	12/29/99	158	34
003	12/29/99	166	18

Injury Table

Worker ID	*Injury ID*	*Injury Date*	*OSHA*	*Employer's First Report*	*Workers' Compensation*
001	A	1/14/99	Y	Y	N
002	B	6/14/99	N	N	Y

Only the hours of workers 001 and 002 will count in the denominator. The injuries in workers 001 and 002 will be counted in the numerator, but worker 003, who is 18 years old will be excluded from the numerator and the denominator.

This has very important implications for programmers who are not used to creating ratio statistics. Even among skilled programmers outside of health sciences, it is very common for rate statistics to be confused with percentages.

Other stratification variables apply only to the health event in the numerator. For example, cases of injury can be subdivided by their nature: sprain and strain, fracture, burn, contusion, etc. The specific rates for sprains and strains, fractures, and burns use the same denominator for hours worked.

Employment Table

Worker ID	*Payroll Date*	*Hours Worked*
001	1/29/99	160
002	1/29/99	158
003	1/29/99	166
001	2/28/99	145
002	2/28/99	160
003	2/28/99	154
. . .	. . .	. . .
001	12/29/99	160
002	12/29/99	158
003	12/29/99	166
Total hours		5808

Worker ID	*Injury ID*	*Injury Date*	*Nature*
001	A	01/14/99	Fracture
002	B	02/08/99	Sprain
003	C	03/27/99	Concussion
004	D	05/05/99	Hernia
005	E	07/11/99	Sprain
006	F	09/14/99	Hernia
007	G	09/19/99	Sprain
008	H	10/02/99	Contusion
009	I	11/16/99	Sprain
010	J	12/10/99	Sprain

The rate of hernias is 2 per 5808 hours; hernias comprise 20% (2/10) of injuries. The overall injury rate is the sum of the individual rates by nature. These rates, too, are often confused by programmers with the percent distribution of injuries in which the total number of injuries is the denominator instead of the hours worked of the population.

Some outcomes follow a natural hierarchical structure, and stratification variables represent a link in a hierarchical chain. For example, an injury rate can be observed for single establishment, multiple establishments of single employer, or all employers in a single industry. This is sometimes called the scalability of a variable.

Make an Inventory of Available Data Sources

An inventory of data sources should include:

- written documentation of databases, policies, and procedures
- description of the physical media (paper, magnetic) and the years of data collection in each format
- data structures, layout of computer records and

paper forms, data dictionaries, coding manuals, and code lists for coded text data
- disposition of archived records that may not be part of an active database; inactive or closed cases
- administrative and physical access
- data security including procedures for authorizing access, confidentiality, and emergency recovery (after floods, earthquakes, fires)

Drawing a diagram of how the information flows is very useful (Chapter 3). This often reveals discrepancies and confusion between official policy and actual field procedures. Chapter 3 also identifies the basic elements of a data quality assurance program.

Information Triage: Sort the Outcomes and Stratification Variables

Information falls along a spectrum, starting with (*1*) unstructured text narratives on paper forms and progressing to (*2*) standardized, coded electronic database files. The purpose of the information triage is to determine where outcomes and stratification variables fall in the two categories, or whether they are not part of any existing data source. Other goals are to assess whether:

- data quality of an information source is so low that it should not be seriously considered to measure an outcome
- the definition of data elements in available sources are compatible with those to define the outcome
- the level of detail is satisfactory to answer the key question
- the data elements in the available data sources aggregate the outcome in a way that answers the key questions

The process of screening outcomes with available data sources is done in two steps: (*1*) range finding for general content, and (*2*) honing in on the operational definition. If the outcome is beyond the scope of any available source, it is a candidate for a new method of data collection or it will have to be omitted. If the general content seems to match, one needs to examine data quality, compatibility of definition, detail, and level of aggregation.

It is a judgement whether data quality makes a source usable or salvageable. There is no automatic threshold, but at some point the validity of the data is legitimately called into question. Missing data may be randomly distributed or systematic. For example, age data may be complete for men, but not for women.

The definition of the outcome and the definitions of data elements in data sources need to be scrutinized very carefully. That data elements match in name or general content is not sufficient; one needs to dig into the definitions to see how they are put into practice. For example, a field called DATE_RETURN_TO_WORK probably deals with some aspect of return to work. However, is DATE_RETURN_TO_WORK the predicted date of return after the physician's initial evaluation and treatment, the date the physician released the worker from temporary disability to return to work, the date the worker physically returned to work, or the latest date in a series of returns to work? If the outcome calls for a data element that is the actual date of return to work, it is important to determine which of available data elements creates the least amount of error, and whether the error will be random or systematic. If it is systematic, will the outcome be overestimated or underestimated?

The level of detail for categorical variables may be inadequate. For example, in many workers' compensation claims databases, carpal tunnel syndrome (CTS) was not identified as a separate category of injury or illness until the mid-1980s. Some systems that coded body part and nature of injury inferred CTS by cross classifying body part (wrist) with nature of injury (nerve disease).

Some data sources aggregate an outcome too much to be of use in answering the key question. For example, a data source that lists total cost for each case will not answer the question of cost per case of low back pain, a specific diagnosis. To answer the question, the data source must list the diagnosis and the costs associated with that diagnosis.

INFORMATION SYSTEM PYRAMID

The result of the information triage is outcomes sorted in three groups: (*1*) stored in existing computerized administrative data; (*2*) not stored in any system, and (*3*) stored as text fields but not coded (Fig. 10.2).

The overall design of the information system is the interplay between the data collection strategies. Several strategies are often necessary to answer the key questions. Data on injury and illness stored in computerized administrative databases are characterized as a mile wide and an inch deep. This is because a large number of cases may be included, but few outcomes or stratification variables. The importance of this tier is that it provides a comprehensive list from which statistical samples can be drawn. The second tier includes outcomes that are not easily coded or part of a sampling strategy where it is not necessary to have data on every case. Information in claims files or medical charts are often part of a second tier for which samples may be appropriate. Data collection may include manual ab-

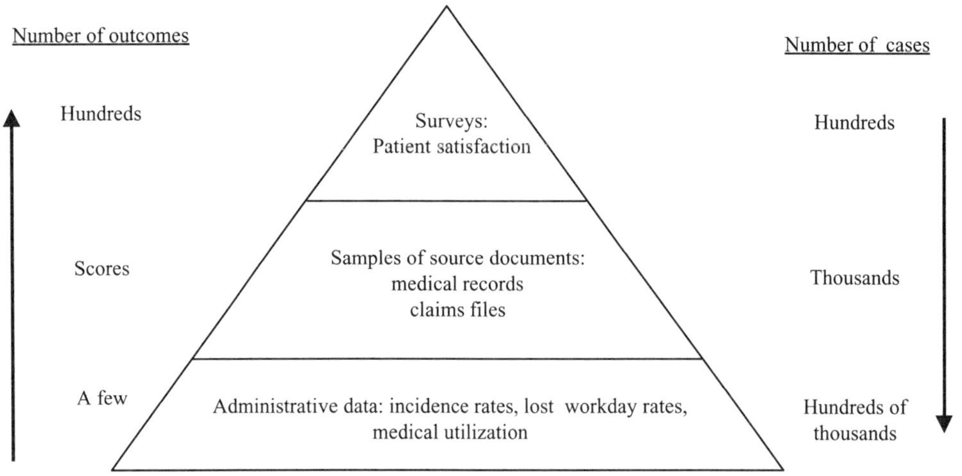

Figure 10.2 Occupational health information systems require several different data collection strategies to answer key questions regarding injury frequency, return to work, costs, timeliness of benefit delivery, patient satisfaction, and other outcomes.

straction, record linkage to other databases, or computer records selected with specific criteria. The rationale for using a sample is to minimize the data collection burden. However, complicated decision rules for selecting cases increases the administrative costs of sampling. The highest tier based on surveys are for outcomes that are only available as opinions, sensitive issues, personal experiences, or too costly to collect otherwise. Examples are satisfaction with medical care, home care provided to an injured worker by a family member, or job discrimination because of a work injury. Because self-administered mail questionnaires or telephone interviews are labor intensive and costly, only several hundred to several thousand interviews are possible at the second and third tiers. Chapter 24 provides an example of how this methodology is applied to the design of a state-based workers' compensation information system.

REFERENCES

1. American National Standards Institute. Accredited Subcommittee X12. *Electronic Data Interchange Standards. Draft version 3 release 5.* Alexandria, VA: Data Interchange Standards Association, 1995. (Transaction sets 148 - First Report of Injury; 837 - Health Care Claim)
2. IAIABC EDI Development Project. *First Report of Injury, Subsequent Report, Medical Bill Payment Report. Release 1.* Daytona Beach: International Association of Industrial Accident Boards and Commissions, September 1995.
3. Health Insurance Portability and Accountability Act. Public Law 104-191. Part F. Administrative Simplification. Section 1173. *Standards for Information Transactions and Data Elements.* Washington, DC: U.S. Government Printing Office, 1996.
4. National Council on Compensation Insurance. *Compendium of States Managed Care Programs.* Boca Raton: National Council on Compensation Insurance, 1995.
5. National Center for Health Statistics. *Occupational Health. Healthy People 2000 Review 1998–1999. National Health Promotion and Disease Prevention Objectives.* Publ. No. DHHS (PHS) 99-1256. Hyattsville, MD: Public Health Service, 1999.

II

CASE STUDIES

11

Lead Poisoning and Elevated Blood Lead

NEIL A. MAIZLISH AND LINDA A. RUDOLPH

Lead is perhaps the most widely recognized neurotoxin in the workplace and human environment. At high doses, lead causes the swelling of the lining of the brain, coma, and death. High doses also cause damage to the kidneys, severe abdominal cramping, and spontaneous abortions. At lower doses over a long period of time lead accumulates in the bones and other tissues. It can cause nerve damage in the hands and feet, alter the development of red blood cells, and affect human behavior in subtle ways. Children are more vulnerable than adults and can be contaminated from lead dust taken home on work clothes of adult household members.[1] During the 1980s, scientific reports that low-level lead exposure alters the mental development of children fueled additional concerns regarding low-level exposures.[2]

Workplace exposures to lead in the United States have been the object of control efforts by states and the federal government for decades, and are currently regulated under a standard issued in 1978 by the federal Occupational Safety and Health Administration (OSHA).[3] The standard established an exposure limit of 50 $\mu g/m^3$ for airborne lead exposures for an 8-hour workday, and requires employers to provide training, respiratory protection, work clothes changes, shower facilities, and a medical surveillance program, including annual physical examinations and periodic blood lead tests to eligible employees. Workers in construction were excluded prior to 1992. The standard requires that workers with blood lead levels exceeding 40 $\mu g/dL$ (1.93 $\mu mol/L$) be retested every other month and those exceeding 60 $\mu g/dL$ (2.90 $\mu mol/L$) or having an average of 50 $\mu g/dL$ (2.41 $\mu mol/L$) on three previous tests be immediately transferred and placed in jobs with low or no exposure. During the 1980s, enforcement was aimed at large employers in battery manufacturing and secondary lead smelting, and the number of reported cases of occupational lead poisoning dwindled to a trickle as measured by passive reporting systems of physicians[4] and employers.[5] Many had concluded that occupational lead poisoning was largely eliminated.

Since the 1970s, blood lead levels in the U.S. population have been monitored periodically as part of a national health survey.[6] Levels have progressively declined over the last decade[7] but there are still pockets of higher levels. To improve surveillance and target prevention activities, 25 state health departments, accounting for over half the U.S. population, have required licensed clinical laboratories that measure lead in blood to report the results to their state health department.[8] Reporting is aimed at the general population and includes children and adults. As part of a surveillance system, state health departments count cases, identify high-risk groups, examine trends, trace and follow-up high-risk children and adults, and for occupational cases target interventions at specific worksites and industries of adult "index" cases.[9–11] Since most adult cases are occupational in nature, the states also report to the National Institute for Occupational Safety and Health (NIOSH), which pools the data and publishes the results quarterly.[8]

This chapter describes the design and initial results of one such surveillance system in the occupational health program of the California Department of Health Services (CDHS).[12] Under a state law in effect since 1987, California medical laboratories that test for blood lead have been required to report personal identifiers and blood lead levels of individuals with tests exceeding 25 $\mu g/dL$, irrespective of age (Table 11.1).

Table 11.1 California Health and Safety Code for Laboratory Reporting of Blood Lead

309.71 Medical laboratories; reports of blood lead findings; confidentiality of information; fines for failure to meet reporting requirements

(a) All medical laboratories shall report to the department each detected case of a blood lead greater than 25 micrograms of lead per deciliter of human blood or the equivalent standard measured in micrograms of protoporphyrin per gram of hemoglobin. The blood lead findings, the names, ages, and addresses of the patients involved in each detected case and any additional information necessary to implement provisions of this article shall be reported to the department in a manner prescribed by the director.

(b) All information reported pursuant to this section shall be confidential . . .

(c) All medical laboratories testing for blood lead levels shall participate in a blood lead and free erythrocyte protoporphyrin (FEP) proficiency testing program.*

(d) All medical laboratories which fail to meet reporting requirements will be assessed fines of up to $500 at the discretion of the director.

*Laboratories are certified as proficient if in 75% of at least 9 reference samples, lead concentrations are reported within 15 percent of target values for concentrations less than 40 μg/dL, or within 6 μg/dL of target values for concentrations greater than 40 μg/dL.

METHODS

Goals, Objectives, and Scope

The goal was to improve the estimates of occupational lead poisoning in California. The scope included both children (take-home exposures) and adults throughout California. For occupationally exposed adults, there was a concern that a laboratory-based surveillance system would not detect the majority of lead-exposed workers, but would focus on two smaller groups:

- employees with low lead levels at larger companies that were complying with the OSHA lead standard
- symptomatic workers with high levels at smaller workplaces with little awareness of the OSHA lead standard

In the latter case, a family physician or local industrial medical clinic would be the most likely to request a test.

The estimate of potential underreporting was addressed in a statewide survey of lead-using employers,[13] which was a unique tool to evaluate the lead registry.

An important additional objective of surveillance was added shortly after case reporting started. Within the first 9 months, over 3000 case reports of elevated blood lead in adults were received. Scores of blood lead tests were greater than 60 μg/dL and several cases exceeded 80 μg/dL. This level not only triggers immediate removal from occupational exposure but merits a label of public health emergency. Telephone follow-up of the first few cases with highly elevated blood lead levels revealed:

- occupation was the source of exposure
- treating physicians were unfamiliar with diagnosis and treatment of lead poisoning
- employers had not controlled the source of exposure, putting additional workers at risk

The surveillance system was rapidly reformulated as a sentinel event notification system in which the state health department played a modest, but active role in coordinating follow-up at specific worksites of urgent cases. The scope of contact was limited to telephone interviews with the worker, physician, and employer to gather information; one-on-one education of workers, physicians, and employers; and referrals to other government agencies such as California's Division of Occupational Safety and Health (Cal/OSHA), professional associations, and university-based occupational health clinics.

Gaining Support

Even though blood lead reporting was a legal requirement, gaining support from the laboratories and other participants was important. First, the laboratories were contacted and informed of their new responsibilities. Based on the state's list of licensed laboratories, a cover letter and a copy of the new law was sent to all the commercial clinical laboratories with copies of the report form (Fig. 11.1). Approximately 40 laboratories carried out blood lead testing. Telephone contact was made with California laboratory directors and arrangements were made for proficiency testing. The tone was collegial rather than legalistic. The appeal for participation was framed in terms of contributing to public health.

Support was also sought from organizations that got referrals from follow-up. When it became apparent that most family physicians and industrial clinics were unfamiliar with clinical management of lead poisoning, physicians at occupational health specialty clinics of the University of California were recruited as back-up consultants for ongoing care. Similarly, the health department made contact with Cal/OSHA's Consultation Services, which visits workplaces and offers free advice to employers on how to comply with the lead standard.

Because children with possible take-home exposures and nonoccupationally exposed adults were occasionally reported, county health officers were also informed of the surveillance activities.

Multidisciplinary Surveillance Team

Active follow-up of urgent cases (> 60 μg/dL) required a mix of skills. The surveillance team at CDHS consisted of a bilingual interviewer (Spanish/English) who doubled at data entry, an occupational health physi-

LEAD REPORTING FORM

Type of print clearly, completing all the questions below / *Laboratory: Use separate card for each sample analyzed.*			DOH Use Only
Patient Name: Last, First, M.I.	Phone no. where patient can be reached		Date Received
Patient Address: Street	Sex: ☐ Male ☐ Female	Date of Birth M D Y	Reporting Source No.
City, State, Zip Code	Age	Social Security No.	Patient No.
Employer at time of Exposure	Occupation		Employer Code
Address	Industry		Occupational Code
Sample Source (Check One) ☐ Lab ☐ Physician ☐ Employer ☐ Hospital	Name		Industry Code
	Address: Street		Date of Test
	City, State, Zip Code		Physician No.
Physician Requesting Test (if different from sample source): Name, City, State, Zip Code			Laboratory No.

Testing Lab Name	Date Sample Taken	Date Sample Rec'd	Lab Sample No.	Date Analyzed

Type of Specimen	Lead	EP by Extraction	EP by Hematofluorometer	Hematocrit
Blood	μg/dL			
Urine				

This report being completed by: ☐ Lab ☐ Employer ☐ Phys. ☐ Hosp. ☐ Check here if you need more report forms

DHS (2/87) See Reverse for Distribution

Figure 11.1 State of California laboratory report form for elevated blood lead.

cian, an industrial hygienist, and a epidemiologist, who doubled as the database manager and coordinator of the lead surveillance program. Each of the four staff worked only part-time on the lead registry for a total of 1.5 full-time equivalents. The annual workload consisted of key entry of 5000 reports, 150–250 telephone interviews, case management of 50–75 priority cases, statistical analysis, and generation of a 10-page report.

Case Definition and Data Collection

A case of reportable blood lead was 25 μg/dL or greater. The mechanism of reporting by laboratories was specially designed form that contained fields for patient identifiers, demographics, blood lead level, and other relevant information (Fig. 11.1). Small laboratories mailed in forms individually and larger ones batch mailed scores of reports. A few large employers voluntarily reported all blood lead results from non-California laboratories, including results below 25 μg/dL. Blood lead level was always reported, but sometimes laboratories did not know or record the age and address of patients. To facilitate reporting, CDHS offered to accept electronic data interchange. However, large commercial laboratories were not inclined to reprogram their computers to accommodate a low volume, specialty test such as blood lead.

Protocol for Follow-up

One or more cases with blood lead reports of 60 μg/dL or greater at a worksite was the threshold for follow-up (Fig. 11.2). This threshold was selected to balance available resources and clinical urgency. This was a difficult decision because adverse health effects below 60 μg/dL are well-documented in the scientific literature. However, at 30 minutes to 2 hours of tracing per case, the part-time staff could not contact hundreds of cases between 40 and 60 μg/dL before they became emergencies.

Cases, their physicians, and employers were traced, and structured telephone interviews were administered to determine: the level of direct medical supervision, if any; work history and source of exposure, occupational or nonoccupational; number of household contacts less

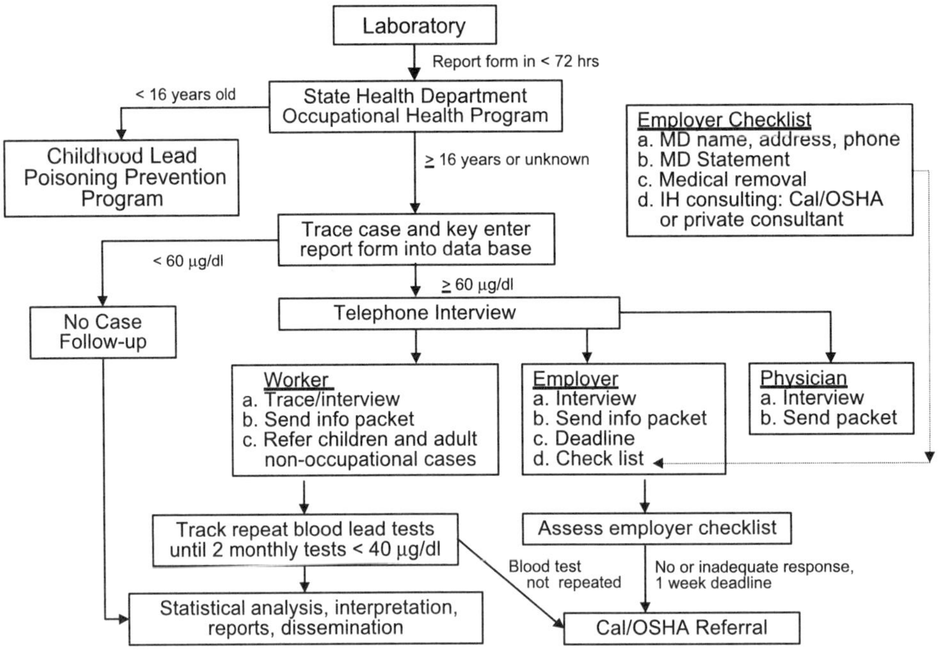

Figure 11.2 Protocol for follow-up of elevated blood lead in California adults.

than 7 years of age; number of coworkers exposed to lead; use of personal protective equipment and hygienic practices at work; and application of medical removal requirements of the federal OSHA lead standard. The questionnaires are presented in Appendix G.

The length of interviews was about 15 minutes for physicians, 30 minutes for workers, and 20 minutes for employers. Employers were always contacted for blood lead reports of 80 μg/dL or greater. Because workers expressed concerns of employment discrimination, at levels between 60 and 79 μg/dL, employers were interviewed if the case did not express reservations, or if any other worker with an elevated blood lead level at the same worksite did not object to contact with the employer. Interviews were often conducted during evenings when workers were at home. This was done to shield workers from reprisals until the employer was formally contacted by CDHS. While on the job, many workers could not come to the telephone, or were wary of explaining the reason for the call.

In addition to questions to confirm and prioritize the case, the questionnaires had short, educational paragraphs. To reinforce this immediate one-on-one education, an information packet was sent to the worker, his or her physician and employer. Both English and Spanish language versions explained the health effects of lead, employer and physician responsibilities under the OSHA lead standard, and how to contact the local offices of Cal/OSHA and workers' compensation.[14–16]

Subsequent blood lead reports of cases were tracked by the surveillance system until two successive tests taken a month a part were below 40 μg/dL. Workers, employers, and physicians were recontacted if a subsequent blood lead abruptly increased, an initial blood lead test over 80 μg/dL was not repeated within 2 weeks, or a monthly follow-up test was missed. An example of tracking an employer's follow-up to prevent further cases is shown in Figure 11.3.[17]

Referrals

When the interviews indicated that take-home exposures were likely or the case was not related to work (e.g., ingestion of folk medicines containing lead), CDHS arranged blood lead testing at county public health clinics for children and nonoccupationally exposed adults.

At the end of each interview, employers were informed of free industrial hygiene services available from Cal/OSHA Consultation Services or were encouraged to seek private consultants. Based on interview responses, employers who did not formally contract with a physician to carry out medical monitoring or did not provide protective equipment, ventilation, or sanitary facilities were sent a certified letter. The letter requested that employers have a contracted physician and industrial hygiene consultant contact CDHS for assistance. If the employer said they would request help from Cal/OSHA Consultation, CDHS called ahead to the local Cal/OSHA Consultation office to confirm the call. Employers who did not respond by a deadline were then referred to enforcement agencies.

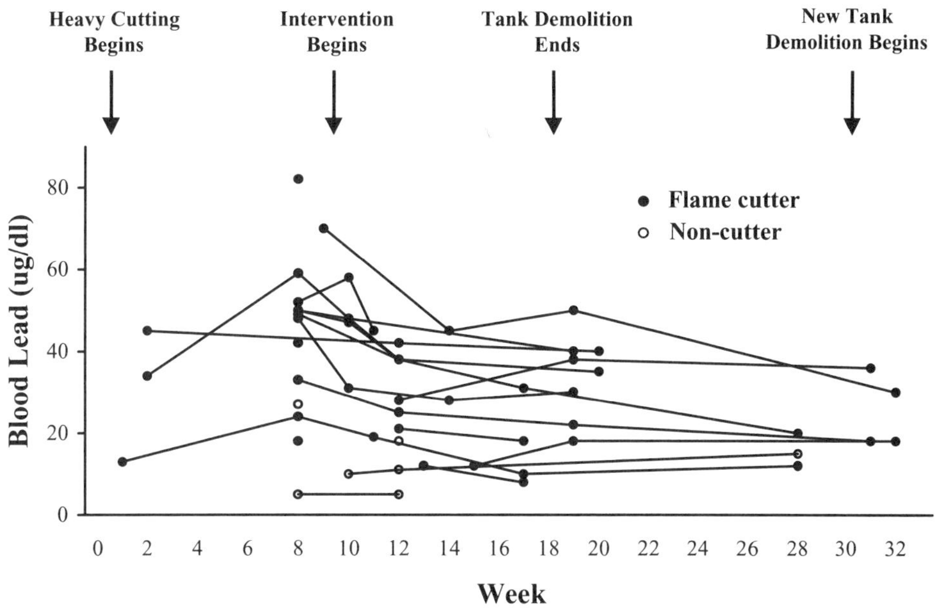

Figure 11.3 Follow-up of an industrial hygiene intervention among tank demolition workers in California's lead registry. The occupational health program in the California state health department tracked blood lead levels in a successful intervention of an employer to reduce lead overexposures in a crew of 29 male demolition workers in 1989. The workers dismantled a two-story metal gas storage tank coated with 10% lead paint by flame cutting square swatches with acetylene torches. Airborne lead exposures were extremely intense with some individual breathing zone samples (8-hour Time-Weighted Average) exceeding 5.0 mg/m^3—over 10 times the then in-effect permissible exposure level. Eight weeks after starting the demolition job and the detection of high airborne levels, the employer put into place a series of control measures that included powered air purifying respirators, hiring a technician to maintain the personal protective equipment, flame cutting from the unpainted tank interior when it was safe to do so, installing showers and portable hand washing stands, laundering and changing work clothes, weekly training on lead, monthly biologic monitoring, and medical removal to noncutting jobs for workers who tested 40 μg/dL or greater. With the encouragement of the state health department, these measures reduced subsequent lead exposure, which was reflected in lower blood lead levels reported to the lead registry. (Waller and Osorio.[23])

The CDHS protocol involved more effort than an automatic referral to OSHA enforcement. Although this was considered, in 1988, California's state OSHA plan reverted to federal jurisdiction. Hundreds of experienced enforcement officers left the agency. Federal OSHA could not rapidly train and hire a sufficient number of personnel to follow-up every significant case (e.g., $>$ 40 μg/dL case). When jurisdiction changed back to California in 1989, Cal/OSHA had difficulties hiring a sufficient number of experienced staff. During this period, CDHS's referrals to OSHA for enforcement were directed to employers who refused to seek assistance voluntarily.

Collect and Code Data

Information from report forms and questionnaires was key-entered on a desktop computer into a simple relational database consisting of two linked files. One file recorded all the fields on the report form and a second file recorded questionnaire responses for the cases $\geq$ 60 μg Pb/dL. Key entry tried to keep pace with incoming reports. Before entering a report, the database was indexed and scanned to determine if the case had prior laboratory reports. If so, the demographic information on the cases was recycled or updated. Many text fields were precoded to facilitate coding. If the gender field was blank, gender was designated on the basis of first name. An additional indicator of Hispanic surname was created, and coded by the key enterer who was Hispanic. The industry of employment was based on an assignment of the four-digit Standard Industrial Classification (SIC)[18] code for reports that identified the employer. Employer name and address on the report form were matched to listings in the California Manufacturers Directory,[19] which gives the SIC code for the primary business activity. Occupation was usually blank.

Manage Cases

The worksite, physician, and individual workers were contacted by CDHS to assure that employers and their physicians were carrying out their responsibilities to prevent and treat overexposures to lead. Interviews and contact notes of the physician, employer, and worker were consolidated into a paper file organized by worker within an employer, and became a case. A case manager was assigned, from the professional staff at CDHS, who was responsible for carrying out the protocol for follow-up.

No one staff member had all the technical skills to carry out follow-up. It was necessary to sequence activities and route case files between the bilingual interviewer who interviewed the worker, the CDHS physician who interviewed the case's treating physician, and the CDHS industrial hygienist who evaluated exposure information from worker and employer interviews. Most treating physicians required clinical assistance and responded favorably when interviewed by a CDHS physician.

A simple, automated case management system generated lists of blood lead tests in date order sorted by worker and employer. This allowed case managers to see the time series of blood lead tests and dates, and whether the target date for the next scheduled monthly test had been missed.

Case managers also checked deadlines by which employers were asked to provide written documentation of a contract with a physician or an industrial hygiene consultant or both. Case management meetings were held at least once a month to discuss developments of specific cases, difficulties with the protocols, cases that made good educational vignettes, and action items for the chief of the program, such as referrals to OSHA and medical emergencies.

Analysis and Interpretation

There were three principal analyses: (*1*) statistical analysis of data on the report forms, (*2*) statistical analysis of questionnaire responses from the smaller set of cases with blood lead levels over 60 μg/dL, and (*3*) case narratives of specific worksites based on all available information, including case contact notes and OSHA investigations. The statistical analyses profiled the demographic, geographic, and occupational distribution of elevated blood lead reports, and distinguished between worksites, individual workers at their peak blood lead level, and laboratory reports. Analysis of questionnaires described the prevalence of ventilation, protective equipment and clothing, hygienic practices, medical monitoring, medical removal, and other concerns such as employment discrimination. The case narratives were half-page vignettes illustrating specific messages such as unprotected high-risk groups in construction and demolition, take-home exposures, and ignorance of the OSHA lead standard.

The time period of analysis was based on the date the report was received during a calendar year (January 1 to December 31), rather than the date the sample was analyzed. This was done to provide data as soon as possible to policy makers, and not wait an additional 3–4 months until all late reports were finally mailed in.

To analyze the distribution of reports and individuals, two different flat files were exported from the database. One file contained all reports (N = 5000–8000 per year), including multiple reports on the same individual. Another file (N = 1000) contained individuals appearing once at their peak blood lead level during the calendar year. The two flat files were imported into commercial statistical analysis package, and batch commands were used to carry out the analysis.

The annual report was a one-page summary, a few case vignettes, and 5–10 tables. File editing, correcting data entry errors by scanning outliers, running batch programs to generate statistical output, and writing up the report usually took about 2–3 weeks.

Feedback

Several types of feedback were carried out by CDHS. The first was one-on-one education to persuade employers to carry out medical monitoring and control lead exposures. This approach was a delicate balance of positive and negative messages, played as a scenario of good cop-bad cop. Employers were told that they had a problem and that solutions were available. If they followed the recommendations in the time prescribed by CDHS—the good cop, they could avoid being referred to OSHA enforcement personnel—the bad cop. The written proof and short deadline that CDHS demanded required the employer to get third parties—the employers' physician and health and safety consultants—to take action. This requirement made it less likely that an employer could engage in an elaborate deception or offer a tepid written response. This also created a paper trail.

Despite appeals to public health, laboratories regarded the new reporting as extra work for staff and potential compliance hassles with the State. There were few incentives that the state could offer to facilitate reporting such as electronic reporting and batch mailing of paper forms. Most laboratories had difficulties with reporting their results within 72 hours after the analysis, as required, and they did not monitor their own timeliness. Educating the laboratories by feeding back their timeliness (days from sample analyzed to date received by the state) compared to the average of the other laboratories, usually spurred improvements in reporting. Threats of fines or removal of their names from the list of certified laboratories were infrequently invoked, but held out as a next step if improvements were not forthcoming.

Second, broader audiences were informed of the findings. Along with a cover letter repeating the key findings, the annual technical report was sent to a mailing list of approximately 150 individuals and organizations. These included those directly in the flow of information or referrals such as the 40 laboratories, the 58 California county health officers, central and regional offices of California OSHA, and the university-based occupational health clinics to whom serious cases

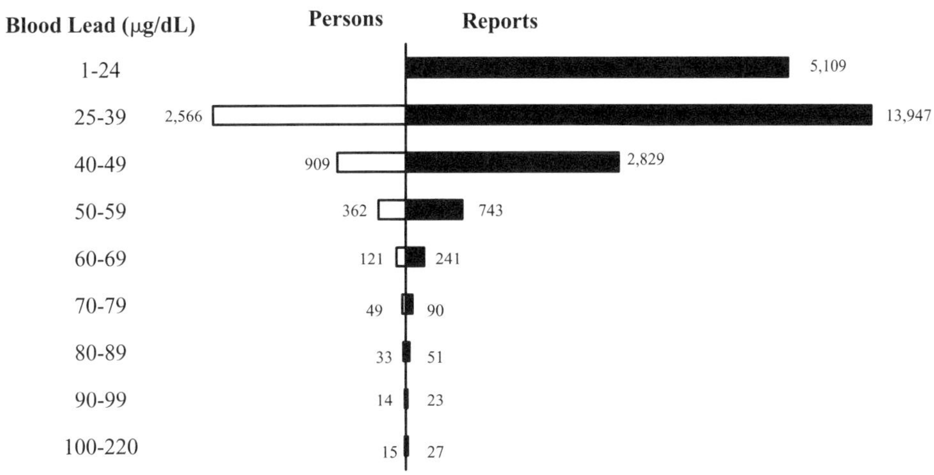

Figure 11.4 Blood lead distribution in California adults, 1988–1990. (Maizlish et al.[11])

were often referred. The state medical association and labor unions, and employer groups were also included. Copies were sent to national organizations such as NIOSH and other state health departments.

Third, a marketing campaign was undertaken. Brainstorming sessions were held to identify organizations with an interest in occupational lead poisoning. The campaign involved scores of grassroots organizations in the medical, labor, university, Latino, and public health communities. A packet of materials was written in nontechnical language and mailed to the organizations. These packets were followed with telephone calls. The CDHS created a press release from the annual report. Press coverage was significant. Reporters requested CDHS to facilitate interviews with lead poisoned workers. A few cases were contacted by CDHS after their medical recovery. The cases were asked if they were interested in having a reporter contact them. This was done without pressure and with the understanding that they could refuse without reprisals. Several lead-poisoned workers agreed to have their stories covered by major California daily newspapers.

RESULTS

Blood Lead Distributions

Between April 1, 1987 and December 31, 1990, CDHS received 23,060 blood lead reports from 38 laboratories for 4069 civilian, noninstitutionalized adults aged 16 years and older. Three thousand twenty-five were received in 1987, 5874 in 1988, 7622 in 1989, and 6539 in 1990. Of these, 17,951 were greater than 25 μg/dL.

Counting individuals once, but at their highest blood lead level, 1503 individuals (37%) had a peak blood lead level of 40 μg/dL or greater; 594 (15%) peaked at 50 μg/dL or greater; 232 (6%) peaked at 60 μg/dL or greater; and 52 (1%) had peak levels at or above 80 μg/dL (Fig. 11.4). Three hundred twenty-eight employers were reported. Individuals with elevated blood lead were overwhelmingly male, and evenly divided among Hispanic and non-Hispanic surnames (Table 11.2). One thousand and eighty-nine

Table 11.2 Demographic Characteristics of California Adults with a Blood Lead Report 25 μg/dL or Greater, 1987–1990

Item	*N*	%
Age*		
16–19	44	2
20–29	574	25
30–39	700	30
40–49	547	23
50–59	311	13
60–69	144	6
70+	21	1
Sex†		
Male	3730	95
Female	199	5
Surname‡		
Non-Hispanic	2009	49
Hispanic	1958	50
Asian	22	1
County of Employer		
Los Angeles	9053	67
Orange	2164	16
San Bernardino	679	5
San Diego	370	3

*Excludes 1728 individuals with reports not stating age.
†Excludes 140 individuals for whom gender was not stated or determined.
‡Excludes 80 individuals for whom surname was not classified.

workers (5240 reports) in 22 battery manufacturing plants and 473 workers (6793 reports) in 10 lead smelters or metal recovery operations accounted for 38% of persons and 67% of reports 25 μg/dL or greater. Persons with the highest peak blood lead levels were employed in mining assay laboratories, construction industries, ceramics manufacturing, explosives manufacturing, brass foundries and castings facilities, lead battery plants, lead smelting, electrical machinery manufacturing, scrap metal recycling, radiator repair shops, and gun firing ranges (Table 11.3). Southern California employers generated the bulk of lead reports followed by central valley counties (Fig. 11.5).[20]

Follow-up of Index Cases with Elevated Blood Lead Levels

Of the 232 incident cases with blood lead levels exceeding 60 μg/dL, 182 (78%) were traced and completed telephone interviews. Two percent refused interview; 3% were secondary cases from the same work site and were not interviewed; and 17% were untraceable or out-of-state referrals.

Table 11.3 Distribution of Persons by Peak Blood Lead Levels by Standard Industrial Classification, 1987–1990

					Peak Blood Lead (μg/dL)‡			
*SIC Code**	*Industry*	*Employers*	*Reports†*	*Persons*	*25–39*	*40–59*	*60–79*	*80+*
3691	Lead batteries	22	5240	1089	726	335	19	9
3341	Secondary lead smelting	8	6793	473	335	131	6	1
3362	Brass/copper foundry	10	449	251	173	57	15	6
7539	Radiator repair	65	306	124	40	53	23	8
7997	Firing ranges—sport	12	203	78	36	26	12	4
3494	Brass pipe/main valves	6	147	65	48	15	2	—
3269	Pottery, nec§	4	181	58	39	14	3	2
3360	Nonferrous foundry	7	104	51	34	17	—	—
9221	Firing ranges—police	10	153	51	28	19	3	1
3264	Porcelain electrical supplies	1	53	35	28	6	1	—
3724	Aircraft engines manufacturing	2	95	35	27	7	1	—
3721	Aircraft manufacturing and assembly	2	40	30	20	9	1	—
3351	Brass/copper rolling	2	112	28	10	11	6	1
1000	Mining	5	69	26	15	8	1	2
3674	Semiconductors	3	45	26	20	5	1	—
3339	Primary smelting	1	66	23	6	11	5	1
3253	Ceramic tile	4	48	18	8	6	4	—
3354	Aluminum extruded products	1	21	17	17	—	—	—
3431	Metal sanitary ware	1	84	16	9	5	2	—
1721	Painting contractors	4	28	15	6	7	—	2
3260	Pottery and related	3	27	15	11	2	1	1
3699	Electrical machinery	1	23	15	9	4	1	1
1629	Heavy construction, nec	3	57	13	3	8	1	1
1795	Construction, demolition	3	34	13	1	3	5	4
3321	Gray iron foundry	1	35	13	9	4	—	—
3714	Motor vehicle equipment	2	21	13	11	2	—	—
3369	Nonferrous castings, nec	5	44	11	1	7	2	1
3432	Brass plumbing fittings	1	12	11	5	6	—	—
3561	Pump manufacturing	2	26	11	7	2	1	1
9711	U.S. Armed Forces	4	18	11	9	2	—	—
3312	Steel mill	1	21	10	—	9	1	—
3364	Nonferrous die-casting	3	24	10	4	4	2	—
Total	All Adults	328	17,951	4069	2566	1271	170	62

*Standard Industrial Classification (SIC) code; categories with fewer than 10 persons are not shown. Data on report forms that precluded their industrial classification was missing for 1292 persons.

†Includes multiple reports on some individuals.

‡1.21 μmol/L = 25 μg/dL; 1.93 μmol/L = 40 μg/dL; 2.90 μmol/L = 60 μg/dL; 3.87 μmol/L = 80 μg/dL.

§nec, not elsewhere classified.

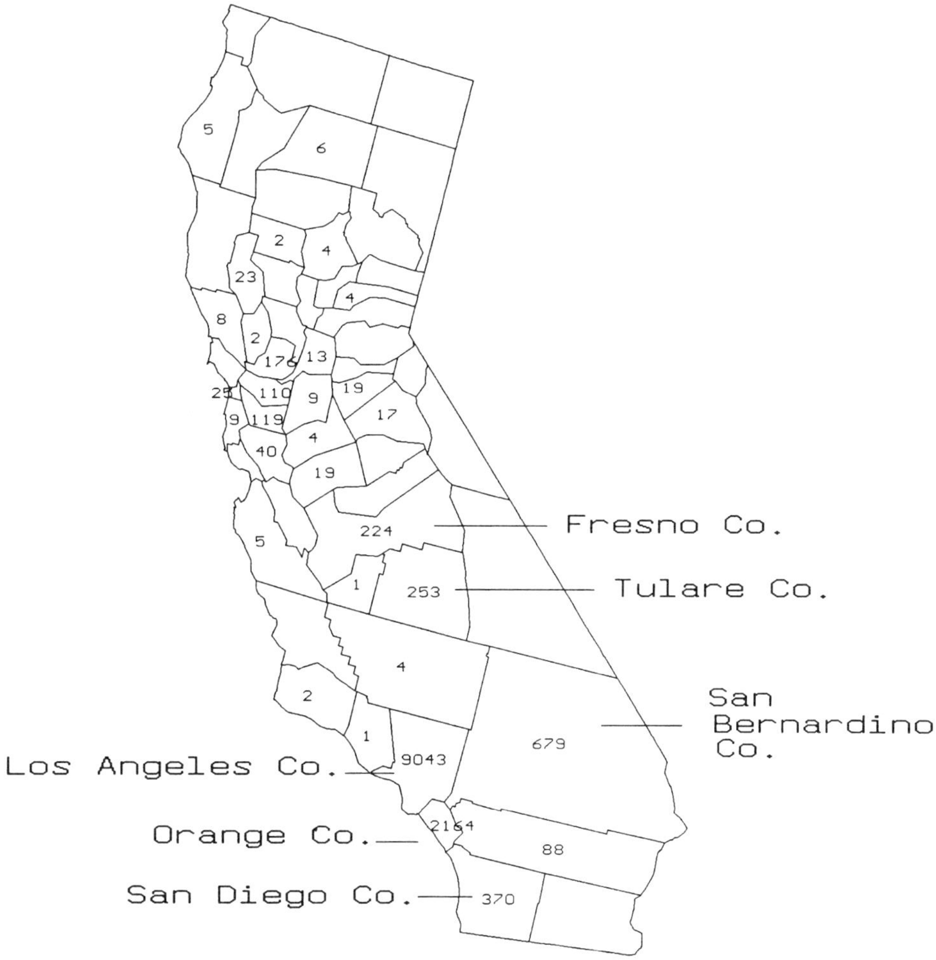

Figure 11.5 Distribution of blood lead reports by county—California, 1987–1990. (California Occupational Health Program.[20])

The index cases were overwhelmingly male (95%), disproportionately Hispanic (46%),[21] and the majority (70%) were 35 years old or older (Table 11.4). Approximately one-third never attended high school. Forty-six percent spoke Spanish or another non-English language at home. Thirty-five percent reported that they resided with at least one child under 7 years of age.

All but 9 of the 149 index cases were employed in industries with well-documented potential for lead overexposure (Table 11.4). Hobbies and other nonoccupational activities with the potential for lead exposure were reported by 16%. The highest blood lead level of 220 μg/dL was in a ceramics tile glaze-sprayer who worked in an unventilated booth. Index cases were mostly employed in radiator repair shops (22%), battery plants (13%), brass and other nonferrous founding and casting operations (13%), gun firing ranges (12%), ceramics and pottery manufacture (8%), painting and demolition (6%), and secondary lead smelting (6%). Twenty-one percent were employed for less than 1 year and 46% had been employed for 5 or more years at the job associated with their blood lead test. Sixty-four percent reported they had never received any training about the health hazards of lead. Half reported that they had not been transferred or medically removed from the job they had when their blood lead test was taken. Thirteen percent reported they had been transferred to lower paying jobs. Cases reported a mean of 10 coworkers employed in their immediate work area.

Fifteen (10%) cases had been hospitalized for treatment of lead poisoning. Nineteen percent reported that they were first informed of their blood lead test results by CDHS staff. Nearly one-third reported that their blood lead tests were taken by a private physician, rather than an employer-sponsored screening program. Fifty-eight percent reported one or more symptoms consistent with lead toxicity. Twenty-nine percent reported not having had a previous blood lead test.

Table 11.4 Profile of 149 Index Cases with Elevated Blood Lead Levels, 1988–1990

Item	*N*	%*
DEMOGRAPHICS		
Age		
<25	18	13
25–44	79	56
45+	44	31
Males	141	94
Race or ethnicity		
Hispanic, White	68	46
Non-Hispanic, White	60	41
Black	13	9
Other	6	4
Less than 9th grade education	55	38
Spanish only spoken at home	60	41
Children < 7 years at home	52	35
MEDICAL CHARACTERISTICS		
Hospitalized	15	10
Blood test not done by employer	44	32
Not transferred from exposed job	61	50
Not informed of test results	27	19
Symptoms at interview		
Fatigue	69	48
Joint pain	58	41
Headache	55	39
Nausea	40	29
Constipation	34	24
OCCUPATIONAL CHARACTERISTICS		
Radiator repair	33	22
Lead batteries	20	13
Brass/copper foundry and castings	19	13
Gun firing ranges (sport and police)	18	12
Ceramic tile and pottery	12	8
Construction	9	6
Secondary lead smelting	5	3
Nonoccupational†	9	6
No hours of training	84	64
No ventilation system	45	36
No or disposable respirator	83	62
No clothing change at work	59	45
No showers at work	78	60

*Missing data excluded in calculating percentages.

†Nonoccupational cases include use of dishes with leaded ceramic glaze (2 cases), probable use of folk medicines containing lead (1 case), and 6 cases of unknown etiology, but not likely due to occupation.

Thirty-six percent reported their worksite did not have a ventilation system for the removal of lead dusts or fumes. Forty-two percent reported not using any respirator, and 20% reported using a disposable respirator. Not changing work clothes before leaving work for home was reported by 45%, and not showering before leaving work for home was reported by 60%. Smoking at work was reported by 14%, and eating at work was reported by 88%.

Seven nonresponsive employers were referred to enforcement agencies. Several employers without a supervising physician contracted directly with medical laboratories to draw blood from employees for analysis. Virtually all of the private physicians and many contract industrial physicians charged with carrying out employer medical monitoring programs were unfamiliar with the OSHA lead standard. A few physicians were totally unfamiliar with normal limits of blood lead in adults.

DISCUSSION AND EVALUATION

Because of mandatory reporting of elevated blood lead, the magnitude of California adults with elevated blood has begun to be documented. Compared to the number of notifiable communicable diseases in California,[22] the roughly 1000 annual adult cases puts elevated blood lead as the 10th most frequent condition (after meningitis, 1356 cases). Using 50 μg/dL as a reference, the registry identified 594 cases of adult lead poisoning, nearly all of which would have otherwise gone undetected or without timely follow-up by CDHS, or enforcement agencies.

During the first 3 years, the proportion of reports by industry remained approximately the same. Compared to reports received in 1987, there was a modest decline in the percentage from secondary lead smelting (59% in 1987 versus 46% overall), a small rise in the proportion of reports from lead battery manufacturing (26% in 1987 versus 35% overall), but a large relative increase from radiator repair shops (0.5% in 1987 versus 2.1% overall). The increase in reports from radiator shops can be tied directly to a targeted intervention by CDHS in 1990 in which 141 Los Angeles County radiator repair shops screened 330 individuals for elevated blood lead (Chapter 25).[23]

The interviews of index cases (Table 11.4) document the clustering of well-known risk factors for occupational lead poisoning, including inadequate ventilation, respiratory protection, personal hygiene facilities and practices, nonexistent or poor training and education, and inadequate medical supervision. Lack of showering and clothing changes also increased the risk of take-home exposures in children and other household contacts of the index cases. While the interview data was not externally validated in every case with air sampling for lead or direct observation by industrial hygienists, when CDHS, OSHA, or employers' consultants performed on-site follow-up, air samples and direct observation confirmed the presence of lead overexposures.

Ethnic and racial minority workers were a disproportionate number of cases compared to the general California population, although they may be representative of the industrial population exposed to lead. Nonetheless, these cases require culturally sensitive follow-up, including bilingual interviews. Other high-risk groups included construction and demolition workers, whose initial blood level levels were often highly elevated.

Limitations

The most important potential bias is the undercounting of lead-exposed individuals with elevated blood lead levels who do not have their blood tested periodically for lead. This prevents the full estimation of the prevalence of elevated blood lead among California adults. The 4069 adults with elevated blood lead was of the same order of magnitude as predicted by a statewide survey of employers, in which only 2.6% (5914) of the estimated 229,000 workers with direct exposure to lead were reported to be in routine blood lead monitoring programs.[13]

Undercounting that affects some subgroups more than others creates a bias. For example, data from the California Employment Development Department[24] indicated that there were approximately 14,500 employees in 2790 radiator repair establishments in 1985. However, only three employers, accounting for 15 reports were found in the lead registry in 1987. Similarly, in lead battery manufacturing where there also is a high probability of direct lead exposure, 11 employers accounting for 496 reports were found in the lead registry. In 1985, California employment data indicated that there were 33 employers with 2500 workers in lead battery manufacturing.

Lack of complete information on age, residence, and occupation occurred in a significant proportion of reports. This limits an accurate profile of subgroups where risk may be concentrated and surveillance needs to be expanded.

The timeliness of reporting is another concern for timely case follow-up, particularly for persons with highly elevated blood lead levels. On average, reports were received by CDHS 22 days after blood lead specimens were analyzed by the laboratory. Only 9% of report forms were received by CDHS within 72 hours of analysis as required by the reporting law.

Perhaps the most serious limitation is strategic. Follow-up of the severely elevated cases and individual case management until blood lead levels fall to below 40 μg/dL was a labor-intensive task, even with automated case management techniques. An overall program to reduce the incidence of occupational lead poisoning needs to balance one-on-one case management with broader community-based interventions that eliminate lead exposures before they cause an elevation in blood lead level (Chapter 25).

CONCLUSION

California's blood lead surveillance program indicated the need for intensified lead poisoning surveillance, education, and enforcement. Workers, employers, physicians and other health care personnel, laboratories, and government agencies would benefit from expanded training and education focused on lead-related health problems. Aided by surveillance data, the state legislature passed a law in 1993 that expanded the program in CDHS to prevent occupational lead poisoning.

ACKNOWLEDGMENTS

The authors acknowledge Elizabeth Abello, Arleen Ervin, Corky Hull, MD, Jeffry Jones, M.P.H., Gina Micarelli, M.S., Patricia Sutton, M.P.H, Ana Osorio, M.D., Jon Rosenberg, M.D., Sarah Royce, M.D., Kirsten Waller, M.D., Kevin Tabb, and Betty Woo for their assistance in case follow-up and database management.

Portions of this chapter were published previously in the *American Journal of Public Health* and have been used with permission.

REFERENCES

1. Fischbein A. Lead. In Rom WR, ed. *Occupational and Environmental Medicine*. Second Edition. Boston: Little Brown & Co, 1990.
2. Needleman HL, Gunnoe C, Leviton A, Reed R, Peresie H, Maheo C, Barreto D. Deficits in psychologic and classroom performance in children with elevated dentine lead levels *New Engl J Med* 1979; 300(13):689–695.
3. Code of Federal Regulations. *Lead*. Occupational Health and Safety Administration. 29 CFR 1910.1025. US Government Printing Office, Washington, DC, 1983.
4. Division of Labor Statistics and Research. *Occupational Disease in California, 1989*. San Francisco. California Department of Industrial Relations, 1992.
5. Division of Labor Statistics and Research. *Work Injuries and Illnesses, California, 1991*. San Francisco. California Department of Industrial Relations, 1992.
6. Annest JL, Mahaffey KR, Cox DH, Roberts J. *Health and Nutrition Examination Survey. Blood Lead Levels for Persons 6 Months-74 Years of Age: United States, 1976–1980*. Advanced Data from Vital and Health Statistics, No. 79. DHHS Pub. No (PHS) 82-1250. Hyattsville, MD: Public Health Service, 1982.
7. Pirkle JL, Brody DJ, Gunther EW, et al. The decline of blood lead levels in the United States: the Health and Nutrition Examination Surveys (NHANES). *JAMA* 1994; 272:284–291.
8. Lofgren JP, Schaller K, Payne S, et al. Adult lead epidemiology and surveillance—United States, Second and third quarters 1998, and annual 1994–1997. *MMWR* 1999; 48:213–223.
9. Tepper A. Surveillance of occupational lead exposure in New Jersey: 1986–1989. *Am J Public Health* 1992; 82:275–277.
10. Baser ME, Marion D. A statewide case registry for surveillance

of occupational heavy metals absorption. *Am J Public Health* 1990; 80:162–164.

11. Maizlish NA, Rudolph LA. California adults with elevated blood lead levels, 1987 through 1990. *Am J Public Health* 1993; 83:402–405.
12. Maizlish NA, Rudolph LA, Sutton P, Jones RJ, Kizer K. Surveillance of elevated blood lead in California adults, 1987. *Am J Public Health* 1990; 80:931–934.
13. Rudolph L, Sharp D, Perkins C, Samuels S, et al. Environmental and biological monitoring for lead exposure in California workplaces. *Am J Public Health* 1990; 80:921–925.
14. Hazard Evaluation System and Information Service (HESIS). *Lead, Medical Guidelines.* California Department of Health Services/Department of Industrial Relations, 2151 Berkeley Way, Berkeley, CA, 1988.
15. Hazard Evaluation System and Information Service. *Lead, Fact Sheet.* California Department of Health Services/Department of Industrial Relations, 2151 Berkeley Way, Berkeley, 1985.
16. Keogh JP. Medical surveillance of lead-exposed workers. *Semin Occup Med* 1986; 1:125–130
17. Waller K, Osorio AM. *Lead Exposure in a Tank Demolition Crew.* California Occupational Health Program Pub. No. FI-90-54. Berkeley: California Department of Health Services, 1990.
18. *Standard Industrial Classification.* Office of Management and Budget, Superintendent of Documents, US Government Printing Office, Washington DC, 1972.
19. *California Manufacturers Directory.* Times-Mirror Press, Inc. Los Angeles, CA, 1987.
20. California Occupational Health Program. *Elevated Blood Lead in California Adults, 1987–1990.* Berkeley, CA: California Department of Health Services, 1991.
21. Bureau of Census: General characteristics of persons by Spanish origin and race, 1980. *General population characteristics, California. 1980 Census of Population.* US Department of Commerce. Vol. 1B(6):57, Table 24.
22. Centers for Disease Control. Summary of notifiable diseases, United States, 1989. *MMWR* 1989; 38(54).
23. Bellows J, Rudolph L. Initial impact of a workplace lead-poisoning prevention project: expanded blood-lead testing improves surveillance and focuses follow-up effort. *Am J Public Health* 1993; 83:406–410.
24. California Employment Development Department. *California Employment and Payrolls, October—December, 1986. Report 127.* Sacramento: California Employment Development Department, 1987.

12

Acute Pesticide Poisoning

NEIL A. MAIZLISH, LINDA A. RUDOLPH, AND KATHY A. DERVIN

Approximately 6 billion pounds of pesticides are introduced into the global environment every year. Hundreds of millions of individuals are potentially exposed, and approximately 1 million acute illnesses occur each year and about 1000 die from acute poisoning.[1] The burden of chronic diseases like cancer, respiratory disease, and birth defects due to pesticides is less well-documented, but may be quite large on a global scale. Much of this health burden occurs as a result of occupational exposures.

Pesticides are a large group diverse chemicals with a function to kill or suppress insects, rodents, weeds, fungi, and other pests. There are over 1000 active ingredients in pesticides registered with the U.S. Environmental Protection Agency and over 10,000 different products marketed in the United States.[2] Acute exposure to toxic organophosphates has received most attention because they are life threatening and antidotes are available for treatment. But there are many other pesticides that are not chemically related to organophosphates. The health effects of pesticides involve different organ systems including the skin, eyes, liver, lungs, nervous system, and reproductive system.[3]

California accounts for approximately 10% of all pesticides used each year.[4] In the 1950s and 1960s, agricultural workers harvesting citrus, stone fruits, and grapes—crops with abundant leaf area—experienced mass outbreaks of poisoning due to parathion and other toxic organophosphates, often affecting a 100 or more workers at a time.[5] California's dry climate allowed these pesticides to persist on leaf surfaces (instead of being washed away by rain), creating risks for harvesters in contact with dense foliage.

To prevent poisonings of both harvesters and the workers who mix, load, and apply concentrated pesticides, California has developed what many consider the most comprehensive and strict system of pesticide regulation in the world.[4,6] Several key features include:

- manufacturers must submit health studies as a condition of registration and label the specific uses by crop and pest
- farmers and professional pesticide applicators must pass written certification tests
- farmers and pest control advisors must apply for permits for specific pesticide applications and then report their use
- farm owners must adhere to mandatory time lags (reentry intervals) from when a pesticide is applied to when a worker may enter the field or greenhouse to harvest
- the use of engineering controls such as closed systems for mixing and loading pesticides as well as personal protective clothing are required for toxic pesticides
- agricultural workers must receive education about the risks of pesticides
- farm owners and pesticide application companies must contract with physicians to provide medical monitoring of mixer, loader, and applicators who work with toxic cholinesterase-inhibiting pesticides
- clinical laboratories must pass state-sponsored proficiency tests before offering cholinesterase analysis
- workers with cholinesterase activity inhibited beyond established thresholds must be medically removed from their jobs with the exposure

- pesticide containers must receive appropriate decontamination and disposal
- any suspect or confirmed pesticide illness must be reported

The last requirement is part of public health and labor laws that have been in effect since the early 1970s. Physicians are required to call their county public health officer within 24 hours of treating a suspect or clinically confirmed pesticide illness case, and then follow up with a one-page written form called a Pesticide Illness Report (PIR). For occupational cases, physicians must mail an additional one-page form known as the Doctor's First Report within 5 days of patient contact to the state's labor statistics agency and the local health department. In many of California's 58 counties, each reported case involving agricultural pesticides is then investigated, usually by county agriculture department personnel who enforce the pesticide regulations.[4] Nonagricultural pesticide illnesses are investigated by California's OSHA or jointly by Cal/OSHA and agricultural agencies.

Although the number of suspected cases reported by California physicians has increased since the 1980s, the number of occupational cases confirmed by agricultural authorities has remained within an annual range of 1100 to 1500, after a marked decline from over 3000 in 1970s.[5,7] Nonetheless, there are persistent concerns that pesticide illness is seriously underreported.[8]

Case reporting by California physicians is the basis for a passive surveillance system that is maintained by the California Department of Food and Agriculture (now part of the California Environmental Protection Agency).[7] Into this preexisting reporting system, the California Department of Health Services (CDHS) developed a targeted and active surveillance system in one California county. This is one of several applications of the SENSOR occupational disease surveillance model,[9] supported by the National Institute for Occupational Safety and Health (NIOSH).

METHODS

Goals, Objectives, and Scope

The goal of this surveillance system was to prevent occupational pesticide illness by following up individual cases reported by a network of physicians recruited by the surveillance system.

The specific objectives of the active surveillance system were to:

- enhance the quantity and quality of case reporting
- identify risk factors and high-risk worksites
- link preventive interventions at specific worksites to the broader community

The first objective was a specific response to the concern that occupational pesticide illness may be underreported. Frequent one-on-one interaction with key providers was designed into the surveillance system to stimulate reporting. The second objective is the central idea of sentinel health events: that each case points to a potential lapse in controlling well-recognized occupational exposures.[10] Lastly, feedback must be in place to ensure that preventive interventions are carried out, and they have the desired effect of reducing exposures and preventing additional cases.

Because state agricultural agencies routinely carried out pesticide enforcement activities at the worksites of cases, another purpose of the active surveillance system was to determine whether a public health model of case follow-up would reveal the same or different risk factors and recommendations as the enforcement model.

Identifying the population of workers at risk for rate-based surveillance of pesticide illness was not part of the purpose, and is a difficult task. A significant percentage of the agricultural work force in California are undocumented workers, and a widely publicized immigration amnesty program occurred during the surveillance program. Moreover, employment statistics are not collected by California state agencies[11] at a level of detail that permit pesticide-, crop-, or job-specific estimates for the large number of harvest workers who have many short-term jobs with multiple employers in a dozen or more different crops that are treated with scores of different pesticides.

Geographic Targeting

The scope was limited to a single county. This was necessary to do because the amount of available resources was not sufficient to maintain an active surveillance system with hundreds of providers in a state as large as California. Several California counties were considered based on (*1*) diversity of exposures including agricultural use, manufacturing, and pesticide formulation, (*2*) proximity to the headquarters to reduce travel time and costs, (*3*) a good working relationship and support of the local county health officer, and (*4*) a meaningful volume of pesticide illness cases. Fresno County met these criteria. It has agricultural work force of more than 60,000 on 7000 farms that produce over 250 crops worth an estimated $2 billion annually. Fresno County also ranks among the top counties in pesticide used and the annual number of reported cases.[12]

Assemble Staff

Seven staff (3.7 full-time equivalents) included an occupational physician, an epidemiologist, a health educator, an industrial hygienist, an outreach worker, a data analyst, and a data technician. Because most workers were anticipated to be of Mexican origin, the outreach worker was both bilingual and bicultural to facilitate interviews and educational programs.

Gaining Support

Introductory and regular meetings were held with representatives of county and state organizations, including the county health department, agricultural commissioner's office, the Occupational Safety and Health Administration (enforcement and consultation), labor organizations and farm worker legal advocates, agribusiness groups, pest control professional associations, and the county medical society. The meetings covered the goals of the project and requested ongoing consultation and feedback. This outreach confirmed that the use of pesticides was a divisive community issue, and because of the polarization between organizations representing farm labor, agribusiness, and pest control professionals, community leaders were consulted individually rather than in a group setting.

Community outreach and education activities were targeted to providers and health care professionals, farm workers, agribusiness, pest control professionals, and university-based experts in integrated pest management (Table 12.1). This was done to create positive working relationships between the surveillance team and local organizations.

Case Definition and Data Collection

A case definition was developed for a range of pesticide illnesses including those due to cholinesterase inhibition, other systemic illness, eye contact, dermatitis, and any other type of pesticide illness (Table 12.2). The certainty of confirmation was classified on a five-point scale: definite, probable, possible, uncertain, and not a case. A work sheet was developed that arrayed the criteria for case classification in a probability grid (see Chapter 3). Cases were first compared to the criteria for possible, and then rose or descended based on the information available. After the case definition was drafted, reporting guidelines for providers were developed that reflected the case definition, but were simpler and aimed to educate as well as guide decisions on reporting.

To reduce additional workload for reporters, Pesticide Illness Reports were taken by telephone and fax by project staff on a 24-hour basis. The preexisting report form, which covered patient demographics, description of illness and exposure, and medical treatment, was expanded to include language spoken at home, occupation, crop, and medical treatment (Fig. 12.1).

Select, Recruit, and Train Case Reporters

Survey of Providers

To identify potential providers for case reporting and to obtain a measure of potential underreporting, a survey of county physicians was conducted in Spring 1988. The methodology was based on two different approaches: traditional epidemiologic survey and a snowball sample within the professional networks of key providers. The traditional survey first identified the medical specialties that are likely to treat pesticide illness. Then, all physicians in Fresno County in those specialties were identified using yellow pages phone di-

Table 12.1 Selected Education and Outreach Activities, 1988–1991

Sector	*Activity*	*Audience*
All*	Quarterly reports and updates; press surveillance	County and region
Providers	Annual reportbacks of cases	102
	Accredited continuing medical education	200
	Newsletter, journal articles	300
Workers	One-on-one education	75
	Annual 3-hour radio show and audio-cassette	25,000
	Migrant parent group presentations	100
Employers	Workshops	30
Pest Control Association	Survey of members	350
	Accredited continuing education	100
University	Continuing education	100
	Integrated pest management consultation	2
County health departments	In-service trainings	30
	Cosponsorship of continuing medical education	

*All also includes safety and health enforcement agencies (Occupational Safety and Health Administration and county agricultural commissioner and state counterparts).

Table 12.2 Case Definition of Work-Related Pesticide Illness for Epidemiologic Surveillance in California SENSOR

Pesticide illnesses and pesticide-related conditions for the purpose of epidemiologic surveillance comprise one or more of the following types of illnesses or conditions:

- acute systemic illness or condition due to cholinesterase inhibitors
- acute systemic illness or condition due to noncholinesterase inhibitors
- dermatitis and other topical illnesses or conditions
- pesticide-chemical eye injury

I. ACUTE SYSTEMIC ILLNESS OR CONDITION DUE TO CHOLINESTERASE INHIBITORS

1. Work history consistent with exposure to an organophosphate or n-methyl carbamate pesticide,

- AND -

2. Two or more symptoms of acute OP/carbamate poisoning

- OR -

3. Physical findings
   a. Signs of OP or carbamate poisoning,

   - OR -

   b. Cholinesterase tests with preexisting baselines indicating:
      i. 30% reduction of red blood cell ChE from baseline, OR
      ii. 40% reduction of plasma ChE from baseline

   - OR -

   c. Cholinesterase tests without preexisting baselines:
      i. at least a 15%–20% increase in plasma cholinesterase activity upon retest within 5 exposure-free days after initial test, OR, at least a 30% increase in RBC ChE activity after 90 exposure-free days in serial retests,[1] OR,
      ii. ChE test result below lower limit of laboratory reference range*

*A cholinesterase test that is within the laboratory reference range but without a prior baseline for comparison cannot be used alone to exclude an individual from being a case.

- AND -

4. Appropriate temporal sequence between exposure and onset of illness
   The time between exposure and onset of symptoms or physical findings needs to be consistent with the work history, work practices, toxicology of putative agent, route of exposure, etc.

- AND -

5. Biologic plausibility
   a. Dose-relatedness: correspondence between the symptoms, signs, biologic response, and level of exposure
   b. Epidemic (case) clustering

II. ACUTE SYSTEMIC ILLNESS DUE TO NONCHOLINESTERASE INHIBITORS

1. Work history consistent with exposure to noncholinesterase inhibiting pesticide(s)

- AND -

2. Symptoms of putative agent(s). Hayes[2] and Morgan[3] can be used as references, or CAL/SENSOR staff consultants

- OR -

3. Physical findings:
   a. Signs specific to clinical toxicology of putative agent(s)
   b. Laboratory tests consistent with known toxic effects (e.g., abnormal liver enzymes, BUN, etc.)

- AND -

4. Appropriate temporal sequence between exposure and onset of illness
   The time between exposure and onset of symptoms or physical findings needs to be consistent with the work history, work practices, toxicology of putative agent, route of exposure, etc.

- AND -

5. Biologic plausibility
   a. Dose-relatedness: correspondence between the symptoms, signs, biologic response, and level of exposure
   b. Epidemic (case) clustering

III. DERMATITIS AND OTHER TOPICAL ILLNESSES

1. Work history consistent with exposure to a pesticide that is a primary contact irritant, or allergic contact irritant. Pesticides cited by Adams[4] can be used as a reference.

Continued

- AND -

2. Symptoms of dermatitis (itching, pain, visible eruptions, self-observation of patient)

- OR -

3. Physical findings
   a. physical examination of skin or conjunctiva, or both
   b. patch test for allergic contact dermatitis

- AND -

4. Appropriate temporal sequence between exposure and onset of illness
   The time between exposure and onset of symptoms or physical findings needs to be consistent with the work history, work practices, toxicology of putative agent, route of exposure, etc.

- AND -

5. Biologic plausibility
   a. Dose-relatedness: correspondence between the symptoms, signs, biologic response, and level of exposure
   b. Epidemic (case) clustering

IV. PESTICIDE-CHEMICAL EYE INJURY

1. Work history consistent with focal, ocular exposure to one or more pesticides.

- AND -

2. Symptoms of chemical eye trauma

- OR -

3. Physical findings
   a. Physical examination of eye
   b. Laboratory tests

- AND -

4. Appropriate temporal sequence between exposure and onset of illness
   The time between exposure and onset of symptoms or physical findings needs to be consistent with the work history, work practices, toxicology of putative agent, route of exposure, etc.

- AND -

5. Biologic plausibility
   a. Dose-relatedness: correspondence between the symptoms, signs, biologic response, and level of exposure
   b. Epidemic (case) clustering

[1]Coye MJ, Barnett PG, Midtling JE, Velasco AR, Romero P, Clements CL, Rose TG. Clinical confirmation of organophosphate poisoning by serial cholinesterase analyses. *Arch Intern Med* 1987; 147:438–442.
[2]Hayes WJ. *Pesticides Studied in Man*. Baltimore: Williams and Wilkins, 1983.
[3]Morgan DP. *Recognition and Management of Pesticide Poisonings*. 4th Edition. USEPA 540-/9-88-001; 1989.
[4]Adams RM. *Occupational Skin Disease*. Philadelphia: WB Saunders, 1990.

rectories as the sample frame. A brief, four-page questionnaire was developed to inquire about the number of pesticide cases the provider treated in the prior calendar year, the number that were occupationally related, and the physicians they referred cases to or received referrals from. The questionnaire also asked about professional education and interest in continuing education in pesticide diagnosis and treatment. Approximately two-thirds of the questionnaires were self-administered by mail and one-third were administered by telephone. Of 491 providers identified, 169 reported treating 342 work-related pesticide illnesses in 1987—compared to 308 in the preexisting reporting system.[7]

The snowball sample identified a handful of prominent physicians, farm worker legal advocates, and community figures. Ten individuals were interviewed using a semistructured, informal telephone format that had the same content as the formal questionnaire. At the conclusion of each interview, the contact (snowball starter) was asked to name another knowledgeable person in their personal and professional network who could also identify prominent physicians or clinics that treat pesticide illnesses and handle referrals. This process was repeated two to three times when no new hospitals, occupational medicine practices, and rural clinics were mentioned. The prominent providers using this approach were largely the same as the traditional survey in which all providers were contacted.

Selection of Providers

The survey results and a few additional case reporters listed in the preexisting passive surveillance system in the 2 previous years were used to identify candidates for a sentinel provider network. Physicians and nurses

State of California – Health and Welfare Agency — Department of Health Services

MODIFIED PESTICIDE ILLNESS REPORT*

PATIENT: Physician Report Date: / /

Name: Age: Sex: M F
Address: City: County:
Phone No.: ( ) Social Security No.:
Occupation: Language: _____English _____Spanish _____Other

INJURY:
At address: City County:
Was injury [ ]1 At home [ ]2 At Work – agriculture [ ]3 At Work – nonagriculture [ ]4 Other exposure
If at work: a) Employer's name and address:

b) Manager or Supervisor

Date of exposure: / / Time of Exposure: Date of Illness: / / Date of death: / /

Is there reason to believe others were exposed? [ ]1 No [ ]2 Yes [ ]3 Don't Know If yes, how many? _____
Is there reason to believe others had symptoms? [ ]1 No [ ]2 Yes [ ]3 Don't Know If yes, how many? _____

PATIENT'S DESCRIPTION OF EXPOSURE:
Activity at time of exposure [ ]1 Applying pesticides [ ]2 Manufacturing pesticides [ ]3 Mixing pesticides
[ ]4 Entering pesticide areas [ ]5 Disposing of pesticides or their containers [ ]6 Eating contaminated food
[ ]7 Other exposure (explain):

Name of pesticide(s): Ingredients of pesticide(s):

Name of crop(s):
Primary route of exposure: [ ]1 Oral [ ]2 Dermal [ ]3 Eye [ ]4 Inhalation [ ]5 Unknown

PHYSICIAN'S DESCRIPTION OF EXPOSURE
Date first seen: / / Time first seen:
Major signs, symptoms, adverse reactions:

Hospitalized? [ ]1 No [ ]2 Yes If yes, hospital name: City:
Hospital phone: ( )
Emergency room only? [ ]1 No [ ]2 Yes
Physician's office only? [ ]1 No [ ]2 Yes
Physician (name and address): Physician phone: ( )

Diagnostic studies orders? [ ]1 No [ ]2 Yes If yes, which studies?
Diagnosis: Treatment:

Brief description of incident (if female, indicate if pregnant):

AGENCY COMPLETING FORM:

Name/Agency/County:

Pesticide illness reporting is required by California Health and Safety Code (See back of this form, Part 1 and Part 2)
Please complete as much information as possible and submit form promptly.

* PIR form modified for Fresno County (1/91)

Figure 12.1 Pesticide Incident Report Form as modified by the Cal/SENSOR Project. California physicians are required to report suspected and confirmed pesticide illness to their county health officer within 24 hours of diagnosis.

Table 12.3 Work-Related Case Reports of California SENSOR Providers by Practice Setting, 1988–1991*

Type of Facility	*Number of Facilities*	*Cases Reported* N	%
Occupational health practice	3	94	49
Hospital emergency room	3	37	20
Rural community health center	4	19	11
County health departments†		40	22
Total	10	190	100

*16 providers in Fresno, Madera, or Tulare County with an agricultural case were included in 1991.

†Excludes 27 cases classified as unlikely.

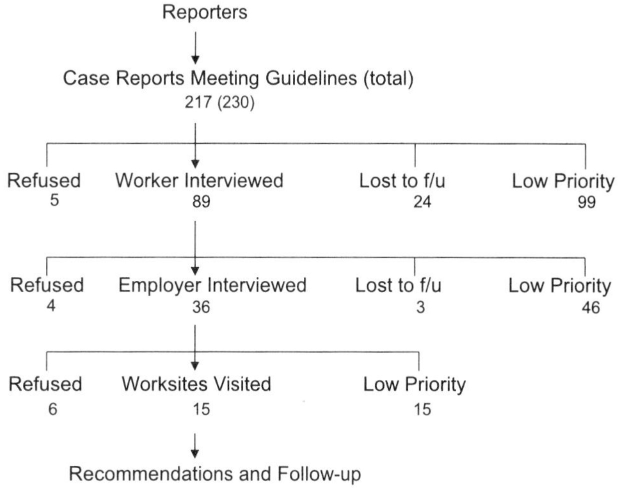

Figure 12.2 Protocol for follow-up of cases of reported pesticide illness, California SENSOR. (Maizlish et al.[17])

from 10 medical facilities were selected by applying criteria of urban and rural distribution and a diversity of practice settings, including emergency, occupational, family practice, and migrant health clinics (Table 12.3).

Recruitment

The 102 members of the medical and clerical staffs were then recruited in face-to-face meetings, starting in mid-1988. Participation in the preexisting passive system was obligatory but participation in the active system was voluntary. All institutions consented to participate. Some providers expressed concern over the confidentiality of patient medical records. This concern was allayed by existing state laws that protect the confidentiality of information requested by public health authorities. The surveillance project had also been approved by the state's institutional review board for the protection of human subjects.

Training

Reporters were given a manual covering reporting requirements, reporting guidelines, report forms, CDHS medical monitoring guidelines,[13] a list of pesticide names, and other educational materials.

To promote reporting, shortly after reporting a case, participants received a recent journal article on the same pesticide implicated in their case report. Interest in reporting was also maintained by organizing continuing education events, providing case summaries, and reports of field investigations triggered by their case reports.

Protocol for Follow-up

A protocol was developed to receive case reports, and to sequence and prioritize follow-up activities based on probable pesticide-relatedness, severity and clustering of cases, and the suitability of agricultural cases for the intervention component of the surveillance model (Fig. 12.2). No fatal cases occurred, but hospitalized cases including those treated in emergency rooms, and mini-clusters of three or cases independent of treatment setting were considered priorities for follow-up.

The prioritized cases were then followed up, first, with a 50-minute telephone or face-to-face standardized interview, and then, conditioned on patient approval, telephone contact with the employer for a 30-minute structured interview. Up to three coworkers, if any, mentioned by the index case were also interviewed. To protect employee confidentiality, workers were offered the choice of being personally identified (or not) in employer interviews. Employers almost always knew the identity of cases before being contacted by CDHS. This occurred because case reports in the passive surveillance system were automatically routed to agricultural enforcement agencies who contacted employers. Employers regarded CDHS's attempts to conceal the identity of cases, especially at small work sites, as coy and evasive. This led to the hostile termination of several initial interviews. The protocol was reevaluated and workers were offered a choice of having CDHS contact their employer or not, and if contact was permitted, an additional choice was offered to maintain anonymity or to allow personal identification. Almost all workers who authorized employer contact did not object to personal identification.

The employee questionnaire consisted of demographics; a narrative of events by the worker; symptoms; treatment setting and payment for medical bills; prior medical conditions and medications; workdays lost, if any; employment history over the past 6 months; activities at the time of the exposure incident or illness; contact with skin or clothing with contaminated work surfaces; use of protective equipment; method of notification of pesticide application; field sanitation and personal hygiene;

training; and number and names of coworkers in the same incident. After completing the interview, cases received written information in English or Spanish.

The employer questionnaire consisted of demographics and business activities; health care provider for pesticide illness; activities of workers during exposure incident; history of pesticide application of fields where workers were present; personal protective equipment provided and used; employer's opinion of why the incident occurred; training frequency and procedures; source of information for pesticide illness prevention; and name of grower's pest control advisor, if any. In agricultural cases, the employer interview included a brief questionnaire on pest control practices. The responses were reviewed by an entomologist from a local university who worked with the surveillance project to help identify alternatives to the pesticide applications.

Worksites that were agricultural pest control companies or farms were prioritized for an on-site visit. Employer permission was requested, and a site visit was scheduled.

Case Management

Data were keyed from case report forms and questionnaires into an automated administrative database to assist case managers track cases through successive stages of follow-up. Cases were reviewed weekly to assure compliance with the protocol, make appropriate referrals, and to identify (*1*) gaps in the protocol, (*2*) missing information to confirm cases, and (*3*) illustrative cases for educational purposes.

Field Investigations and Community Interventions

Field investigations were carried out on-site by surveillance staff. The investigations consisted of a walk-through of operations and confidential interviews of employers and workers to evaluate engineering controls, equipment maintenance, training, medical monitoring, work practices, administrative practices, hazard communication, and personal protective equipment. The investigations took place independently of and immediately after enforcement inspections, in which Cal/SENSOR staff would observe, but not participate. The on-site inspection was followed up with a written 7- to 10-page report sent to the employer who was requested to disseminate the report to employees. Summaries in English or Spanish were sent to cases.

To broaden this traditional health hazard evaluation model, university-based pest management professionals were brought to selected worksites to identify the reasons for using the pesticide implicated in a case. These pest management professionals also offered growers consultation in alternative strategies to minimize future pesticide use based on integrated pest management (IPM) principles.[14] At 6-month to 1-year intervals, employers were contacted by telephone to determine if the recommendations were implemented.

Analysis and Interpretation

Frequency distributions of data reported by providers in case reports were summarized on a quarterly basis. Industry was coded using Standard Industrial Classification codes.[15] Pesticides were classified into functional use categories and chemical classes, using standard references.[2,3,16]

Cases were confirmed into the categories of definite, probable, possible, uncertain, and not pesticide related (Table 12.2). Case confirmation was done quarterly, using standardized forms and procedures and all available information, including case reports, interview data, and, reports of field investigations done by project staff or enforcement agencies, when available. Final analysis of interview data excluded cases judged not pesticide related.

Feedback and Recommendations

Providers were visited each year for a personalized project update. They also received summaries of their cases and follow-up, journal articles of cases similar to those reported, a newsletter, and annual accredited continuing medical education (Table 12.1). In addition to one-on-one education of workers as cases, annual 3-hour radio shows featuring local panelists on pesticide recognition, treatment, and prevention were aired on a local bilingual radio station at prime listening times. A tape of the radio shows was edited into a cassette that was distributed to farmworkers by the local outreach worker. A 20-minute video that tied pesticide health and safety and integrated pest management was developed for farmers. The video featured local farmers and information from the active surveillance system.

Annual updates were held with community leaders. Staff monitored local newspapers for pesticide and agriculture-related stories to improve awareness and sensitivity to local viewpoints.

Worksite-specific recommendations of field investigations were disseminated to providers, employers and employees, enforcement and other government agencies, and to employer trade groups. Final recommendations were a product of annual project evaluation, which helped define areas in which the surveillance system and intervention model were working or not and needed change.

Evaluate Functioning of System Model

Changes in provider reporting were evaluated using data from the preexisting reporting system that contains data from both Pesticide Illness Reports and Doctor's First Reports. Cal/SENSOR providers were name- and/or institution-matched and compared to non-Cal/SENSOR providers in the same county from 1986 through 1990. Data in the preexisting reporting system were used to calculate frequencies and means to examine temporal trends in reporting and to assess representativeness of cases based on age, sex, industrial classifications, and other variables. To eliminate distortions in reporting due to large epidemic clusters, secondary cases of clusters with five or more case reports were excluded from analysis for both Cal/SENSOR and non-Cal/SENSOR providers.

Field investigations were compared to enforcement activities by searching the text of respective reports for matching recommendations, if present.

RESULTS

Forty-five of 102 providers employed in four rural clinics, three occupational health practices, and three hospital-based emergency departments, each reported a case from October 1988 through 1991 (Table 12.3). Of 230 cases reported, 217 cases from 80 worksites met reporting guidelines for suspect, work-related cases. Applying the case definition to these cases, 142 (66%) were confirmed as definite, probable, or possible, 48 (21%) were uncertain because of missing information, and 27 (13%) were unlikely to be pesticide related, though most of these were work-related exposures to fertilizers or other agricultural chemicals. Excluding unlikely cases, three occupational health practices accounted for 49% of all work-related cases. The 230 Cal/SENSOR case reports comprised 28% of all cases reported in Fresno county from 1988 to 1990, during which 243 providers reported 827 cases using Pesticide Illness Reports, Doctors First Reports, or both.

Of 116 cases selected for follow-up, 89 (77%) completed interviews, 5 refused, and 24 (21%) were lost to follow-up (Fig. 12.2). Three workers objected to contacting their employers after the interview. Of 40 cases whose employers were selected for additional follow-up, 36 employers (90%) completed interviews and 4 refused to do so. Of 21 worksites selected for field investigations, 15 were visited, and 6 (29%) employers refused. In median days, reports were received 1 day after treatment, worker interviews were completed 5 days later, employer interviews were completed 7 days afterwards, and worksite visits were completed 19 days after the employer interview. Written reports were available 66 days after the site visit.

Case Report Demographics and Occupational Characteristics

Excluding 27 reports classified as unlikely, cases (N = 190) were on average 35 years old (standard deviation, 11; range 18 to 61), mostly male (3:1), and Spanish-surnamed. Nearly half spoke Spanish at home, and half were employed in agriculture (Table 12.4). Cholinesterase-inhibiting organophosphates or carbamates were identified in 40% of case reports, and con-

Table 12.4 Demographic and Occupational Characteristics of 190 Work-Related Cases Reported by California SENSOR Providers, 1988–1991*

Item	N	%†
Men	139	75
Spanish surname	137	73
Language spoken at home		
English	67	51
Spanish	65	49
Industry (SIC Code)‡		
Agriculture (01–09)	91	47
Grape farm	16	
Aerial spraying/dusting	15	
Deciduous tree fruit farm	12	
Manufacturing (20–39)	44	23
Poultry slaughtering	23	
Corrugated and solid fiber boxes	10	
Pesticide formulation	8	
Services (70–89)	13	7
Wholesale trade (50–51)	11	5
Transportation, utilities (40–49)	7	4
Public administration (91–97)	4	2
Construction (15–17)	2	1
Retail trade (52–59)	1	1
Agent§		
Organophosphate	71	36
Sulfur	36	18
Chlorine, hypochlorites	33	17
Pyrethrins	9	5
Propargite	9	5
N-methyl carbamates	7	4
Organochlorines	5	3
Others	27	14
Functional Use Category§		
Insecticide	97	49
Antimicrobial disinfectant	34	17
Fungicide	34	17
Miticide	10	5
Herbicide	5	3
Other	19	9

*Excluding 27 cases classified as unlikely.
†Missing data excluded in calculation of percentages.
‡Standard Industrial Classification code.
§More than one pesticide in some case reports.

tact irritants such as sulfur and propargite were identified in approximately one-quarter. Insecticides were nearly half of all identified agents; antimicrobial disinfectants and fungicides each comprised 17%. There were no fatalities and four cases were hospitalized for 7 days. There were 3 large epidemic clusters, involving 10 workers exposed to pyrolysis products of pesticides during a fire at an adjacent pesticide formulation plant; 23 poultry processing workers exposed to a chlorine gas; and, 15 office products workers exposed to a pyrethrin-containing insecticide after a structural pest control treatment.

Worker and Employer Interviews

Excluding eight unlikely cases, interviewed workers ($N = 81$) were demographically similar to those not interviewed. Educational attainment was lowest among agricultural workers, only 13% of whom completed high school (Table 12.5). Illnesses were characterized by symptoms of headache and dizziness (72%), nausea (59%), skin rash (64%), or eye irritation (73%). Fifty-one percent lost none or 1 workday due to their illness, and 36% lost between 4 and 16 days. Eleven workers (14%) reported being required to work while becoming ill, lacking prompt medical care, or being required to pay for medical treatment. Twenty-nine percent of interviewed index cases reported that coworkers in the same exposure episode did not seek medical treatment.

A majority of workers, both agricultural (51%) and nonagricultural (54%), reported not receiving any training in pesticide hazards by their employers. Agricultural cases were distributed among 31 field workers and 22 workers who either mixed, loaded, or applied pesticides as farm employees or employees of agricultural pest control companies. Among agricultural cases, 70% of mixer-loader-applicators and 33% of field workers recalled having read or seen the label of the pesticide they were exposed to or were working with. Lack of toilets at the worksite were reported by roughly one-third of cases. Eight of 53 agricultural workers (15%) reported urinating or defecating in the fields. The proportion of cases reporting the lack of hand washing facilities (34%), drinking water (43%), and showering facilities (79%) was greatest among agricultural workers. Only 19% of agricultural workers changed out of their work clothes at the end of their shift.

All nonagricultural workers and all mixer-loader-applicators had heard of workers' compensation before their illnesses. However, nearly 40% of all workers reported that workers' compensation was not the expected source of payment for medical bills. Among the field workers, 20% had not heard of workers' compensation, and only 47% reported it as the source of payment of their medical bills for the pesticide illness.

Eighteen (50%) of 36 interviewed employers attributed the illness to carelessness of the worker, and 9 (25%) attributed the illness to workers not wearing personal protective equipment, or to environmental conditions (19%). Virtually all respondents reported having a safety training program using written materials (89%), a training video (74%), a hands-on demonstration (95%), or a slide show (17%).

Table 12.5 Characteristics of 81 Interviewed Cases Reported by California SENSOR Providers, 1988–1991*

	Agricultural†		*Nonagricultural*	
Item	*N*	%‡	*N*	%
Educational attainment				
Grade school	34	67	1	4
Some high school	10	20	2	8
High school graduate	7	13	21	88
Coworkers not seeking medical treatment	14	26	6	25
Medical bills paid by workers' compensation	30	57	15	65
Field sanitation provided				
Toilet	32	60	16	67
Hand washing facilities	35	66	18	75
Drinking water available	30	57	21	88
Showers at worksite	11	21	9	38
Change clothes after work	10	19	7	29
No training	27	51	13	54
Shown or read label	20	38	4	17

*Excluding 8 cases classified as unlikely.

†Agricultural workers were made up of 31 field workers and 22 workers who mixed, loaded, or applied pesticides as employees of farms or pest control companies.

‡Missing data were excluded in calculating percentages.

Table 12.6 Field Investigations at Index Case Worksites in California SENSOR Surveillance System, 1988–1991

Type of Worksite	*N*	*Activity at Exposure*	*Pesticides*
Farm*	8	Application	Methomyl, diazinon, glyphosate
		Drift	Azinphos-methyl, propargite
		Field work	Cryolite
		Equipment maintenance	Methidithion
Pest control service†	3	Mixing, loading application	Azinphos-methyl, mevinphos, naled profenphos, endosulfan
Packing shed‡	2	Sorting	Chlorine
		Fumigation	Sulfur dioxide
Formulation	1	Clean-up	Dimethoate
		Bagging	Carbofuran
School	1	Application	Glyphosate, Surflan

*Citrus, grapes, stone fruit, walnuts, and vegetables.
†Two aerial and one ground application services.
‡Citrus and grapes.

Field Investigations

Field investigations were carried out at eight farms, three pest control companies, two packing sheds, one pesticide formulation facility, and one school yard (Table 12.6). Most involved exposure to toxic organophosphates and carbamates. Industrial hygienists of CDHS identified risk factors for pesticide illness including inadequate safety training, nonexistent or inadequate medical monitoring, lax supervision, inadequate personal protective equipment, engineering flaws in aerial application equipment, improper respirator use and a lack of respirator fit testing. Integrated pest management specialists were brought on-site or provided consultation at three worksites. In total, 117 specific recommendations were made to employers that reflected routine and serious inadequacies in their health and safety program (Table 12.7). Of these, only seven were identified in enforcement reports of the same worksites. Nineteen recommendations, however, were related to regulations of the state Occupational Health and Safety Administration (OSHA) and 20 (17%) were related to pesticide use reduction using integrated pest management, areas not included in pesticide use enforcement. The local agricultural enforcement agency cited two employers for violations of the agricultural safety code, and made one recommendation that was not made by Cal/SENSOR.

Table 12.7 Comparison of Recommendations of CAL/SENSOR and Agricultural Enforcement Agencies at Worksites Visited by CAL/SENSOR, 1988–1991

	CAL/SENSOR		*Agricultural Enforcement**
Agency Item	*N*	*%*	*N*
Administrative practices	24	21	0
Medical monitoring	16	14	2
Respiratory protection	15	13	0
Other personal protective equipment	15	13	2
Training	10	9	1
Equipment maintenance	3	2	0
Engineering controls	3	2	1
Posting or entry	3	2	0
Pesticide use reduction	20	17	—
Other	8	7	1
Total	117	100	7

*Agricultural enforcement agency issued two citations for violations of the agricultural safety code, and made one recommendation not made by Cal/SENSOR.

Evaluation of Reporting

The number of reports of Cal/SENSOR providers doubled between 1987 and 1988, and plateaued during 1989 and 1990 (Fig. 12.3). Increased reporting among two of the three occupational health practices, and one of the two hospital emergency rooms accounted for most of the increase. While reporting of antimicrobial disinfectants such as chlorine, sodium hypochlorite, and quaternary ammonium compounds increased for both Cal/SENSOR and non-Cal/SENSOR providers after 1987, Cal/SENSOR providers had proportionately more of these reports (Table 12.8). During 1989 and 1990 (years in which data for age, sex and Standard Industrial Classification were coded in the preexisting reporting system), Cal/SENSOR cases had the same mean age (35 years), a slightly higher proportion of women, and proportionately more agricultural employment compared to non-Cal/SENSOR cases. The number of reports of non-Cal/SENSOR providers peaked in 1987, decreased slightly in 1988, and then fell to levels above the 1986 baseline for 1989 and 1990.

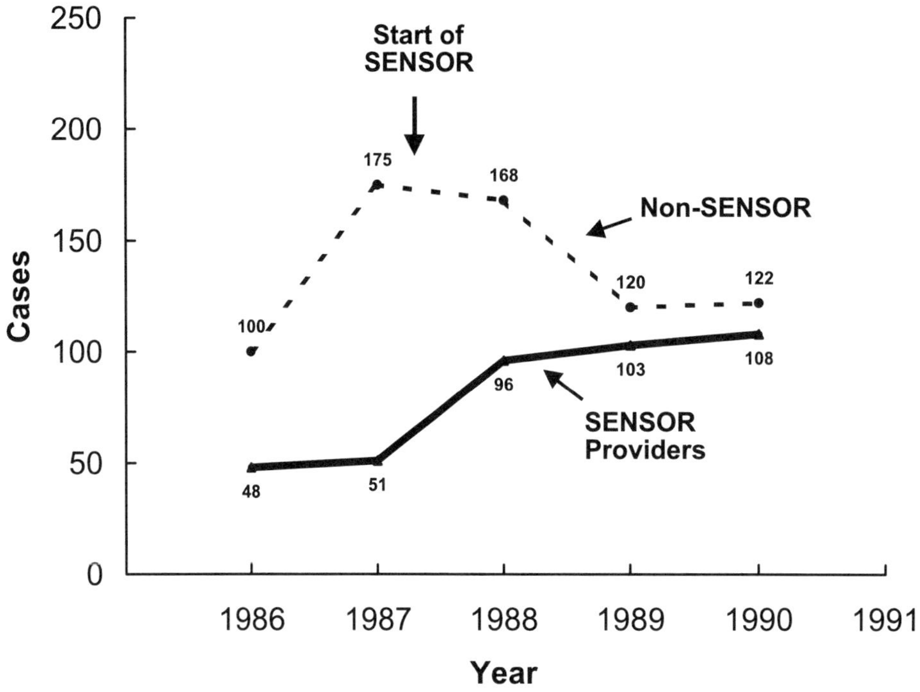

Figure 12.3 Reporting of pesticide illness by Cal/SENSOR and non-Cal/SENSOR health care providers as detected by the preexisting, mandatory reporting system, 1986–1990. (Maizlish et al.[17])

Table 12.8 Characteristics of Cases Reported by Cal/SENSOR and non-Cal/SENSOR Providers

	CAL/SENSOR†		*Non-CAL/SENSOR*	
Item	N	%*	N	%
Men	169	80	216	89
Industry‡ (Standard Industrial Classification) [SIC]				
Agriculture (01–09)	96	48	102	40
Manufacturing (20–39)	33	17	63	25
Services (70–89)	33	17	54	21
Transportation, utilities (40–49)	11	5	11	4
Wholesale trade (50–51)	10	5	10	4
Retail trade (52–59)	8	4	8	3
Public administration (91–97)	7	4	7	3
Construction (15–17)	2	1	2	1
Primary pesticide implicated§				
1986–1987				
Organophosphate and carbamates	16	40	40	34
Sulfur, propargite, glyphosate	10	25	23	19
Chlorine, hypochlorites, NH_4	0	0	5	4
Others	14	35	50	42
1988–1990				
Organophosphate and carbamates	37	22	38	22
Sulfur, propargite, glyphosate	26	15	50	28
Chlorine, hypochlorites, NH_4	40	24	28	16
Others	65	39	60	34

*Missing data excluded in calculation of percentages.
†Includes all suspect and confirmed cases.
‡Age, sex, and SIC coded only for 1989–1990 data.
§Based on California Environmental Protection Agency data for which primary pesticide was determined.

DISCUSSION

This is an example of an active surveillance system that linked case-reporting in real time to worksite follow-up. The specific objectives were realized: the quality and quantity of reports were increased compared to the passive reporting baseline. Case interviews revealed a clustering of risk factors for pesticide illness among index cases that was verified by direct observation at selected worksites, but that went undetected by enforcement agencies.

These findings need to be placed in context of strengths and weaknesses of the surveillance system and its setting. The surveillance methodology was not population-based, so the magnitude of the problem was not estimated in terms of the rates of illness.

Much infrastructure for reporting and follow-up was already in place before the active surveillance program started. The existing legal requirement for reporting made participation more attractive for physicians. The protection of confidentiality was another potential barrier to participation. Preexisting laws and approval by a human subjects committee helped allay concerns about disclosure of patient information.

Fresno County is among the most developed settings for pesticide illness prevention activities in California. Resources are frequently available for continuing medical education and it is the site of the regional poison control center. Universities and state colleges offer active programs in integrated pest management and safety training. Relative to other counties, Fresno County has a large agricultural enforcement program with personnel trained in standardized data collection, and an automated system to track pesticide use. This suggests that counties and states with less infrastructure and fewer resources would not fare as well in case detection and follow-up.

Of note, during the active surveillance project, Fresno County experienced the worst draught in modern times resulting in agricultural water rationing and scaled back planted acreage. In 1990, Fresno County experienced an unusual winter frost that heavily damaged fruit trees, threw thousands of farm workers out of work, and diminished the population of some overwintering pests. The net result of all these environmental factors was to reduce pesticide use and farm worker exposure. Cal/SENSOR providers' increased reporting may be a conservative estimate had normal environmental conditions prevailed.

Enhancing the Quantity and Quality of Reports

Providers participated and doubled their reporting from 50 to about 100 cases per year compared to the pre-Cal/SENSOR baseline. No Cal/SENSOR provider dropped out. The increase in reports was primarily due to mild and moderate cases exposed to antimicrobial disinfectants and other nonorganophosphate pesticides. This was probably the direct consequence of distributing educational materials to each provider that included a list of antimicrobial disinfectants. The percentage of reports that were not related to pesticides (13%) and were uncertain (21%) was about the same as the passive system.[7]

The active surveillance program was able to collect data of broader scope and depth than that available through the preexisting passive surveillance system. Some of this information shed light on possible underreporting. For example, in interviews, approximately 30% of cases reported that coworkers involved in the same exposure incident did not seek medical treatment. This is the minimum interaction with the health care system in either the active or passive surveillance systems. Workers were extremely reluctant to provide their coworkers' names, limiting the ability to verify this finding. Nonetheless, other questionnaire responses suggest there are several barriers to complete case ascertainment. Interviewed workers reported knowing about workers' compensation, but a significant percentage, especially among field workers, did not indicate workers' compensation as the expected source of payment for medical bills. A significant percentage of workers also alleged incidents of employment discrimination because of their illnesses, some of which directly involved responsibility for payment of medical bills. Low-income workers, especially those with only seasonal work and limited English language skills, would not be expected to jeopardize their jobs except for treatment of the most serious illness. In contrast to the early 1970s when widespread lack of knowledge of workers' compensation among agricultural workers was documented,[8] claim discouragement and threats of discrimination may be more significant issues in the 1980s and 1990s.

Identification of Worksite Risk Factors

Compared to the Cal/SENSOR approach, traditional enforcement had a low yield for identifying and controlling risk factors at specific worksites. Although receiving training related to enforcement, agricultural personnel are not trained health and safety specialists. Crop inspection activities often preempted all but the most urgent pesticide illness investigations. Moreover, none of the inspectors worked full-time on pesticide health and safety. At the worksites visited by Cal/SENSOR, no agricultural inspector was fluent in Spanish. Inspectors do not have direct responsibility for enforcement of nonpesticide occupational health safety. That responsibility lies with the Occupational Safety and Health Administration.

Linking Case Finding to Worksites and Broader Interventions

Part of the feedback was in the form of questioning the effectiveness of existing prevention strategies in a population of workers that has many barriers such as low literacy, limited English language skills, cultural and racial differences from their employers, high work demands in hot climates, and night work. This led the surveillance system to promote ways to eliminate and reduce exposure by bringing integrated pest management professionals to worksites where pesticide illnesses had been reported. This was not a mandate of enforcement authorities, but well within a public health model. An important element of acceptance by employers was distancing participation in the Cal/SENSOR program from the enforcement activities. Employers were receptive to this kind of consultation as a follow-up to a pesticide illnesses.

CONCLUSIONS

The active Cal/SENSOR surveillance system was an independent evaluation of the 2 decade-old passive surveillance system linked to a traditional enforcement approach. Given that California's system is a model for other states and countries, the Cal/SENSOR project suggests that there are many unmet challenges in occupational pesticide illness prevention.

The preexisting system of passive surveillance and follow-up, largely based on regulation and enforcement, has played an important role in reducing acute, serious work-related pesticide illness from historical highs in the 1970s. During the 1980s, occupational pesticide illness became endemic with an annual incidence of 1000 to 2000 cases. Further reduction will require a change in strategy by enforcement agencies, changes in pest management practices, or both. An expansion of integrated pest management practices that are sensitive to worker health and safety is an avenue for further pesticide illness prevention. Officials in California's Department of Pesticide Regulation have acknowledged that the observations made by the active surveillance system helped spur efforts to improve their enforcement activities.

ACKNOWLEDGMENTS

The authors acknowledge the participating health care providers, workers, and employers, without whom this project would not have been possible. Financial support and technical assistance was provided through a cooperative agreement with the National Institute for Occupational Safety and Health, and consultation in project evaluation was provided by the Public Health Practice Program Office, Centers for Disease Control and Prevention. Feedback and technical support was provided by the staff of the Fresno, Madera, and Tulare County Health Departments; Fresno County Department of Agriculture; Fresno County Farm Bureau; California Rural Legal Assistance; Madera-Fresno Medical Society; California State University (Fresno); University of California Statewide IPM Programs and Kearney Field Station; University of California Cooperative Extension Agricultural Labor Management Program; the California Public Health Foundation; and the Worker Health and Safety Branch, California Environmental Protection Agency. Lupe Ortiz, Kate Cummings, Jim Bellows, Barbara Materna, Arleen Ervin, Elizabeth Abello, and Susan Payne are acknowledged for their valuable assistance in data collection and analysis.

Portions of this chapter were published previously in the *American Journal of Public Health* and have been used with permission.

REFERENCES

1. WHO/UNEP Working Group. *Public health impact of pesticides used in agriculture.* Geneva: World Health Organization; 1990.
2. *Farm Chemicals Handbook, 1991.* Willoughby, Ohio: Meister Publishing; 1991.
3. Hayes WJ. *Pesticides Studied in Man.* Baltimore: Williams and Wilkins, 1983.
4. Stimmann MW. Pesticide use and regulation. In: Scheuring AF, ed. *A Guidebook to California Agriculture.* Berkeley: University of California Press, 1990:272–279.
5. Maddy KT, Edmiston S, Richmond. Illness, injury, and deaths from pesticide exposures in California, 1949–1988. *Rev Environ Contam Toxicol* 1990; 114:57–123.
6. California Code of Regulations. *Title 3. Agriculture.* Pest Control Operations, 1993.
7. Mehler L. *Summary of Illness and Injuries Reported by Physicians as Potentially Related to Pesticides, 1995.* Sacramento: California Department of Pesticide Regulation, 1997 (and preceding years).
8. Kahn E. Pesticide illness in California. *J Occup Med* 1976; 18: 693–696.
9. Baker EL. Sentinel Event Notification System for Occupational Risks (SENSOR): the concept. *Am J Public Health* 1989; 79(suppl):18–20.
10. Rutstein DD, Mullan RJ, Frazier TM, Halperin WE, Melius JM, Sestito JP. Sentinel events (occupational) for physician recognition and public health surveillance. *Am J Public Health* 1983; 73:1054–1062.
11. *Labor Market Information Division.* Sacramento: California Employment Development Department, 1997.
12. Insalaco C. *Annual Crop and Livestock Report, 1989.* Fresno, CA: Fresno County Department of Agriculture, 1989.
13. California Development of Health Services. *Guidelines for Physicians: Medical Monitoring of Pesticide Exposed Workers.* Berkeley, CA: California Development of Health Services, 1989.
14. Flint ML, van den Bosch R. *Introduction to Integrated Pest Management.* New York: Plenum Press, 1981.
15. Office of Management and Budget. *Standard Industrial Classification Codes.* 1987 Rev., Washington, D.C.: U.S. Government Printing Office, 1989.
16. Morgan DP. *Recognition and Management of Pesticide Poisonings.* 4th Edition. USEPA 540-/9-88-001; 1989.
17. Maizlish NA, Rudolph LA, Dervin KA. Surveillance of work-related pesticide illness: an application of the Sentinel Event Notification System for Occupational Risks (SENSOR). *Am J Public Health* 1995; 85:806–811.

13

Carpal Tunnel Syndrome

NEIL A. MAIZLISH, LINDA A. RUDOLPH, AND KATHY A. DERVIN

Carpal tunnel syndrome (CTS) is a disorder of the median nerve as it crosses an anatomical tunnel in the wrist formed from bone, ligament, and tendon. Forceful and repetitive motions over time, especially when done in an awkward hand posture, damage soft tissues that swell and entrap the median nerve. The severity of illness ranges from reversible mild symptoms of pain, cramping, numbness and tingling in the thumb and adjacent fingers to irreversible nerve damage, atrophy of the fleshy thumb muscle, and permanent disability.[1–3]

Carpal tunnel syndrome is one of several cumulative disorders (CTDs) of the upper extremities that include tendinitis, tennis elbow (epicondylitis), trigger finger, thoracic outlet syndrome, and Reynaud's disease (white finger). State[4,5] and national[6] data in the United States show a 14-fold increase in the incidence of work-related CTDs over the last 2 decades—from 23,800 in 1972 to 332,000 in 1994. High rates of cumulative trauma disorders associated with repetition or force have been found in the garment industry, automobile manufacturing, meat packing, and electronics assembly (Table 13.1).

This chapter illustrates active surveillance using a sentinel events model at the California Department of Health Services (CDHS). Sentinel applies in two ways. First, the outcome—CTS—is a sentinel health event/occupational (SHE/O), a preventable condition that is occupational in a significant proportion of cases.[7] Second, CDHS recruited a network of physicians and other health care professionals to report cases. This is a sentinel network. The National Institute for Occupational Safety and Health (NIOSH) played a pivotal role in promoting experimentation among states to improve surveillance in its Sentinel Event Notification System for Occupational Risks (SENSOR).[8] Work-related CTS was selected because it was one of the priority conditions identified by NIOSH, and a growing problem in California (Fig. 13.1).[5]

This chapter contrasts with those of lead (Chapter 11) and pesticide poisoning (Chapter 12), where the existence of standards and a history of enforcement strongly influenced the follow-up strategy. (This surveillance project was done before the passage of the California ergonomics standard in 1997.) A passive surveillance system was already in place.[5] This formed the legal basis of case reporting for physicians, who are required to report all work-related illness within 5 days of the patient visit using a mailed Doctor's First Report form (Appendix A).

METHODS

Goals, Objectives, and Scope

The objectives were to:

- enhance the quantity and quality of case reporting
- identify risk factors and high-risk worksites
- link preventive interventions to specific worksites
- extend the interventions to the broader community

The scope was brought in line with the available resources by geographic targeting of a single county. The criteria used for selecting the county were proximity to the surveillance center, diversity of industries and occupations, a population large enough to generate a meaningful number of cases for follow-up, and a sympathetic local health officer. Santa Clara County—home of the Silicon Valley—met the criteria and has a

Table 13.1 Private Sector Industries with the Highest Incidence Rates of Injuries and Illnesses from Repetitive Motion Resulting in Days Away from Work, 1994

*Industry**	*SIC† code*	*1994 annual average employment (in thousands)*	*Incidence rate (per 10,000 workers)*	*Number of cases*
Knit underwear mills	2254	25	165.6	370
House slippers	3142	3	146.3	48
Men's and boy's work clothes	2326	42	117.2	463
Textile bags	2393	11	115.7	117
Potato chips and similar snacks	2096	35	115.2	406
Motor vehicles and car bodies	3711	335	113.9	4058
Hats, caps, and millinery	235	21	103.9	202
Meat packing plants	2011	138	98.5	1402
Bras, girdles, and allied garments	2342	12	96.2	111
Wood products, not elsewhere classified	2499	58	92.8	515
Men's and boy's suits and coats	231	40	89.1	320
Electronic coils and transfers	3677	17	87.0	142
Men's footwear (excluding athletic)	3143	28	84.9	221
COMPARISON INDUSTRIES				
All manufacturing	2, 3	18,319	27.0	49,278
All private industry		94,146	11.5	92,576
Finance, insurance, and real estate	6	6707	8.1	5046

*The high-risk industries listed are in the manufacturing sector not the service sector.
†SIC, Standard Industrialization Code.
Source: Bureau of Labor Statistics.[6]

diverse industrial base of old and new industries (e.g., semiconductor and computer manufacturing), and a large service economy.

Gain Support

Introductory and regular meetings were held with representatives of county and state organizations, including the county health department, the state Occupational Safety and Health Administration (OSHA), labor organizations, large and small business associations, ergonomics professionals, and the county medical society. The meetings covered the goals of the project and requested ongoing consultation and feedback. These representatives were consulted individually rather than in a group setting (Table 13.2).

Assemble Multidisciplinary Staff

Seven staff (3.7 full-time equivalents) of the Cal/SENSOR Project included a physician, an epidemiologist, a health educator, an ergonomist, a data analyst, a data technician, and an English/Spanish bilingual interviewer.

Case Definition and Data Collection

The case definition combined symptoms, signs, and laboratory tests for the medical diagnosis of CTS with evidence of work-related risk factors such as a job with repetition, force, awkward hand posture, vibration, or pressure (see Chapter 3 and Table 13.3).[9]

Because case reporters did not always conduct complete physical examinations or report their results, questions arose whether compelling cases that had missing exclusion criteria would meet the definition. Practical problems such as these were resolved by building levels of probability into the case definition: definite, probable, possible or suspect, and not a case (Chapter 3). Even though probability levels made the definition more complex, it also made classifying more rapid and consistent.

A data collection form was designed to capture information needed for the case definition and prioritizing follow-up (Fig. 13.2). To minimize the workload to physician reporters, the half-page report form was designed to supplement the preexisting Doctor's First Report form (Appendix A). The form covered patient demographics, general description of illness and exposure, medical treatment, coworkers at risk, presence of specific symptoms, signs, laboratory findings, and work-related risk factors.

Mail and manual data abstraction were the mechanisms for reporting. Reporters were provided with business reply envelopes and nearly all mailed in their reports. One hand surgeon and a health maintenance

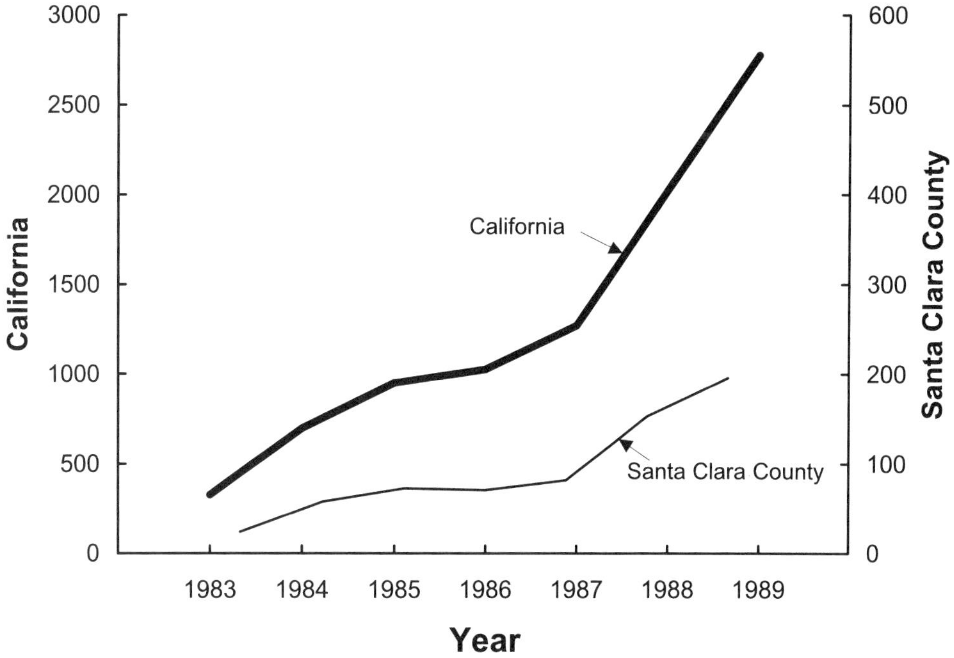

Figure 13.1 Cases of work-related carpal tunnel syndrome reported by California physicians, 1983–1989, using Doctor's First Reports, California and Santa Clara County. (Division of Labor Statistics and Research.[5])

organization found mailing too burdensome, and the surveillance staff visited their offices periodically and manually abstracted case files onto the data collection form.

Selecting, Recruiting, and Training Providers

Two different approaches were used to identify potential case reporters: (*1*) a countywide survey[9] based on contacting every health care provider, and (2) a survey of a sample of community leaders and their professional network.

Traditional Survey

Medical specialties likely to treat CTS were identified. Using the yellow pages of county telephone directories as a listing source, 1698 health care personnel, practices, and hospitals in these specialties were key entered into a database. A 17-item questionnaire was developed that asked about the number of work-related and

Table 13.2 Selected Education and Outreach Activities, 1989–1991

Sector	*Activity*	*Audience*
All*	Quarterly reports and updates	County and region
	Press surveillance and coverage	
Providers	Annual reportbacks of cases	54
	Newsletter	200
Workers	One-on-one education	120
	Union stewards trainings	300
	Radio shows—Spanish and English	10,000s
	Targeted outreach at community clinic for monolingual Spanish workers	100
Employers	Conference on ergonomics	100
	Survey of members of business association	300
Safety professionals Ergonomists	Bimonthly roundtable of scientific and practical exchanges	50
	Presentations	100
Government	U.S. Congressional hearings	10,000s

*All also includes safety and health enforcement agencies (OSHA regional and state counterparts).

Table 13.3 Case Definition for Work-Related Carpal Tunnel Syndrome for Epidemiologic Surveillance, California SENSOR Project, 1987–1992

For the purpose of epidemiologic surveillance, cases of work-related carpal tunnel syndrome must match the following criteria:

1. Work history consistent with risk factors of carpal tunnel syndrome.
   a. Frequent, repetitive use of the same hand or similar movements of the hand or wrist on the affected sides(s)

   - or -

   b. Regular tasks requiring the generation of high force by the hand on the affected side(s)

   - or -

   c. Regular or sustained tasks requiring awkward hand position on the affected side(s) (i.e., extreme extension, flexion of wrist; radial, ulnar deviation; various pinch grips)

   - or -

   d. Regular use of vibrating hand tools or contact with vibrating surfaces

   - or -

   e. Frequent or prolonged pressure over the wrist or base of palm on the affected side(s).

AND

2. Physical findings consistent with carpal tunnel syndrome
   a. Abnormal nerve conduction velocity or latency for the distal median sensory nerve. Abnormal is defined as values falling outside the laboratory range, or, in the absence of laboratory normals, abnormal is
      i. nerve conduction velocities of less than 38 meters per second
      ii. sensory nerve latency greater than 3.5 milliseconds
      iii. motor nerve latency greater than 4.4 milliseconds

   - or -

   b. Positive Tinel's or Phalen's sign or decreased or absent sensation to pin prick in the median nerve distribution or evidence of thenar atrophy

   - or -

3. Symptoms of pain or tingling or numbness affecting at least part of the median sensory nerve distribution of the hand. Symptoms must have lasted more than a week or occurred on multiple occasions (> 1 episode of symptoms)

AND

4. Appropriate consideration of associated and mimicking conditions:
   a. Absence of acute trauma in the recent past

   - AND -

   b. Clinical exclusion of mimicking conditions:
      i. cervical nerve root compression
      ii. generalized peripheral neuropathy
      iii. thoracic outlet syndrome
      iv. pronater teres syndrome

   - AND -

   c. Clinical exclusion of associated conditions:
      i. rheumatoid arthritis
      ii. insulin-dependent diabetes
      iii. documented hypothyroidism
      iv. gout
      v. pregnancy
      vi. oophorectomy

AND

5. Logical Temporal Sequence
   a. Symptom onset after date of hire
   b. Symptoms become worse after date of hire (exacerbation)

State of California – Department of Health Services
California Occupational Health Program

INSTRUCTIONS TO PROVIDERS

SENSOR Project
01/91

Please fill out this form when you see a case of carpal tunnel syndrome that meets our reporting guidelines. If accompanied by a Doctor's First Report (DFR) please staple the two forms together.

PATIENT INFORMATION
Please complete all blanks including addresses and phone numbers. If a DFR is attached, there is no need to complete the shaded portion.

SUBJECTIVE COMPLAINTS
These complaints refer to symptoms in the distribution of the median nerve. The number of co-workers with similar symptoms can include those co-workers in the same worksite who do not perform exactly the same tasks as the patient.

MEDICAL HISTORY
Check all that are present.

JOB CHARACTERISTICS
Based on the information the patient provides
Repetition: Does the job consist of performing repetitive tasks of the upper extremities during the workday?
Unnatural Wrist Posture: Is the wrist used in a posture other than neutral, i.e., lateral deviation, flexion, extension, rotation/wringing motion?
Force: Does the job require much hand and upper limb strength or generation of force to perform?
Palm/Wrist Pressure: Is there direct pressure to the wrist or palm during work, i.e., pressure points on the wrist, tool handles digging into palm?
Prolonged Constrained Postures: Does the patient hold one posture for long uninterrupted periods of time throughout the workshift?
Vibration: Does the work involve exposure to vibration of the upper limb (i.e, use of vibrating hand tools, contact with vibrating surfaces)?
Pinch Grip: Are the thumb and finger opposed in a forceful closed grip?

OBJECTIVE FINDINGS
Circle + for positive or – for negative or ND for not determined for those physical tests. For NCV indicate if velocity or latency, and specify lab normals

CAL/SENSOR - CARPAL TUNNEL SYNDROME CASE REPORT

Today's Date ___/___/__
mo dy yr

____
Provider Name (please print)

SUBJECTIVE COMPLAINTS
(Circle all that apply)

pain	R	L
paresthesia	R	L
numbness	R	L
weakness	R	L

Symptoms awaken at night? _Y _N
Symptoms present ≥ 1 week? _Y _N
Did symptoms start with acute trauma? ? _Y _N
Date of symptom onset ___/___/___

__# lost work days
__# co-workers w/similar symptoms

PAST MEDICAL HX OR HX
(Check all that apply)
__ cervical root nerve compression
__ generalized peripheral neuropathy
__ thoracic outlet syndrome
__ pronator teres syndrome
__ rheumatoid arthritis
__ hypothyroidism
__ diabetes (ID)
__ gout
__ bilateral oophorectomy

Currently pregnant? __Y __N

JOB CHARACTERISTICS
(Check all that apply)
__ repetition
__ force
__ unnatural wrist posture
__ palm/wrist pressure
__ prolonged constrained posture
__ vibration
__ pinch grip

Date of hire: ___/___/___
Diagnosis work-related? Y N DK
__# co-workers w/similar job duties
Hours/shift___

OBJECTIVE FINDINGS
(Circle all that apply)

	R			L		
Tinel's	+	-	ND	+	-	ND
Phalen's	+	-	ND	+	-	ND
Pinprick	+	-	ND	+	-	ND
Thenar Atrophy	+	-	ND	+	-	ND

Median Sensory Conduction
___Distal Latency ____ ____
___Velocity(m/sec) R L
___ pending ___ND
Motor Nerve Conduction
___Distal Latency (msec) ____ ____
___Velocity (m/sec) R L
___pending ___ND
Please specify laboratory normal ranges: Sensory ____-____/ Motor ____-____

PATIENT INFORMATION

PATIENTNAME: ____________________
Last First MI
SSN ____-___-____ Chart # ____________
Race/Ethnicity: _White _Black _Hisp. _Asian _Other__
Specify

Address ____________________
____
City State Zip
Phone (___)________ DOB __/__/__ Sex: _F _M
Occupation ____________________
Tasks ____________________
Employer ____________________
Employer Phone (_____)____________
Worksite address ____________________
Street
____
City State Zip
Industry ____________________

Comments ____________________

Date Received ___/___/___ DHS Case # ____
mo dy yr

Figure 13.2 Attachment used to report cases of carpal tunnel syndrome. This was used in combination with the Doctor's First Report (Appendix A).

nonwork-related CTS cases seen in their offices during 1987, the names of specific health care providers that referred cases, the names of providers to whom they referred cases, and the sources of information to diagnose and treat occupational health problems. The questionnaire was administered using a combination of the telephone and mail. Approximately 25% of the list was contacted by telephone and the rest were contacted by mail. The list was randomized so that each specialty would have a representative number of telephone interviews. However, in specialties with fewer than 20 contacts, each provider was interviewed by telephone.

The response rate was 40% for the telephone interviews, and 30% overall. Of 1698 providers, 489 reported treating 7214 cases of CTS in 1987 (Table 13.4). Of these, 3413 (47%) were believed by the respondents to be work-related. In 1986, only 82 cases of work-related CTS were officially reported in the preexisting passive reporting system. Moreover, a dozen providers, mostly in specialties of hand surgery, neurology, and occupational medicine, were remarkable for their high numbers of cases. Also, a few physicians were consistently named as referrals for occupational health expertise. These popular providers were considered potential candidates for recruitment into the sentinel network.

Informed Network Sample

An alternative method to identify high volume providers was based on sampling within the social and professional networks of opinion leaders. Using their own experience, project staff identified a short list of persons they believed to be highly knowledgeable about occupational health or cumulative trauma disorders in Santa Clara County. These included prominent members of university-based occupational health clinics, private practitioners in occupational medicine, workers' compensation insurers, and ergonomics consultants. Each person was interviewed by telephone using an informal but structured questionnaire that asked about the number of cases he or she treated and referral patterns. At the conclusion of the interview each was asked to name several other persons in their professional network that the project staff should interview. These second-level contacts were then interviewed. Because so many of the names overlapped at the second level, third-level contacts were not pursued. Thirty-one individuals were interviewed, 11 of whom reported treating 315 cases of work-related CTS.

The two different surveys provided not only overlapping names of potential candidates for the sentinel network, but also information about health care services for patients with CTS. In particular, the large proportion of cases seen by chiropractors influenced the decision to include chiropractors in the sentinel network, even though the median number of cases per chiropractor was low (Table 13.4). Besides the number of cases, additional criteria for selection included geographic distribution in the county and a *diversity* of settings and specialties. These included hand surgery, neurology, occupational health, family medicine, vocational rehabilitation, occupational therapy, and chiropractic.

Fourteen different institutions were selected as the sentinel network, and the 54 members of their staffs were then recruited in face-to-face meetings. All institutions consented to participate. Reporting of work-related CTS was mandatory for physicians but participation in the Cal/SENSOR Project was voluntary.

Table 13.4 Reported Cases of Carpal Tunnel Syndrome by Health Care Provider—Santa Clara County, California, 1988

		All CTS	*Work-Related CTS Cases*	
Specialty	*Providers*	*Cases*	N	*Median*
Chiropractic	95	1659	759	4
Neurology	22	1032	515	28
Internal medicine	116	1352	413	2
Family practice	65	627	346	2
Hand surgery	6	378	315	38
Occupational/industrial medicine	11	300	281	12
Orthopedics	39	592	272	5
Physical therapy	19	199	169	3
Rheumatology	12	384	107	6
Rehabilitation medicine	2	50	25	25
Emergency medicine	10	53	21	3
Other	92	588	190	—
Total	489	7214	3413	—

Source: Cummings et al.[9]

Confidentiality of patient medical records was assured under existing state laws. Reporters were given a manual covering reporting requirements, specific SENSOR reporting guidelines (Chapter 3), report forms, and educational materials including journal articles on the clinical and occupational aspects of CTS.[10]

Protocols for Follow-up

Cases classified initially as possible were followed up if symptomatic coworkers or a large number of coworkers with similar work were also reported on the report form. Follow-up consisted of telephone interviews and worksite visits (Fig. 13.3). Employers of cases in manufacturing or service industries also had priority. Cases associated with computer keyboards and terminals were not accorded a high priority for worksite visits by the surveillance team. Because prevention measures were already available,[11] they were provided with information and referred to consultants for controlling these ergonomic hazards.

When data provided by the employer indicated high CTS rates or clustering of cases, the employer was requested in writing to seek the assistance of the Cal/SENSOR project or an outside consultant by a deadline. High rates of CTS were defined as:

- a worksite- or department-specific annual period prevalence of 5% or greater, or
- an incidence ratio of 2 or more based on the observed number of surgical or workers' compensation cases

The expected number of cases was based on the number of workers at the workplace or the case's department and a background rate of 1 case per 1000 person-years.[12] If the employer was not responsive, a certified letter was sent proposing a referral to enforcement agencies. No referrals to Cal/OSHA had to be made.

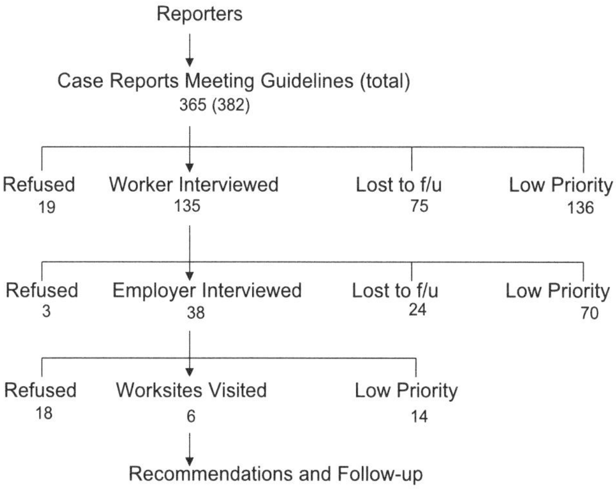

Figure 13.3 Protocol for carpal tunnel syndrome case follow-up, California Sentinel Event Notification System for Occupational Risks.

Interviews

Prioritized cases were first followed up with a 50-minute standardized telephone interview, and then, conditional on the worker's approval, telephone contact with the employer for a 30-minute structured interview. Up to three coworkers mentioned by the index case were also interviewed by telephone. The worker questionnaire consisted of demographics; symptoms; treatment setting and payment; workdays lost; prior medical conditions, medical treatment history; employment history; and employment status and social reaction to the illness. After completing the interview, cases were mailed educational materials in English or Spanish.

The employer questionnaire consisted of company demographics and business activities; number of known cases, including those involving surgery and workers' compensation; number of workers in the same job and department as the reported cases; presence of jobs involving hand repetition and force, tools, and other ergonomic risk factors; and, training frequency and procedures. At the conclusion of the interview, employers were asked if they would like the ergonomist in the CDHS surveillance project to conduct a voluntary and free evaluation of the work areas of the case and other problem areas suggested in the interview. If employer permission was obtained, a site visit was scheduled.

Employers who had a worksite visit were contacted by telephone at 6-month intervals to follow-up worksite visits. Using a standardized questionnaire, the recommendations from site visits were reviewed to determine which had been implemented and the barriers experienced by employers.

Collect and Code Data

Case report forms, questionnaires of workers and employers were entered into separate database files and relationally linked with a common identifier. Four-digit Standard Industrial Classification (SIC) codes were used to describe the industry,[13] and five-digit Standard Occupational Classification (SOC) codes were used for the occupation.[14]

Case Management

The original report form, questionnaires of worker and employer, correspondence, and contact notes collectively made up a paper case file. Each case that met the criteria for follow-up was assigned to a member of the surveillance team who was responsible for carrying out the follow-up protocol. An automated administrative database assisted managers track cases through successive stages of follow-up. Case management meetings were held at approximately monthly intervals with the entire surveillance team to make appropriate referrals, and to identify difficulties in the protocol, missing information to confirm cases, and case studies for educational purposes.

Field Investigations and Broader Interventions

Field investigations were on-site investigations conducted by an ergonomist-led team to identify uncontrolled risk factors and recommend preventive interventions at the index cases' workstation and other work areas. Investigations usually lasted up to 4 hours, and were walk-throughs of operations and confidential interviews of employers and workers. Investigations used simple instruments, such as measuring tapes, stopwatches, goniometers, or Wagner scales to evaluate repetition, force, posture, and contact stresses. The team examined the design of workstations, tools, work practices, administrative practices, hazard communication, medical department records, and training. The site visit was followed up with a written 7- to 10-page report containing recommendations. The report was sent to the employer who was requested to disseminate the report to employees. A sample report is shown in Appendix H.

Broader interventions based on community outreach and education were also targeted among health care professionals, workers' organizations, business associations, and ergonomists and other safety professionals. These activities were designed to maintain reporting, facilitate community liaison, and provide education (Table 13.2).

Analyze and Interpret Data

Data reported by providers in case reports were summarized on a quarterly basis using simple descriptive statistics (means, frequencies). Descriptive statistics were analyzed for worker and employer questionnaires annually. Analyses included demographics and occupational characteristics of workers, medical characteristics and treatment of CTS, risk factors for CTS, training, and social consequences of their illness. Cases were confirmed into the categories of definite, probable, possible, uncertain, and unlikely, based on the case definition. Case confirmation used all available information, including case reports, interview data, and reports of field investigations done by project staff. Final analysis of interview data excluded the unlikely cases.

Feedback and Recommendations

Providers received annual summaries of cases and their follow-ups, and a newsletter. In addition to one-on-one education of cases, group training sessions were provided to union stewards representing workers in the local food industry. Radio shows aimed at monolingual Spanish-speaking workers were aired on local radio stations at prime listening times. Cal/SENSOR conducted an ergonomics needs assessment survey for members of a key 300-member business association, and followed up by cosponsoring a conference that featured national, state, and local experts, including Cal/SENSOR providers. Staff monitored local newspapers to gain awareness of local viewpoints.

Worksite-specific recommendations of field investigations (without identifying the employer or cases) were disseminated to providers, employers, employees, government agencies, and employer trade groups. Final recommendations were a product of annual project evaluations that helped define areas in which the surveillance system and intervention model were working or not and needed change.

Evaluation of the Surveillance Model

Several different evaluations were carried out during the 5-year project. These addressed the questions of impact, effectiveness, and technical efficiency:

- To what degree was the surveillance project contributing to solving the health problem?
- Was the surveillance project achieving its goals?
- Was the project running efficiently?
- What impact was the project having?

Evaluation and planning started with analyzing the problem. This was done to make sure that the surveillance system was useful and focused on solving the central problem—the high incidence of work-related CTS. The technique used was a logic tree of the determinants and contributing factors to work-related CTS (Chapter 9). This was done at an early stage in the project, and the causal web was examined periodically for opportunities to insert surveillance and surveillance data as part of a broad intervention strategy. For example, as a response to the contributing factor of "the lack of knowledge of available solutions" Cal/SENSOR convened an ongoing roundtable of local ergonomic experts to share solutions among themselves and their clients.

Formal evaluations were done in week-long retreats each project year. The content of the evaluation coincided with the life cycle of the project: establishing the sentinel network and case reporting (years 1–2), linkage to worksites and follow-up (years 3–4), and broader interventions and impact (year 5). Frank discussions among project staff examined the degree to which each project goal was being met, and whether the major activities were positive, negative, and which program elements needed change. For example, although identifying cases through the sentinel network was met as a goal, promoting preventive interventions at the worksites had limited success. Most employers declined access to project staff. At worksites where the surveillance team had conducted site visits, employers were generally unable to implement the recommendations. This type of effectiveness evaluation spurred midcourse changes in strategy to promote employer education.

Periodic analysis of surveillance data was also used to evaluate whether the cases reported by the sentinel network were representative. In midproject, analyses suggested that Latino workers were underrepresented compared to the general county work force. Lack of access to health services among Latinos is widely documented, but it was unknown to what degree this played a role in the sentinel network. To explore this possibility, a new member of the sentinel network was added—a primary care clinic that served a large blue-collar Latino community. Clinic staff were trained and other clinics in the sentinel network became referral centers. As part of a broader educational campaign on CTS in the Latino community, this clinic was identified as a gateway to CTS diagnostics and referral services.

Evaluation of the technical efficiency of the project was an ongoing activity in response to specific problems. Some high volume case reporters found case reporting burdensome. In response, project staff manually abstracted cases at their offices periodically. The additional workload was offset by the large volume of cases. Some aspects of technical efficiency were evaluated using descriptive statistics, such as the time steps between successive parts of the surveillance system (case reports, worker interview, employer interview, worksite visit, report with recommendations).

Technical attributes of surveillance systems mentioned by Klauke et al.[15] were evaluated: sensitivity, positive predictive value, representativeness, and timeliness. Sensitivity of the *preexisting* passive surveillance system was evaluated using a capture-recapture technique (Fig. 13.4).[16] The overlap of cases in the preexisting reporting system and Cal/SENSOR cases was evaluated for cases during 1987, 1988, 1989. The Cal/SENSOR cases were matched using name, social security number, and date of birth as matching criteria. Nonmatches were inspected manually, which yielded a small number of additional matches. Positive predictive value (false-positive case reports) was the percentage of reports that were either uncertain or were noncases. To examine representativeness, case reports from each source (Cal/SENSOR and Doctor's First Reports) were compared on their distribution of age, sex, and industrial classifications.

List 1: SENSOR	List 2: DLSR Yes	List 2: DLSR No	
Yes	19 (a)	(b)	141 (L)
No	403 (c)	(d)	
	422 (M)		N (a+b+c+d)

Formula	Example
$\text{Expected(a)} = \frac{L \times M}{N}$	$19 = \frac{141 \times 422}{N}$
$N = \frac{L \times M}{\text{Expected(a)}}$	$3132 = \frac{141 \times 422}{19}$

Figure 13.4 Example of capture-recapture technique to estimate the prevalence of work-related carpal tunnel syndrome in Santa Clara County. For the same time period, List 1 from Cal/SENSOR had 141 cases and List 2 from the Division of Labor Statistics (DLSR) had 422 cases. Nineteen (19) cases overlapped on the two lists. In general, the expected value of overlap (a) is given by the product of the marginal values (L, M) divided by the total prevalence, N. In this sample, an estimate of the overlap (a) is 19. Rearranging the terms to solve for N, we estimate the prevalence at 3132 cases. Because of variability in small samples, a more exact formula is $N = [(L + 1) \times (M + 1)/(a + 1)] - 1$, which gives a slightly smaller estimate of 3002. There are several assumptions that must be met to give accurate estimates: the lists are independent, all the true matches have been identified (no false positives or false negatives on either list), and the population from which the cases are drawn is closed. *Closed* implies that the population is not increasing or decreasing in time and there are no cases entering from other geographic areas. Seldom are all these assumptions met.[16]

RESULTS

From January 1989 to December 1991, 54 providers in 14 Santa Clara County facilities sent 382 case reports to Cal/SENSOR. Of these, 365 reports from 195 worksites met reporting guidelines for suspect, work-related cases. Eighty percent were classified as definite, probable, or possible, 20% were classified as uncertain, and 2 cases were classified as unlikely. One hand surgeon reported 45% of all cases (Table 13.5).

Table 13.5 Work-Related Case Reports of California SENSOR Providers by Practice Setting, 1989–1991—Santa Clara County

Type of Practice	*No. of Providers*	*No. of Facilities*	*Cases Reported* N	*Cases Reported* %
Hand surgeon*	4	2	170	47
Physical therapy clinic	5	2	45	12
Health maintenance organization	~20	1	40	11
Vocational rehabilitation	2	1	25	7
Neurologist	1	1	22	6
Occupational health	12	2	21	6
Primary medicine clinic	5	1	21	6
Union stewards	1	1	8	2
Chiropractor	2	2	4	2
Community clinic	2	1	3	1
Total†	54	14	359	100

*One hand surgeon alone reported 45% of all cases

†Note: Excludes 4 cases with missing provider and 2 reports classified as unlikely.

Table 13.6 Demographic, Occupational, and Medical Characteristics of Work-Related Cases Reported by California SENSOR providers, 1989–1991

	Cases		*Employers*	
Item	N	%*	N	%
Total Work-Related Cases†	363	100	195	100
Demographics				
Women	270	79		
Spanish surname	70	21		
Black	15	9		
Industry (SIC Code)				
Manufacturing (20–39)	104	35	58	30
Electronic computers (357)	39		17	
Semiconductors (367)	13		9	
Services (70–89)	67	23	56	29
Medical and surgical hospitals (8062)	10		8	
Retail trade (52–59)	48	16	28	14
Grocery stores (5411)	34		14	
Public administration (91–97)	34	11	18	9
Police, public order, safety	10		4	
Transportation and utilities (40–49)	14	5	8	4
Construction (15–17)	11	4	11	6
Agriculture (01–09)	10	4	8	4
Finance, insurance, real estate (60–67)	5	1	5	3
Wholesale trade (50–51)	4	1	3	2
Symptoms				
Pain	260	79		
Numbness	231	69		
Parethesia	194	58		
Nocturnal symptoms	170	51		
Weakness	146	44		
Signs				
Phalen	177	53		
Tinel	156	47		
Pin prick	40	19		
Thenar atrophy	20	6		
Abnormal Nerve Conduction	25	8		

*Missing data excluded from percentages.

†Excludes 2 cases meeting reporting guidelines but classified as unlikely.

Of 200 cases prioritized for follow-up, 135 (68%) completed interviews, 19 refused (10%), and 46 (23%) were lost to follow-up (Fig. 13.3). Twenty-four workers objected to having their employer contacted. Of 41 cases whose employer was selected for additional follow-up, 38 employers (93%) completed telephone interviews and 3 (7%) refused. Of 24 worksites selected for field investigations, 6 were visited, and employers at 18 (75%), refused to participate.

Case Reports

Cases were on average 40 years old (standard deviation = 10; range: 19–68) and mostly female (4:1); 21% were Spanish-surnamed and 9% were African-American (Table 13.6). There were 105 different 4-digit Standard Industrial Classification codes distributed among 195 different employers. Multiple cases from the same worksite were reported among 35 employers (18%). Manufacturing accounted for nearly one-third of cases, and services for one-fifth. Multiple cases were reported among computer and electronic equipment manufacturing, semiconductor manufacturing, retail grocery stores, and public service and governmental agencies.

Cases had a high prevalence of symptoms of pain, numbness, paresthesia, nocturnal pain, and weakness in the distribution of the median nerve (Table 13.6). Phalen and Tinel signs were positive in a majority of cases. Thenar atrophy was found among 6% of cases, and abnormal slowing of nerve conduction was reported in 8% of cases.

Interviewed workers ($N = 135$) were demographically similar to those not interviewed. Educational attainment was high (Table 13.7). However, only 6% reported receiving any training from their employer on job-related ergonomics hazards; 63% of cases reported knowing of at least one additional symptomatic coworker. A high proportion of cases characterized their jobs as repetitive, excessively forceful, and involving pinch grips, or awkward postures.

Cases received a wide range of treatments (Table 13.7): 57 cases (42%) reported undergoing surgery, 16 (12%) went on medical leave (range 2–480 days; median 22 days), and 83 (65%) reported a work restriction (range 1–365 days; median 2 weeks). Median workdays lost was 12, and 69% reported losing 1 or more workday due to their illnesses. Twenty-five percent of cases reported that symptoms appeared within 1 year of hire or starting the job that was associated with their case of carpal tunnel syndrome. Median latency—time between start of the job and physician treatment—was 4.0 years. Among 57 surgical cases, median time between start of the problem job and surgery was 5.0 years. Thirteen (9%) workers reported quitting their jobs, 6 (4%) reported being fired due to their illnesses, and 24 (18%) reported being transferred to another job, which resulted in a loss of wages for 9 of them. In 52% of cases, the known or expected source of payment for medical bills was employer-paid health insurance. Workers' compensation was reported as the source of payment for only 29%.

Interviewed employers ($N = 38$) had the same industrial distribution as noninterviewed employers. Nearly all employers were familiar with the CTS, and nearly all reported knowing of other symptomatic workers besides the index case (Table 13.8). At least 15 employers reported workers' compensation cases of CTS in the last 12 months, and 7 reported a case involving surgery. Only 8 employers (21%) had a health care provider on site, 13 (39%) had a regular physical

Table 13.7 Characteristics of 135 Interviewed Cases Reported by California SENSOR Providers, 1989–1991*

Item	N	%
High school graduate	116	86
Received job training in ergonomics	6	14
RISK FACTORS		
Repetition	134	99
Wrist bent for most of day	114	86
Workstation not adjustable	89	66
Pinch grip	81	61
Excessive force	65	49
Pressure on hand or wrist	48	37
Vibration	18	14
TREATMENTS		
Splints	118	91
Analgesics	114	88
Physical therapy	88	65
Work restriction	83	65
Exercise	71	57
Rest	70	56
Surgery	57	42
Steroid injections	46	36
Chiropractic	16	12
TIME BETWEEN INITIAL JOB EXPOSURE AND DEVELOPMENT OF SYMPTOMS		
< 6 months	12	11
6 months–1 year	15	14
1–4 years	27	25
4–10 years	35	32
10+	20	18
SOURCE OF PAYMENT FOR MEDICAL BILLS		
Employer-paid health insurance	57	52
Workers' compensation	32	29
Employee-paid health insurance	7	6
Employee out-of-pocket	4	4
Other	10	10

*Missing data excluded from percentages.

Table 13.8 Characteristics of 38 Interviewed Employers of Cases Reported by California SENSOR Providers, 1989–1991

Item	N	%*
Number of Employees		
1–9	3	9
10–99	8	24
100–499	8	24
500+	14	42
Health and safety committee	28	76
Familiar with carpal tunnel syndrome (CTS)	34	90
Aware of symptomatic workers besides index case	36	95
Worksite evaluated for CTS risks	12	32
Hazard reduction activities in response to cases		
Administrative change	19	53
Job rotation	10	29
Training	5	15
Engineering change	15	44

*Missing data excluded from percentages.

therapist for referrals, and 17 employers (47%) claimed to have a specialist to provide ergonomics consultation. Only one-third had carried out an ergonomics evaluation for risk factors of CTS. Approximately half of employers reported instituting administrative changes to reduce risks. Nearly half of the administrative changes involved job rotation. Forty-four percent of employers reported making engineering changes, including automation, or physical changes to the workstation.

Field Investigations

Field investigations were carried out at six worksites, including three manufacturing facilities, two governmental agencies, and one service firm (Table 13.9). Cal/SENSOR identified risk factors, including repetitive and forceful hand motions, awkward postures, contact stresses, and nonexistent or inadequate medical monitoring, engineering problems in production equipment

Table 13.9 Field Investigations at Index Case Worksites in California SENSOR Surveillance System, 1988–1991*

No. of Workers	*Industry or Department*	*Occupations*	*Cases of CTS*	*Risk Factors Observed*	*No. of Specific Recommendations*
100	Public safety, Police department	Clerical staff; key enterers, indexers, transcribers (*N* = 100)	9	Contact stress from sharp edges of workstation; severe neck flexion; glare from video display terminal (VDT); unadjustable desks; lack of detachable keyboard; pinch grip in handling multiple copies of forms; high force handling thick files; telephone positioned between head and shoulder	8
83	Public sector social service agency	VDT clerks (*N* = 18) and case workers (*N* = 65)	7	High force, extended reach with pinch grip to handle case files; contact stress on edge of desks; pinch grips to tear off computer output and remove staples; contact stress on palms using stapler	8
205	Frozen food manufacturing	Inspectors and machine operators (*N* = 95)	6	High repetition of 20,000 motions per 8-hour shift; contact stress from conveyor guards and trays; awkward posture in extended reaches and wrist flicks and in loading and unloading racks; pinch grips in loading and unloading trays; cold exposure in handling frozen food; long hours with seasonal heavy demand	13
159	Pharmaceutical manufacturing	Bottle and medical kit assemblers and packagers (*N* = 90)	2	High repetition due to assembly line speed, 20,000 repetitions/8-hour shift; rapid elbow flexion and continual pinching of cartons; confined space required extended reaches; contact stress to forearm and wrist on hard edges of conveyor guards	14
75	Industrial gas supply service	Truck drivers; gas cylinder loaders and unloaders (*N* = 26)	1	Forceful exertions to open valves; wrist bending to open and close valves; awkward postures involving elbows above midtorso; contact stress on palm to open valves; lifting and moving 140–200 lb. cylinders	5
620	Computer integrated manufacturing systems manufacturing plant	Electro-mechanical assemblers (*N* = 70)	1	Contact stress against palm using needle-nose pliers; sharp edges of work stations; high hand force using crimping tools; repetitive pinch grips to handle small parts; awkward postures in reaching for parts; prolonged seating without back support; forceful forearm rotation with screwdrivers	20

*CTS, carpal tunnel syndrome; VDT, video display terminal.

and process layout, improper use of splints, and lack of training. In total, 68 specific recommendations and 5 general recommendations were noted that reflected inadequacies in health and safety programs.

Evaluation of Reporting

Sensitivity

Of 141 cases of SENSOR providers with a date of first treatment during 1987, 1988, or 1989, Doctor's First Reports (DFR) were found for only 19 (Fig. 13.4). During these 3 years, 422 DFRs for carpal tunnel syndrome were filed in Santa Clara County. The estimate of countywide prevalence was 3132 cases (422 DFRs × 141 SENSOR cases)/19 overlap) based on capture-recapture methods (Fig. 13.4). The sensitivity of the passive reporting system based on DFRs is approximately 14% (422/3132).

Representativeness

The age and industrial distribution of cases of Cal/SENSOR providers was nearly the same as cases reported by DFR (Table 13.10). The Cal/SENSOR cases tended to be proportionately comprised of more women than men.

Positive Predictive Value

Of all cases reported, 80% were definite, probable, or possible. Nearly all of the remaining 20% were generally uncertain due to missing data. Of note, the percents of the statistical distributions did not differ whether these uncertain cases were included or excluded.

Timeliness

In median days, reports were received 49 days after the patient visit, worker interviews were completed 34 days later, employer interviews were completed 26 days afterwards, and worksite visits were completed 50 days after the employer interview. Reports were available 24 days after the site visit.

DISCUSSION

This is an example of an active surveillance system that linked cases reported by a sentinel network to worksite follow-up. Interviews of cases and their employers revealed a clustering of occupational risk factors among index cases that was confirmed by direct observation at selected work sites. The sentinel network captured a significant number of cases of CTS not reported through the preexisting, legally mandated reporting system.

There are several important limitations to the surveillance system and the data it generated. The sentinel network was a nonrandom sample that was chosen to help the surveillance team learn the advantages and pitfalls of working with both physicians and nonphysicians. Although the demographics and industrial char-

Table 13.10 Characteristics of Cases Reported by Cal/SENSOR and non-SENSOR Providers

	Cal/SENSOR, 1989–1991		*Doctor's First Reports, 1987–1989*	
Item	N	%	N	%
Women*	90	82	253	63
Age (years)*				
< 20	4	6	4	1
20–29	16	22	100	25
30–39	26	36	150	38
40–49	17	24	86	22
50–59	7	10	49	12
60+	2	3	8	2
Industry (SIC)†				
Manufacturing (20–39)	104	35	67	37
Services (70–89)	67	23	22	12
Retail trade (52–59)	48	16	28	16
Public administration (91–97)	34	11	24	13
Transportation, utilities (40–49)	14	5	8	4
Construction (15–17)	11	4	12	7
Agriculture (01–09)	10	4	0	0
Finance and real estate (60–67)	5	1	7	4
Wholesale trade (50–51)	4	1	13	7

†Standard Industrial Classification; includes 297 Cal/SENSOR cases with nonmissing SIC codes.

*Restricted to 122 Cal/SENSOR cases with first treatment dates 1987–1989 and not reported on DFRs.

acteristics of cases in the sentinel network and in DFR are similar, random samples are a surer means of having a representative group of cases. The network was not designed to find all the cases in Santa Clara County. Only when the sentinel network's cases were matched to those reported in the preexisting passive using DFRs was an estimate of the total number of cases possible. While the geographic focus of surveillance was restricted to Santa Clara County, there is no reason to believe that the results would be different for counties of similar demographic and industrial composition.

There has been a discussion as to whether only electrodiagnostically confirmed cases should be used for surveillance purposes.[17] While these data are ideal, the Cal/SENSOR experience highlights barriers that makes this impractical. In the early stages of the disease process there may not be striking electrodiagnostic changes. Providers in managed care organizations (which dominate medical care in northern California) may be less inclined to do electrodiagnostic testing. These factors potentially introduce biases that may diminish the sensitivity by restricting the number of true cases and skewing their severity. The probability levels used in case confirmation used information about nerve conduction velocity when it was available.

Case Reports

Cases were distributed among a wide variety of industries and occupations with multiple cases occurring at 18% of worksites and among industries with previously documented risk factors.[1] Cases also revealed a profile of disability, disruption of work life, and exposure to risk factors. Despite the presence of health and safety committees (Table 13.8), ergonomics training was largely absent. As in other states,[4,18] the distribution of cases by industry probably reflects both the distribution of local industries and actual risks. Nearly half of all cases were reported by a single hand surgeon. Because the maintenance of reporting through feedback to providers and community liaison was a labor intensive process, targeted reporting by high-yield providers appears to be cost-efficient, especially when considering that cases reported by hand surgeons and neurologists were often documented with electrodiagnostic testing, and were consequently easier to confirm as probable or definite.

Worksite Investigations

Employers were willing to complete telephone interviews, but generally refused worksite visits. Site visits were clearly described as a voluntary and nonenforcement consultation that offered expensive services, free-of-charge, by highly qualified occupational ergonomists. Although the Cal/SENSOR Project had legal authority to enter worksites for epidemiologic investigations, this was not done because of concerns that it would alienate health care providers and the business community. High refusal rates were encountered early on, and persisted even with outreach to the business community. In contrast, with the identical approach and staff, *low* refusal rates (25%) were encountered in nearby Fresno County involving surveillance of pesticide illness (Chapter 12).[19] Differences in enforcement presence may have affected employer behaviors and consequently the access to the worksites. Unlike Santa Clara County employers, Fresno County employers with a reported pesticide illness expected enforcement personnel to visit their workplaces because of a statewide policy that requires *every* reported case of pesticide illness to be investigated. Among Santa Clara County employers, the expectation of enforcement activity was probably lower, because a relatively small number of OSHA inspectors had to cover a large number of employers, and a specific ergonomics standard had not been approved.

Long-term telephone follow-up of worksite investigations revealed the difficulties that employers faced in taking corrective action. While most plant safety and medical personnel were sympathetic to the Cal/SENSOR aims and were eager to control ergonomic hazards, they encountered a higher management blockade. Some employers were phasing out old, uncompetitive operations and could not justify an ergonomics initiative except at new production facilities. Public sector employers often found recommendations put on hold because of low budgetary priority. Most employers lacked in-house expertise to follow up recommendations with an engineering component. Most employers indicated that job rotation was used for dealing with the problem (Table 13.8). This is frequently the least effective intervention, especially when jobs in the rotation share risk factors similar to those that produced the index case.

The lack of improvements at worksites and lack of access by the Cal/SENSOR Project showed that for ergonomics hazards, the promotion of control measures cannot be accomplished through one-time-only consultation by outside experts. The control of risk factors for work-related CTS is ongoing, and involves considerable organizational commitment by the company. This observation motivated a midcourse strategy change in which volunteer worksites were sought to help Cal/SENSOR develop educational materials for a model ergonomics program.

Evaluation of Reporting

There are several observations that support the principal finding that underreporting is significant. Two similar estimates of prevalence were: (*1*) 3413 cases from a countywide survey[9] based on recall by physicians and other providers (Table 13.3), and (*2*) 3132 cases from the capture-recapture estimate from Cal/SENSOR and Doctors' First Reports (Fig. 13.4). While both methods have limitations and assumptions, they gave similar estimates of the magnitude of the problem. Using either estimate, the number of cases reported in the preexisting passive surveillance reporting system is low (14%).

A Doctor's First Report is a frequent adjunct to filing a workers' compensation claim. Therefore, it is important that a majority of interviewed workers reported that employer-paid health insurance, rather than workers' compensation was the source of payment for their medical bills. Shifting payment to employer-paid health insurance and the underreporting of CTS has been shown in other surveillance projects (Chapter 18).[20] Several estimates of direct costs per case from employers and insurers were in a range of $12,000 for nonlitigated cases and $60,000 for litigated cases. In California, annual direct costs for work-related CTS cases could conservatively range from $33 million to $165 million, based on the 2775 cases officially reported in 1989 alone. If these cases represent only 14% of the actual number, the estimate would range from $235 million to over $1 billion.

Anecdotal reports by workers and providers illustrate several reasons for underreporting. Workers reported that they were pressured by their employers not to file a workers' compensation claim, and expressed disenchantment with "company doctors" whom they claimed were biased. Several workers also reported that the administrative process in the workers' compensation system imposed delays and excessive paperwork, and that having medical bills paid by employer-sponsored health insurance was faster and less adversarial, even if they would lose indemnity benefits.

Several providers expressed concerns that employers became adversarial when work-related cases were identified. In one case, a Cal/SENSOR provider was told by an employer to stop participating in the project or face the cancellation of the contract to provide medical services. The sentinel physician initially responded by reporting cases without patient or employer personal identifiers, but later dropped out. The employer's misplaced concern that the Cal/SENSOR Project was enforcement-oriented raises important issues for surveillance systems linked to enforcement activities in a way that drives reporting underground.

As to representativeness of cases, there was a high degree of similarity in frequency distributions of demographic and industrial characteristics between Cal/SENSOR and Doctor's First Reports. As previously reported,[21] cases were disproportionately women. There may be biological differences, but other plausible explanations include employment practices that select women to perform certain jobs that are higher risk. Smaller stature persons, a greater percentage of which are female, may be exposed more frequently to awkward reaches and physical exertion because of ill-suited dimensions of work stations.[22]

CONCLUSION

The Cal/SENSOR Project revealed that the magnitude of work-related CTS is much larger than indicated by official case reporting, especially by relying on cases reported by hand surgeons and related specialists. Workers, physicians, and employers lack awareness and training, and employers appear to lack organizational commitment and expertise to reduce ergonomic hazards effectively.

In 1997, California became the first state to adopt an ergonomics standard (California Code of Regulations, Title 8, Section 5110). During the standards development, the results of the Cal/SENSOR project were entered into the official record along with hundreds of other studies. Business, labor, academic, and public health officials debated whether the scientific evidence was strong enough to merit taking action and whether the costs of implementation would be prohibitive. The California standard requires a worksite evaluation, control measures, and employee training.

ACKNOWLEDGMENTS

The authors acknowledge the participating health care providers, workers, and employers, without whom this project would not have been possible. Financial support and technical assistance was provided through a cooperative agreement with the National Institute for Occupational Safety and Health, and consultation in project evaluation was provided by the Public Health Practice Program Office, Centers for Disease Control and Prevention. Technical assistance and feedback were provided by staff of the Peninsula Industrial and Business Association; Division of Labor Statistics and Research, Department of Industrial Relations; the Labor Occupational Health Program, University of California, Berkeley; Central Labor Council, Santa Clara County; Santa Clara County Medical Association; and the Santa Clara County Coalition for Occupational Safety and Health.

Dr. Barbara Silverstein is gratefully acknowledged for her recruitment of key providers and worksite inspections. Mukund Sankaranarayan, Kate Cummings, Arleen Ervin, Fidel Dolorier, Francisco Curiel, Elizabeth Abello, and Susan Payne are acknowledged for their valuable assistance in data collection and analysis. Administrative assistance was provided by the Public Health Institute, Berkeley, California.

Portions of this chapter were published previously in the *American Journal of Industrial Medicine* and have been used with permission.

REFERENCES

1. Kuorinka I, Forcier L, eds. *Work-Related Musculoskeletal Disorders (WMSDs): A Reference Book for Prevention.* Bristol, PA: Taylor and Francis Ltd., 1995.

2. Committee on Human Factors of the National Research Council. *Work-Related Musculoskeletal Disorders: A Review of the Evidence.* Washington, DC: National Academy Press, 1998.
3. Bernard B (ed). *Musculoskeletal Disorders (MSDs) and Workplace Factors: A Critical Review of Epidemiologic Evidence for Work-Related Musculoskeletal Disorders of the Neck, Upper Extremity, and Low Back.* Cincinnati: National Institute for Occupational Safety and Health, July 1997.
4. Hanrahan LP, Higgins D, Anderson H, Haskins L, Tai S. Project SENSOR: Wisconsin surveillance of occupational carpal tunnel syndrome. *Wisconsin Med J* 1991; 90:80–83.
5. Division of Labor Statistics and Research. *Cases of Carpal Tunnel Syndrome from the Occupational Disease File, 1983–1989.* San Francisco: California Department of Industrial Relations; 1983–1989.
6. Bureau of Labor Statistics. *Annual Survey of Occupational Injuries and Illnesses, 1994 Case and Demographic Resource Tables.* Washington, DC: U.S. Department of Labor, 1995.
7. Rutstein DD, Mullan RJ, Frazier TM, Halperin WE, Melius JM, Sestito JP. Sentinel events (occupational) for physician recognition and public health surveillance. *Am J Public Health* 1983; 73:1054–1062.
8. Baker EL. Sentinel event notification system for occupational risks (SENSOR): The concept. *Am J Public Health* 1989; 79(suppl): 18–20.
9. Cummings KC, Maizlish NA, Rudolph LA, Dervin KA, Ervin A. Occupational disease surveillance: carpal tunnel syndrome. *MMWR* 1989; 38:485–489.
10. Silverstein B, Fine L, Armstrong TJ. Carpal tunnel syndrome: causes and a preventive strategy. *Sem Occup Med* 1986; 1:213–221.
11. National Institute for Occupational Safety and Health. *NIOSH Publications on Video Display Terminals (Revised).* NTIS No: PB 92-109-230/A6, Cincinnati, OH: National Institute for Occupational Safety and Health, June 1991.
12. Stevens JC, Sun S, Beard CM, O'Fallon WM, Kurland LT. Carpal tunnel syndrome in Rochester, Minnesota, 1961 to 1980. *Neurology* 1988; 38:134–138.12.
13. Office of Management and Budget. *Standard Industrial Classification Codes. 1987 Rev.,* Washington, DC: U.S. Government Printing Office;1989.
14. Bureau of Labor Statistics. *Standard Occupational Titles, 1980.* Washington, DC, Department of Labor, 1977.
15. Klauke DN. Evaluating public health surveillance. In: Tuetsch SM, Churchill R, ed. *Principles and Practice of Public Health Surveillance.* New York: Oxford University Press, 1994:158–174.
16. Stroup DF. Special Analytic Issues. In: Tuetsch SM, Churchill R, eds. *Principles and Practice of Public Health Surveillance.* New York: Oxford University Press, 1994:136–149.
17. Katz JF, Larson MG, Fossel AH, Liang MH. Validation of a surveillance case definition of carpal tunnel syndrome. *Am J Public Health* 1991; 81:189–193.
18. Franklin G, Haug J, Heyer N, Checkoway H, Peck N. Occupational carpal tunnel syndrome in Washington State, 1984–1988. *Am J Public Health* 1991; 81:741–746.
19. Maizlish NA, Rudolph LA, Dervin KA. Surveillance of work-related pesticide illness: an application of the Sentinel Event Notification System for Occupational Risks (SENSOR). *Am J Public Health* 1995; 85:806–811.
20. Park R, Nelson NA, Silverstein MA, Mirer FE. Use of medical insurance claims for surveillance of occupational disease. An analysis of cumulative trauma in the auto industry. *J Occup Med* 1992; 34:731–737.
21. Armstrong TJ, Chaffin DB. Carpal tunnel syndrome and selected personal attributes. *J Occup Med* 1979; 21:481–486.
22. Silverstein BA, Fine LJ, Armstrong TA. Hand wrist cumulative trauma disorders in industry. *Brit J Ind Med* 1986; 43:779–784.

14

Silicosis

KENNETH D. ROSENMAN AND MARY JO REILLY

Quartz, the crystalline form of silicon dioxide (SiO_2), is the most common constituent of the earth's crust and workers exposed to quartz all over the world are at risk of developing silicosis. High-risk industries include: mining; quarrying; tunneling; abrasive blasting; monument engraving; working in a foundry; manufacturing ceramic products, including sinks, toilet bowls, and bathtubs; and fire brick manufacturing. Less common exposures to silica have been reported including the manufacture of slate-pencils, gemstones, and glass.

Lung disease secondary to exposure to dusty work conditions among miners was first described over 2000 years ago by Hipprocrates. The presence of silica in the lungs was first described in the 1860s and the fibrotic lung disease was first called silicosis in 1870. The term silicosis was derived from the Latin word *silex*, which means flint.

Silicosis is a chronic, irreversible illness that may cause progressively debilitating symptoms as well as increasing an individual's likelihood of developing other serious conditions. Silicosis has three clinical presentations:

- the typical slow-developing chronic form that develops 20 or more years after exposure
- a more accelerated form from more intense exposure that develops within years of exposure
- and an acute form that develops within months or even weeks of initial exposure to airborne respirable silica particles

Chronic and accelerated silicosis are characterized by small opacities in the upper zones of the lungs. There is a distinctive silicotic nodule present in pathological specimens. Acute silicosis has different x-ray and pathological features as compared to chronic or accelerated silicosis and is more similar to the disease alveolar proteinosis. With more advanced silicosis there is a conglomeration of the smaller nodules and the presence of large opacities, termed progressive massive fibrosis. An individual with silicosis finds it increasingly difficult to breathe as the scarring in the lungs increases.

Traditionally silicosis has been considered to cause restrictive changes on pulmonary function testing, however there is both clinical and pathological evidence that silica also causes obstructive disease.[1]

Silicosis has long been noted to increase an individual's risk of developing tuberculosis.[2] More recently, individuals with silicosis have been shown to be at increased risk of developing connective tissue disease such as scleroderma,[3] kidney disease,[4] and lung cancer.[5]

The source for data on the incidence of silicosis and other work-related illnesses in the United States has typically been the state agencies responsible for administering workers' compensation.[6] With the advent of the Occupational Safety and Health Administration (OSHA) in 1970 the primary source of data on the incidence of silicosis and other occupational diseases shifted to the Bureau of Labor's annual survey of employers. Both the workers' compensation system and the Bureau of Labor's system are known to markedly under count the true number of cases of occupational illnesses, including silicosis. For example, for the years 1984 and 1985, the four states of California, New Jersey, New York, and Wisconsin reported more cases of silicosis than were reported by the Bureau of Labor Statistics for all 50 states combined and by the workers' compensation bureaus in 23 states combined.[7] Indeed, studies in Michigan and New Jersey have documented that less than 50% of individuals with silicosis apply for workers' compensation.[8,9]

New Jersey received funds from the National Institute for Occupational Safety and Health (NIOSH) in 1982 to develop a comprehensive surveillance system for silicosis. Based on the success of this system, federal funding from NIOSH was expanded in 1987 to fund surveillance systems in three additional states: Michigan, Ohio, and Wisconsin and then expanded again in 1992 to include Illinois, North Carolina, and Texas. These surveillance systems were called Project SENSOR, or the Sentinel Event Notification System for Occupational Risks. Funding from NIOSH for silicosis surveillance was cut back in 1997; only New Jersey and Ohio still receive funding, although Michigan has continued its surveillance system for silicosis using state resources.

Historically, Michigan has been one of the leading states in the foundry industry in terms of production and work force. Accordingly, the foundries in Michigan were thought to be at significant economic risk because of the large number of workers who might develop silicosis. In the 1930s, to protect the foundries, a monetary cap was placed on the workers' compensation award amount that a worker could receive. This cap was less than what a worker would receive for other work-related injuries. In 1966, the cap was removed. However, in order to continue to protect the foundry industry, an annual special assessment was instituted for all insurance companies and self-insured employers who provide workers' compensation to foundries and other manufacturing facilities where harmful dusts are present. The funds from this special assessment are used to limit the liability of foundries and the insurance companies that provide their workers' compensation insurance while allowing workers with silicosis to receive benefits equivalent to those paid for other work-related injuries. The assessment is under the control of a special branch of Michigan's workers' compensation program, called the Michigan Silicosis, Dust Disease and Logging Industry Compensation Fund.

By the 1960s Michigan had the largest number of foundry employees (42,000) and produced more grey iron (24,000 tons in 300 foundries) than any other state. Because of increased automation, the number of foundries and the size of the work force decreased both in Michigan and nationwide. The foundry work force in Michigan dropped by 70% by the end of the 1980s.

METHODS

Define Goals, Objectives, and Scope

The purpose of the Michigan silicosis surveillance system was to identify workplaces where preventive activity might be useful and to develop better estimates of the incidence of disease.

The surveillance system for silicosis was based on an existing state law that requires hospitals, clinics, physicians, and employers to report all known or suspected occupational disease or workplace-aggravated health conditions to the state within 10 days of the discovery of the disease or condition (Part 56 of Public Act 368 of 1978). The failure to report cases can result in a $50 fine per individual not reported, although no nonreporter has been fined since the introduction of the law in 1978. Compliance with the law relied more on professional responsibility rather than on the threat of monetary punishment. The reporting law relieved the health practitioner of any liability for releasing confidential patient information to the state.

Assemble Multidisciplinary Team

In 1988, a multidisciplinary surveillance team was formed from the staff at the Michigan Department of Consumer and Industry Services (MDCIS) (formerly the Michigan Department of Public Health) and the staff from the College of Human Medicine at Michigan State University (MSU). Staff at MSU provided the medical and epidemiologic expertise for surveillance whereas staff at the MDCIS fulfilled the industrial hygiene and enforcement role of the intervention efforts. Michigan has a state enforcement plan and operates the OSHA program in Michigan. As one of the NIOSH funded Project SENSOR states, Michigan was unique in that it had the legal authority to collect the surveillance data as well as intervene through enforcement inspections in workplaces that were identified by sentinel cases.

Staff at MSU under contract to the MDCIS included an occupational physician, an epidemiologist, and office support staff. Staff at the MDCIS included 25 industrial hygienists located at 6 district offices across the state, an administrator acting as a codirector of the surveillance program along with MSU's occupational physician, and two MDCIS/MSU liaisons—one for administrative issues and one for issues related to enforcement inspections. The personnel at the MDCIS provided in-kind support for the program, whereas all new funds were used for the surveillance staff at MSU.

Geographic Targeting

All known or suspected cases of silicosis were targeted in case finding efforts and potentially acted as the basis for intervention. The tremendous support of staff at the MDCIS allowed available monetary resources to be directed to case-finding in the entire state of Michigan. Although certain counties in Michigan have more silica-using industries and therefore generate a greater number of cases of silicosis, resources were available to monitor the entire state and thus satisfy one of the goals of the program—to document the extent of the problem.

Gain Support

An advisory committee was developed that consisted of seven physicians:

- an occupational medicine physician from each of the other three medical schools in the state besides the College of Human Medicine at MSU
- an occupational medicine physician representing the labor unions
- an occupational medicine physician representing the Michigan Occupational and Environmental Medicine Association
- a pulmonary physician representing the Michigan Thoracic Society
- a physician representing the Michigan Allergy Society

At the same time that the surveillance system was initiated for silicosis, a similar system was being developed for work-related asthma (Chapter 16). The advisory committee was also responsible for advising on this latter system, which explains the inclusion of the allergist on the committee. The group's major role was to be a sounding board if physicians around the state had questions or concerns about the reporting system. The advisory board also reviewed educational material sent out to practicing physicians.

By directing the focus of the surveillance activity from a medical school rather than a state agency, physicians identified the reporting system as being more of a collegial and consultative type of medical service rather than a less personal and more bureaucratic regulatory activity. However, the medical school staff acted as the gateway to the regulatory activity that ensured effective follow-up after the identification of cases.

Case Definition and Data Collection

The silicosis case definition was developed in conjunction with NIOSH and the other states conducting similar silicosis surveillance.[9] The silicosis case definition was:

1. a history of occupational exposure to airborne silica dust
2. a chest radiograph, a lung histopathology, or both interpreted as characteristic of silicosis

All chest radiographs were reviewed by a physician who was a NIOSH-certified "B" reader. This designation means the physician has special training and accreditation to interpret chest radiographs for all the pneumoconioses, including silicosis. A chest radiograph needed to be interpreted as having a profusion of rounded opacities of 1/0 or greater per the International Labor Office (ILO) classification system to be considered characteristic of silicosis.

Michigan has had an occupational disease reporting law since 1978. Reporting of cases could be done by mail, electronic mail, telephone, or fax. The standard occupational disease reporting form was used for any known or suspected occupational disease or work-aggravated condition and collected demographic information on the employee affected, information about the employer, illness information, and information on the person, clinic, or other such entity submitting the report. Hospitals were also requested to submit the discharge summary. To determine if reported cases met the case definition for silicosis a recent chest x-ray was obtained on all individuals reported. If the medical record noted that a lung biopsy had been performed or if the individual or next of kin indicated a biopsy had been done, the pathology report of the biopsy was requested and reviewed. The Michigan law (Part 56 of Public Act 368 of 1978) indicated specific items required to be included on the reporting form such as name and address but also gave the state broad discretion on the types of information it could request (". . . and other information required by the department.").

Select, Recruit, and Train Providers

Based on the New Jersey silicosis surveillance experience, key reporting sources of silicosis cases were expected to be:

- hospitals
- physicians
- workers' compensation
- death certificates

Prior work in New Jersey showed that the greatest number of reports of silicosis (approximately 80%) could be obtained from reviewing hospital discharge records.[8] All acute care hospitals in Michigan, including Veteran Administration Hospitals, were requested in January or February of each year to submit information on all individuals discharged with a primary or secondary diagnosis of silicosis (International Classification of Diseases [ICD]502), or pneumoconiosis not otherwise specified (ICD505). The information requested included the hospital discharge summary, a recent chest x-ray and available pulmonary function tests. In order to verify the completeness of reporting by hospitals, a computerized listing of all hospital discharges, which was available approximately 2 years later, was reviewed and any discharges for ICD 502 or 505 not previously reported by a hospital were obtained from the hospital.

Although all 25,000 physicians who practice medicine in Michigan were required to report occupational disease, including silicosis, a special effort was made to inform allergists, pulmonologists, occupational physicians, and selected internists and family practitioners about the reporting law. Again, the allergists were included because of a simultaneous effort to encourage the reporting of work-related asthma. Members of the Michigan Allergy Society, the Michigan Occupational and Environmental Medicine Association, the Michigan Thoracic Society and the full-time and adjunct faculty at the Departments of Family Practice and Medicine at the four medical schools in the state received a letter announcing the program. For four organizations the letter was sent by the chair of the department, and for seven from the director of the state health department. All three specialty organizations officially supported the program and this support was highlighted in the letter. Approximately 3000 physicians received the introductory mailing. These targeted physicians then continued to receive a four-page quarterly newsletter that contained reviews of pertinent diagnostic issues, case reports, and abstracts of selected articles. Both silicosis and work-related asthma were covered in the newsletter. In addition, these physicians received an annual report on silicosis that summarized the demographics, type of industries, x-ray and pulmonary function test results, and industrial hygiene follow-up activity. In more recent years the annual report and newsletter became available on an MSU website. The targeted physicians received a letter notifying them of the website and announcing the availability of the annual reports, along with a postage paid post card that allowed them to request a printed copy of the reports. Although the newsletter was also posted on the website, it continued to be mailed out quarterly to the targeted physicians.

To encourage physicians to report cases of all occupational diseases including silicosis, and to remind them of the reporting law, a display booth was set up at the Annual Michigan State Medical Society Scientific Meeting, the Annual Michigan Thoracic Society Scientific Meeting, the Annual Michigan Occupational and Environmental Association Meeting, and selected continuing medical education meetings. Similar to displays set up by pharmaceutical companies, educational materials and small novelty items such as pens, pencils, magnets, and rulers with the telephone number to report occupational diseases were distributed.

An additional group of physicians that was targeted was the 15–20 physicians in the state who were certified by NIOSH as "B readers." These are physicians who have had special training and passed a test on interpreting chest radiographs for the pneumoconioses. They are required to be recertified and pass a test every 4 years. Each year the Michigan silicosis surveillance program sent them a survey asking them how many B-reading interpretations they performed in the previous year and how many were positive for pneumoconiosis. They were also reminded of their obligation to report occupational diseases. Any x-ray with 1/0 profusion or greater, or pleural thickening or both was considered to meet the state's legal definition of a suspected occupational disease.

Two other sources used to identify persons with silicosis were: (*1*) death certificates where silicosis (ICD 502) or pneumoconiosis not otherwise specified (ICD 505) was the underlying or contributing cause of death; and (*2*) claims to the Michigan Silicosis, Dust Disease and Logging Industry Compensation Fund (the special workers' compensation program for silicosis discussed in the background section). Both these administrative data systems were accessed once per year. Death certificates were identified by a computer search of deaths from the previous year with ICD codes 502 or 505, and the actual death certificate was then obtained and reviewed. The medical records of all claims filed with the special silicosis compensation fund from the previous year were manually reviewed once per year.

Protocol for Follow-up

When a report of unknown or suspected silicosis was received, the individual was administered a standardized medical and work history questionnaire by a trained interviewer over the phone. The interviews were typically performed by second-year medical students. The interview took approximately 30 to 45 minutes and consisted of the following:

- lifetime work history
- cigarette smoking history
- onset, frequency, and temporal pattern of respiratory symptoms
- medical care history
- medication history

The only part of the questionnaire that was necessary for an individual to meet the surveillance criteria for silicosis was the lifetime work history. The collection of the other historical information allowed the surveillance team to describe the epidemiology of silicosis in Michigan, including the severity of disease.

All workplaces where a confirmed case was exposed to silica were inspected if they met the following criteria:

- the company was located within the state
- the company was still in operation
- the Michigan OSHA program had jurisdiction
- the company had not been inspected for silica in the past 3 years

If the company was out of state or the Michigan OSHA program did not have enforcement jurisdiction (i.e., mining or transportation) the company's name was forwarded to the appropriate agency that did have enforcement jurisdiction.

Case Management

Data from the occupational disease reports for silicosis and data from the case interviews were entered into a tracking database. The database was used to track the progress of case interviews and the status of inspections and to analyze the information collected through the telephone administered questionnaires.

Field Investigations

Companies that were still in operation and where a recent inspection had not been conducted, were considered for inspections. Certain industries in Michigan are not covered by the Michigan OSHA laws. These include mining, agriculture, transportation, and oil and gas well drilling and servicing.

After the investigation was completed, a report of the inspection results and any recommendations were sent to the company and to the union (or designated labor representative if the company did not have a union), as well as to the reporting physician. If the company was cited for violations of any regulations, a copy of the citations was posted at or near the location of the violations for a minimum of 3 days or until the items were corrected, whichever was later.

A copy of the report was also sent to the physician who reported the original index silicosis case that prompted the field investigation. The cover letter to the physician indicated that the investigation was conducted in response to their case report and the physician was thanked for initiating this public health activity to prevent other similarly exposed workers from developing silicosis.

Analyze and Interpret Data

On a quarterly basis, progress reports detailing the numbers of cases identified, numbers of inspections completed, and other related information were written and submitted to the funding agency. On a yearly basis, an overall report on the surveillance data was developed. This annual report summarized the history of the surveillance project, the elements of surveillance, and a summary of the data obtained including questionnaire data and inspection report summaries.

Feedback and Recommendations

The annual reports were distributed to the approximately 3000 targeted physicians, to administrative personnel in the MDCIS, and to other government officials. After the first 5 years of funding, a website was developed that posted the newsletters, annual reports, reporting law, and other educational information.

Industrial hygiene inspections conducted by Michigan OSHA were enforcement inspections. Any violations of Michigan's silica standard were required to be corrected and proof of such corrections was required to be submitted to Michigan OSHA. In addition to possible violations, individual industrial hygienists would make recommendations regarding work practices, medical screening, and engineering controls. These recommendations would be part of the report shared with the company and if present, the union.

Evaluation of the Surveillance System

With review of the computerized records of hospital discharge data and followback to the hospitals, the system was successful in obtaining complete hospital reporting. Because it is to the employers' benefit to make sure all workers' compensation claims for silicosis are handled by the special fund for silicosis, the system is presumed to have received complete reporting on individuals who filed workers' compensation claims.

Reporting of nonhospitalized individuals with silicosis is incomplete. In a given year only 1.7% of Michigan physicians submit a report on any type of occupational disease to the state.[10] A previous study in New Jersey estimated that their system missed two-thirds of the cases of silicosis.[11] Capture–recapture analyses (described in Chapter 13) were carried out on the Michigan data for the years 1987–1995 using the overlap of cases reported from multiple reporting sources to estimate the number of cases not received by any reporting source.[10] This analysis suggested that over this 9-year period 77% of cases were not being reported.

Reporting of silicosis from death certificates is also incomplete. In a follow-up mortality study of deaths among confirmed cases of silicosis from the Michigan and New Jersey surveillance systems, 42 deaths listed emphysema as the cause of death and had no mention of silicosis.[12]

Despite the known underreporting, the system has been effective in identifying problem worksites and improving the working conditions in these workplaces. Field investigations revealed violations of the exposure standard for silica in 12 (38.7%) of the 31 facilities where sampling was performed.[10] Another 7 (22.5%) of the facilities were above the NIOSH recommended silica exposure standard. Follow-up inspections of these

Table 14.1 Among 13 Companies Reinspected Comparison of Air Sampling Results at Initial and Follow-up Inspections*

Type of Industry	Initial Inspection: Above OSHA TLV	No. of air samples	Range (mg/m³)	Average (mg/m³)	Follow-up Inspection: Above OSHA TLV	No. of air samples	Range (mg/m³)	Average (mg/m³)
Malleable iron foundry	Y	10	0.34–1.71	0.83	N	2	0.03–0.06	0.05
Grey iron foundry	Y	15	0.13–1.63	0.62	N	2	0.03–0.05	0.04
Pottery	Y	3	0.47–0.97	0.57	N	1	0.03	—
Grey iron foundry	Y	17	0.09–16.64	1.94	N	1	0.03	—
Copper foundry	Y†	2	0.37–0.50	0.44	N	0	—	—
Grey and ductile iron foundry	N‡	5	0.20–4.5	1.01	N‡	4	0.3–0.5	0.04
Fabricated metal production	Y	10	ND–0.98	0.21	N	2	ND	0
Dental equipment and supplies	Y§	7	0.008–0.37	0.16	N	3	ND	0
Grey and ductile iron foundry	Y	6	0.05–3.85	1.04	Y	—	Requested variance	—
Ferrous foundry	Y	11	0.20–5.77	1.17	N	3	ND–0.05	0.02
Ferrous foundry	Y	11	ND–3.87	1.00	N	2	0.20–0.60	0.40
Ferrous foundry	Y	5	0.89–6.45	2.76	Y	4	0.50–1.00	0.73
Grey and ductile iron foundry	Y	25	ND–0.12	0.01	N	2	0.01–0.08	0.04

*OSHA, Occupational Safety and Health Administration; TLV, Threshold Limit Value; Y, yes; N, no; ND, none detected.

†This facility was within silica TLV but had air samples for beryllium above the OSHA TLV of 2μg/m³; number of samples 2, range 5.7–7.6; repeat testing for beryllium, number of samples 4, none detected.

‡Respirable dust not silica was measured.

§Over TLV for cristobalite.

same companies several years after the initial inspection revealed a marked decrease in the air concentrations of silica (Table 14.1). In the two companies still not in compliance, the workers were using respirators. New Jersey has documented similar efficacy with their surveillance system in identifying deficiencies among silica-using industries. Nonenforcement follow-up inspections in New Jersey revealed less than 75% of companies had adequate control programs including medical surveillance and engineering controls.[8]

RESULTS

Demographic and Occupational Characteristics

The following section highlights the main findings of the Michigan surveillance system, from 1985 to 1998. Table 14.2 shows the primary reporting source of the 746 persons confirmed with silicosis for the years 1987–1998. The cases identified for 1997 and 1998 are not complete, primarily because of the typical lag in identification of cases through the hospitals. Hospital reports are the primary source of identification of patients, with 58% of silicosis patients identified solely through the hospitals. Often a patient will be reported to the system by more than one source. Figure 14.1 shows the overlap of reporting sources for the most complete reporting years of 1987 through 1997.

The following statistics are based on the 746 cases of silicosis confirmed from 1987 to 1998. Seven hundred twenty-nine (97.7%) of the persons with silicosis were men. Three hundred twenty-five (43.9%) of the persons with silicosis were African-American, 392 (53.0%) were white, one (0.1%) was of Asian ancestry, and 22 (3.0%)

Table 14.2 Number of Confirmed Individuals with Silicosis by Year and Reporting Source*

Reporting Source	Year: < 1987	1988	1989	1990	1991	1992	1993	1994	1995	1996	1997	1998	All Years
PR	—	—	7	5	5	16	6	7	27	28	13	9	123
HDC	68	57	41	44	36	54	31	36	3 5	36	24	0	462
DC	34	5	8	0	1	6	0	3	0	0	1	0	58
DL	42	7	4	6	6	2	4	28	0	0	0	0	99
ICFU	—	—	3	1	0	0	0	0	0	0	0	0	4
Total	144	69	63	56	48	78	41	74	62	64	38	9	746

*PR, physician referral; HDC, hospital discharge data; DC, death certificate; DL, Department of Labor; ICFU, index case follow-up.

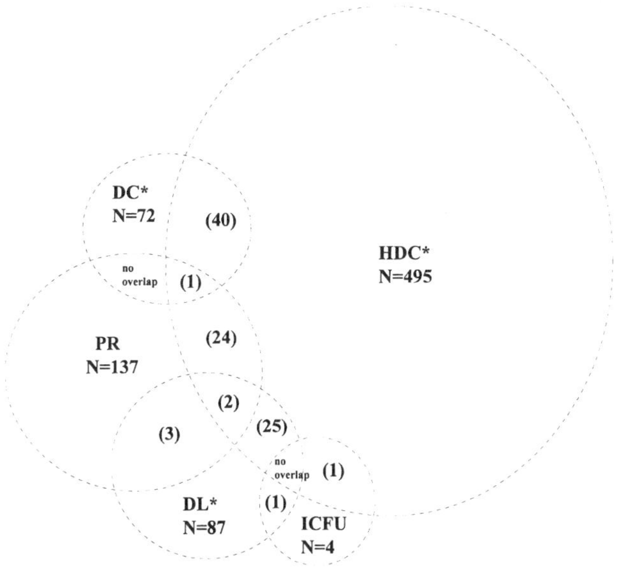

Figure 14.1 Overlap of reporting sources for confirmed individuals with silicosis, Michigan, 1987–1997. Six hundred eighty-nine individuals initially reported from 1987–1997. Numbers in parentheses represent the overlap of reporting sources. HDC, hospital discharge data; DC, death certificate; PR, physician referral; DL, Department of Labor; ICFU, Index Case Follow-up. N, the total number for that source. *There was also an overlap of HDC-DC-DL for three individuals.

were listed as other ancestry. The race on six individuals was unknown. The distribution of the decade of birth is shown in Figure 14.2. The average year of birth was 1919, ranging from 1888 to 1959.

The distribution of the decade of first exposure to silica is shown in Figure 14.3. The average year of first exposure to silica was 1946, ranging from 1910 to 1985. The distribution of years worked at a silica exposed job is shown in Figure 14.4. The average number of years worked was 27.6.

The cases were clustered in three counties in Michigan: Muskegon, Saginaw, and Wayne (Fig. 14.5). The overall average annual incidence rates for silicosis among African-American men was 14.8 cases per 100,000, and for white men was 2.1 cases per 100,000. Figure 14.6 shows the average annual incidence rate of silicosis among African-American men aged 40 and greater in each county. Figure 14.7 shows the annual average incidence rate of silicosis among white men aged 40 or greater by county.

Table 14.3 describes the primary type of industry where the silica exposure occurred. The predominant industry where individuals developed silicosis in Michigan is iron foundries (78.9%). One hundred seventy-nine (25.6%) people stated they had done sandblasting as part of their work.

Overall 516 (69.2%) of the people with silicosis had simple silicosis and 188 (25.2%) had progressive massive fibrosis. Twenty-two (2.9%) silicotics had normal x-rays with biopsy evidence. Twenty (2.7%) individuals had x-ray reports that were consistent with silicosis but because we did not have a standardized "B" reader interpretation of them they could not be classified.

Two hundred three (27.6%) of the people with silicosis never smoked cigarettes, 428 (58.2%) had quit,

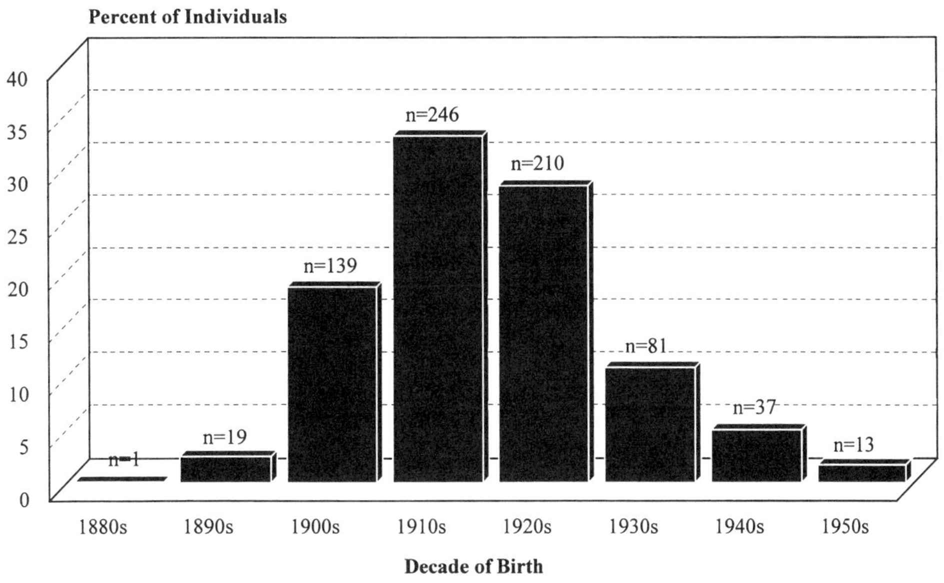

Figure 14.2 Distribution of decade of birth for individuals confirmed with silicosis, Michigan, 1985–1998. Total number of individuals: 746.

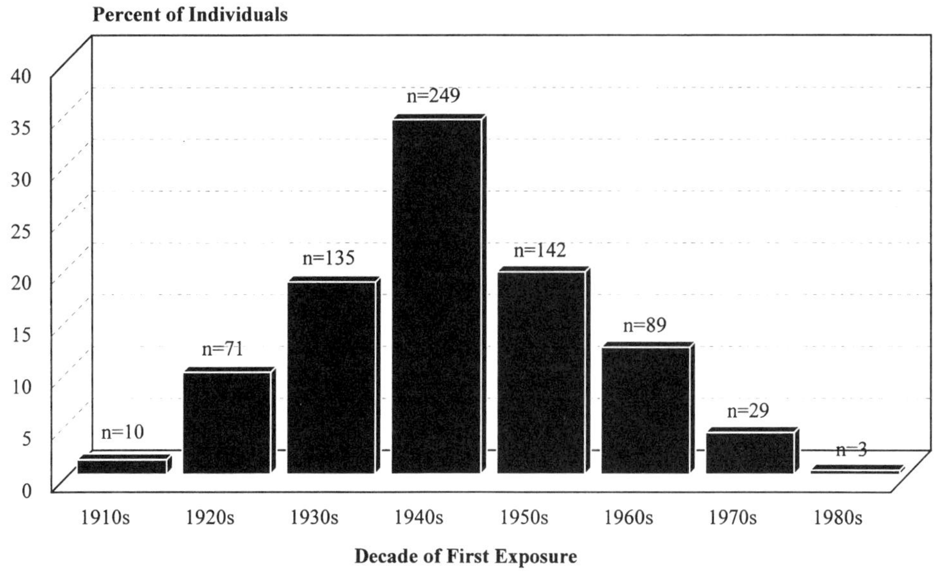

Figure 14.3 Distribution of decade when silica exposure began for individuals confirmed with silicosis, Michigan, 1985–1998. Total number of individuals: 728. Unknown decade for 18 individuals.

105 (14.3%) were still smoking, and no information was available on 10 individuals. Figure 14.8 shows the distribution of x-ray results according to the ILO classification and smoking status. Nonsmokers tended to have more severe silicosis. The greater percentage of nonsmokers with progressive massive fibrosis was statistically significant (29.6% nonsmokers versus 20.0% current smokers versus 24.8% exsmokers) (X^2 = 26.45, p = 0.003). This latter finding may be an artifact of the reporting system that is based on mainly reports of hospitalized individuals. Nonsmoking individuals with simple silicosis are less likely to be symptomatic and less likely to be hospitalized and therefore less likely to have been reported.

Tables 14.4 and 14.5 show the distribution of forced vital capacity (FVC) and the ratio of forced expiratory

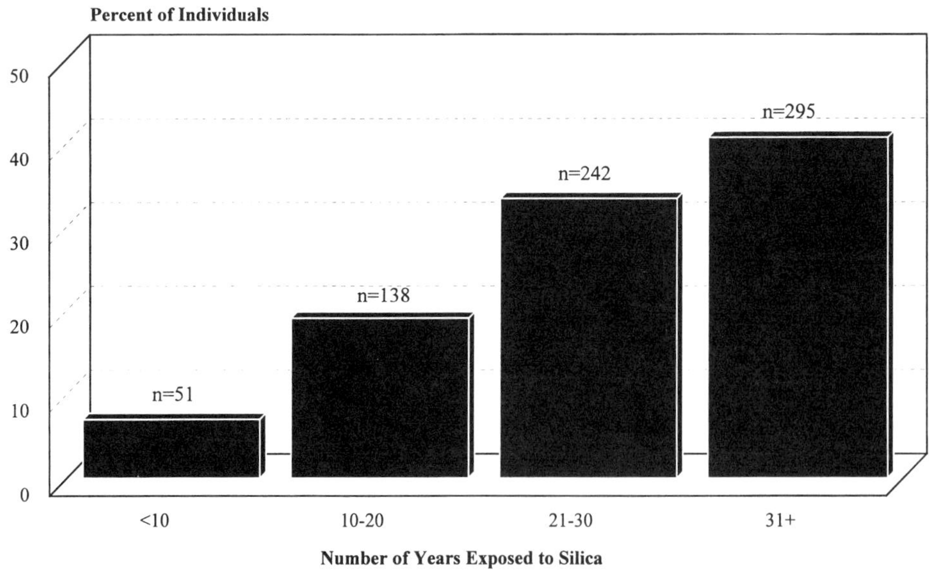

Figure 14.4 Distribution of years worked at silica-exposed job for individuals confirmed with silicosis, Michigan, 1985–1998. Total number of individuals: 726. Unknown years for 20 individuals.

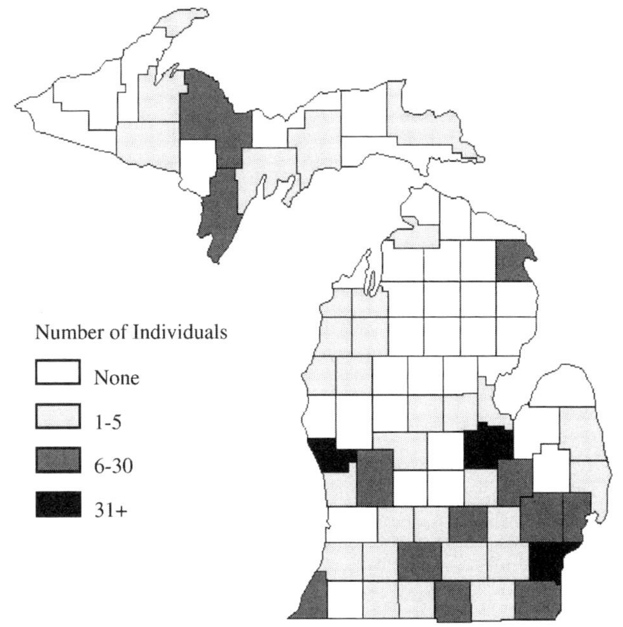

Figure 14.5 Distribution of confirmed silicosis in individuals by county of exposure, Michigan, 1985–1998. Total number of Michigan individuals: 686. Fifty-five were exposed out-of-state, and five individuals had an unknown county of exposure. Muskegon, Saginaw, and Wayne counties had the highest number of silicosis cases with 181, 118, and 188 individuals, respectively.

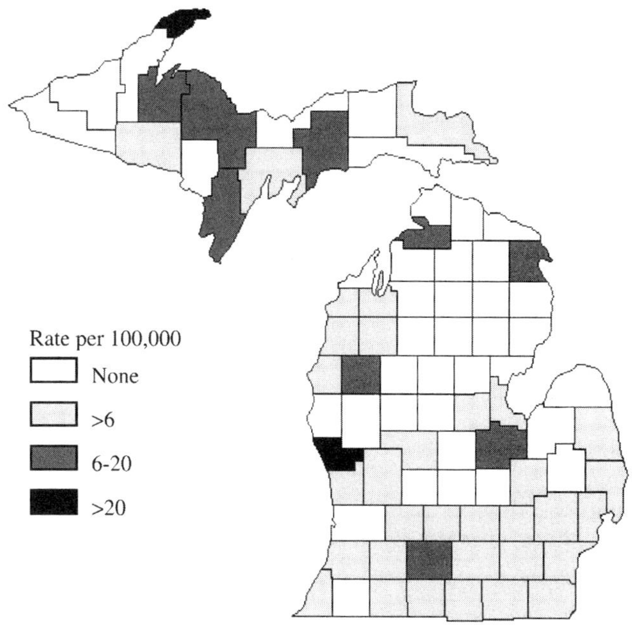

Figure 14.7 Average annual incidence rate of silicosis among white males by county of exposure, Michigan, 1987–1996. Rate per 100,000 among white men aged 40+. Numerator is the average number of individuals for the years 1987–1996; denominator is the 1990 U.S. Census population data for white men aged 40 and older, by county. In 1990, there were 1,410,341 white males 40 years and older living in Michigan.

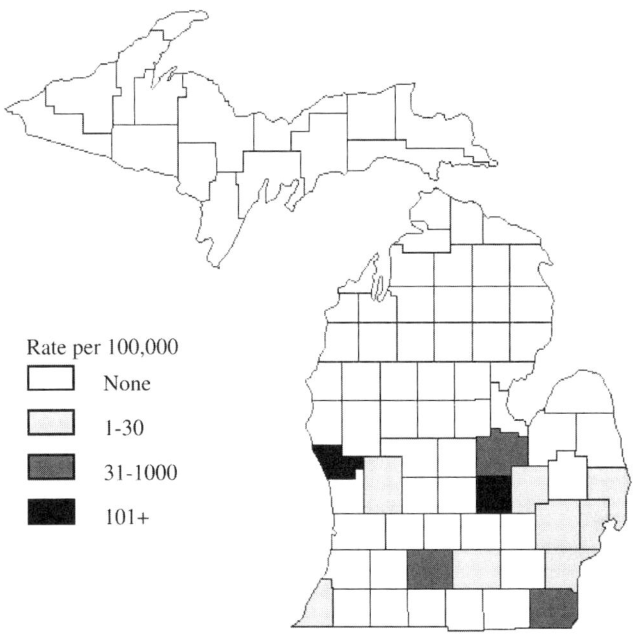

Figure 14.6 Average annual incidence rate of silicosis among African-American males by county of exposure, Michigan, 1987–1996. Rate per 100,000 among African-American men aged 40+. Numerator is the average number of individuals for the years 1987–1996; denominator is the 1990 U.S. Census population data for African-American men aged 40 and older, by county. In 1990, there were 174,325 African-American males 40 years and older living in Michigan.

volume in one second (FEV_1) to FVC by x-ray and cigarette smoking status. Approximately 60% of the people with silicosis had reduced breathing function, either restrictive ($FVC < 80\%$) or obstructive (FEV_1/FVC ratio less than 76%). Obstructive changes were found in two-thirds of the individuals who had ever smoked cigarettes and half of the individuals who had never smoked cigarettes.

Only 278 (44.3%) of the individuals with known filing status with silicosis or their next of kin applied for workers' compensation. Three hundred fifty (55.7%) had not applied. It was unknown whether the remaining 118 people with silicosis applied for compensation. There was no association between severity of disease and whether or not a person applied for workers' compensation. Of those known to apply, 227 (81.7%) received compensation, 17 (6.1%) were denied, and 34 (12.2%) were pending.

Industrial Hygiene Results

The 746 individuals with silicosis were exposed to silica in 278 facilities. Inspections were performed at 68 (24.5%) of these facilities. One hundred five (37.8%) facilities were no longer in operation, 43 (15.5%) were

Table 14.3 Primary Industry Where Silica Exposure Occurred for Individuals Confirmed with Silicosis for the Years 1985–1998

*Industry (SIC code)**	*Number of Individuals*†	*Percent*
Manufacturing		
Primary metal industries (33)	586	78.9
Includes iron, steel, gray, and ductile iron foundries		
Stone, clay, glass, and concrete products (32)	37	5.0
Transportation equipment (37)	27	3.6
Includes auto bodies and boat building		
Fabricated metal products (34)	10	1.3
Industrial machinery (35)	8	1.1
Miscellaneous (25, 26, 28, 30, 36, 38)	10	1.3
Includes chemicals and allied products, rubber parts, metalworking machinery and dental equipment		
Mining (10–14)	19	2.6
Construction (15–17)	35	4.7
Transportation, communication, services (40–49)	5	0.7
Wholesale trade (50)	1	0.1
Business and repair services (73,76)	2	0.3
Dental laboratory (80)	3	0.4
Total	743	100.0

*Standard Industrial Classification.
†For three workers, the industrial classification was not known.

located out of state, 19 (6.8%) facilities no longer used silica, 26 (9.4%) had worked at multiple construction sites as building trade workers, 1 (0.4%) was referred to the Mine Safety and Health Administration since the company was out of MIOSHA jurisdiction, and 15 (5.4%) were unknown.

Air sampling was conducted in 48 of the 68 facilities inspected (Table 14.6). Thirty of 48 (62.5%) fa-

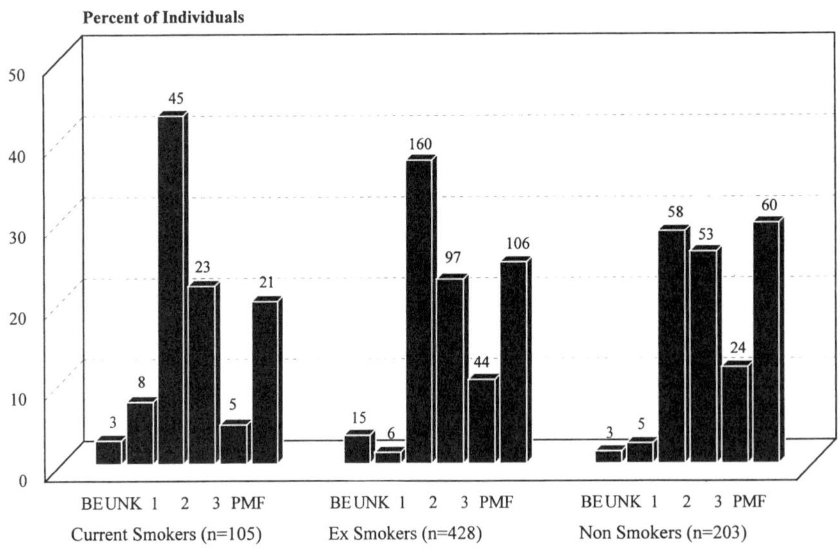

Figure 14.8 Severity of x-ray results by smoking status for individuals confirmed with silicosis, Michigan, 1985–1988. BE, biopsy evidence; UNK, unknown; 1–3 International Labor Organization categorization system for grading pneumoconioses; Category 1: 1/0, 1/1, 1/2; Category 2: 2/1, 2/2, 2/3; Category 3: 3/2, 3/3, 3/3+; PMF, progressive massive fibrosis. Total number of individuals: 736. Unknown smoking status for 10 individuals.

Table 14.4 Percent Predicted Forced Vital Capacity by X-Ray Results and Cigarette Smoking Status for Individuals* Confirmed with Silicosis for the Years 1985–1998

	Percent FVC†					
	< 60%		*60%–79%*		*> 80%*	
X-Ray Results	*Ever Smoked (%)*	*Never Smoked (%)*	*Ever Smoked (%)*	*Never Smoked (%)*	*Ever Smoked (%)*	*Never Smoked (%)*
Biopsy evidence	5 (31.3)	0 (—)	8 (50.0)	1 (33.3)	3 (18.8)	2 (66.7)
Unknown severity	3 (27.3)	1 (33.3)	4 (36.4)	1 (33.3)	4 (36.4)	1 (33.3)
Category 1	37 (23.9)	14 (33.3)	53 (34.2)	10 (23.8)	65 (41.9)	18 (42.9)
Category 2	28 (31.5)	14 (38.9)	27 (30.3)	11 (30.6)	34 (38.2)	11 (30.6)
Category 3	9 (30.0)	10 (62.5)	12 (40.0)	3 (18.8)	9 (30.0)	3 (18.8)
Progressive massive fibrosis	31 (35.6)	13 (31.7)	30 (34.5)	15 (36.6)	26 (29.9)	13 (31.7)
Total	113 (29.1)	52 (36.9)	134 (34.5)	41 (29.1)	141 (36.3)	48 (34.0)

*Total number of individuals: 529. Information was missing for 217 individuals.

†Percentages represent the proportion of individuals in each of the x-ray result categories within smoking status category (ever or never).

Table 14.5 Ratio of Forced Expiratory Volume in 1 Second Divided by Forced Vital Capacity by X-Ray Results and Cigarette Smoking Status for Individuals* Confirmed with Silicosis for the Years 1985–1998

	FEV_1/FVC†							
	< 40%		*41%–59%*		*60%–74%*		*> 75%*	
X-Ray Results	*Ever Smoked (%)*	*Never Smoked (%)*	*Ever Smoked (%)*	*Never Smoked (%)*	*Ever Smoked (%)*	*Never Smoked (%)*	*Ever Smoked (%)*	*Never Smoked (%)*
Biopsy evidence	2 (12.5)	1 (33.3)	3 (18.8)	0 (—)	5 (31.3)	2 (66.7)	6 (37.5)	0 (—)
Unknown severity	0 (—)	0 (—)	0 (—)	0 (—)	1 (12.5)	2 (66.7)	7 (87.5)	1 (33.3)
Category 1	16 (10.4)	2 (4.8)	33 (21.4)	3 (7.1)	58 (37.7)	12 (28.6)	47 (30.5)	25 (59.5)
Category 2	3 (3.6)	2 (5.6)	18 (21.4)	5 (13.9)	36 (42.9)	9 (25.0)	27 (32.1)	20 (55.6)
Category 3	1 (3.4)	0 (—)	4 (13.8)	0 (—)	5 (17.2)	5 (31.3)	19 (65.5)	11 (68.8)
Progressive massive fibrosis	13 (15.5)	4 (9.8)	24 (28.6)	9 (22.0)	26 (31.0)	13 (31.7)	21 (25.0)	15 (36.6)
Total	35 (9.3)	9 (6.4)	82 (21.9)	17 (12.1)	131 (34.9)	43 (30.5)	127 (33.9)	72 (51.1)

* Total number of individuals: 516. Information was missing for 230 individuals.

†FEV_1, forced expiratory volume in 1 second; FVC, forced vital capacity. Percentages represent the proportion of individuals in each of the x-ray result categories within smoking status category (ever or never).

Table 14.6 Results of Industrial Hygiene Inspections of 68 Facilities Where Individuals Confirmed with Silicosis for the Years 1985–1998 Were Exposed to Silica

Inspection	*No. of Companies*	*Percent*
Air sampling performed*	48	
Above NIOSH recommended standard for silica	30	62.8
Above MIOSHA enforceable standard for any exposure	21	43.8
Above MIOSHA enforceable standard for silica	20	41.7
Medical surveillance evaluated	59	
Periodic chest x-rays with B reader	5	8.5
Periodic chest X-rays without a B reader	2	3.4
Preemployment testing only	19	32.2
No medical surveillance	22	37.3
Periodic pulmonary function testing	15	35.4

*NIOSH, National Institute for Occupational Safety; MIOSHA, Michigan Occupational Health and Safety Administration.

cilities were above the National Institute for Occupational Safety and Health (NIOSH) recommended exposure level for silica. Twenty of the 48 (41.7%) were above the enforceable Michigan Occupational Health and Safety Administration (MIOSHA) standard for silica. Another one (2.1%) company was above the MIOSHA standard for beryllium and one company was above the MIOSHA standard for silica and silver.

Only 5 of the 59 (8.5%) facilities where the medical surveillance program was evaluated provided medical screening for silicosis for its workers that included a periodic chest x-ray interpreted by a "B" certified reader, whereas two companies provided periodic chest x-rays that were not interpreted by a "B" certified reader. Nineteen (32.2%) performed only preemployment testing, 22 (37.3%) provided no medical surveillance, and 15 (25.4%) performed annual or biannual pulmonary function testing without chest x-rays.

DISCUSSION

Michigan has had a surveillance system for silicosis since 1988. Similar to the New Jersey system that began in 1982, reports are received from hospitals, physicians, death certificates and the workers' compensation system. In Michigan, 60% of the reports are received from hospitals as compared to New Jersey where 80% are received from hospitals.[8,13] Workers' compensation is a minor source of case reports in both states since the majority of workers with silicosis do not apply for workers' compensation. Death certificates and physician reporting also account for a small percentage of the cases (10.4%, and 19.9% respectively) and act as the initial reporting source of cases in only 7.8% and 16.5%, respectively.

The Michigan surveillance system has proved useful in describing the epidemiology of the disease and directing prevention activity despite the underreporting of cases, which may be as high as 80%.

Silicosis occurred mainly among men born before 1940 who began working in a ferrous foundry in the 1930s or 1940s and were exposed to silica sand for over 25 years. Forty-four percent of the patients were African-American. The overall annual average incidence rate of silicosis among African-American males (14.8 cases per 100,000) was seven times higher than white males (2.1 cases per 100,000). The rates within specific counties ranged between 2.2 and 25.4 times higher for African-American males than for white males. The reason for the higher rates among African-Americans is that historically the foundries hired large numbers of African-Americans who were given the higher silica-exposure jobs.[14]

The patients identified with silicosis generally had severe disease. Twenty-five percent had progressive massive fibrosis (PMF) and another 33.4% had advanced simple silicosis. Only about one-third of all patients had normal breathing tests. Twenty-three percent had been told they had tuberculosis (includes both clinical disease and a positive skin test). Individuals in Michigan with silicosis have an increase of over 300% in the likelihood of dying from nonmalignant respiratory disease, both restrictive and obstructive, and an 80% increase in the likelihood of dying from lung cancer.[11] Despite the severity of disease, 56% of the patients with known filing status had not applied for workers' compensation.

Although silicosis typically occurs after a long duration of exposure to silica, there continues to be patients who develop silicosis after a relatively short time because of the severity of exposure. Three patients developed silicosis who began working with silica in the 1980s, 29 in the 1970s, and 89 in the 1960s. These cases could be classified as having accelerated silicosis.

Exposure to silica is still occurring in foundries and other silica-using industries, although working conditions have clearly improved from the 1930s and 1940s. Industrial hygiene inspections revealed violations of the exposure standard for silica in 38.7% of the facilities where sampling was conducted. However, follow-up inspections of these same companies showed a significant decrease in airborne silica levels (Table 14.1). Those companies not in compliance with the silica standard required their workers to use powered air purifying respirators or air line respirators.

CONCLUSION

Silicosis remains an ongoing problem in Michigan with former foundry workers continuing to develop severe disease. Further, some Michigan workers will continue to be at risk of developing silicosis because of inadequate controls at foundries currently in operation. In addition, sandblasting continues to be a high-risk operation. Silica is inexpensive and abundant in Michigan. Given the ready availability of nonsilica abrasives, further educational and regulatory efforts are needed to encourage the replacement of silica in blasting operations or at the minimum ensure that silica is used properly. Continuation of the silicosis surveillance system is important to direct intervention activity, monitor trends, and maintain a level of concern among silica users about the importance of good industrial hygiene practices. Because the disease typically occurs after 20 years or more of exposure to silica, the data from the surveillance system and the dissemination of that information about individuals with silicosis highlights the consequences of inadequate work practices and controls. Current theories on health behavior support the importance of personalizing the consequences of not implementing preventive action to motivate such action.[15] Although more complete reporting would presumably identify more problem worksites, even with marked underreporting, the system has been successful in meeting its objectives of estimating the burden of disease, describing the epidemiology, and directing effective preventive interventions.

ACKNOWLEDGMENTS

The authors acknowledge the office and interview staff who handle the reports of silicosis on a daily basis: Amy Allemier, Amy Krizek, Tracy Murphy, and Ruth VanderWaals as well as the numerous medical students who conducted interviews throughout the years of surveillance efforts. The authors also acknowledge the tremendous support of the program by Michigan's OSHA inspectors and administrative staff. This project was partially funded by the National Institute for Occupational Safety and Health, under cooperative agreement number U60-CCU502998.

REFERENCES

1. Begin R, Filion R, Ostiguy G. Emphysema in silica and asbestos exposed workers seeking compensation, a CT scan study. *Chest* 1995; 108:647–655.
2. Snider DE. The relationship between tuberculosis and silicosis. *Am Rev Resp Dis* 1978; 118:455–460.
3. Rosenman KD, Reilly MJ, Moore-Fuller M. Connective tissue disease and silicosis. *Am J Ind Med* 1999; 35:375–381.
4. Kallenberg CGM. Renal disease—another effect of silica exposure? *Nephrol Dial Transplant* 1995; 10:1117–1119.
5. Smith AH, Lopipero PA, Barroga VR. Meta-analysis of studies of lung cancer among silicotics. *Epidemiology* 1995; 6:617–624.
6. Trasko VM. Some facts on the prevalence of silicosis in the United States. *AMA Arch Ind Health* 1956; 14:379–386.
7. Windau J, Rosenman KD, Anderson H, Hanrahan L, Rudolph L, Stanbury M, Stark A. The identification of occupational lung disease from hospital discharge data. *J Occup Med* 1991; 33: 1061–1066.
8. Valiante D, Rosenman KD. Does silicosis still occur? *JAMA* 1989; 262:3003–3007.
9. Maxfield R, Alo C, Reilly MJ, Rosenman KD et al. Silicosis surveillance, 1993—Illinois, Michigan, New Jersey, North Carolina, Ohio, Texas and Wisconsin. *MMWR* 1997; 45(SS-1):13–28.
10. Rosenman KD, Reilly MJ, Kalinowski DJ. 1998 Annual report on silicosis in Michigan. Lansing, Michigan: Michigan State University; February 26, 1999.
11. Rosenman KD, Trimbath L, Stanbury M. Surveillance of occupational lung disease: comparison of hospital discharge data to physician reporting. *Am J Public Health* 1990; 80:1257–1258.
12. Rosenman KD, Stanbury MJ, Reilly MJ. Mortality among persons with silicosis reported to disease surveillance systems in Michigan and New Jersey in the United States. *Scand J Work Environ Health* 1995; 21(suppl 2):73–76.
13. Rosenman KD, Reilly MJ, Kalinowski DJ, Watt FC. Silicosis in the 1990's. *Chest* 1997; 111:779–786.
14. Rosenman KD, Reilly MK, Rice C, Hertzberg V, Tseng CY, Anderson HA. Silicosis among foundry workers. *Am J Epidemiol* 1996; 144:890–900.
15. Witte K. Putting the fear back into fear appeals: the extended parallel process model. *Communication Monogr* 1992; 59:329–349.

15

Noise-Induced Hearing Loss

MARY JO REILLY AND KENNETH D. ROSENMAN

Occupational noise-induced hearing loss (NIHL) is an insidious, irreversible condition. The slow development of hearing loss over time detracts from its being noticed by workers exposed to noise at work, and downplays the immediacy of the problem and the need to address noise issues. The perception that hearing loss is only or primarily due to aging also works to minimize the recognition of noise at work as a real threat to one's hearing health. Hearing loss affects more than a person's hearing; it affects an individual's job performance and the likelihood of accidents at work and home; it has significant social and emotional consequences, and affects physical and psychosocial function in the elderly.[1,2]

In Michigan a minimum estimate of the number of workers exposed to noise at or above an 8-hour time-weighted average (TWA) of 85 dBA (the action level) by general industry categories is: 145,000 manufacturing production workers; 20,700 construction workers; 500 miners; 27,200 blue-collar workers in wholesale and retail trade; and, 12,100 workers in noisy service industry environments (Table 15.1). Based on data from the National Health Interview Survey, one would expect approximately 86,000 individuals in Michigan to have noise-induced hearing loss related to workplace exposures.[3]

Nationally, it is estimated that 30 million individuals are exposed to excessive levels of noise at work,[4] whereas one million workers are estimated to have work-related hearing loss, primarily from exposures to noise in manufacturing.[5]

Work-related hearing loss is one of the top ten priority occupational safety and health objectives for targeted efforts at the reduction of its incidence in the Healthy People 2000 report,[6] as well as a priority in the Healthy People 2010 objectives of the U.S. Public Health Service. In addition, the reduction of the prevalence of significant hearing impairment is one of the top ten objectives for chronic disability conditions in the Healthy People 2000 report. The National Institute for Occupational Safety and Health (NIOSH) has recently reevaluated their recommendations for hearing conservation and published a revised criteria document outlining recommendations for the prevention of occupational noise-induced hearing loss.[4] Further, recent research directions at NIOSH through its National Occupational Research Agenda (NORA) initiative are aimed at research and prevention of occupational NIHL.[7]

In 1993, Michigan received funding from NIOSH to develop and implement a surveillance system for occupational NIHL. Michigan was the only state funded for surveillance of occupational NIHL, as part of the Sentinel Event Notification System for Occupational Risk program (Project SENSOR).

Occupational NIHL was chosen for surveillance in Michigan for several reasons:

- the condition had a known cause-and-effect relationship between exposure and disease
- it had serious consequences not only at work but in nonwork arenas
- it was easily identified through audiometric testing
- it was preventable
- a well-defined and accepted enforcement standard for workplaces existed
- there was a well-defined and easily identifiable target population of sentinel health providers (i.e., audiologists and otolaryngologists)
- it affected a large number of workers

Table 15.1 Estimates of the Number of Blue-Collar Workers in Michigan Exposed to Excessive Levels of Noise, by Industry Type

*Industry (SIC)**	*No. of Workers†*	*No. of Noise-Exposed‡*	*% Noise-Exposed Workers*
MINING			
Oil and gas extraction (13)	2100	485	23.1
CONSTRUCTION			
General building contractors (15)	26,100	4124	15.8
Heavy construction (16)	11,700	2808	24.0
Special trade contractors (17)	88,700	13,837	15.6
MANUFACTURING			
Food (20)	32,300	9335	28.9
Textiles (22)	400	170	42.6
Apparel (23)	16,400	2280	13.9
Lumber and wood (24)	13,700	5658	41.3
Furniture (25)	25,900	7330	28.3
Paper (26)	15,600	5273	33.8
Printing (27)	24,900	5329	21.4
Chemicals (28)	22,000	3806	17.3
Petroleum and coal (29)	900	179	19.9
Rubber and plastics (30)	50,700	11,560	22.8
Leather (31)	3300	215	6.5
Stone, clay, and glass (32)	12,400	2666	21.5
Primary metals (33)	28,400	9287	32.7
Fabricated metals (34)	101,600	29,769	29.3
Machinery (35)	86,200	12,844	14.9
Electrical machinery (36)	24,500	1985	8.1
Transportation equipment (37)	198,600	36,145	18.2
Instruments (38)	10,500	914	8.7
Miscellaneous manufacturing (39)	5100	479	9.4
TRANSPORTATION			
Freight (42)	38,800	2716	7.0
TRADE			
Wholesale durable goods (50)	110,600	23,115	20.9
Wholesale nondurable goods (51)	58,600	3106	5.3
Retail (52)	70,500	987	1.4
SERVICES			
Business (73)	228,100	3422	1.5
Automotive Repair (75)	49,600	5258	10.6
Health (80)	581,800	3491	0.6

*Office of Management and Budget. Standard Industrial Classification, 1987 Manual. Washington, DC: U.S. Government Printing Office, 1989.

†Bureau of Labor Statistics, Michigan Employment Security Commission, Current Employment Statistics. 1996 Annual Report of Michigan Production/Non-supervisory Workers. Detroit, MI: Michigan Department of Labor; 1996.

‡National Institute for Occupational Safety and Health, Criteria for a Recommended Standard, Occupational Noise Exposure Revised Criteria 1998. June 1998, DHHS (NIOSH) Publication No. 98-126, Table 2.1. Percentages are estimates based on data collected in the National Occupational Exposure Survey (NOES). Excessive noise is defined as at or above 85 dBA.

- Michigan had an existing reporting system for occupational diseases that included occupational NIHL
- an infrastructure to conduct occupational disease surveillance already existed, which facilitated the addition of a new condition for surveillance

METHODS

Define Goals, Objectives, and Scope

The goal of the surveillance system for occupational NIHL was to prevent Michigan workers from developing hearing loss from exposure to noise at their jobs.

The system was designed to identify sentinel cases of individuals with occupational NIHL through the state's hearing health professionals (audiologists and otolaryngologists). After identifying cases, the system then provided for intervention in the workplace when interviews with the sentinel cases indicated an ongoing problem with exposure to noise at work and the absence of regular hearing testing. In addition, the surveillance system sought to increase and expand the number of reports of hearing loss from noise at work in order to better document and describe the magnitude of the problem. Work-related NIHL was considered to be an under-reported condition based on various estimates of the prevalence of occupational NIHL in the state and the almost total lack of reporting of the condition by any of the state's 150 otolaryngologists or 400 audiologists.

Geographic Targeting

All known or suspected cases of work-related NIHL were targeted in case-finding efforts and acted potentially as the basis for intervention. The tremendous in-kind support of staff at the Michigan Department of Consumer and Industry Services, MDCIS, (formerly the Michigan Department of Public Health) allowed available monetary resources to be directed to case-finding in the entire state of Michigan. Although certain counties in Michigan are more industrial and therefore might be expected to generate a greater number of cases of occupational NIHL, resources were available to cover the entire state and thus satisfy one of the goals of the program—to document the extent of the problem.

Assemble Multidisciplinary Team

The structure of the multidisciplinary surveillance team was based on the ongoing working relationship between personnel at the MDCIS and personnel in the College of Human Medicine at Michigan State University (MSU). Since 1988, the MDCIS and MSU have conducted surveillance and intervention of occupational asthma and silicosis. Staff at MSU provided the medical and epidemiologic expertise for surveillance whereas staff at the MDCIS fulfilled the industrial hygiene and enforcement role of the intervention efforts. Michigan has a state enforcement plan and operates the Occupational Safety and Health Administration (OSHA) program, which is part of the MDCIS. The state therefore had the legal authority to collect the surveillance data and intervene in workplaces where sentinel cases were identified.

Surveillance staff were in place prior to the initiation of the surveillance program for occupational NIHL, as part of other funded SENSOR surveillance conditions (occupational asthma and silicosis). Staff at MSU under contract to the MDCIS included an occupational physician, an epidemiologist, and office support staff. Staff at the MDCIS included 25 industrial hygienists located at 6 district offices across the state, an administrator acting as a codirector of the surveillance program along with MSU's occupational physician, and 2 MDCIS/MSU liaisons, 1 for administrative issues and 1 for issues related to enforcement inspections. The personnel at the MDCIS acted as in-kind support for the program.

Gain Support

In addition to hired staff, an advisory committee was assembled, which included an otolaryngologist from the Michigan Otolaryngology Society, an audiologist representative from the Michigan Speech Language and Hearing Association, a nurse representative from the Michigan Occupational Health Nurses' Association, an audiologist representative from the Michigan Academy of Audiology, and two audiologists from two of the major universities in the state that had graduate audiology programs. This group helped develop the working definition of hearing loss that was distributed to the state's hearing health professionals, helped identify barriers and ways to overcome the obstacles to reporting, and acted as a guide and sounding board for the direction of surveillance efforts.

One of the major strengths of the program was the multidisciplinary nature of the organizations involved in the surveillance efforts. This was a key component of the program, providing a variety of expertise and insights into effective ways to promote the new surveillance initiative and a variety of levels of intervention possibilities in the workplace and among the health professionals targeted as key reporters of sentinel cases.

Case Definition and Data Collection

The case definition was developed with the help of the advisory committee and was defined as an individual with:

1. audiometric findings consistent with NIHL and
2. history of exposure to noise at work sufficient to cause hearing loss

The interpretation of audiometric findings and association of such findings with work exposures was left to the professional judgement of the hearing health professional submitting the report. When more specific audiometric criteria were requested, the advisory committee developed the following suggestions as indicative of a minimum hearing loss:

1. a standard threshold shift (STS) of 10 dB or more in either ear at an average of 2000, 3000, and 4000 Hz, which reflects the Michigan OSHA noise standard definition for occupational NIHL, or
2. a fixed loss (suggested definitions: a 25 dB or greater loss in either ear at an average of 500, 1000, and 2000 Hz; or 1000, 2000, and 3000 Hz; or 3000, 4000, and 6000 Hz; or a 15 to 25 dB or greater loss in either ear at an average of 3000 and 4000 Hz)

No correction for age was suggested, and no audiograms with actual testing results were required to be reported with the occupational disease reporting form.

The above recommendations were developed because many private practice hearing clinics not associated with a particular company would only have one hearing test result and would therefore only be able to evaluate a patient's fixed loss rather than an STS, which requires a baseline and subsequent audiometric test results.

Mechanism for Reporting and Reporting Guidelines

The standard occupational disease reporting form was used for any known or suspected occupational disease or work-aggravated condition and collected demographic information on the employee affected, information about the employer, illness information, and information on the person, clinic, or other such entity submitting the report.

The surveillance system for occupational NIHL hinged on an existing state law for the reporting of all known or *suspected* occupational diseases. The word *suspected* was an important qualifier for the state's audiologists and otolaryngologists, who repeatedly voiced concerns about their ability to determine what part of a patient's hearing loss was due to work. A hearing loss in the higher frequencies (typically around 4000 Hz) is typically viewed as noise-related hearing loss. The state's hearing health professionals were instructed to report patients with such a noise notch, and, who in their professional judgement were exposed to sufficient noise at work to cause any part of the hearing loss. In Michigan, if any portion of an individual's hearing loss is due to workplace noise exposures, the loss is considered work-related. These criteria helped to sideline discussions about recreational noise causing or contributing to an individual's hearing loss and keep the focus of reporting on patients with sufficient workplace noise exposures.

The Michigan law, Part 56 of Public Act 368 of 1978, as amended, states that a physician, hospital, clinic, or employer must report known or suspected cases of occupational diseases or workplace-aggravated health conditions to the Michigan Department of Consumer and Industry Services (MDCIS) within 10 days after the discovery of the disease or condition. The failure to report cases can result in a $50 fine per individual not reported, although no health care provider who failed to report a patient has ever been fined since the introduction of the law. Compliance with the law relies more on professional responsibility rather than on the threat of monetary punishment. The reporting law relieves the health practitioner of any liability for releasing confidential patient information to the state.

Identify, Select, and Recruit Reporters

Prior to the initiation of the surveillance program, an examination of the nature of the reports of hearing loss submitted to the MDCIS revealed that nearly all the cases were being reported by company or contract medical services, and were being reported by the companies as part of the requirements of the companies' hearing conservation programs. There were almost no reports of hearing loss from private practice audiologists or otolaryngologists not associated with a particular company.

Through discussions with respected audiologists in the state, key reporters were expected to be:

- audiologists
- otolaryngologists
- speech and hearing clinics
- mobile van hearing testing units
- occupational health nurses

A strong adversarial relationship existed between the mobile testing vans and hearing aid dealers not associated with hearing clinics, especially those from out-of-state doing business in Michigan, and the audiologists and otolaryngologists associated with hearing clinics in the state. Mobile testing vans and hearing aid dealers were viewed as having poor quality control and taking away business from the more reputable hearing clinics that provide more comprehensive hearing testing, evaluation, and follow-up services.

Through the Michigan Speech, Language and Hearing Association (MSHA), the Michigan Otolaryngology Society, the Michigan Occupational Health Nurses' Association, and several hearing health professionals in the Lansing, Michigan area, members of each of these associations were identified as potential key reporters of individuals with work-related noise-induced hearing loss. Few, if any of these members were expected to be aware of the occupational disease reporting law, although at least one of the state's four university graduate audiology programs regularly reviewed the reporting law and form with their students prior to the initiation of Project SENSOR's outreach efforts. In order to introduce the surveillance project to these groups of hearing health professionals and encourage the reporting of known and suspected cases of work-related NIHL, several outreach and education efforts were instituted. An introductory mailing was tailored to the members of each of these groups, which included a cover letter from the state health director, and a copy of the occupational disease reporting law and form.

To ease the burden of reporting, a fact sheet on how to report was developed and distributed at conferences attended by hearing health professionals. Reporting of cases could be done by mail, electronic mail, telephone, or fax.

Protocol for Follow-up

Case reports received by the MDCIS were followed up if reported by hearing health professionals not associated with a particular company. The logic behind such follow-up was that cases reported by company or contract medical groups were being reported as part of a company's compliance with Michigan's noise standard, and would therefore provide less of an opportunity for meaningful intervention compared to cases reported by private practice hearing health professionals not associated with a particular company.

A common concern of the audiologists and otolaryngologists was the potential for nonnoise exposures contributing to the patient's hearing loss. These hearing health professionals were directed to report patients if any part of the patient's hearing loss was due to noise at work, regardless of the potential contribution of recreational noise or presbycusis (hearing loss due to aging) to the loss.

When a case was identified as known or suspected occupational NIHL, and reported by a noncompany hearing health professional, an interview with the case was conducted. A standardized telephone-administered questionnaire consisted of demographic information and information on up to three most recent workplaces where the case was exposed to noise.

Workplaces were referred to the Michigan OSHA program for inspection if:

- the case was exposed to noise recently (within the last 5 years)
- no regular hearing testing was provided
- no hearing protection devices (ear plugs or muffs) were available
- no inspection had been conducted recently (within the last 5 years)
- the industry was covered by the Michigan OSHA noise standard

Michigan's major automotive manufacturing facilities were automatically excluded from consideration of being inspected because the state and university staff were aware that these companies had hearing conservation programs. Prior to initiating an inspection, the industrial hygiene inspector in the district where the company was located reviewed Michigan OSHA files to ensure that no prior inspections had been conducted at the facility, particularly if noise issues had been addressed. An inspection was then scheduled.

Case Management

Data from the occupational disease reports on occupational NIHL and data from the case interviews were entered into a tracking database. The database was used to track the progress of case interviews, the status of inspections, and to analyze the information collected through the telephone-administered interviews.

Field Investigations

Companies where a recent inspection had not been conducted, where the sentinel case worked within the last 5 years, and where no regular hearing testing had been provided were considered for inspections. Certain industries in Michigan are not covered by the Michigan OSHA laws, or are not covered as completely such as mining, agriculture, transportation, and oil and gas well drilling and servicing. Construction is covered, but the standard for construction workers is not as comprehensive as that for workers in manufacturing.

Enforcement inspections were carried out by the state's industrial hygienists and consisted of an evaluation of noise levels and compliance with the elements in Michigan's noise standard. The Michigan OSHA rules require employees exposed to noise levels at or greater than the action level of 85 dBA, 8-hour time-weighted average (TWA) be included in a hearing conservation program. If employees are exposed to noise levels at or greater than the permissible noise exposure limit of 90 dBA, 8-hour TWA, feasible administrative or engineering controls must be utilized and hearing protection required. The elements of a Hearing Conservation Program (HCP) as outlined by the state are:

Monitoring

Representative personal monitoring must be conducted to identify all affected employees for inclusion in a hearing conservation program and to determine the appropriate level of hearing protection.

Training
The employer must provide a training program regarding noise and hearing protection for employees exposed at or above the action level of 85 dBA. It is important that employees understand that extended exposure to high noise levels can cause permanent hearing loss. Training must include instruction on fitting and use of hearing protective devices. Training must include information on the purpose of audiometric testing and an explanation of the test procedures.

Hearing Protection
The employer shall, at no cost to the employees, make hearing protectors available to all employees who are exposed to noise at or above the action level of 85 dBA. Hearing protection is required for employees who have not had a baseline audiogram or who show an STS.

Baseline Audiograms
Employees who have had audiograms administered by the company shall have their first such audiogram designated as their baseline. Baseline audiograms must be provided within 6 months of the exposure for all employees exposed at or above the action level of 85 dBA.

Annual Audiograms
Audiometric testing must be performed at least once per year on all individuals in work areas where noise levels are determined to be above the action level. The results of these annual audiograms must be compared to the employee's baseline audiogram to determine if an STS has occurred.

Rules
The employer must make copies of the rules available to employees and must post a copy in the workplace.

While the enforcement inspections evaluated the company's compliance with the noise standard, issues such as the quality of the compliance with the standard were not as easily addressed. After the investigation was completed, a report of the inspection results and any recommendations was sent to the company and union (or designated labor representative if the company did not have a union), as well as to the reporting audiologist or otolaryngologist. If the company was cited for violations of any regulations, a copy of the citations was posted at or near the location of the violations for a minimum of 3 days or until the items were corrected, whichever was later.

Analyze and Interpret Data

On a biannual basis, progress reports detailing the numbers of cases identified, number of inspections completed, and other related information were submitted to the funding agency. On a yearly basis, a report on all the surveillance data was developed. This annual report summarized the history of the surveillance project, the elements of surveillance, and a summary of the data obtained including questionnaire data and inspection report summaries.

Feedback and Recommendations

The annual reports were distributed to the state's audiologists and otolaryngologists, to hearing clinics, to the mobile vans conducting hearing tests, to administrative personnel in the MDCIS, and to other government officials. In the 5th year of surveillance, a website was developed, which posted the newsletters, annual reports, reporting law, and other educational information.

Industrial hygiene inspections conducted by Michigan OSHA were enforcement inspections. Any violations of Michigan's noise standard were required to be corrected and proof of such corrections were required to be submitted to Michigan OSHA.

Evaluate the Surveillance System

Each year, a meeting was held with the advisory committee to review the successes and difficulties faced during the year. To evaluate the success of the model, statistics comparing reports submitted by companies to reports submitted by private practice hearing health professionals were reviewed. Major gaps especially in the types of industries identified by the two reporting sources highlighted the importance of encouraging reporting by the noncompany hearing health professionals (Table 15.2). Companies reporting cases were primarily large manufacturing facilities; private practice health professionals reported workers from smaller facilities, and from a wider range of industries including agriculture, mining, construction, trade, service, and government.

Case demographics (i.e., an older population of workers and retirees reported by private practice hearing health professionals) also highlighted the importance of obtaining reports from both sources (Table 15.2). The increase in the number of noncompany reports since the initiation of the occupational NIHL surveillance program from 5 in 1992 to 374 in 1998 provided an indicator of the success of outreach and education efforts directed at sentinel providers (Table 15.2). The ability of the Project SENSOR-initiated workplace enforcement inspections to identify workplaces with excessive noise and no hearing conserva-

Table 15.2 Occupational and Demographic Characteristics of Noise-Induced Hearing Loss Cases Reported in 1998

	Company Reports		*Private Practice HHPs*[a]	
Item	N	%	N‡	%
INDUSTRY				
Agriculture	—		7	2
Mining	—		1	< 1
Construction	—		30	10
Manufacturing	1209	96	148	51
Transportation	—		22	8
Trade	—		6	2
Finance	—		3	1
Services	47	4	48	17
Public administration	—		24	8
Total	1256	100	289[b]	100
EMPLOYER SIZE, BY NUMBER OF EMPLOYEES				
< 25	—		9	7
25–99	15	1	7	5
100–499	17	1	12	9
500+	1224	98	108	79
Total	1256	100	136[c]	100
AGE				
20–29	73	6	8	2
30–39	156	13	24	7
40–49	479	39	73	20
50–59	409	33	104	29
60–69	94	8	87	24
70–79	14	1	54	15
80+	—	—	12	3
Total	1225[d]	100	362[e]	100
YEAR REPORTED				
1992	1425	> 99	5	< 1
1993	1937	99	12	1
1994	1683	85	307	15
1995	1231	72	488	28
1996	1589	80	406	20
1997	1313	73	484	27
1998	1256	77	374	23

[a]HHP, hearing health professionals.
[b]Industry was unknown for 46 individuals.
[c]Company size unknown for 238 patients.
[d]Age unknown for 31 patients.
[e]Age unknown for 12 patients.

tion programs is another demonstration of the success of the model (Table 15.3).

However, an examination of the number of sentinel providers not reporting cases (only 16% of the state's audiologists and otolaryngologists reported at least one case in 1998) highlighted the difficulties in encouraging health providers to comply with reporting despite continued outreach efforts and the existence of a state law requiring such reports. Discussions with the advisory committee shed some light on the reasons for lack of compliance with the reporting law, including:

- concern about releasing confidential patient information
- the exact wording of the reporting law not mentioning audiologists per se
- concern about the loss of business by reporting patients from a particular company

Table 15.3 Sixty Companies Inspected Where Patients with a Fixed Loss Reported No Audiometric Testing: Michigan 1993–1998

	Total Inspections		*Hearing Conservation Program Required*		*OSHA Citations Issued*				
					No Hearing Conservation Program		*Deficient Hearing Conservation Program*		*No. of Employees Exposed to Noise*
Industry	N	%	N	%	N	%†	N	%†	
Construction	1	2	1*	0	1	100	0	0	562
Manufacturing	45	75	27	60	9	33	10	37	2891
Transportation	2	3	0	0	—	—	—	—	—
Trade	5	8	1	20	1	100	0	0	14
Services	4	7	3	75	2	67	0	0	29
Government	3	5	3	100	0	0	2	67	700

*Construction has separate regulations that require a less comprehensive program.
†Percentage of companies in which a hearing conservation program was required.

- the perceived extra amount of work for office staff to submit case reports
- uncertainty about the work-relatedness of the hearing loss (i.e., the inability to distinguish the relative contributions of recreational and occupational noise exposures to the patients' hearing loss)
- general distrust of government

Another issue related to lack of reporting was a tendency for health professionals to treat symptoms rather than address the underlying causes of diseases, especially diseases that were occupational.

RESULTS

Demographics and Occupational Characteristics

About 10% of Michigan's approximately 20,000 occupational disease reports received each year are for occupational noise-induced hearing loss. Prior to the initiation of Project SENSOR surveillance for occupational NIHL in 1993, almost none of the reports of hearing loss submitted to the MDCIS were from audiologists or otolaryngologists in private practice. The first year of focused surveillance on occupational NIHL was dedicated to informing the targeted health professionals about the reporting law and their responsibility to report patients with known or suspected work-related hearing loss.

In 1994, the first jump in hearing loss reporting by private practice hearing health professionals was noted (Table 15.2). Since that time, Michigan has had approximately 400 reports of work-related NIHL reported yearly by these private practice hearing health professionals. The other 1500 or so cases of work-related hearing loss are reported each year by companies. Most of the reports from both companies and hearing health professionals in private practice are for white men in the 30–60 age range from large manufacturing facilities (Table 15.2).

Worker Interviews

Between 1993 and 1998 a total of 1845 interviews were conducted of the 1905 (97%) adults with noise-induced hearing loss who were reported by private practice health professionals to the Michigan surveillance system.

The telephone-administered interviews were conducted by trained interviewers and took 5–10 minutes to complete. The standardized questionnaire elicited patient demographics, military history, and detailed information about up to three of the individual's most recent noisy workplaces. The work-related questions asked about noisy machinery and equipment used, other noise-related work practices, the availability and use of hearing protection, access to audiometric testing, information on the numbers of other workers potentially exposed to noise at the facility, and whether the facility was still in business.

Most of the workers interviewed were men (93%), white (91%), and born between 1920 and 1959 (86%). Over 57% of the 2586 companies where the 1845 patients ever worked were in manufacturing (Table 15.4). For the most recent company where each patient was exposed to noise, 45% did not regularly test their employees' hearing (Table 15.5). The absence of testing

Table 15.4 Industry at Any Company Where Patients with a Fixed Loss Were Exposed to Noise: Michigan, 1993–1998

Industry	*No. of Companies*	%
Agriculture	82	3
Mining	14	1
Construction	251	10
Manufacturing	1484	57
Transportation	179	7
Trade	69	3
Finance	10	< 1
Services	256	10
Public administration	241	9
Total	2586	100

Table 15.5 Industry, Employer Size, and Regular Hearing Testing at Companies Where Patients with a Fixed Loss Were Exposed to Noise: Michigan, 1993–1998

Item	*Companies*	*No Hearing Test* N	%
INDUSTRY			
Agriculture	58	38	66
Mining	8	2	25
Construction	144	109	76
Manufacturing	1013	393	39
Transportation	129	47	36
Trade	49	34	69
Finance	8	4	50
Services	198	110	56
Public Administration	192	69	36
Total	1799*	806	45
EMPLOYER SIZE BY NO. OF EMPLOYEES			
< 25	251	189	75
25–99	203	148	73
100–499	255	127	50
500+	768	278	36
Total	1477†	742	50

*Industry was unknown for 46 individuals.
†Number of employees was unknown for 368 individuals.

Table 15.6 Total Duration of Years Worked and Decade of First Exposure in Noise for Patients with a Fixed Hearing Loss: Michigan, 1993–1998

Item	N	%
YEARS WORKED		
1–9	234	17
10–19	239	17
20–29	428	30
30+	513	36
Total	1414*	100
DECADE OF FIRST EXPOSURE		
1910s	3	< 1
1920s	4	< 1
1930s	24	2
1940s	156	11
1950s	249	17
1960s	445	31
1970s	321	22
1980s	164	11
1990s	91	6
Total	1457†	100

*Duration exposed to noise was unknown for 421 individuals.
†Decade was unknown for 388 individuals.

was greater in companies employing smaller numbers of workers (Table 15.5). Thirty-four percent of interviewed workers reported by noncompany health professionals worked in noise for fewer than 19 years (Table 15.6). Some patients had very early exposures to noise; however, over 17% had first exposures to noise from the 1980s onward (Table 15.6).

Table 15.7 shows the decade when the interviewed patients with fixed hearing loss most recently worked, and whether they were provided with ear plugs or muffs, by industry type. Over time, the percentage of workers provided with hearing protection increased in all industries. The percentage of workers in manufacturing given hearing protection improved the most of all industry types, from only 10% of workers given hearing protection in the 1940s to 91% of workers given hearing protection in the 1990s.

Table 15.8 shows the decade when the interviewed patients with fixed hearing loss were most recently exposed to noise by industry. The percentage of individuals at companies with regular hearing tests generally increased over time within the industries required by OSHA (since 1972) to provide such testing. Construction and agriculture had the greatest percentages of workers with no regular hearing tests; these industries are not required by MIOSHA or OSHA to provide regular hearing tests.

An underprotected group identified through the surveillance program and worker interviews was construction workers. Interviews with workers who developed NIHL from construction noise exposures indicated they were almost never provided with hearing testing (96% never received testing), and that only approximately 40% were provided with hearing protection devices (ear plugs or muffs). Workers exposed to noise in construction in more recent decades, however, were more likely to be given hearing protection than workers exposed to noise before the 1980s.

Table 15.7 Prevalence of Regular Hearing Protection in Patients with a Fixed Loss by Most Recent Industry Where Noise Exposure Occurred and Decade Most Recently Worked, Michigan, 1993–1998

	%					
*Industry**	*1940s*	*1950s*	*1960s*	*1970s*	*1980s*	*1990s*
Agriculture	—	—	0	0	40	59
Mining	—	—	—	—	—	—
Construction	—	0	0	33	50	76
Manufacturing	10	25	28	53	77	91
Transportation	—	—	50	37	64	69
Trade	—	0	0	0	33	61
Finance	—	—	—	0	—	67
Services	—	—	—	—	28	77
Public administration	—	—	75	60	91	81

*Either industry or decade exposed was unknown for 379 patients.

Table 15.8 Prevalence of Regular Hearing Testing in Patients with a Fixed Loss by Most Recent Industry Where Noise Exposure Occurred and Decade Most Recently Worked, Michigan, 1993–1998

	%					
*Industry**	*1940s*	*1950s*	*1960s*	*1970s*	*1980s*	*1990s*
Agriculture	0	0	50	0	20	11
Mining	—	—	—	—	0	75
Construction	—	0	0	33	11	11
Manufacturing	20	19	4	26	54	67
Transportation	—	—	50	37	36	63
Trade	—	0	—	—	33	14
Finance	—	—	—	0	—	0
Services	—	—	0	—	11	38
Public administration	—	0	0	40	64	36

*Either industry or decade exposed was unknown for 379 patients.

Some workers were interested in the potential for receiving workers' compensation for their hearing loss. However, in Michigan the workers' compensation laws do not pay a monetary amount for the loss itself. Rather, the system is designed to cover medical visits and the costs of medical equipment (i.e., hearing aids). A worker would typically not have lost work time due to a hearing loss unless the loss was from an acute exposure to noise, for example, from an explosion at work.

Because there is little potential for a monetary settlement for workers' compensation cases of hearing loss, there is no incentive for lawyers to represent individuals with such claims. Anecdotally, the experience of workers attempting to have hearing aids and medical visits paid for by workers' compensation in Michigan has shown extreme resistance on the part of companies to cover any expenses for hearing loss among its workers, regardless of the health professionals' judgement of the work relatedness of the hearing loss. The companies often attribute recreational noise as the cause of the worker's hearing loss. Without legal representation, a worker seeking reimbursement for medical-related costs or hearing aids would have great difficulty appealing a denied workers' compensation claim.

Even in a state with more comprehensive workers' compensation laws for occupational NIHL, researchers in the state of Washington who examined workers' compensation claims from 1984 to 1991 demonstrated that occupational NIHL is underreported and underrecognized, especially in older retired individuals.[8,9]

Field Investigations

A total of 60 workplace inspections took place between 1993 and 1998, based on information obtained during interviews with sentinel cases of work-related hearing loss. Of the 60 inspections, 35 (58%) were identified by the enforcement inspectors as being required to have a hearing conservation program because some of their workers were exposed to noise at or greater than the action limit of 85 dBA. The other 25 companies were determined to have noise levels below 85 dBA and therefore were not required to institute a hearing conservation program (HCP). Table 15.3 lists the characteristics of the 60 companies inspected as part of the surveillance efforts.

Of the 35 companies required by the Michigan OSHA noise standard to have an HCP, 25 had no program or a program deficient in at least one of the areas covered by the standard. These 25 companies had at least 4200 workers who would benefit from a comprehensive HCP.

Evaluation of Reporting

Severe underreporting exists in the state for occupational noise-induced hearing loss as well as for other work-related diseases and work-aggravated conditions. A substantial percentage (typically around 90%) of the reports to the MDCIS each year are from manufacturing facilities, particularly the major automotive manufacturing plants. Although reporting is less than ideal, it has improved especially with respect to private clinics. Repeated updates and outreach efforts to the state's hearing health professionals and other providers likely to treat patients with work-related diseases were necessary to maintain interest among the state's reporters.

Since the initial large increase in reports from private practices across the state in 1994, the number of reports by private practice hearing health professionals has not increased substantially. Continued and new efforts were needed to increase compliance with the reporting law. One way the surveillance program sought to increase reporting was through the hire of an audiologist to contact the clinics and graduate programs to encourage these groups to report cases.

DISCUSSION

Michigan was the only state funded by NIOSH to institute a surveillance program for occupational NIHL, under Project SENSOR. Since 1993, a multidisciplinary team consisting of individuals from Michigan OSHA and the College of Human Medicine at Michigan State University worked to identify companies in the state with excessive noise and no hearing conservation program to protect workers' hearing. To this end, the program worked to encourage the state's key reporters to submit sentinel cases of work-related NIHL to the MD-

CIS. The cases reported from private practice hearing health professionals were interviewed to determine the status of their work conditions. Michigan OSHA enforcement inspections at 60 companies sought to identify deficiencies in or complete lack of hearing conservation programs in those companies with excessive noise levels (i.e., noise levels at or greater than 85 dBA). In the 25 companies that were found to have no or a deficient HCP, at least 4200 workers exposed to noise were thus potentially protected from further exposures to excessive levels of noise at work.

Approximately 11% of the interviewed patients were exposed to noise in construction. Yet, construction is an industry that is minimally covered by MIOSHA and OSHA regulations. Interviews with these construction workers revealed that almost none were given regular hearing testing and approximately half were provided with ear plugs or muffs. Construction is one industry not adequately covered by the hearing conservation regulations and employers are not voluntarily providing audiometric testing to their employees.

Enhancing the Quantity and Quality of Reports

When the surveillance initiative began in 1993 for occupational noise-induced hearing loss, there was much resistance among the state's hearing health professionals in reporting any cases of known or suspected occupational NIHL. An important lesson and success story learned from this initiative is the value of persistence and the development of personal relationships. By attending conferences and meeting with some of the state's key hearing health professionals, the audiologists and otolaryngologists learned to trust that there would be no negative repercussions for reporting their patients to the state.

The state's hearing health professionals received repeated mailings about the importance and need for reporting, and learned about the status and progress of the surveillance efforts through the surveillance staff's presentations at the hearing health professionals' annual meetings and conferences. The development of a quarterly newsletter, a website, and the addition of a paid audiologist consultant in the second phase of funding all worked to solidify and maintain the relationships developed with this group of health professionals who were initially very suspicious of the surveillance efforts and consequently very reluctant to report any cases to the state.

Although the infrastructure for reporting occupational diseases already existed when the surveillance efforts for occupational NIHL first began, the key reporters of sentinel cases for NIHL were completely out of the reporting loop. Almost all of the state's audiologists and otolaryngologists had no knowledge of the reporting law prior to 1993.

Identification of Worksite Risk Factors

Companies that were more likely to be cited for violations of the noise standard were those that were smaller manufacturing facilities in the state. Smaller companies often lacked the resources to dedicate an individual's time to workplace health and safety, or to hire an outside consultant to provide those services. Workers from industries that were not required to have a comprehensive hearing conservation program such as agriculture and construction were less likely to be part of any audiometric testing or to be provided with hearing protection. There were similar findings for workers exposed to noise in earlier decades (prior to the 1980s).

CONCLUSION

Future directions of the surveillance program could include:

- reinspection of workplaces to determine the level of continued compliance with the noise standard
- reinterviews of sentinel cases to determine the work experiences and hearing health status of those individuals
- targeting of manufacturers of noisy equipment to work toward the development of better warning labels on machines about the effects of noise, and to work to decrease the noise levels emitted by this machinery itself
- targeting of professional groups likely to have large numbers of members exposed to excessive levels of noise, such as professional lawn management groups or farmers through their trade association journals
- assessing the potential contribution of other causes of hearing loss such as chemicals at work and cigarette smoke[10,11]
- continued encouragement of reporting by the state's key hearing health professionals by continuing to refine ways to make reporting a less disruptive and more agreeable activity

The surveillance program provides an example of some of the issues related to occupational disease surveillance and the hurdles that must be overcome if workers are to be protected at their jobs.

ACKNOWLEDGMENTS

The authors acknowledge the office and interview staff who handle the reports of occupational NIHL on a daily basis: Amy Allemier,

Amy Krizek, Tracy Murphy, and Ruth VanderWaals. The authors also acknowledge the tremendous support of the program by Michigan's OSHA inspectors and administrative staff. This project was funded by the National Institute for Occupational Safety and Health, under cooperative agreement number U60-CCU502998-12.

REFERENCES

1. Hetu R, Getty L, Quoc HT. Impact of occupational hearing loss on the lives of workers. *Occup Med* 1995; 10:495–512.
2. Bess FH, Lichtenstein MJ, Logan SA, Burger MC, Nelson E. Hearing impairment as a determinant of function in the elderly. *J Amer Geriatrics Soc* 1989; 37:123–128.
3. Ries PW. Prevalence and characteristics of persons with hearing trouble: United States 1990–1991. *Vital Health Stat* 1994; 10(Mar):1–75.
4. National Institute for Occupational Safety and Health. Criteria for a Recommended Standard Occupational Noise Exposure Revised Criteria 1998. DHHS (NIOSH) Publication No. 98–126. Cincinnati, OH: National Institute for Occupational Safety and Health, June 1998.
5. Weeks JL, Levy BS, Wagner GR, eds. *Preventing Occupational Disease and Injury.* Washington, DC: American Public Health Association, 1991.
6. Public Health Service. *Healthy People 2000 Midcourse Review and 1995 Revisions.* Washington, DC: US Department of Health and Human Services, 1995.
7. National Institute for Occupational Safety and Health. National Occupational Research Agenda (NORA). Cincinnati, OH: National Institute for Occupational Safety and Health, 1996.
8. Daniell WE, Fulton-Kehoe D, Smith-Weller T, Franklin GM. Occupational hearing loss in Washington State, 1984–1991: I. Statewide and industry specific incidence. *Am J Ind Med* 1998; 33:519–528.
9. Daniell WE, Fulton-Kehoe D, Smith-Weller T, Franklin GM. Occupational hearing loss in Washington State, 1984-1991: II. Morbidity and associated costs. *Am J Ind Med* 1998; 33:529–536.
10. Morata TC. Assessing occupational hearing loss: beyond noise exposures. *Scand Audiol* 1998; 48(Suppl):111–116.
11. Cruickshanks KJ, Klein R, Klein BE, Wiley TL, Nondahl DM, Tweed TS. Cigarette smoking and hearing loss: the epidemiology of hearing loss study. *JAMA* 1998; 279:1715–1719.

16

Asthma

KENNETH D. ROSENMAN AND MARY JO REILLY

Asthma was first described by Hippocrates, and the word asthma means panting in Greek. Physicians in the 1700s recognized that asthma was more common in certain trades such as bakers or grain handlers. Beginning in the early 1900s specific workplace exposures were recognized as causes of asthma and since then approximately 250 agents have been described as causing asthma via an immunological mechanism. Many other workplace exposures are known to either aggravate preexisting asthma or cause a nonimmunological form of asthma after exposure to an irritating substance. Some of the more commonly recognized agents associated with work-related asthma include isocyanates, flour (baker's asthma), laboratory animal dander, and wood dust.

Work-related asthma can be a debilitating lung disease that manifests itself with symptoms of chest tightness, cough, shortness of breath, wheezing, or any or all of the above in relation to exposures to chemicals or other substances at work. An individual who develops work-related asthma typically will not see a complete resolution of their symptoms, especially if they continue to be exposed to the substance causing their symptoms for a prolonged period of time after their symptoms develop (i.e., months to years).

There is no unique diagnostic code for work-related asthma; this condition is included in the larger diagnostic category of asthma (International Classification of Diseases, 9th revision [ICD-9], 493). Work-related asthma can be divided into two categories based on the mechanism involved in the development of disease: that which occurs after a latency period of symptomless exposure; and that which has an acute onset after initial exposure. An immunological mechanism has been described for a number of the 250 substances that cause asthma after a period of symptomless exposure.[1] It has been suggested recently that a period of symptomless low level exposure to irritants not documented as capable of causing asthma by an immunological mechanism may cause a similar clinical picture.[2] Work-related asthma, which develops without a latency period of symptomless exposure includes: Reactive Airways Dysfunction Syndrome (RADS), which occurs after significant exposure to an irritating substance, causes acute respiratory symptoms and persists as a chronic respiratory problem[3]; and aggravated asthma, where individuals who already have asthma experience an increase in symptoms requiring increased breathing medication and frequently an increased use of medical care facilities.

Colorado, Michigan, and New Jersey received funds from the National Institute for Occupational Safety and Health (NIOSH) in 1988 to develop a comprehensive surveillance system for work-related asthma. Based on the success of this system, federal funding from NIOSH was expanded in 1987 to fund surveillance systems in two additional states: California and Massachusetts. These surveillance systems were called Project SENSOR, or the Sentinel Event Notification System for Occupational Risks. Funding from NIOSH for work-related asthma was cut back in 1997; only California, Massachusetts, and Michigan still receive funding. New Jersey however, has continued its surveillance system for work-related asthma using state resources.

METHODS

Defining the Goals, Objectives, and Scope

The purpose of the Michigan work-related asthma surveillance system was to identify workplaces where preventive activity might be useful, to identify new causes of work-related asthma, and to develop better estimates of the incidence of disease. Additionally, the creation of this surveillance system was intended to develop a model for other states wishing to conduct surveillance of occupational diseases including work-related asthma. The development of this system was intended to fill a gap in the identification of occupational disease, given the documented inadequacies of state workers' compensation records and employer-maintained logs collected by the Bureau of Labor Statistics.[4] Through the development of an occupational disease surveillance infrastructure, other states could learn from the successes and lessons learned in the SENSOR states, and incorporate elements of these newly developed surveillance systems into their own state plans.

Geographic Targeting

All known or suspected cases of work-related asthma were targeted in case finding efforts and potentially acted as the basis for intervention. The tremendous in-kind support of staff at the Michigan Department of Consumer and Industry Services (MDCIS) (formerly the Michigan Department of Public Health) allowed available monetary resources to be directed to case-finding in the entire state of Michigan. There was no reason to suspect at the initiation of the project that any region of the state would generate more cases of work-related asthma than any other region.

Assemble Multidisciplinary Team

In 1988, a multidisciplinary surveillance team was formed from staff at the MDCIS and staff from the College of Human Medicine at Michigan State University (MSU). The staff and their roles were the same as for the silicosis surveillance initiative that began at the same time as the work-related asthma initiative (see Chapter 14).

An advisory committee was developed that consisted of seven physicians who were part of the silicosis surveillance project. The advisory committee's major role was to be a sounding board if physicians around the state had questions or concerns about reporting occupational diseases including their legal obligation to participate in this system. The pulmonary physician member of the advisory board also reviewed a quarterly newsletter sent to the targeted practitioners.

The focus of the surveillance activity was directed from a medical school rather than from a state agency; to encourage physicians to consult with the university-based part of the surveillance team was less threatening to these health care professionals than a state government institution. This was particularly useful for work-related asthma, which can be a difficult disease to diagnose. Practicing physicians have repeatedly consulted over the phone or referred patients for examination to the SENSOR occupational medicine physician. However, the medical school staff were still responsible to direct referrals for regulatory activity that ensured effective workplace follow-up after the identification of cases.

Case Definition and Data Collection

The work-related asthma case definition was developed in conjunction with NIOSH and the other states conducting similar work-related asthma surveillance.[5] The work-related asthma case definition was:

1. a diagnosis of asthma; and
2. an association between symptoms and work

Work-related asthma cases were classified into work-aggravated asthma, RADS, and occupational asthma with or without exposure to a known causal agent and with or without pulmonary function evidence of work-relatedness. The flow diagram in Figure 16.1 presents the case classification scheme.[5]

Mechanism for Reporting and Reporting Guidelines

The surveillance system for work-related asthma in Michigan was based on an existing state law for occupational disease reporting that since 1978 has required hospitals, clinics, physicians, and employers to report all known or suspected occupational diseases or workplace-aggravated health conditions to the state within 10 days after the discovery of the disease or condition (Part 56 of Public Act 368 of 1978). The failure to report cases can result in a $50 fine per individual not reported, although no nonreporter has ever been fined since the introduction of the law in 1978. Compliance with the law relied more on professional responsibility rather than the threat of monetary punishment. The reporting law relieved the health practitioner of any liability for releasing confidential patient information to the state.

The standard occupational disease reporting form was used for any known or suspected occupational disease or work-aggravated condition and collected demographic information on the employee affected, information about the employer, illness information, and information on the person, clinic, or other such entity submitting the report. Hospitals were also requested to submit the discharge summary and any pulmonary function tests. To determine if reported cases met the case definition for work-related asthma, the reported patient was interviewed and any pulmonary function tests that were performed were reviewed. If the reported

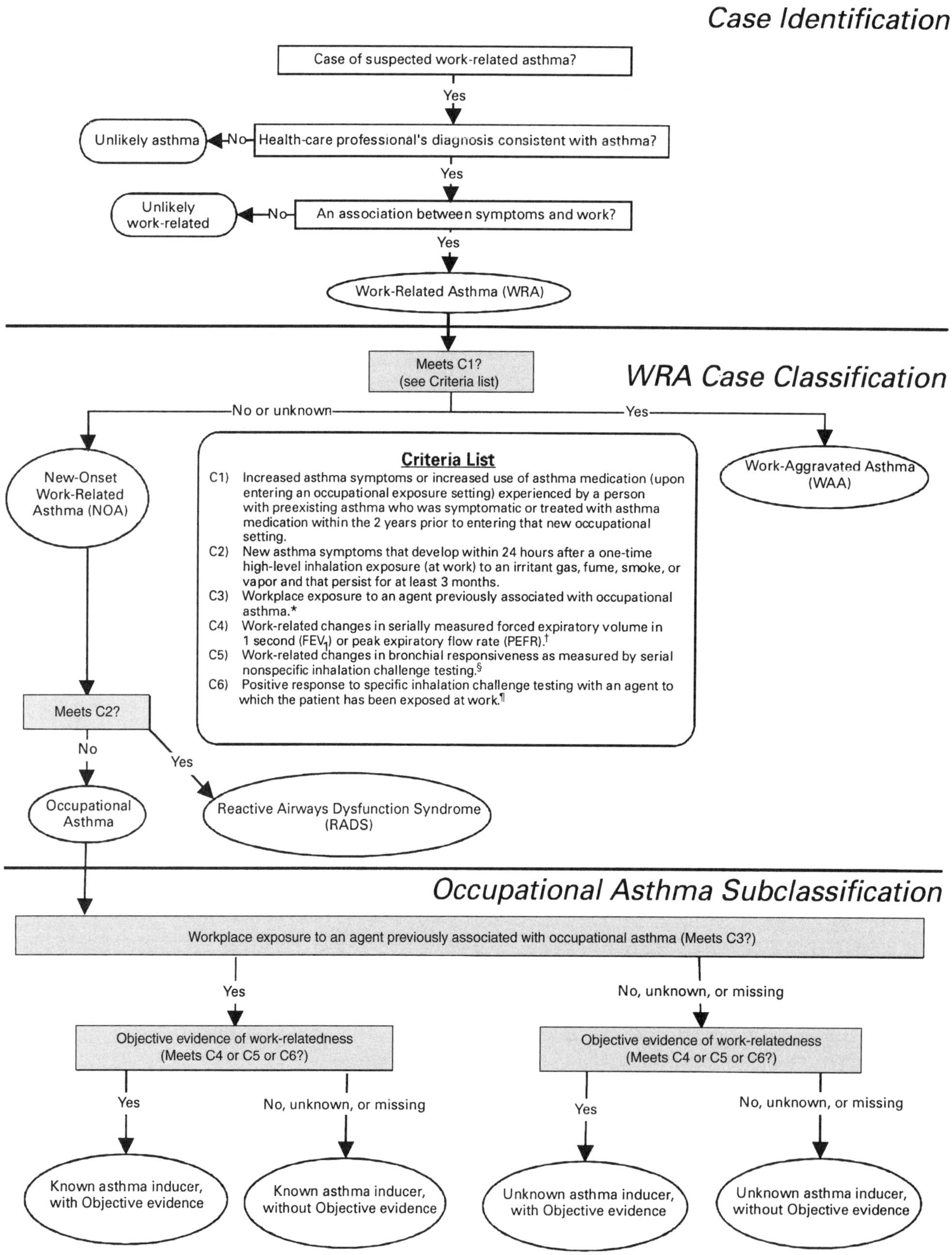
Case Identification
Case of suspected work-related asthma?
Yes
Unlikely asthma
No
Health-care professional's diagnosis consistent with asthma?
Yes
Unlikely work-related
No
An association between symptoms and work?
Yes
Work-Related Asthma (WRA)
Meets C1? (see Criteria list)
WRA Case Classification
No or unknown
Yes
New-Onset Work-Related Asthma (NOA)
Work-Aggravated Asthma (WAA)
Criteria List
C1) Increased asthma symptoms or increased use of asthma medication (upon entering an occupational exposure setting) experienced by a person with preexisting asthma who was symptomatic or treated with asthma medication within the 2 years prior to entering that new occupational setting.
C2) New asthma symptoms that develop within 24 hours after a one-time high-level inhalation exposure (at work) to an irritant gas, fume, smoke, or vapor and that persist for at least 3 months.
C3) Workplace exposure to an agent previously associated with occupational asthma.*
C4) Work-related changes in serially measured forced expiratory volume in 1 second (FEV1) or peak expiratory flow rate (PEFR).†
C5) Work-related changes in bronchial responsiveness as measured by serial nonspecific inhalation challenge testing.§
C6) Positive response to specific inhalation challenge testing with an agent to which the patient has been exposed at work.¶
Meets C2?
No
Yes
Occupational Asthma
Reactive Airways Dysfunction Syndrome (RADS)
Occupational Asthma Subclassification
Workplace exposure to an agent previously associated with occupational asthma (Meets C3?)
Yes
No, unknown, or missing
Objective evidence of work-relatedness (Meets C4 or C5 or C6?)
Objective evidence of work-relatedness (Meets C4 or C5 or C6?)
Yes
No, unknown, or missing
Yes
No, unknown, or missing
Known asthma inducer, with Objective evidence
Known asthma inducer, without Objective evidence
Unknown asthma inducer, with Objective evidence
Unknown asthma inducer, without Objective evidence

Figure 16.1 Decision logic and case classification scheme for work-related asthma (Jajosky et al.[5]).

*Many agents can induce occupational asthma via a specific hypersensitivity mechanism. A comprehensive list of these asthma inducers (*a, b, c*, see Sources below) is used for this criterion. Known asthma inducers have been integrated into the Association of Occupational and Environmental Clinics' (AOEC) coding scheme and have been flagged with the letter "A" (*d*).

†Spirometric measurements (e.g., FEV_1) can be obtained after a person's work shift (i.e., cross-shift spirometry). However, many cases of occupational asthma can fail to demonstrate a significant cross-shift reduction in FEV_1, either because of a delayed bronchoconstrictor response or because of intermittent exposure patterns. Cross-shift spirometry testing on multiple days might help confirm the association with work. Alternatively, PEFRs can be measured serially throughout the day using a portable peak flow meter.

§Changes in bronchial responsiveness can be measured by serial inhalation challenge testing with nonspecific agents (e.g., using methacholine or histamine). Evidence for work-relatedness is manifested by increased bronchial responsiveness (i.e., bronchoconstriction at lower inhaled doses of methacholine or histamine) following work exposures and decreased or normal bronchial responsiveness after a period away from work.

¶Specific inhalation challenge testing has distinct objectives, including the following: (*1*) identifying previously unrecognized causes of occupational asthma, (*2*) confirming the diagnosis of occupational asthma, and (*3*) identifying the causative agent when more than one allergen is present in the occupational environment and identification of the causative agent is essential for management. Specific inhalation challenge testing is potentially dangerous and should be performed by experienced personnel in a hospital setting where resuscitation facilities are available and frequent observations can be made over sufficient time to monitor for delayed reactions. Specific inhalation challenge testing is usually not necessary for clinical diagnosis of occupational asthma.

Sources:

a. Chan-Yeung M, Malo J-L. Compendium 1: table of the major inducers of occupational asthma. In Berstein IL, Chan-Yeung M, Malo J-L, eds. *Asthma in the Workplace.* New York: Marcel Dekker, Inc; 1993:595–623.

b. Chan-Yeung M, Malo J-L. Aetiological agents in occupational asthma. *Eur Respir J* 1994; 7:346–371.

c. Malo J-L, Chan-Yeung M. Occupational agents. In: Barnes PJ, Grunstein MM, Leff AR, Woolcock AJ, eds. *Asthma.* Philadelphia, PA: Lippincott-Raven Publishers; 1997:1217–1244.

d. Hunting KL, McDonald SM. Development of a hierarchical exposure coding system for clinic-based surveillance of occupational disease and injury. *Appl Occup Environ Hyg* 1995; 10:317–322. The exposure coding scheme is available on the Internet at http://occ-env-med.mc.duke.edu/oem/aoec.htm. Accessed February 26, 1999.

patient could not be interviewed, then medical records, typically progress notes and the initial history and physical as well as the pulmonary function tests, were requested from the physician or hospital reporting the case. It was possible to obtain more information on patients than on the initial reporting form because the Michigan law (Part 56 of Public Act 368 of 1978) gave the state broad discretion on any additional types of information it could request (" . . . and other information required by the department.").

Reporting of cases could be done by mail, electronic mail, telephone, or fax. Numerous ways to report cases were available to be as accommodating as possible for physicians, and to help make reporting as simple as possible for medical offices already over burdened with paperwork.

Select, Recruit, and Train Reporters

Key reporting sources of work-related asthma cases were expected to be physicians and hospitals. Physicians were targeted as the main source of work-related asthma case reporting for several reasons: there is no ICD-9 diagnostic code for work-related asthma so hospital reporting, which relies on these codes to identify cases, could not be the primary reporting source; and, physician reports would serve as a more timely source of work-related asthma case reports, enabling more immediate workplace follow-up activities than hospital-based reports that typically lag 1–2 years after the initial diagnosis of work-related asthma.

Hospitals were anticipated to be the second major source to identify cases. A prior study in New Jersey demonstrated that 39% of hospital discharges for the International Classification of Diseases—9th revision (ICD-9) diagnostic code 506, respiratory conditions due to chemical fumes and vapors, were work-related.[6] Accordingly, all of the individuals discharged with this diagnostic code either as a primary or secondary diagnosis, as well as the diagnostic code for asthma (ICD-9 493) only when workers' compensation was the payor, were identified in addition to direct physician reporting. The results in Michigan were similar to New Jersey in that 35% of patients with an ICD-9 code of 506 had a work-related etiology[7] and overall that 60% of the work-related cases reported from hospitals, also including an ICD-9 code of 493 where workers' compensation was the payor, were confirmed with work-related asthma.

All acute care hospitals in Michigan, including Veterans' Administration Hospitals, were requested in January or February of each year to submit information on all individuals regardless of payor discharged with a primary or secondary diagnosis of respiratory disease secondary to chemical fumes or vapors (ICD-9 506) and all individuals where workers' compensation was the payor, who had a discharge diagnosis of asthma (ICD-9 493). The information requested included the hospital discharge summary and pulmonary function test results. In order to verify the completeness of reporting by hospitals, a computerized listing of all hospital discharges, which was available approximately 2 years after the hospitalization, was reviewed and used for followback when necessary to obtain reports on patients not previously reported by the hospitals. Both physician and hospital-based reporting were important in order to identify the full spectrum of disease—from a milder new-onset asthma to more severe cases of asthma. Hospitalized patients would typically represent a more severely affected group of workers whereas physician-based reports of patients would be able to help identify workers with relatively new-onset asthma with symptoms that might not yet be as severe.

Although all 25,000 physicians who practice medicine in Michigan were required to report any known or suspected occupational disease including work-related asthma, most of these physicians were unaware of the reporting law and the requirements. A special effort was made to inform those physicians most likely to see patients with work-related asthma about the reporting law: allergists, pulmonologists, occupational physicians, and selected internists and family practitioners. These physicians were targeted with a simultaneous effort to encourage the reporting of silicosis. After the initial mailing to these groups, these targeted physicians then continued to receive a four-page quarterly newsletter that contained reviews of pertinent diagnostic issues, case reports, and abstracts of selected articles. The intent of continued informational mailings to these groups was to maintain a level of awareness and interest about the reporting of occupational diseases, including work-related asthma. Both silicosis and work-related asthma were covered in the newsletter. Further, these physicians received an annual report on work-related asthma that summarized the demographics, type of industries, pulmonary function test results and industrial hygiene follow-up activity. In more recent years the annual report and newsletter became available on an MSU website. The targeted physicians received a letter notifying them about the website and announcing the availability of the annual reports, along with a postage-paid post card that allowed them to request a printed copy of the reports. Although the newsletter was also posted on the website, it continued to be mailed out quarterly to the targeted physicians.

To encourage physicians to report cases of all occupational diseases including work-related asthma, and remind them of the reporting law, an educational and informational display booth was exhibited at the Annual Michigan State Medical Society Scientific Meeting, the Annual Michigan Thoracic Society Scientific Meeting, the Annual Michigan Occupational and Environmental Association Meeting, and selected continuing medical education meetings. Similar to displays exhibited by pharmaceutical companies, educational materials and small novelty items such as pens, pencils, magnets, and rulers with the telephone number to report occupational diseases were distributed. Again, these efforts were intended to help maintain interest and awareness about occupational diseases.

The surveillance system in New Jersey used a similar reporting system as Michigan. California used an existing mandatory state-physician reporting system directly linked to physician reimbursement, called "Doctor's First Reports of Occupational Injury or Illness" (Appendix A). Massachusetts's surveillance was based on an English system, Surveillance of Work-Related and Occupational Respiratory Disease (SWORD) where a group of approximately 100 targeted occupational and pulmonary physicians received a monthly mailing requesting reports of patients with work-related asthma who were seen in the previous month.[8]

Protocols for Follow-up

When a report of work-related asthma was received, the individual was administered a standardized medical and work history questionnaire over the telephone by a trained interviewer. The interviews were typically performed by second-year medical students. Each interview took approximately 30 to 45 minutes and consisted of the following:

- lifetime work history
- cigarette smoking history
- onset, frequency, and temporal pattern of respiratory symptoms
- medical care history
- medication history

The parts of the questionnaire that were necessary for an individual to meet the surveillance criteria for work-related asthma were the lifetime work history; onset, frequency, and temporal pattern of respiratory symptoms; and medical care history regarding any previous diagnosis of asthma. The collection of the other historical information allowed the surveillance team to describe the epidemiology of work-related asthma in Michigan, including the severity of disease.

All workplaces where a case was confirmed were inspected if they met the following criteria:

- the company was located within the state
- the company was still in operation and the suspected exposure(s) were still occurring
- the Michigan OSHA program had jurisdiction (mining, agriculture, transportation—oil and gas well drilling are not covered by Michigan OSHA laws)

- it was *not* a possible indoor air exposure in an office or school type setting
- it was *not* a case of aggravation of preexisting asthma
- it had *not* been inspected for a similar type of exposure

If the company was out of state or the Michigan OSHA program did not have enforcement jurisdiction (i.e., mining or transportation) the company's name was forwarded to the appropriate agency that did have enforcement jurisdiction.

Case Management

Data from the occupational disease reports for work-related asthma and data from the case interviews were entered into a tracking database. The database was used to monitor the progress of case interviews, the status of inspections, and to analyze the information collected through the telephone administered questionnaires.

Field Investigations

All investigations performed were enforcement inspections. In addition to addressing the standard components of a regular enforcement inspection, workers in the suspect area were administered a short 5–10 minute medical symptom questionnaire. The ability to administer these questionnaires was based on the inspector's regulatory authority to conduct private interviews with workers during an inspection on paid company time. Although some questionnaires were administered individually, most were administered in groups of 10–25 workers. Groups of workers were brought into conference rooms and were told that an inspection was taking place because a doctor had reported a case of lung disease from this workplace and the questionnaire results would be used as part of the Michigan OSHA inspection to assess if other similarly exposed workers had similar breathing problems. The results would be used to help determine the magnitude of the problem. All workers were assured of the confidential and voluntary nature of the questionnaire.

All workers who reported daily or weekly symptoms of wheezing, chest tightness, or shortness of breath were sent letters to their home addresses. Their addresses were obtained from the questionnaires and neither the company nor the union was told who received letters. The letters advised them to see a physician to determine the cause of their breathing symptoms but that there were no funds available from the project to pay for this medical evaluation. They were given the name and telephone number of the physician who reported the index case. The reporting physician was given the names of all individuals who received the letters. The rationale behind giving the reporting physician's name to the symptomatic workers was that:

- the reporting physician already had an awareness of work-related asthma
- the reporting physician had some familiarity with the specific workplace being inspected and types of exposures that would be encountered at that workplace
- if the reporting physician diagnosed additional cases of work-related asthma it was likely these cases would be reported to the surveillance system
- this was positive feedback to the reporting physician to demonstrate that their compliance with the Michigan occupational disease reporting regulations did make a difference in helping to prevent work-related asthma

After the investigation was completed, a report of the inspection results and any recommendations were sent to the company and union (or designated labor representative if the company did not have a union). The report included a summary of the number of completed questionnaires and the number of workers who had developed asthma since beginning to work at the facility or who had daily or weekly symptoms of chest tightness, shortness of breath, or wheezing. If the percentage of workers with new onset asthma and daily or weekly respiratory symptoms was 20% or greater, then it was recommended that the company initiate a medical surveillance program and the outline of such a program including a questionnaire to be used annually was attached to the report (Appendix I). If the company was cited for violations of any regulations, a copy of the citations was posted at or near the location of the violations for a minimum of 3 days or until the items were corrected, whichever was later.

A copy of the inspection report was also sent to the physician who reported the original index work-related asthma case that prompted the field investigation. The cover letter to the physician indicated that the investigation was conducted in response to his or her case report and the physician was thanked for initiating this public health activity to prevent other similarly exposed workers from developing work-related asthma.

Analyze and Interpret Data

On a quarterly basis, progress reports detailing the numbers of cases identified, numbers of inspections completed, and other related information were submitted to the funding agency. On a yearly basis, an overall report on the surveillance data was developed that summarized the history of the surveillance project, the elements of surveillance, and a review of the data obtained including questionnaire data and inspection report summaries.

Feedback and Recommendations

The annual reports were distributed to the approximately 3000 targeted physicians, to administrative personnel in the MDCIS, and to other government officials. After the first 5 years of funding, a website was developed that posted the newsletters, annual reports, reporting law, and other educational information.

Industrial hygiene inspections conducted by Michigan OSHA were enforcement inspections. Any violations of any applicable Michigan standards were required to be corrected and proof of such corrections was required to be submitted to Michigan OSHA. In addition to possible violations, individual industrial hygienists would make recommendations regarding work practices, medical screening, and engineering controls. These recommendations would be part of the report shared with the company and if present, the union.

Evaluation of the Surveillance System

Reporting of individuals with work-related asthma is incomplete. In a given year only 1.7% of Michigan physicians submit a report on any type of occupational disease to the state.[9]

Reporting of work-related asthma from hospitals is also incomplete. There is no ICD-9 code for work-related asthma. A survey of three hospitals in Michigan found that 3%–20% of adults hospitalized for asthma (ICD-9 493) met the criteria for a confirmed case. This represents 330–2222 of the 11,000 adults discharged with asthma each year from Michigan hospitals.[10] We have received only 250 confirmed cases from Michigan hospitals for the years 1988–1998. Capture–recapture analyses (see Chapter 13) were carried out on the Michigan data for the years 1988–1995 using the overlap of cases reported from multiple reporting sources to estimate the number of cases not received by any reporting source.[11] This analysis suggested that over this 8-year period 53%–87% of cases were not being reported.

In addition and related to underreporting of work-related asthma cases, physicians who examine these patients in their practices and surveillance staff who handle the case reports to direct intervention efforts often have difficulty in defining work-related asthma and in proving that the patient has work-related asthma. Several newsletter issues by the Michigan SENSOR project have addressed these concerns and there have been numerous discussions and meetings among surveillance staff from all the work-related asthma states to define these issues and to provide some guidelines for states attempting to conduct surveillance of work-related asthma. Unlike other chronic occupational diseases such as silicosis where there is one agent (silica) responsible for the condition and few nonoccupational exposures, asthma and especially work-related asthma is a condition that can be caused by many different substances and in many different work and nonwork situations. Sometimes in occupational disease surveillance, proof of the work-relatedness is less than ideal. Yet, despite these limitations, surveillance staff have been able to develop meaningful guidelines and definitions for work-related asthma, and prevent others with similar exposures from developing diseases.

Despite the known underreporting and difficulties faced with trying to define or confirm a case of work-related asthma, the system has been effective in identifying problem worksites,[9] identifying problems with existing workplace standards[12,13] and new allergens.[14,15] Field investigations revealed violations of an exposure standard in 19 (7%) of the 286 facilities where sampling was performed.[9] Another 16 (6%) of the facilities were above the NIOSH recommended exposure standard.

RESULTS

Demographics and Occupational Characteristics of Cases

The following section highlights the main findings of the Michigan surveillance system, from 1988–1998 and is based on the 1336 cases of work-related asthma confirmed during this time. Table 16.1 shows the number

Table 16.1 Number of Confirmed Cases of Work-Related Asthma in Michigan by Year and Type

	Year											
*Disease Status**	*1988*	*1989*	*1990*	*1991*	*1992*	*1993*	*1994*	*1995*	*1996*	*1997*	*1998*	*Total*
OA	23	43	87	55	81	75	65	56	58	43	33	619
POA	7	12	35	29	37	69	59	35	59	64	49	455
AA	0	3	14	14	14	13	15	19	24	16	12	144
RA	1	5	8	16	18	19	13	17	11	9	1	118
Total	31	63	144	114	150	176	152	127	152	132	95	1336

*OA, occupational asthma after latency period with known agent; POA, occupational asthma after latency period to agent not previously known to cause asthma; AA, aggravated asthma; RA, reactive airway dysfunction syndrome.

of persons confirmed with work-related asthma for the years 1988–1998 by type of work-related asthma. For 80% of the confirmed cases of work-related asthma there was a latency period between onset of exposure and onset of symptoms. The majority of these individuals (58%) had been exposed to an agent that was known to cause work-related asthma via an immunologically mediated mechanism. The remaining 42% were exposed to substances that have not been documented in the medical literature as causing work-related asthma. Among the 20% of the confirmed cases of work-related asthma that did not occur after a latency, half were RADS and half were aggravation of preexisting asthma. The cases identified for 1997 and 1998 are not complete, primarily due to the typical lag in identification of cases through the hospitals. Since hospitals admit thousands of patients each year, the most feasible way for the hospitals to report patients was after the close of the calendar year, usually by generating a computerized listing of all adult patients discharged with and ICD-9 diagnostic code of 506 or the ICD-9 code of 493 where the payor was workers' compensation. This lag in reporting cases did not detract greatly from surveillance activities, especially in light of all the other cases requiring follow-up efforts and since hospital reports are a minor source of identification of patients, with only 18% of work-related asthma patients identified solely through the hospitals. Often a patient will be reported to the system by more than one source. Figure 16.2 shows the overlap of reporting sources for the most complete reporting years of 1988 through 1997.

Six hundred seventy (50%) of the persons with work-related asthma were women. One thousand twenty-two (77%) of the persons with work-related asthma were white, 250 (19%) were African-American, 34 (3%) were Hispanic, 11 were Alaskan or Native American (1%), 5 (0.4%) were of Asian ancestry, and 11 (1%) were listed as other ancestry. The race on three individuals was unknown. The average year of birth of the cases reported was 1951, ranging from 1905 to 1976.

The cases were clustered in the most populous counties in Michigan with relatively little variation in the average annual incidence rates by counties (Fig. 16.3). The two counties that had appreciably higher rates were rural counties with small populations and most likely had better reporting by a single physician within the county.

Table 16.2 shows the types of Michigan industries where the exposures to the occupational allergens occurred. The predominant industries for the total number of cases identified between 1988 and 1998 were in the manufacturing sector: automobile (43%), industrial and commercial machinery and computer equipment

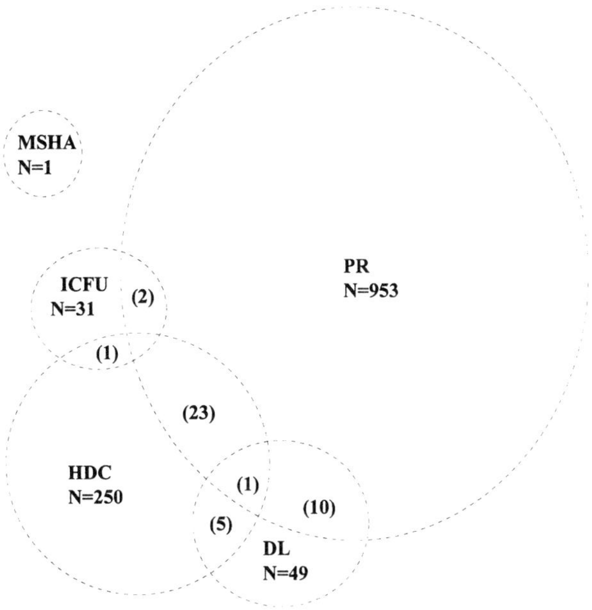

Figure 16.2 Overlap of reporting sources for confirmed work-related asthma patients, 1988–1987. The diagram represents 1241 individuals initially reported from 1988–1997. N, the total number for that source. Numbers in parentheses represent the overlap of reporting sources. HDC, hospital discharge data; PR, physician referral; DL, Department of Labor; ICFU, index case follow-up; MSHA, Mine Safety and Health Administration.

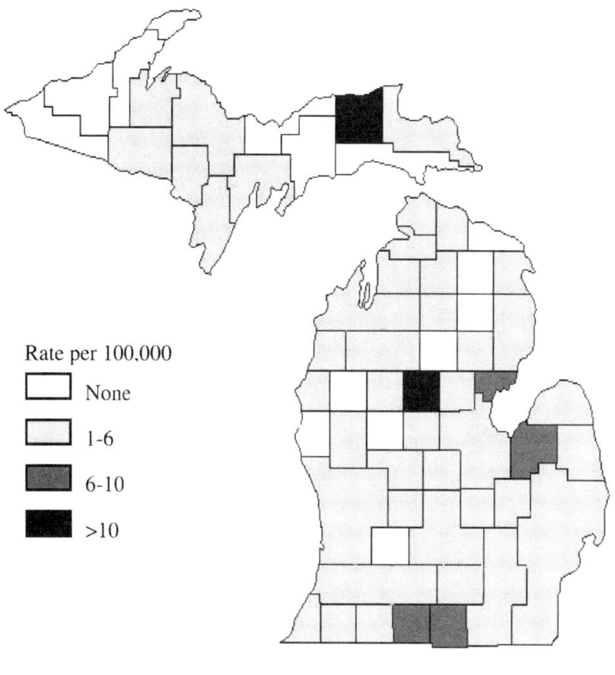

Figure 16.3 Average annual incidence rates of work-related asthma among Michigan workers by county of exposure, 1989–1996. Rate is per 100,000 Michigan workers. In 1992, there were 3,928,000 Michigan workers. (Source: Michigan Employment Security Commission. 1992 Annual average labor statistics for employment by place of work. Detroit, MI: Michigan Department of Labor, 1992.)

Table 16.2 Primary Industrial Exposure for Confirmed Work-Related Asthma Patients in Michigan, 1988–1998

*Industry (SIC Code)**	*No. of Cases, 1988–1998*	%	*No. of Employees*†	*Annual Incidence Rate, 1989–1996*‡
MANUFACTURING (20–39)				
Automobile (37)	572	42.8	272,000	20.8
Industrial and commercial machinery and computer equipment (35)	55	4.1	115,000	5.3
Fabricated metal products (34)	63	4.7	114,000	5.5
Rubber and miscellaneous plastic products (30)	57	4.3	52,000	11.1
Foundries (33)	46	3.4	37,000	13.9
Food and kindred products (20)	27	2.0	44,000	6.8
Printing and publishing (27)	13	1.0	45,000	3.3
Paper and allied products (26)	13	1.0	21,000	7.1
Lumber and wood (24)	10	0.7	15,000	8.3
Electrical equipment (36)	12	0.9	30,000	2.9
Furniture and fixtures (25)	4	0.3	34,000	1.5
Apparel made from fabric (23)	2	0.1	19,000	1.3
Other durables (32, 38, 39)	30	2.2	41,000	7.6
Other nondurables (22, 28, 29, 31)	56	4.2	50,000	11.3
WHOLESALE AND RETAIL TRADE (50–59)				
Wholesale nondurable goods (51)	10	0.7	71,000	1.4
Food stores (54)	11	0.8	100,000	1.1
Eating and drinking places (54)	7	0.5	256,000	0.3
Wholesale durable goods (50)	10	0.7	126,000	0.7
Automotive dealers and gasoline services (55)	3	0.2	75,000	0.5
General merchandise stores (53)	4	0.3	118,000	0.3
Home furniture and furnishings (57)	1	0.1	27,000	0.5
Building materials (52)	1	0.1	30,000	—
SERVICES (70–89)				
Health (80)	111	8.3	324,000	2.9
Education (82)	43	3.2	37,000	10.5
Automotive repair (75)	8	0.6	33,000	2.7
Business (73)	9	0.7	188,000	0.6
Social services (83)	7	0.5	69,000	1.1
Engineering, Accounting, etc. (87)	6	0.4	80,000	0.8
Other services (70, 72, 76, 79, 81, 86, 89)	31	2.3	249,000	1.4
CONSTRUCTION AND MINING (10–17)				
Special trade construction (17)	23	1.7	87,000	3.0
Other construction (15–16)	9	0.7	42,000	2.7
Mining (10)	4	0.3	9,000	5.6
MISCELLANEOUS INDUSTRIES				
Government (91–97)	46	3.4	639,000	0.8
Transportation and utilities (40–49)	22	1.6	154,000	1.7
Finance, insurance, and real estate (60–67)	5	0.4	191,000	0.3
Agricultural production and services (01, 02, 07)	3	0.2	90,000	0.3
Unknown	2	0.1	—	—
Total	1336	100	3,928,000	3.4

*Office of Management and Budget. Standard Industrial Classification, 1987 manual. Washington, DC: U.S. Government Printing Office, 1989.

†Source: Bureau of Labor Statistics, Michigan Employment Security Commission, Current Employment Statistics. 1992 Annual Report of Michigan Production/Nonsupervisory Workers. Detroit, MI: Michigan Department of Labor, 1992.

‡Average annual incidence rate. Rates are based on average number of cases from 1989–1996 per 100,000 adult workers in each industrial category.

(4%), foundries (3%), fabricated metal products (5%), and rubber and miscellaneous plastic products (4%). Workers in the health field also accounted for a high percentage of the total number of patients (8%).

Overall, by broad industrial classification, there were 13.3 cases per 100,000 workers in the manufacturing industry; 3.3 cases per 100,000 workers in the construction and mining industry; and 1.3 cases per 100,000 workers in the service producing industry. The incidence rate of work-related asthma by industry type ranged from 0.3 cases per 100,000 in agriculture, to a high of 20.8 cases per 100,000 in the manufacture of transportation equipment. The industries with the highest annual average incidence rates besides the manufacture of transportation equipment included foundries with 13.9 cases per 100,000 workers; the manufacture of rubber products with 11.1 cases per 100,000 workers and the manufacture of other nondurables with 11.3 cases per 100,000 workers (Table 16-2).

Table 16.3 shows the predominant exposures causing work-related asthma in Michigan. The most frequent exposures were to isocyanates (19%), metal working fluids (12%), vehicle exhaust (6%), welding fumes (5%), and solvents (3%). The agent had not yet been identified for 179 patients (13%), occurring 92 times in the manufacturing sector and 87 times in an office setting. These agents not identified highlight the difficulty in determining a causative agent in many workplace exposure settings.

One thousand eighty-three of the patients identified with work-related asthma had persistence of their asthma symptoms (Table 16.4). This was true for 373 of 390 (95.6%) of those still exposed as well as 710 of 860 (83%) no longer exposed to the substance causing their asthma. Among those no longer exposed, 51% stated their symptoms were less severe compared to 35% among those still exposed who reported their symptoms were less severe. Similarly, 84% of those still exposed were continuing to take asthma medications whereas 75% of those no longer exposed were still tak-

Table 16.3 Occupational Allergens Identified for 1336 Confirmed Work-Related Asthma Patients in Michigan, 1988–1998

Allergen	N	%	*Allergen*	N	%
Isocyanates	255	19.1	Amines	9	0.7
Metal-working fluids	163	12.2	Caustics	8	0.6
Unknown (manufacturing)	92	6.9	Grain dust	7	0.5
Unknown (office)	87	6.5	Pickling ingredients	6	0.4
Exhaust, smoke, fumes	73	5.5	Animals	6	0.4
Welding fumes	66	4.9	Fiberglass	5	0.4
Cleaning solutions	58	4.3	Meat wrappers' asthma	5	0.4
Solvent	41	3.1	Rose hips	4	0.3
Epoxy	35	2.6	Sulfonate	4	0.3
Formaldehyde	34	2.5	Sulfur dioxide	4	0.3
Rubber	32	2.4	1,1,1 Trichloroethane	4	0.3
Acrylates	30	2.2	Cement dust	4	0.3
Acids	25	1.9	Colophony	3	0.2
Chlorine	24	1.8	Cosmetology chemicals	3	0.2
Paint fumes	22	1.6	Nitrogen	3	0.2
Styrene	19	1.4	Photo developing fluids	3	0.2
Cobalt	19	1.4	Nickel	3	0.2
Wood dust	14	1.0	Phthalic anhydride	3	0.2
Plastic fumes	14	1.0	Glutaraldehyde	3	0.2
Flour	12	0.9	Cadmium solder	3	0.1
Ammonia	12	0.9	Enzymes	2	0.1
Chromium	11	0.8	Other*	85	6.4
Herbicide, pesticide	11	0.8	Total	1336	100
Printing inks	10	0.7			

*Includes x-ray developing fluids, chemicals used in the construction industry, freon, sulfite, gas and oil refinery exposures, maleic anhydride, solder fumes, vinyl acetate, ozone, zinc, textile lint, 1,3-dichloro-2-propanol, pepper gas, exercise, weeds, soda ash, asbestos, limone, coal dust, ethylene oxide, trichloroethylene, iodine, polyvinyl butyrate, lime dust, polyester, methyl ethyl ketone (MEK), nylon-polyhexamethyleneadipamide, potassium aluminum fluoride, ammonium hydroxide, methanol, naphtha, drywall dust, paper dust, zinc oxide, methylene chloride, ethylene glycol monobutyl ether, sewage, tar fumes, monoammonium phosphate, potassium hydroxide, ethyl alcohol, heptane, stress, sodium hydroxide, platinum, phosgene, cyanide, heat, polyethylene, perchloroethylene, hydraulic oil, blood, 1,3-dichloro 5 5-dimethyl hydrantoin, ninhydrin, cigarette smoke, azodicarbamide, and lactase.

Table 16.4 Persistence of Symptoms and Medication Use in Confirmed Work-Related Asthma Patients in Michigan, 1988–1998

		Symptoms		*Asthma Medications*	
Exposure Status	*Total**	*Yes (%)*	*Less (%)*	*Yes (%)*	*Less (%)*
Still exposed	390	373 (95.6)	138 (35.4)	329 (84.4)	86 (22.1)
No longer exposed	860	710 (82.6)	435 (50.6)	646 (75.1)	268 (31.2)
Total	1250	1083	573	975	354

*Information is missing on 86 individuals.

ing asthma medications. Among those no longer exposed, 31% stated they were taking fewer medications whereas only 22% of those still exposed were taking fewer medications (Table 16.4). So, although removal from exposure was associated with a greater percentage of cases having their symptoms resolved or decreased, the fact that many cases continued to experience symptoms and needed to take medication highlights the chronic nature of this disease and underscores the importance of primary prevention for conditions such as this.

Five hundred seventy-eight of 1232 (47%) patients with known workers' compensation status had applied for workers' compensation. Cases were pending for 282 (49%) of those who applied, whereas 206 (36%) had received awards and 90 (16%) had been denied. Anecdotally, many of the patients who pursued workers' compensation for their work-related asthma faced a very difficult, drawn-out uphill battle. Many workplaces attempted to attribute the patient's symptoms to other nonwork exposures, to cigarette smoking or to deny that the patient was truly sick. Along with these struggles, physicians themselves often disagree on the diagnosis of work-related asthma. Many of the cases identified faced serious financial trouble since manufacturing jobs are often well-paying and it was difficult to find other unskilled labor jobs that would be comparable to manufacturing jobs.

Field Investigations

The 1336 people with work-related asthma worked at 888 different facilities. Inspections were performed at 430 of these facilities. In addition, because of inadequate resources to conduct inspections at all the identified facilities, 45 facilities received letters notifying them that a disease report had been received and asking them to investigate potential exposures causing the respiratory problem, including indoor air problems.

Air sampling for allergens was conducted during 285 of the inspections. Thirty-five of the 285 (12%) facilities were above the National Institute for Occupational Safety and Health (NIOSH) recommended exposure limit (REL). Nineteen of the 285 (7%) were above the enforceable Michigan Occupational Health and Safety Administration (MIOSHA) permissible exposure limit (PEL) (Table 16.5).

Interviews of coworkers were performed at 322 of the 430 inspections. Workers had daily or weekly breathing symptoms in 230 of the 322 (71%) companies. The average percentage of workers with symptoms in these 230 companies was 22%, ranging from 2% to 100%. Interviews conducted in 92 companies found no coworkers with symptoms. One thousand ninety-seven of the 6153 (18%) coworkers interviewed had symptoms consistent with occupational asthma (new onset asthma or bothered at work by daily or weekly shortness of breath, wheezing or chest tightness) (Table 16.6).

Three hundred sixty-one workers from 70 companies were listed by employers on the Occupational Safety and Health Administration (OSHA) Injury and Illness log as having asthma or asthma-like symptoms.

Table 16.5 Results of 430 Industrial Hygiene Inspections in 389 Facilities in Michigan Where Patients with Confirmed Work-Related Asthma Were Exposed to Allergens: 1988–1998*

Inspection Results	N	%
Air-Sampling—NIOSH Standard		
Above NIOSH standard	35	8.1
Below NIOSH standard	244	56.7
No NIOSH standard	6	1.4
Unknown (no report yet)	16	3.7
Did not sample for an allergen	8	1.9
Did not sample	121	28.1
Total	430	100
Air-Sampling—MIOSHA Standard		
Above MIOSHA standard	19	4.4
Below MIOSHA standard	265	61.6
No MIOSHA standard	2	0.5
Unknown (no report yet)	16	3.7
Did not sample for an allergen	7	1.6
Did not sample	121	28.1
Total	430	100

*NIOSH, National Institute for Occupational Safety and Health; MIOSHA, Michigan Occupational Health and Safety Administration.

Table 16.6 Symptomatic Coworkers of the 1336 Confirmed Work-Related Asthma Patients in Michigan

	Disease Status of Index Patient[a]				
Source	*All (%)*[b]	*OA (%)*	*POA (%)*	*AA (%)*	*RA (%)*
Symptomatic workers interviewed by SENSOR[c]	1097 (17.8)	857 (18.3)	202 (16.6)	4 (16.0)	34 (15.3)
OSHA Log[d]	362 (16.2)	298 (20.0)	53 (9.6)	2 (12.5)	8 (5.6)
Total	1458[e]	1155	255	6	42

[a]OA, occupational asthma; POA, possible occupational asthma; AA, aggravated asthma; RA, reactive airways dysfunction syndrome.

[b]Number of individuals with symptoms; percentages are in parentheses. The denominator for calculating percentages was the number of workers interviewed.

[c]Symptoms reported = daily or weekly shortness of breath, wheezing, or chest tightness.

[d]Numerator for calculating percentages was the number of companies with an employee other than the index patient on the OSHA log.

[e]Eight individuals were identified both on the questionnaire and the OSHA log.

Eight workers had both daily or weekly breathing symptoms and were listed on the OSHA log. Therefore, a total of 1450 symptomatic workers were identified during the 430 inspections.

Comparison of Work-Related Asthma in Michigan with Other Geographic Areas

The results of the surveillance system in Michigan can be compared to information generated by surveillance systems in other geographic areas that use different surveillance approaches. The annual rate of 3.4 cases per 100,000 received in the Michigan surveillance system is similar to the rates reported in other surveillance systems. In England, the rates reported vary from 2.0 to 4.3 cases per 100,000 with rates as high as 6.3 per 100,000 reported in some regions.[8,16,17] Similarly in Michigan there is regional variation with rates in some counties as high as 65.0 cases per 100,000.[18] The system in England is voluntary, and is based only on reports received from pulmonary and occupational physicians.[18] This differs from Michigan's surveillance system, which is mandatory and covers physicians of all specialties. In Michigan, 54% of the reports are from occupational and pulmonary physicians, 7% are from allergists and the remaining 38% are from other specialties. Finland has a national mandatory reporting system that is connected with their workers' compensation system; their reported rate is 15.2 cases per 100,000.[19] Isocyanates are typically the most common cause of work-related asthma reported in other surveillance systems.[18,20] However, when farmers were included in the workers' compensation system in Finland, cow dander became the most commonly reported allergen in that county.[21]

A more recent report from a study that was based on interviewers of patients at an HMO in Massachusetts estimated the annual rate of work-related asthma at 71 cases per 100,000.[22] Possible reasons for this much higher rate reported in the study from Massachusetts include:

- less restrictive case criteria in the HMO study
- more intense case-finding in the HMO study
- increasing incidence of work-related asthma between the time of the more recent HMO study and previous studies
- the fact that the annual estimates from the HMO study were extrapolated from cases identified during the 3-month period of July, August, and September

DISCUSSION

Michigan has had a surveillance system for work-related asthma since 1988. Similar to the New Jersey system, reports are received from physicians and hospitals. In Michigan, over 80% of the reports are received from physicians.[12]

The Michigan surveillance system has proved useful in describing the epidemiology of the disease and directing prevention activity despite the underreporting of cases, which may be as high as 80%.

Although most facilities where the patient developed asthma were not in violation of exposure standards, there were high percentages of symptomatic fellow workers in facilities using occupational allergens. The presence of symptomatic coworkers suggests that some of the occupational health standards are not sufficiently protective to ensure a safe workplace, and provides some insight into the magnitude of the problem.

Reevaluations of allowable exposure standards are needed. These reevaluations should consider comprehensive workplace controls that address not only daily average exposures but exposures during spills and leaks and provision of medical surveillance for potentially exposed workers. Medical monitoring is particularly relevant to reducing the burden of work-related asthma; the longer a person with symptoms remains exposed, the more likely his or her asthma will become a chronic problem.[1]

CONCLUSION

Work-related asthma remains an ongoing problem in Michigan and worldwide. Work-related asthma surveillance systems are critical to direct primary prevention and intervention activities, monitor trends, and identify new workplace allergens. Without continued surveillance of work-related asthma and other occupational diseases, workers will be unnecessarily subjected to exposures that jeopardize their health and livelihood. The Michigan surveillance system has been useful in identifying problems with existing workplace standards and providing data to justify revision for these standards that will provide greater protection to workers. Although more complete reporting would presumably identify more problem worksites, even with marked underreporting the system has been successful in meeting its objectives of estimating the burden of disease, describing the epidemiology, and directing effective preventive interventions.

ACKNOWLEGMENTS

The authors acknowledge the office and interview staff who handle the reports of silicosis on a daily basis: Amy Sims, Amy Krizek, Tracy Murphy, and Ruth VanderWaals as well as the numerous medical students who conducted interviews throughout the years of surveillance efforts. The authors also acknowledge the tremendous support of the program by Michigan's OSHA inspectors and administrative staff. This project was partially funded by the National Institute for Occupational Safety and Health, under cooperative agreement number U60-CCU502998.

REFERENCES

1. Chan-Yeung M, Malo JL. Occupational asthma. *New Engl J Med* 1995; 333:107–112.
2. Brooks S, Hammad Y, Richards I, Grovinco-Barbas J, Jenkins K. The spectrum of irritant-induced asthma. Sudden and not-so-sudden onset and the role of allergy. *Chest* 1998; 113:42–49.
3. Brooks SM, Weiss MA, Bernstein I. Reactive airways dysfunction syndrome (RADS): persistent asthma syndrome after high level irritant exposures. *Chest* 1985; 85:376–384.
4. National Research Council. *Counting Injuries and Illnesses in the Workplace: Proposal for a Better System.* Washington, DC: National Academy Press; 1987.
5. Jajosky RA, Harrison R, Reinisch F, Flattery J, Chan J, Tumpowsky C, Davis L, Reilly MJ, Rosenman KD, Kalinowski D, Stanbury M, Schill DP, Wood J. Surveillance of work-related asthma in selected U.S. states using surveillance guidelines for state health departments—California, Massachusetts, Michigan and New Jersey, 1993–1995. *MMWR* 1999; 48(SS-3):1–20.
6. Kipen HM, Gelperin K, Tepper A, Stanbury M. Acute respiratory diseases in hospital discharge data. *Am J Ind Med* 1991; 19:637–642.
7. Reilly MJ, Rosenman KD. Use of hospital discharge data for surveillance of chemical related respiratory disease. *Arch Environ Health* 1995; 50:26–30.
8. Meredith SK, Taylor VM, McDonald JC. Occupational respiratory disease in the United Kingdom 1989: a report to the British thoracic society and the society of occupational medicine by the project group. *Br J Ind Med* 1991; 48:292–298.
9. Rosenman KD, Reilly MJ, Kalinowski DJ. *1998 Annual Report on Work-Related Asthma in Michigan.* Lansing, Michigan: Michigan State University; February 24, 1999.
10. Timmer S, Rosenman KD. Occurrence of occupational Asthma. *Chest* 1993; 104:816–820.
11. Henneberger PK, Kreiss K, Rosenman KD, Reilly MJ, Chang Y-F, Geidenberger CA. An evaluation of the incidence of work-related asthma in the United States. *Internat J Occup Environ Health* 1999; 5:1–8.
12. Rosenman KD, Reilly MJ, Kalinowski DJ. State-based surveillance system for work-related asthma. *J Occup Environ Med* 1997; 39:415–425.
13. Rosenman KD, Reilly MJ, Kalinowski D. Work-Related Asthma and Respiratory Symptoms Among Workers Exposed to Metal-Working Fluids. *Am J Ind Med* 1997; 32:325–331.
14. Kwaselow A, Rowe M, Sears-Ewald D, Ownby D. Rose hips: a new occupational allergen. *J Allergy Clin Immunol* 1992; 85:704–708.
15. Rosenman KD, Hart M, Ownby DR. Occupational asthma in a beet sugar processing plant. *Chest* 1992; 101:1720–1722.
16. Gannon PFG, Burge PS. A preliminary report of a surveillance scheme of occupational asthma in the West Midlands. *Br J Ind Med* 1991; 48:579–582.
17. Meredith S. Reported incidence of occupational asthma in the United Kingdom, 1989-1990. *J Epidemiol Community Health*; 1993; 47:459–463.
18. Gannon PFG, Burge PS. The SHIELD scheme in the West Midlands Region, United Kingdom. *Br J Ind Med* 1993; 50:791–796.
19. Keskinen H. Epidemiology of occupational lung disease: asthma and allergic alveolitis. In: Kerr JW, Ganderton MA, eds. *Proceedings of XI International Congress of Allergy and Clinical Immunology, London.* London: MacMillan; 1982:403–407.
20. Lee HS, Phoon WH, Wang YT, et al. Occupational asthma in Singapore. A review of cases from 1983–1990. *Singapore Med J* 1991; 32:398–402.
21. Reijula K, Patterson R. Occupational allergies in Finland in 1981–1991. *Allergy Proc* 1994; 15:163–168.
22. Milton DK, Solomon GM, Rosiello RA, Herrick RA. Risk and incidence of asthma attributable to occupational exposure among HMO members. *Am J Ind Med* 1998; 33:1–10.

17

Injury Surveillance at Ford Motor Company

GORDON R. REEVE

There are several types of occupational injury surveillance. The most traditional approach is surveillance using vital records at the federal- or state-level. Many, but not all states require occupational injuries or illnesses to be reported as part of their public health reporting system that has historically focused on communicable diseases. Other systems try to capture all injuries seen at the emergency rooms in community- or statewide networks with information about the situation surrounding the injury event, including occupational factors. Finally, there is the surveillance conducted by the health and safety staff of a company as part of its routine operation or as part of a short-term research project conducted by university researchers.

Of these types of surveillance systems, the company-based surveillance systems are most likely to result in significant changes in injury prevention and risk reduction efforts. The workplace has a structure that is much more controllable than that in the public arena where injury prevention advocates must deal with behavioral factors and broader political issues. Company management is required by statute to provide a safe workplace and comply with existing standards, but is free to implement more stringent safety measures. The company also has control of how the work processes are designed, what skill level is needed to perform these work processes, and how to train these workers. In unionized workplaces, a union's advocacy for safety and health further enhances the level of control over injury risk.

Despite this level of control over the workplace environment, company-based injury surveillance and its impact on injury prevention and intervention efforts are rarely described to others outside of a particular company or industry. More importantly, the inability of most companies to conduct injury surveillance and to use its data effectively is one of the greatest missed opportunities in public health. Most company personnel responsible for health and safety know very little about the use of surveillance data, even when it is available. Many companies view OSHA record keeping as a chore to be done at a minimal level, e.g., we hate OSHA so we'll only so the minimum level of record keeping, and do it as poorly as possible. More interestingly, plant management routinely measures and analyzes every critical aspect of their operations, but they generally limit the analysis of health and safety process to a summary view of plantwide injury statistics. These plantwide frequency data are of little value in guiding prevention efforts. In addition, a common reaction to using plantwide safety statistics to evaluate manager's performance is adulterating the data itself.

This chapter describes the experiences of the epidemiologist for a major U.S. manufacturer over the past 10 years in the struggle to improve the company's existing injury surveillance system and to have the data be used to drive the injury prevention and intervention. Although the challenges of conducting injury surveillance will vary with the size, structure, and business of each company, many issues discussed here are applicable across many different company environments. The discussion includes (*1*) how to establish or improve your plant's injury surveillance system; (*2*) the road blocks put in your way by people who want to steal your resources and by well-intentioned bunglers whose efforts can also stop your progress; (*3*) the constant struggle to keep the surveillance system viable; and, (*4*) the toughest of all, how to get people to use the surveillance data to drive health and safety processes.

METHODS

Define Goals, Objectives, and Scope

If your company or plant has 11 or more employees, you have or should have the basis of an injury surveillance system. It's called the OSHA Log (Appendix A). This record keeping process was mandated by the Occupational Health and Safety Administration (OSHA) in the early 1970s. The system is driven by the OSHA Log (OSHA Form 200), which is a line listing of each occupational injury or illness meeting a set of criteria that indicates that the disorder is more serious that those requiring only first aid. A minimal level of information (name and age of worker, type of illness or injury, date and time of event or diagnosis, job function of the worker) is collected and recorded on the Log. For each case listed there is a one-page form (OSHA 101) that is completed and provides detailed information about the factors associated with the injury or illness.

The record keeping process required by OSHA has not changed much over the last 25 years. It is still a paper-driven process for most companies or plants. Many moderate to large companies use computerized software to keep their OSHA records. The rules for determining which injury or illness cases to add to the Log are tedious and difficult to apply consistently. When the record keeping rules are properly applied, only 30%–40% of all first time occupational medical visits (FTOVs) will be added to the log. An OSHA log and the OSHA 101s maintained on paper do not readily lend themselves to analysis of injury patterns by relevant organizational levels within a plant, such as department or supervisor unit. Despite these shortcomings, the OSHA log provides a place to start and eliminates the need to justify the need for even the most basic injury surveillance system.

The first challenge is to build on the OSHA record keeping process so it meets your plant's needs to identify and describe injury events. Many companies view OSHA and anything associated with it as a nuisance. Consequently, such companies approach the basic record keeping process as a chore to be dispatched with just enough effort to keep the company out of regulatory trouble. Unfortunately, this mind set squanders a significant opportunity to turn a regulatory requirement into a valuable tool critical to the prevention of occupational injuries. In companies with this mind set, the battle to improve surveillance will be an uphill one, but the section of this chapter on marketing surveillance provides suggestions to turn this thinking around.

If your company's or plant's OSHA record keeping process is not automated, this should be the leading priority. There are several commercially available software packages to support the OSHA record keeping process and that greatly reduce the effort required to analyze injury data. Larger plants with their own inplant medical departments should consider a software package that includes an automated or electronic medical record directly linked to the OSHA record keeping process (Fig. 17.1).[1] The software selected should also have the ability to review each occupational medical visit and all of its follow-up visits to determine whether a injury should be recorded on the OSHA log. This process of having the medical staff enter abbreviated diagnosis and treatment codes and then having the software run the OSHA decision algorithm is much more reliable than having medical staff make that decision and mark or flag the case as OSHA recordable. All plants, regardless of size, should also make sure that the software they buy or develop has the ability to capture the most basic information about all FTOVs; otherwise, they will be miss minor injuries that could have been severe ones under slightly different circumstances. Stated differently, by limiting analysis of injury to the OSHA recordable cases, you completely miss the opportunity to analyze the risk factors associated with 50%–70% of the cases seen by your medical care providers.

Two significant enhancements should be made to a basic record keeping system to really make the data more useful for injury prevention. One is to link the system to each supervisor, preferably through their PC linkage to the plant engineering or payroll system or to their plant e-mail. When an injury visit is documented in the medical department, the supervisor of the injured worker is notified electronically and requested to complete a case investigation. Once entered to the supervisor's PC, the information from the investigation is combined with the medical data in the health and safety database.

The second enhancement is to analyze injury data by specific plant organizational units. The software should have the ability to provide case counts by department down to the smaller organizational units, such as supervisor's area. It should also facilitate analysis of injury rates for the whole plant as well as the smaller organizational units. This requires the attachment of hours worked to the specific plant areas from the plant's payroll system. Analysis of rates will prevent all the attention from being focused on the largest de-

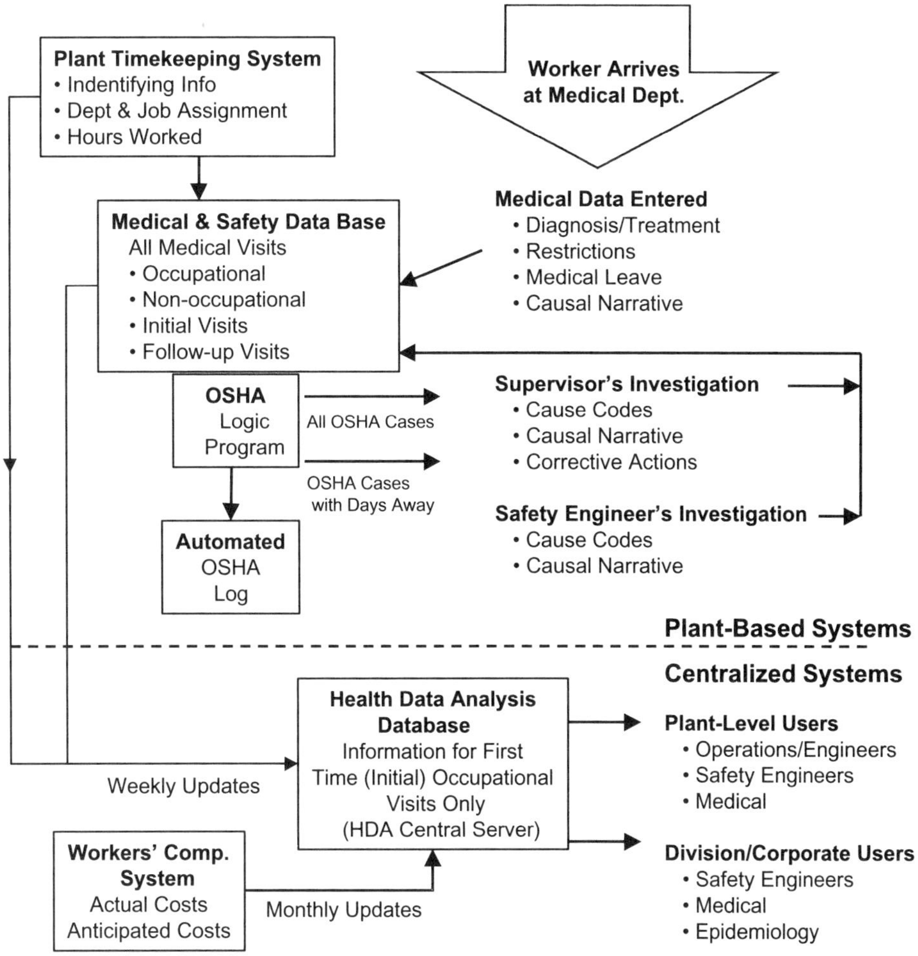

Figure 17.1 Occupational health and safety data system: Ford Motor Company System. (Sorock et al.[1])

partments that may indeed have the largest number of injuries, but have much lower injury rates than smaller departments or functional units (see Chapters 4 and 5, Appendices D and E).

If your plant is small enough that you know every worker by first and last name, you probably will do fine with a well-organized paper system. Still, you should try to distinguish between case counts and case rates to pinpoint problem areas. You should also involve the first-line supervisor in the investigation of all occupational injuries.

Gain Support

The basic product of a surveillance system is reliable information to reduce injuries and their associated costs and to improve manufacturing processes. Surveillance data can identify the manufacturing processes and equipment with elevated injury rates. Further investigation of problem areas can highlight the underlying factors associated with the injury events, such as poorly maintained machinery, use of equipment not suited to the task, or inadequate training of the operator.

Eliminating the underlying causes of occupational injury produces multiple benefits. Some are obvious and other are not so obvious, but each has its own level of marketability. A list of benefits begins with:

- reducing the risk of acute trauma to the affected worker groups
- reducing medical costs and those associated with workers' compensation payments and rehabilitation
- reducing the plant's exposure to regulatory actions either from record keeping fines or for not recognizing injury patterns that could have been significantly reduced
- improving the quality of the product and productivity of the plant by making the product easier and safer for the workers to produce

Of these four benefits, the reduction of injuries, reduction in costs, and not getting fined by OSHA are the obvious and expected outcomes of an injury surveillance system. The last factor, improvement of product quality is not tremendously obvious. Still, all four benefits of injury surveillance are difficult to document. In addition, management may have little interest in injury prevention for at least two reasons: (*1*) they do not understand the business of injury prevention as well as the other aspects of the plant's business, and (*2*) they regard injury prevention and the reduction of injury rates as a process that one cannot control. After all, isn't that why the events leading up to an unintentional injury are referred to as an accident.

This leads to the basic concepts of marketing where you have a good product but an uneasy or uninterested consumer. First, you have to create a market for your product. This requires identifying your customers and getting them interested. Second, you need to show them what the product will look like using data they can relate to. Third, to secure the commitment of resources (staff and money), you will need a definite and realistic time frame for delivery of useful surveillance data.

Building Interest

In situations where your company has already been cited or fined by OSHA, there is opportunity. For example, The Ford Motor Company was cited by OSHA for record keeping violations at two different plants within a 5-year period. The Occupational Safety and Health Administration fined the company $1.9 million. The fine was reduced on the condition, spelled out in a binding settlement agreement, that the company would correct all OSHA records at its 60 U.S. locations for the prior 3 years and conduct third-party audits to demonstrate compliance. The final cost was $1.2 million for the fine and $13 million for the record cleanup.

Part of the internal marketing effort at our company was: we did not want to do this again so we needed to fix our record keeping system, and, while we were at it, we should make it useful to the injury prevention process. Of course, any given plant's odds of being inspected by OSHA are remote, given the number of OSHA inspectors and number of plants. The odds of a fine for record keeping violations are even more remote because the rules for OSHA record keeping are not always fully understood by OSHA inspectors. Therefore, you can not count on OSHA to present you with a survivable crisis that you can turn into a surveillance system. Even with an OSHA situation, marketing efforts based on "we better do this or big bad OSHA will get us, again" did not go very far. We used OSHA to set up some meetings, but our marketing efforts were based on what the system could do to protect our workers, and, in turn, make our plants more efficient.

A successful marketing campaign is built on knowing your data and how the operations and safety people could use it. If you do not have a computer-based surveillance or record keeping system, you will need to assemble, organize, and analyze your plant's data from paper into a very basic PC spreadsheet (Appendix E).

You need to study at least one year's worth of data in detail. You should pick one plant or very large operation within a plant with at least 300 workers, preferably choosing a plant with a history of real or perceived safety problems.

The analysis should proceed from the most general organizational level (plantwide) to the supervisor unit or specific job type. Start with case counts and injury rates by the plant and then by the individual departments. Do not limit yourself to OSHA recordable cases. Plot injuries by all FTOVs as well as OSHA cases and OSHA cases with days away from work. Display them by month for the 12-month study period. You should see variation by month and by department. Examine the data looking at department rankings by case counts and case rates. There should be some smaller departments with high rates that would never be seen if you had looked only at the top 10 departments in terms of number of cases. These small but high-risk departments may lend themselves to a more targeted prevention effort not possible in a large department with relatively low case rates.

Continue to look for variation in the cases that can be turned into real world marketing examples. Look for changes over time, by month or quarter, to see if a department with stable rates actually had a change in injury pattern. Did the top five injury types change? For example, did the first two quarters of the year show more sprains and strains than the 3rd quarter? Did finger lacerations increase? We found such a case in our preliminary analysis of our data, which was traced to an overly zealous newly assigned worker controlling the glove-use program. Workers who needed to replace damaged gloves could not do so easily, so they continued to use their damaged gloves with a corresponding increase in the rate of lacerations.

Look for peaks or spikes in injury rates by department or supervisor. From the time period where rates sharply increased, look at the prior 3 or 6 months to see what changed in terms of injury type or body part affected. If the rate returned to normal also look for changes in patterns. From here, study the narratives of the first report of injury and see if there are any clues in the written report. If not, talk to the supervisor from the effected area for clues, what he or she may have done to correct the situation, and whether the changes worked.

One of the most effective marketing examples for us was to look at a difference between shifts in the same production department. Initially I had assumed (incorrectly) that the night shift would always have higher rates. I also (naively) thought that if one shift figured out how to do a job better or make a tool to do the job better, they would share it with the other shift. Our analysis of injury rates by shift negated both of these assumptions. In fact, there was tremendous variation by shift. In some cases the injury rates would increase or decrease in unison. Inevitably, one shift would show an increase. However, it could be either the night or day shift. Short-lived differences were probably normal variations, but two shifts making the same product having vastly different rates for weeks or months indicates an opportunity to identify a problem and a best practice at the same time. Try to incorporate information in your analysis on the number of restricted days and days away from work. If this is really difficult, do this only for the major departments with the highest rates. Talk to a mid-level person in the plant's workers' compensation group and try to get a rule of thumb about the daily cost of having a worker away from the job. Apply their algorithm, e.g., $246 per day, to the number of days away and apply 20% of it to the restricted days. Use the financial information in your marketing to lay out the actual workers' compensation costs and a corresponding estimate for costs per day away. Use these cost measures to show the maximum cost target than needs to be reduced. Let your customers suggest a realistic percentage of reduction if the plant could be more effective using data to drive its injury prevention efforts. Then translate this cost-savings estimate into your marketing efforts for the surveillance system.

Once armed with the wisdom and insight from studying your plant's data, talk to a sample of your most competent front-line supervisors and their supervisors, but only go up one level. You will want to stay off the radar screen of the plant big shots until you know what the shop floor thinks. Show them the data. Ask them what they think. Would this kind of information be useful to them? Do they have any theories to account for the spikes in the injury rates or for any time the injury rate dramatically decreased? Ask them which process is their biggest headache in terms of injury. Did their worst jobs show up in the data as a worst job? If not, why?

After assimilating the information from the data and feedback from those who actually make the plant run, you are ready to convince the leadership of the plant to support development of an injury surveillance system or improvement of the one you have.

The marketing presentation for establishing or improving your plant's or company's injury surveillance system should be able to show the customers and sponsors what form the surveillance data would take. You should use the flashiest real-world examples that you discovered with your detailed inspection of data and conversations with the people in the plant. Do not be shy about mocking up data charts using your PC's graphics software using real data. If you propose buying an off-the-shelf surveillance package, have the vendor feed your plant's data through their package so you can demonstrate the look and feel of their product.

Finally, you need to frame the presentation in terms of the your plant's need for a competent injury surveillance system. Lower injury rates will lower production costs and increase the quality of the product. Fewer injuries will reduce the amount of rotation into critical jobs where nonveteran workers will not be able to obtain the highest output than a person who has perfected their technique in that job. Mention the regulatory requirements more in the scope of "we have to do something like this anyway, so we may turn this regulatory requirement to a competitive advantage."

Bumps Along the Road

As you move through the steps of approval to run the surveillance system, be aware that you will be competing for precious resources especially if your are doing this in a moderate to large company. The usual and obvious adversaries will be other departments competing for systems and staff resources. Always remember, a key part of a finance person's job description is to say "No." However, the bigger surprises will come from unexpected places such as people you always thought understood the need for good injury data and even people who strongly support health and safety.

"We Don't Need No Surveillance System." During the marketing phases at Ford, one of the toughest issues was the perception that a computer-based injury surveillance system was not needed. The conventional wisdom of this position is that all one needs to do is to make a list of the bad jobs and fix each one. This was a difficult notion to dispel because the company and its union had standing safety and ergonomic committees in each of the company's 60 manufacturing locations in the United States. These committees were comprised of safety engineers, union health and safety representatives, and plant engineers. These people should certainly know where the hazards are and how to fix them. With the exception of small and simple operations, the number of bad jobs will always exceed the resources needed to fix them. Without the benefit of a surveillance system, these committees spent most of their time arranging and rearranging the job priority list. This left little time to actually fix problems. This never-ending priority setting favored jobs that were easy to fix or helped manage situations where the complaints about a job were the loudest, despite other jobs with higher injury rates and more severe injury types.

Proactive versus Reactive. Another problem is the argument about being proactive or being reactive. You probably will encounter opposition from allies in the health and safety ranks who want to put all their resources into proactive approaches. They consider injury surveillance a low priority because it is based on injuries that have already happened. While it is true that an injury surveillance system cannot change the fact that the injuries have happened, careful study of these injuries can lead to measures to prevent future injuries. This makes surveillance a proactive process based on experience. The best description of how surveillance should be turned into a proactive process was provided by a crusty senior manufacturing manager in one of Ford's most productive assembly plants. My first-person account of this discussion follows:

> I was meeting with a group of senior manufacturing managers at one of the company's most productive and profitable assembly plants back in 1992. The design team and I were describing the injury surveillance project and presenting data that we had assembled and analyzed from their plant. After the formal presentation, we asked if this type of data would meet their needs and was there anything else we should add. Mind you that up to this point at some other plants, a typical comment was "you know that report (a line listing of medical visits) we get on Thursday every week, if I could get it on Monday that would be all I want."
>
> The most senior manager and oldest of the group gets up and goes over to a chalk board in the room. He looked like an Air Force colonel from an old black and white World War II movie. He looks me right in the eye and says, "Son (mind you, I was 41 at the time), here's what I want." He began to draw on the board a set of three interconnected loops (Fig. 17.2). Pointing to the first loop he said, "Here I want to know who got hurt, what they were doing and what type of tool they were using so I can get that job fixed so no one else gets hurt." Pointing to the middle loop, he said, "Then I want to be able to look at the engineering system and see where else in the plant that tool is being used or where similar processes are being performed. I want those jobs inspected for safety risk, I also want to go to this system you guys are talking about and look at the injury rates of those jobs." He pointed to the third loop. "Are they the same as the job where people had been injured? If they are different, let's say—lower, then maybe we can figure out why one process is going right in that area and put that process in place where the worker was hurt. If your system can do that or make it a lot easier for us to do that, then I am all for it."

In retrospect, our injury surveillance system made it easy to identify high-risk injury areas and to look at other areas with similar processes. The key element that is still missing and must be done manually, is linking the surveillance system to the plant engineering systems by specific job and tool usage. Any system that could do this will increase the value of traditional injury surveillance efforts greatly.

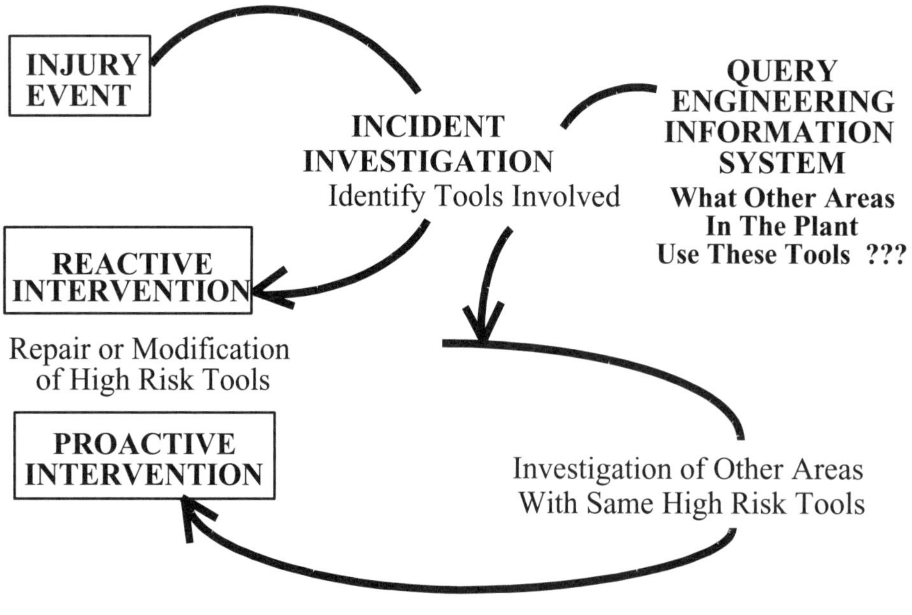

Figure 17.2 Reactive and proactive injury interventions.

Keep It (relatively) Simple. One insidious thing to look out for goes under the heading "Do not let the perfect be the enemy of the good." In particular you have to have a realistic scope of a surveillance system and its purpose. It must identify jobs or processes that have elevated injury rates or ones that could be used in best practice models because their rates are so low. Developing injury prevention or intervention strategies usually requires a detailed analysis of the data that are beyond the scope of a surveillance system. Well-intentioned customers who want the surveillance system to do both surveillance and detailed injury analysis are setting up the surveillance system to fail. One very clear example is the level of detail of the data and how they are coded. Resist overly elaborate coding schemes for the risk factors associated with the injury. Some commercial systems spend an extraordinary amount of effort fixing blame for the injury in terms of proper training, noncompliance issues, and certain intangibles like plant leadership.

Project Sponsor Investment. Be sure the project is developed with strong input and guidance from someone who knows and genuinely represents the people who will ultimately use the system. So many of these projects fail even when they have the right level of funding and resources. This occurs because the health and safety sponsors turn the project over to an information systems team. To avoid failure, the health and safety staff must maintain a high level of involvement. We referred to this as *sweat equity.* Our sweat equity was the near full-time commitment of one middle-level staff person with a high degree of knowledge about the occupational health processes who served as the customer advocate. He led the project team through the critical customer interviews and also brought along the information system specialists so they could hear for themselves the needs and thinking of the customers. As the hundreds of decisions and compromises were made in the development process, the customer advocate was there for all the discussions. Even though compromises were made, they had a small negative effect on the customer and were not driven by the easiest design for the programmers. If you are the customer advocate, it will seem like a war of attrition, but if you disengage from the surveillance project, it will fail—whether it is an in-house development project or an off-the-shelf software package.

Beating the Finance Group and Your Departmental Resource Competition. There are two weapons in your arsenal for battling these potential detractors. One is learning the finance dialect and using their definitions for estimating the total costs of injuries. If you have to play the game of cost savings, look at the cost target you developed and pick a low percentage of savings that can potentially be achieved by using the surveillance system. Try never to exceed 5% as the estimated cost savings, and always discuss your projection with the credible finance person before your presentation. Mention that he or she helped you with the projections.

Finally, battling the finance group and fighting for departmental priority is the place to play the OSHA card. In most project ranking schemes, one of the critical ranking criteria asks: "Is this required by statute or regulation?" If you can answer yes you will be able to move the project well ahead of other projects that are not regulatory requirements. A well-functioning surveillance system can lower the plant's vulnerability to fines by making record keeping more accurate and comply with OSHA rules. It can identify injury and health risks more quickly than the current system and allow the plant to fix hazards before an OSHA inspection may be requested by a worker or worker representative. This line of reasoning usually convinces the heads of Personnel or Human Resources. The key here is to just get a check mark on the priority ranking sheet for your project so it is seen as having regulatory impact. In all of this, be careful not to oversell the OSHA threat.

Maintaining Support

Once you have survived the battles of getting a surveillance system installed or an existing one improved, you begin the difficult tasks of getting the right people to use it as a tool in their injury prevention activities, and of maintaining and improving the system over time.

One of the most unappreciated facts involving a surveillance systems is that they adhere rigidly to the second law of thermodynamics. That is, without constant input of energy, surveillance systems, like all systems, will tend toward entropy (i.e., fall apart). Energies and activities that must be continually provided to surveillance efforts are:

- management support for data driven processes
- monitoring the quality of the data
- training efforts for people who enter and those who analyze the data
- systems support to maintain and improve the system

The following discussions are based on our experiences at Ford. We still fight the war of attrition, occasionally losing some battles.

Management Support. For an injury surveillance system to be maintained and used, plant operations management must clearly demonstrate that they support it by using surveillance data in their operational decisions. This takes the form of weekly reviews of the injury data coupled with concise presentations from selected supervisors. Some will discuss the progress made in their areas to reduce injuries. Others will need to describe issues that they are still struggling with to determine the underlying causes of injury problems in their areas. Projects to improve production processes should incorporate surveillance data so that new projects can be prioritized relative to outstanding injury issues.

Using data to drive and evaluate injury prevention efforts also requires management to accept the risks of using surveillance data. With increased emphasis on injury surveillance and analysis, the injury rates are certain to go up, at least temporarily. Data will identify issues that seem impossible to solve or that require a major change in the manufacturing processes. These are never popular or politically safe situations.

In some companies where performance of staff is tied to outcomes measured by a injury surveillance system, attempts to distort or falsify data must be minimized with the full and active involvement of senior management. If cheating is allowed, then the data will become suspect. The plants and departments that have correctly reported their injury data will be demoralized, while other areas with more serious injury problems will slide through the management reviews without a scratch. Without reliable data, injury prevention efforts fall back to the ever popular "program-of-the-month." These types of safety programs are based on subjective criteria that cannot be evaluated for effectiveness. You should be aware that there might be groups in your plant who want to go back or stay with the program-of-the-month approach. They are often the same detractors who berate data quality or actively contribute to poor data quality.

Management also needs to support the system with the appropriate resources such as computers and staff for data entry. To send the message that the surveillance system will be supported, management needs to place appropriate priority on data collection by medical staff, front line supervisors, and safety engineers. One way to do this is to make the surveillance data activities an integral part of their jobs, and structuring their jobs so it is not something they do when they get around to it. The collection of high quality surveillance data should be one of the items on which their job performance is rated.

Data Quality Reviews. Those assigned to oversee and guide the injury surveillance process must periodically review the completeness and quality of the data being entered into the system. Most coding systems have a category called Other or Unknown to account for unusual cases. Other and Unknown codes should be checked at least once a quarter or after new medical or supervisory staff are hired. A marked increase in these codes indicates: (*1*) the people entering data are doing it poorly; or, (*2*) there is a new situation that does not lend itself to classification by the existing set of codes. Reading the case narratives and comparing them to the codes helps determine the proper course of action. For those entering marginal investigation reports, their performance needs to be brought to their attention. A bar chart counting the number of Unknown and Other codes for each data entry person should be part of the feedback. If improvement is not immediate then this should be brought to the attention of plant management. In the second case, interviews with the people struggling to describe injury events that do not exactly fit the existing coding scheme should be conducted to gain insight for new codes. New codes should be developed and training provided to all system users when the new codes are activated.

Some data fields in the surveillance system will not lend themselves to a fixed code structure. Instead, the specific job or manufacturing process may be described by a code that is entered in a free text field where alpha and numeric characters can legitimately be entered, but cannot be verified against a preestablished set of codes. These situations require special attention. For example, an investigation of an injury involving a worker installing the left tail light on a vehicle might list the job or process number as A10739 at a particular vehicle assembly plant. Although the job number is part of the plant's engineering system, there is no linkage between the plant engineering system and the injury surveillance system. In such situations, it is not uncommon for inappropriate codes to be entered into a required data field by some supervisors who just want to get the investigation request off of their screens. By entering codes such as *n/a* (not available), 999999, 123456, they greatly reduce the utility of the surveillance system and the data properly entered by others. At several Ford plants during the early days of the surveillance system, the most hazardous job or manufacturing process was *n/a*. Periodically, analyses should be run on such free-field codes and the counts of inappropriate codes (n/a, 99999, 123456, 222222) should be displayed by the supervisor identifier. Again, if improvement does not follow feedback to the guilty party, the situation should be brought to the attention of plant management.

Training in Use of the Surveillance System. There are two levels of training for the surveillance system. One is for data entry. It should include not only how to enter the required data, but some explanation of why these data are needed and how they will be used. Training should be implemented when the system is launched, and training should also be available for newly hired staff long after the system has been in place. Depending on the number of people using the surveillance system and the number of data items being collected, the training may be fairly informal or may require structured classes. Periodic quality checks of the data should also be reviewed with the idea that certain issues with data quality might be due to shortcomings of the training. Training must be a job requirement for those who enter data.

The other training involves the actual use of the data from the surveillance system. It should not be assumed that the people motivated to tackle safety issues automatically know how to look at data. This training should cover the basics of looking at descriptive data and how it changes over time. The importance of looking at counts and rates together must be emphasized. Injury rates that show significant increases and decreases must be examined in detail to learn of the causes behind the changes in the rates. In the case of increasing rates, it is important to look at the types of injuries. Did one type of injury account for the increase, and, if so, what might be the underlying cause(s)? If the rate decreased, then what type of injury accounted for the decrease and were there changes in the operation that could have been associated with the reduction. If these changes can be identified, they should be brought to the attention of other manufacturing areas or shifts within the same worksite or company. The surveillance system can also be used to document the impact of a particular injury intervention by comparing the injury rates before the intervention, during its implementation, and for a defined period after the intervention has been in place.

Information Systems Support. As mentioned earlier, a surveillance system needs the ongoing input of energy and resources, especially if it serves many plants. All too often, the surveillance system is purchased from an outside vendor and installed by the information systems group. As soon as installation is completed, the support is radically reduced, and over time it may not be available to keep the surveillance system in good working order. If performance problems develop, the death of the surveillance effort is not far away. Support is needed for the inevitable software upgrades to the basic operating system, hardware, and applications that run the computerized parts of the surveillance system.

As the users become familiar with surveillance, they usually request improved coding schemes and new data for analysis. If the surveillance system, even if it were a good one when installed, does not grow with the users' needs, the more inventive users will begin to produce homegrown data systems to augment the shortcomings of the existing surveillance system. With every auxiliary system, the risk grows that the core system will fall into disuse.

Data Analysis, Interpretation, and Feedback

The examples that follow are based on many different experiences at the Ford Motor Company. Although Ford is a very large company with a well-developed safety and health process that is strongly supported by the United Auto Workers Union, these examples are applicable to most manufacturing situations and plants of various sizes.

More Accurate Reporting of Injury Statistics

Without a standardized computer surveillance system, certain departments or even whole plant locations at Ford had developed unique ways to calculate the safety statistics that they presented to their plant operating committees. Prior to the installation of the computer-based surveillance system, injury surveillance was based on calculations made by the Plant Safety Engineer using copies of the current and prior editions of OSHA logs assembled by the plant medical department. At the end of each month, the case counts and lost workdays appearing on the OSHA log were transferred to a safety statistics spread sheet and adjusted by the Safety Engineer. The number of injury cases might have been inaccurately added to the spreadsheet. The number of hours worked in certain administrative categories might be inappropriately included in the plant's injury rate calculations. This resulted in a reduction in the plant's injury and severity rates. For years, one particular plant location reported nearly the best safety statistics for its division while at the same time posting the highest workers' compensation costs.

With the installation of the computerized safety system, there were several complaints about the quality of the data, mainly that the injury rates from the new system were much too high. Audits of the computerized system and comparisons with the official OSHA log and the plant medical records repeatedly demonstrated that the new system was functioning correctly. Over time the computerized system became the standard for injury statistics. This meant that more attention was paid to solving injury problems that manually adjusting the injury surveillance data.

Justification and Support of Process Improvements to Reduce Injury Risk

When elevated injury risks are linked to specific jobs, changes to the manufacturing processes are often recommended. They may cost a few thousand dollars to well over \$100,000. While it would be desirable to make every job optimal for the worker performing its tasks, financial justification for job improvement is a fact of life in all manufacturing environments. The critical issues are how much will the process change the cost and what is the reasonable expectation that there will some tangible return on investment.

One example involved the installation of a wiring harness in the full-sized truck. The wiring loom is a massive tangle of wires that runs underneath the dashboard and into the vehicle doors. It supports electric door locks and windows, and all the functions that are controlled through fixtures on the dashboard. This is a tough job in terms of ergonomic risks as well as finger lacerations and contusions from threading the wiring harness through the vehicle frame and plugging the electrical connectors together. In recent years the harnesses have grown thicker as more electronics were added to what used to be a plain old pick-up truck. As tough as this job is in the warm summer months, it becomes much more difficult in cold weather when the plant is difficult to heat. Workers in these jobs had elevated injury rates. To make the job easier, overhead heaters had been installed in this particular assembly line to heat the harnesses and make them more pliable. Unfortunately, the line speed was such that there was not enough time for the overhead heaters to warm the harnesses that were further down in the shipping containers.

The safety engineer and union ergonomic representative were convinced they had a solution. The heaters could be replaced with ones that would heat the wiring harness from the bottom of the shipping container. Then all the harnesses in a particular container would be pliable and easier to install, especially when the plant was cooler. To accomplish this, a series of six special heaters were needed. Each heater would cost $25,000 making the cost of the improvement approximately $150,000. By assembling the surveillance data and linking to the workers' compensation costs for this job station, the safety engineer and the union ergonomic representative were able to make the economic case that the improvement would pay for itself in fewer than 2 years. Without data and injury cost information from a reliable surveillance system the project would have not been approved.

Data-Driven Decisions of Policy Issues

In other instances, surveillance data are critical to make the appropriate decisions regarding program initiatives that are well-intentioned but may not produce the intended result.

The corporate Occupational Health and Safety staff was requested to recommend the expansion of a new-hire orientation and physical conditioning program that had been implemented recently at a particular plant. It was thought to be beneficial by both local plant management and by the union. Using the injury surveillance system, occupational injury cases were examined that occurred during the period 6 months before the program and occurring during the 6-month period after the initiation of the program. Case counts were assembled and case rates were computed by seniority: fewer than 3 months, 3–4 months, 5–12 months, and 1 year or more.

The rate for all First Time Occupational Medical Visits among the lowest seniority groups showed a 14% increase after the implementation of the program. This could be attributed to a greater awareness that new hires could and should seek medical attention for injuries. The rate for cases with days away from work increased from 14 prior to the program to 22 cases per 200,000 hours after the program was started. Of greatest concern was that the number of ergonomically related back and shoulder injuries had increased from four to nine during the first 6 months of the program.

The physical training regimen was reviewed and was found to be inappropriate for conditioning or strengthening. The physical conditioning portion of the program was eliminated. The time to evaluate this situation and make data-driven policy recommendations was 10 working days. Without a surveillance system in place, a program that seemed like a good idea could have resulted in significantly increased injury rates as it was implemented through the company.

These examples represent some of the successes in using an injury surveillance system. However, implementing and maintaining the use of such a system is an ongoing process. No one wins every battle with the many and varied issues involving a surveillance system. But those who persevere have the best chance of creating a system that helps make their workplaces safer.

REFERENCES

1. Sorock GS, Smith GS, Reeve GR, Dement J, Stout N, Layne L, Pastula ST. Three perspectives on work-related injury surveillance systems. *Am J Ind Med* 1997; 32:116–128.

18

Health and Disability Insurance

ROBERT M. PARK

Employers with modern data systems and employee benefits programs can perform surveillance for occupational heath problems. Although work-related health problems involving medical treatment or lost time should be handled by workers' compensation, experience suggests a large burden of work-related illness is actually processed through medical insurance and disability insurance systems.[1–4] This results from failure to identify work-related problems. In addition, there are financial incentives such as delays in payments for both the affected worker and medical providers that occur with workers' compensation. Several projects undertaken by the United Auto Workers Union (UAW) with cooperation from the Chrysler Corporation (now DaimlerChrysler) and Blue Cross Blue Shield of Michigan shed light on the role of medical insurance in work-related illness and reveal possibilities and limitations for occupational disease surveillance. Likewise, the UAW and General Motors (GM) Corporation jointly investigated the utility of the GM Sickness and Accident benefit system by examining the experience over a 4-year period at a large automotive stamping and assembly complex in Lordstown, Ohio.

GROUP HEALTH INSURANCE

Methods

Define the Goals, Objectives, and Scope
A series of group health insurance projects examined:

- musculoskeletal outcomes to evaluate feasibility and compare findings with known ergonomic hazards in the automotive industry[3]
- heart disease at an assembly plant among skilled trades workers
- respiratory and cardiac outcomes in machining plants with a special focus on tool grinders (unpublished studies)

The first project served as a model and is presented in this chapter. Five specific musculoskeletal disorders (MSDs) that could result from repetitive trauma were studied at five automotive manufacturing plants located in Indianapolis, Indiana (foundry) and Detroit, Michigan (machining, trim [interior parts such as seats], stamping, and assembly plants).

Explicit identification of the Blue Cross-covered population was not possible. Thus, rate-based surveillance was not possible. However because insurance records identify many different medical conditions besides MSDs, it was possible to use a case-control study design. This study design uses odds ratios (see Chapter 5) to examine associations between claims for MSDs and types of production processes.

Gaining Support
The surveillance effort was initiated by union researchers. Blue Cross Blue Shield of Michigan supported this effort, perhaps motivated by interest in the cost burden of work-related diseases.

Case Definition and Data Collection
Through their collective bargaining contract, UAW Chrysler workers get medical insurance from Blue Cross Blue Shield for nonwork-related health problems involving hospitalization, surgery, and visits to doctors' offices. This is an indemnity type of health insurance where doctors and hospitals who treat UAW Chrysler

workers get reimbursed for medical services by submitting a bill. These bills are called claims by the group health insurance industry. (In contrast, in the workers' compensation insurance industry, medical bills, payments for temporary or permanent disability, and other benefits are collectively called a claim.)

Blue Cross claims for the entire Chrysler corporation were accessible because a nationwide claims processing network has been in place since mid-1984. Medical claim information included diagnostic codes based on the 9th Revision of the International Classification of Diseases[5] (ICD) and procedure codes based on the Current Procedural Technology (CPT-4).[6] Appendix A has a health insurance claim form of the type used in the study. Details of the prior medical history or the onset of the medical conditions under study were not available from insurance records.

Case Definition. Cases of musculoskeletal disease were identified among active union members over a 3.5-year period using the ICD- and CPT-codes on the insurance claims (Table 18.1). Claims were selected for about one hundred conditions thought to encompass most work-related episodes likely to be of interest together with a set of relatively common conditions thought unlikely to be work-related for use as controls. The predefined conditions together with appropriate diagnostic and procedure codes were compiled by several consulting physicians. Work-related traumatic musculoskeletal injuries were unlikely to be included, having been intercepted by the workers' compensation system.

The first available claim for a case was used to define the date of onset. This was a reasonable choice because 84% of MSD cases had all of their claims within 6 months of the first available claim. For controls—conditions thought not to be work-related—the onset date was set to a random year of a worker's tenure during the study period.

Work History and Other Data. The study used a work history database linked with the Blue Cross Blue Shield claims. Plant location and department assignments were available annually for all UAW employees of Chrysler after 1966 as were skill status and age. Information was either incomplete or unavailable for gender, race, and job classifications. Exposure categories were defined on broad process distinctions specific to plant type, based on department assignment. (Exposure categories did not reference job classifications.) Only departments performing repetitive production tasks were assumed to have ergonomic risk factors. Exposure was based on the most recent annual department assignment at onset. Real-time work history, available in virtually all personnel databases, could have provided a considerably enhanced level of detail. In this study, a secondary work history consisting of OSHA 200 log entries was also linked to claim information.

Confidentiality of claims information was preserved by having Blue Cross perform the record linkage to the work history file provided by the investigators. Each claim extract had appended to it a compact work history record (approximately 300 characters). The resulting file was stripped of identifiers except for an encrypted Social Security Number.

Analysis

Case-control studies were constructed with the work history–medical claims database (Box 18.1). Classification of cases and controls on exposure was performed by defining categories of interest, mapping departments to those categories (usually as unexposed/exposed) and, when required, calculating cumulative exposures over time.

Table 18.1 Medical Insurance in Surveillance: Musculoskeletal Outcomes Studied with Defining Diagnostic and Procedure Codes*

Condition	*Diagnostic Codes (ICD-9)*	*Procedure Codes (CPT-4)*
Carpal tunnel syndrome	354.0X	64721
Other upper extremity	354.1X,354.3X,726.30,726.33, 726.4X,727.03,727.05,727.2X, 840.XX,841.XX,842.XX	25005,25115,25116, 25295,26055,26440, 26445,26449
Rotator cuff syndrome	726.1X	
Cumulative trauma, neck	721.0X,721.1X,722.0X,722.4X, 722.71,722.91,723.XX,847.0X	22550,22552,22555,22 600,22615,62293, 6302X,6303X
Cumulative trauma, lower back	721.2X,721.3X,721.4X,722.1X, 722.5X,722.72,722.73,722.92, 722.93,724.XX,846.XX	22560,22561,22565, 22640,22655,22670, 22680,22700,22720

*ICD, International Classification of Diseases; CPT, Current Procedural Terminology.[6]
Source: Park et al., 1992.[1]

Box 18.1 The Case-Control Study Design: Two by Two Tables

In case-control studies, a rule is specified for identifying cases—individuals with some specific health condition—and also for selecting controls (or referents) who are individuals without the condition but who are otherwise very comparable to the cases on nonexposure risk factors.

A basic approach to analysis in a case-control study where individuals can be simply classified as exposed or not exposed is the two by two table, as follows:

Numbers of Case-Control Study Subjects

	Cases	Controls	Total
Exposed	a	b	n_{exp}
Unexposed	c	d	n_{unexp}
Total	n_{case}	n_{cntl}	N

where n_{case} is the number of cases, n_{cntl} is the number of controls, a is the number of cases classified as exposed, etc., and $N = a + b + c + d = n_{case} + n_{cntl} = n_{exp} + n_{unexp}$. A measure of association between being a case and exposure is called the odds ratio (OR): OR = $(a/c)/(b/d)$, where a/c is the odds that a case is an exposed individual, whereas b/d is the odds that a control is an exposed individual. In the absence of a true association between the exposure and the health condition, the odds ratio observed for study populations should fluctuate around 1.0. However, if exposed individuals are twice as likely to experience the condition, the odds ratios should center around 2.0.

From the musculoskeletal study in five Chrysler plants, here are the observed odds ratios separately for men and women for carpal tunnel syndrome (CTS) comparing the Trim/Chassis departments with unexposed workers in the assembly plant:

Men

	CTS Cases	Controls	Total
Trim/Chassis	38	290	328
Unexposed	10	108	118
Total	48	398	446

OR = 1.42

Women

	CTS Cases	Controls	Total
Trim/Chassis	22	68	90
Unexposed	1	15	16
Total	23	83	106

OR = 4.85

In this example, female workers in Trim/Chassis appeared to have higher risk than men (probably because of performing higher risk jobs) but the interpretation was complicated by (*1*) small numbers of unexposed cases (only one for women) and (*2*) possible confounding by age (the prevalence of CTS could depend on age and maybe ages differed across exposure groups so that the effect of exposure might really just be an effect of age).

Logistic regression models were fit on the entire 5-plant study population adjusting for age (two levels) and gender to identify plant exposure categories with statistically significant elevations in odds ratio (Box 18.2). These odds ratios represented the relative frequency (odds) that a study subject in a specific exposure category was a case versus a noncase, compared to the odds for subjects in unexposed or other categories found not to be elevated.

Box 18.2 Logistic Regression Models

The two by two table has limitations when there are multiple exposures of interest or confounding risk factors such as age and gender and especially when exposures are better described as continuous variables rather than all or none. One approach is to use statistical methods that can combine many two-by-two tables into a single analysis. Another statistical approach is to model the various effects using a method such as logistic regression. In this approach, the odds that an individual is a case is said to be a product of several factors, each representing one of the predictors under study:

$$p/(1 - p) = b_0 \,.\, b_1 \,.\, b_2 \,.\, b_3 \ldots = \exp(a_0 + a_1.X_1 + a_2.X_2 + a_3.X_3 + \ldots)$$

where p is the probability that an individual is a case, $p/(1 - p)$ is the *odds* of being a case (ratio of probabilities of being and not being a case), b_0 is the baseline odds, taking other effects into account, i.e., for the unexposed comparison group, and the other b_i are factors that modify the baseline odds related to exposures or other risk factors. For the purpose of mathematically estimating the b_i from the observed data, it is very convenient to express the model in terms of a sum of exponents, $a_0 + a_1.X_1 + a_2.X_2 + a_3.X_3 + \ldots$, where the a_i are coefficients to be estimated for the variables X_i which might be indicators of exposure or categories of age, gender etc. Logistic regression is a statistical procedure that picks a set of a_i that result in the best fitting model; the a_i produce the model that makes the actual data observed the most likely outcome for the class of models represented by a_i.

In the CTS analysis, the logistic regression model was applied to the entire 5-plant population, thus combining the unexposed groups from all plants to obtain a more stable background estimate of CTS prevalence. A general effect of age (greater than 40) across all plants was included and exposure effects from all five plants were tested for statistically significant associations. The procedure that estimates the a_i also allows hypothesis testing, that is each a_i can be tested to see if it contributes to model fit more than just by chance. If an a_i doesn't significantly improve fit, that predictor is excluded from the model. Thus individuals in an exposure group that doesn't improve model fit are added back into the unexposed comparison group. For example, in Table 18.2 the comparison group in the final model for CTS consisted of all men under age 40 in the five plants who were not exposed to Trim/Chassis or Spray Painting in the assembly plant, to Sewing in the Trim plant, etc.

Results

Over 3200 episodes of MSDs were identified. Associations were observed within specific process categories in all plants except the foundry, which had generally elevated rates (Table 18.2). For carpal tunnel syndrome, statistically significant odds ratios ranging 3 to 4 were observed in Trim/Chassis and Spray Paint departments of the assembly plant, in Sewing Operations at the trim plant, and among Large Press workers in the stamping plant. Other MSDs showed somewhat similar distributions of excess across plant process categories, with the assembly plant (trim/chassis), stamping plant (large press) and axle-machining plant (assembly) groups showing elevations in most MSD categories. Lower back problems were elevated with smaller odds ratios, ranging 1.5–1.7, but representing more attributable cases.

Table 18.2 Medical Insurance in Surveillance: Adjusted Odds Ratios and Attributable Cases for Selected Cumulative Trauma Conditions in Automotive Manufacturing Plants*

	Risk Factors	*Relative Risk*			*Attributable Cases*	
Plant Type	*Age, Gender, and Industrial Process*†	*No. of Exposed Cases*	*OR*‡	*95% CI*	*No. of Cases*	*95% CI*
		CARPAL TUNNEL SYNDROME				
	Age	—	1.1			
	Gender	—	2.3	1.6,3.3		
Assembly	Trim/chassis	60	3.1	2.1,4.6	41	31,47
	Spray paint	3	3.6	0.99,13.1	2	0,3
Trim	Sewing	21	2.0	1.1,3.6	10	2,15
Axle	Assembly	9	4.2	1.9,9.4	7	4,8
Stamping	Large press	29	2.9	1.8,4.7	19	13,22
		OTHER UPPER EXTREMITIES				
	Age	—	0.89			
	Gender	—	0.98			
Assembly	Trim/chassis	97	2.1	1.5,2.8	51	32,62
	Other paint	18	2.0	1.1,3.5	9	1,13
	Frame/body	26	1.9	1.1,3.0	12	2,17
Trim	Sewing	27	2.0	1.2,3.4	13	4,19
Foundry	All	29	5.6	3.3,9.5	24	20,26
Axle	Assembly	10	2.3	1.1,4.8	5	1,8
Stamping	Large press	55	2.2	1.5,3.3	30	18,38
	Assembly/finishing	26	1.6	1.0,2.7	9	0,16
	Small press	14	1.6	0.87,3.0	5	0,9
		ROTATOR CUFF SYNDROME				
	Age	—	2.1	1.5,2.9		
	Gender	—	1.1			
Assembly	Frame/body	13	2.0	1.1,3.8	6	1,9
	Trim/chassis	36	1.7	1.1,2.6	5	3,22
Trim	Sewing	23	2.5	1.4,4.5	14	6,18

Table 18.2 (Continued)

Plant Type	Risk Factors: Age, Gender, and Industrial Process†	Relative Risk: No. of Exposed Cases	Relative Risk: OR‡	Relative Risk: 95% CI	Attributable Cases: No. of Cases	Attributable Cases: 95% CI
		ROTATOR CUFF SYNDROME				
Stamping	Large press	39	3.3	2.1,5.1	27	20,31
	Assembly/finishing	19	2.1	1.2,3.7	10	3,14
		CUMULATIVE TRAUMA OF THE NECK				
	Age	—	1.4	1.2,1.7		
	Gender	—	1.1			
Assembly	Spray paint	10	2.3	1.0,5.1	5	0,8
	Other paint	41	2.1	1.4,3.2	21	12,28
	Trim/chassis	136	1.4	1.1,1.8	39	12,60
	Material	18	1.5	0.80,2.6	6	0,11
Trim	Sewing	75	2.1	1.5,3.1	39	25,51
Axle	Assembly	19	1.7	0.95,3.0	8	0,12
Stamping	Large press	100	2.0	1.5,2.6	50	33,61
		CUMULATIVE TRAUMA OF THE LOWER BACK				
	Age	—	1.3	1.1,1.6		
	Gender	—	1.1			
Assembly	Frame/body	93	1.5	1.1,2.1	31	8,48
	Other paint	62	1.5	1.0,2.2	20	0,34
	Trim/chassis	265	1.3	1.1,1.6	61	24,99
Trim	Sewing	123	1.7	1.2,3.2	50	20,84
Foundry	All	31	1.2	0.72,1.9	5	0,14
	Assembly	34	1.5	0.89,2.4	11	0,20
Stamping	Large press	186	1.7	1.4,2.2	76	53,101
	Small press	59	1.4	1.0,2.0	17	0,29

*OR, odds ratio; CI, confidence interval.

†Industrial process is based on worker's department assignment at first available insurance claim for condition under study, Age: 0 = (≤40), 1 = (>40); Gender: 0 = men, 1 = women.

‡By unconditional logistic regression; controls: selected conditions thought not work-related, evaluated at random year of worker tenure during study period.

Discussion

The experience from this study implies that systematic evaluations of acute or subacute health effects are very feasible. Priority issues in the automotive industry might include respiratory, neurological, musculoskeletal, or other concerns in welding, painting, assembly, or injection molding processes, for example. It is necessary that a large number of workers are exposed and routine administrative work histories are sufficient to distinguish relevant exposures. However, interplant variance, job rotation, exposure changes in response to adverse health effects, and limitations in the data sources pose potential methodological obstacles. The findings also imply that simplistic surveillance approaches, e.g., comparisons on current job, could easily miss important chronic disease associations.

Compared to other plants, the foundry population appeared to have substantially elevated risk for upper extremity (including CTS) disorders. Failure to identify specific foundry exposures with elevated risk may have resulted from widespread ergonomic hazards at the plant. However, this plant was the only non-Michigan plant studied and had an unexpectedly small number of control conditions for its size suggesting, as one possibility, a relative underutilization of health care for the control conditions. The absence of elevated odds ratios for MSDs of the back, neck, and shoulder was attributed to thorough workers' compensation activity by persons familiar with this foundry.

Although limited by crude exposure classification and subject to the severe assumption that work-related MSDs were absent in nonrepetitive, production-support departments, this study nevertheless identified attributable risk fractions among exposed workers (fractions of cases in excess of expected) ranging from 0.32 (lower back) to 0.68 (CTS), which were likely to be underestimates. The process associations were consistent with well-known hazards of assembly plants and represented plausible ergonomic hazards in other plants. A comparison with OSHA 200 log reporting from the study plants[3] revealed that many MSDs estimated to be work-related were not reported on OSHA logs. For all but the assembly plant, there was relatively little overlap between the two sources. Only 9% of medical insurance MSD cases also appeared on OSHA logs in the same time period.

Although this database offers a wealth of medical information linked with unbiased work history, as with any source of administrative data, there are concerns. Errors in the way diagnosis is coded on the medical claim is expected to produce misclassification that is *nondifferential.* That is, misclassification should be the same across exposure groups because it is most likely caused by financial or random factors. Workers' health coverage choices are possibly health status-related, although unlikely to depend on exposure history. An exception might be publicized problems (such as asbestos-related) for which some health care options may be more beneficial than others. The benefit package itself imposes limitations related to severity (routine doctor visits may not be covered). Other errors might be related to the specificity of coding. The absence of an onset date is a concern. The first claim in an episode for acute complaints such as for some musculoskeletal disorders is likely to be captured over a multiyear observation period. However, claims for chronic irreversible conditions such as cardiac or respiratory could have begun many years prior to observation.

Race, as a surrogate for socioeconomic status, a possible health services utilization indicator, and a marker for past exposure differences, is essential for meaningful interpretation. Skill status among exposed workers may be an important determinant of study feasibility for some exposures. For both acute and chronic conditions, medical claims for diagnostic tests interpreted as negative represent a potentially overwhelming false-positive threat, although observing an excess of diagnostic activity associated with an exposure may itself be a useful indicator of work-related morbidity.

Follow-up

Although sponsors of a comprehensive joint ergonomics program for the past 10 years, neither the company nor the union has advocated steps to utilize medical insurance records for routine identification of high-risk groups across the company or for assessing the efficacy of ergonomic interventions. In the course of designing a state-of-the-art integrated employee information system for the next century, Chrysler management declined to discuss surveillance design or epidemiological capabilities with jointly appointed outside occupational health experts or the union. Blue Cross Blue Shield of Michigan continued to cooperate on surveillance activities.

Conclusions

This study found that patterns of work-related MSDs were observable with a medical insurance record system using a minimalist exposure classification. Associations were consistent with known ergonomic risk factor distributions. A detailed work classification history over the period of study perhaps could have identified specific classes of high-risk jobs for priority ergonomics evaluation. In principle, time trends in attributable case rates could be assessed.

GROUP DISABILITY INSURANCE

A medical disability benefit or sick-leave system is another database available for surveillance at most large employers. Disability systems have a medical component for certifying leave and return-to-work. They differ in the details of eligibility (such as minimum time off work before the benefit can be claimed), documentation of the medical condition, and interactions with the workers' compensation system. Like medical insurance, there are incentives for employees with work-related conditions to be processed within the disability system contrary to the intent and procedures of workers' compensation. Thus, disability insurance records offers another large database for occupational disease surveillance, with the advantage that the information resides with the employer.

Methods

Define the Goals, Objectives, and Scope

Several health outcomes were of interest based on complaints of workers about chemical exposures and the presence of ergonomic risks. Workers employed at two assembly plants and a metal stamping plant in Lordstown, Ohio had a history of complaints associated with the vehicle painting operations. Respiratory problems and complaints consistent with multiple chemical sensitivity (MCS) were the chief concerns. In addition, musculoskeletal outcomes were of inherent interest. Cardiac outcomes were included for exploratory purposes. Because the population-at-risk was known (nearly 10,000 workers), it was possible to carry out rate-based surveillance.[4]

Gain Support

The UAW and General Motors Corporation (GM) jointly investigated the utility of the GM Sickness and Accident (S&A) benefit system by examining the experience over a 4-year period.

Data Inventory, Case Definition, and Data Set

The GM S&A system is managed by Metropolitan Life Insurance Company but the database is accessible to GM. United Auto Workers GM employees are eligible for an S&A leave benefit immediately when they have a disabling injury or hospitalization, or after 8 days of illness that does not result in hospitalization. Claims judged to be work-related within 2 weeks of onset are transferred to the workers' compensation system leaving no S&A record. Cases qualifying as work-related after 2 weeks are also transferred but an S&A record remains. The medical condition justifying S&A leave is coded (since 1989) using up to four ICD-9 diagnostic codes. Multiple consecutive claims are tied to an initial claim unless the period since termination of the last claim exceeds 3 months.

Case Definition. Cases of respiratory disease, asthma, heart disease, carpal tunnel syndrome, back disorders, and musculoskeletal disorders were defined by grouping individual ICD-9 codes (bottom of Table 18.3). Only the first occurrence of a specific medical condition was analyzed for an individual worker.

Work History. A work history from the GM personnel data system consisted of employee department and job classification assignments and periods of leave, which were coded for the reason for leaving. Exposure classification (exposed versus nonexposed) was based on current department as well as cumulative duration (years) in exposure categories. Additionally, worker follow-up was classified on whether the worker had been in their present assignment for fewer or more than 6 months.

Exposure categories were based on broad process distinctions and for relevance to respiratory health outcomes and possibly also to multiple chemical sensitivity issues. Work history files were consolidated to produce single records per worker and linked to similarly consolidated S&A files.

Analysis

Incidence rates of S&A claims were calculated for each exposure classification. These rates were also adjusted for age, gender, race, and skilled trade status using Poisson regression methods (Box 18.3). The reference category for rate ratios in the regression model was nonexposed, nonskilled, white men, aged 25–40 years with a current work assignment longer than 6 months.

Table 18.3 Outcomes and Numbers of Sickness and Accident Claims at Stamping and Assembly Plants 1989–1992*

	Lower Respiratory	*Upper Respiratory*	*Asthma*	*Heart Disease*	*CSS*	*Back*	*CTS*	*Upper Extremity*	*Neck*	*Shoulder*
Assembly Plants										
Total episodes	73	74	46	377	219	1057	214	593	463	153
Incident claims (No WC)†	57	61	31	294	198	651	176	376	324	111
Stamping Plant										
Total episodes	42	21	18	176	76	398	25	102	134	38
Incident claims (No WC)	30	17	12	124	69	235	19	75	98	29

* International Classification of Disease (ICD-9-CM) codes used to select claims (X: accept any character):
Lower respiratory (nonasthma): 491.X,492.X,496.,786.0X,786.2
Upper respiratory: 472.X,473.X,476.X,478.1,478.4,784.7
Asthma: 493.X
Heart disease: 410.X,411.X,412.,413.X,414.X,786.50
CSS, Chemical sensitivity syndromes: 300.0X,346.9,477.X,493.X,714.XX,780.XX,786.2
Back: 721.2,721.3,721.4X,722.1X,722.5X,722.72,722.73,722.92,722.93,724.XX,846.X,847.2,847.3,847.4,847.9
CTS, Carpal tunnel syndrome: 354.0
All upper extremity musculoskeletal: 353.0,354.X,443.0,726.3X,726.4,726.9X,727.03,727.04,727.05,727.2,727.4X
Neck: 721.0,721.1,722.0,722.4,722.71,722.91,723.X,847.0
Shoulder: 726.0,726.1X,726.2

†Sickness and Accident Claims without associated workers' compensation activity.

Box 18.3 Modeling Rates with Poisson Regression

When a well-defined population is under observation and specific events are being recorded, it is possible to calculate rates in various categories of experience, such as in age levels within exposure groups. Furthermore, when there are multiple risk factors, it is useful to model rates (using Poisson regression) just as odds of being a case was modeled using logistic regression. In Poisson regression, a rate (e.g., no. of incident cases per 100 person-years of observation) can be modeled as follows:

$$\text{Rate} = b_0 \,.\, b_1 \,.\, b_2 \,.\, b_3 \ldots = \exp(a_0 + a_1.X_1 + a_2.X_2 + a_3.X_3 + \ldots)$$

where b_0 is the baseline rate, taking other effects into account, i.e., for the unexposed comparison group, and the other b_i are factors (rate ratios) that modify the baseline rate related to exposures or other risk factors. As for logistic regression, it is convenient to express the model in terms of a sum of exponents, $a_0 + a_1.X_1 + a_2.X_2 + a_3.X_3 + \ldots$, where the a_i are coefficients that the Poisson regression procedure picks to produce the best fitting model.

For the model of lower respiratory disability rate (Model 1, Table 18.5) at a GM assembly plant, the background rate was estimated at 0.03 per 100 person-years among white nonskilled men age 25–40 and in last job assignment more than 6 months. Being in a last job assignment less than 6 months predicted a 2.5-fold increase in disability rate and being in Paint or Final Assembly for fewer than 6 months further increased the predicted rate by a factor of four.

Results

In the two assembly plants, the major exposure categories were Body, Hard Trim, and Chassis, each with more than 5000 person-years of observation. The smaller stamping plant contributed about 10 thousand person-years of observation. Over 4 years from all three plants there were 886 back problems, 87 lower respiratory problems, and 418 cardiac problems resulting in S&A claims with no apparent workers' compensation involvement (Table 18.3). Based on crude rates, respiratory, cardiac and back problems all appeared to be more frequent among short-tenure workers—those in their most recent assignment for fewer than 6 months—and exhibited elevations in several exposure categories (Table 18.4). Adjusted rates for lower respiratory complaints indicated possible trends with Paint and Final Assembly duration. Workers with short-tenure assignment in Paint had a fourfold elevation of claim rate for respiratory problems (rate ratio [RR] = 4.1, 95% CI = 1.48,11.3, p = 0.007) [Table 18.5]. Patterns of elevated risks were observed for upper respiratory, some cardiac, and most upper extremity MSD associations. Heart disease claims were elevated for long assignment tenure in Body (RR = 2.2, 95% CI = 1.29,3.67, p = 0.004) and short tenure in Final Assembly (RR = 2.48, 95% CI = 1.47,4.2, p = <0.001). In assembly plant Body, Hard Trim, and Chassis Departments, short-tenure workers had highly significant, fivefold elevated rates for all upper extremity musculoskeletal disability. An attempt to group medical outcomes to correspond to *multiple chemical sensitivity* was not particularly revealing although it did not negate the feasibility of such an approach.

Review of OSHA log entries during a 1-year period (1992) for the assembly plants identified no lost-time respiratory cases. For back problems, there were 70 log entries of which 27 were for workers who also had S&A claims, which was close to the estimated number of attributable cases from the regression analysis (N = 36), suggesting that most work-related back problems resulting in lost time were recorded on the log. In contrast, of the 38 lost-time OSHA log entries for all upper extremity musculoskeletal conditions in 1992, only 7 had corresponding S&A claims but 47 S&A upper extremity cases had been estimated to be work-related.

Discussion

This analysis of a routine administrative database identified work-related respiratory, musculoskeletal, and possibly cardiac medical conditions. The somewhat surprising observation of a short assignment tenure effect requires further investigation but implies that changes in worker job assignments introduce critical complexity into exposure–response relations. At the time of this study, virtually all workers had been employed at this facility more than 5 years and thus were not responding to a new employment experience. More than half of all work time occurred with fewer than 6 months in assignments. This churning of the work force could distribute high hazard jobs among many workers.

Mechanisms that could explain the tenure effect include: (*1*) some specific job assignments have hazardous chemical or physical exposures; workers tend to remove themselves from these jobs at first opportunity and few remain in these jobs for more than 6 months but during that time they are at high risk; (*2*) workers developing a work-related disability are sometimes able to change to another assignment, but not soon enough avoid a subsequent medical leave commencing in their

Table 18.4 Unadjusted Rates for Respiratory and Other Outcomes by Current Exposures and Tenure at the Assembly Plant (per 100 Person-Years)

	Current, Short Tenure			*Current, Long Tenure*		
Exposure Category	N	*Rate*	*95% CI**	N	*Rate*	*95% CI*
			Lower Respiratory			
Body	5	0.15	0.05–0.36	0	0.00	0.00–0.13
Paint	9	0.48	0.22–0.92	1	0.07	0.00–0.36
Hard trim	9	0.27	0.12–0.50	4	0.16	0.04–0.40
Soft trim	0	0.00	0.00–1.00	0	0.00	0.00–0.65
Chassis	9	0.28	0.13–0.53	3	0.11	0.02–0.31
Tooling	0	0.00	0.00–2.26	0	0.00	0.00–1.00
Maintenance skilled	1	0.14	0.00–0.76	4	0.28	0.08–0.72
Maintenance nonskilled	2	0.32	0.04–1.17	1	0.13	0.00–0.71
Material handling	1	0.12	0.00–0.66	2	0.27	0.03–0.97
Final	6	0.59	0.22–1.29	0	0.00	0.00–0.34
Quality control	0	0.00	0.00–3.33	0	0.00	0.00–1.24
Other	0	0.00	0.00–0.58	0	0.00	0.00–0.73
Total	42	0.26	0.19–0.36	15	0.10	0.06–0.17
			Heart Disease			
Body	35	1.09	0.76–1.51	25	1.13	0.73–1.67
Paint	25	1.36	0.88–2.01	13	0.85	0.45–1.46
Hard trim	37	1.11	0.78–1.53	19	0.74	0.45–1.16
Soft trim	1	0.34	0.01–1.86	0	0.00	0.00–0.65
Chassis	21	0.66	0.41–1.02	18	0.64	0.38–1.01
Tooling	2	1.57	0.19–5.65	3	1.02	0.21–2.99
Maintenance skilled	5	0.69	0.22–1.61	9	0.64	0.29–1.21
Maintenance nonskilled	13	2.17	1.15–3.71	10	1.30	0.63–2.39
Material handling	10	1.20	0.58–2.22	8	1.08	0.47–2.13
Final	23	2.33	1.48–3.50	9	1.02	0.47–1.94
Quality control	0	0.00	0.00–3.33	0	0.00	0.00–1.24
Other	6	1.17	0.43–2.56	2	0.49	0.06–1.78
Total	178	1.13	0.97–1.30	116	0.81	0.66–0.96
			Back			
Body	104	3.38	2.73–4.03	38	1.73	1.22–2.37
Paint	47	2.61	1.92–3.47	14	0.93	0.51–1.55
Hard trim	119	3.71	3.05–4.38	43	1.70	1.23–2.29
Soft trim	6	2.11	0.77–4.59	6	1.31	0.48–2.85
Chassis	97	3.22	2.58–3.86	53	1.91	1.39–2.42
Tooling	2	1.55	0.19–5.59	0	0.00	0.00–1.00
Maintenance skilled	13	1.83	0.97–3.13	17	1.22	0.71–1.95
Maintenance nonskilled	11	1.81	0.91–3.25	9	1.16	0.53–2.21
Material handling	15	1.84	1.03–3.04	11	1.49	0.75–2.67
Final	16	1.63	0.93–2.65	14	1.60	0.87–2.69
Quality control	1	1.14	0.03–6.31	2	0.83	0.10–3.01
Other	13	2.55	1.36–4.36	0	0.00	0.00–0.74
Total	444	2.92	2.65–3.19	207	1.46	1.26–1.66

CI, confidence interval.

Table 18.5 Adjusted Rate Ratios for Selected Disabilities at the Assembly Plant by Poisson Regression with Exposure: Current by Tenure

Risk Factors	*Rate Ratio*	*95% CI**	p
	1. LOWER RESPIRATORY†		
(Adj rate: 0.03)‡			
Short tenure	2.50	0.80–7.84	0.117
Paint: short	4.10	1.48–11.3	0.007
Paint: long	1.40	0.15–12.9	0.769
Hard trim: short	2.36	0.85–6.53	0.099
Hard trim: long	3.42	0.81–14.4	0.094
Chassis: short	2.49	0.90–6.89	0.079
Chassis: long	2.28	0.49–10.7	0.297
Material handling: short	0.95	0.11–7.83	0.958
Material handling: long	5.19	0.91–29.6	0.064
Final: short	4.25	1.38–13.2	0.012
	2. UPPER RESPIRATORY†		
(Adj rate: 0.18)‡			
Short tenure	1.11	0.49–2.55	0.798
Gender (0 = men, 1 = women)	1.67	0.81–3.43	0.166
Body: short	1.43	0.58–3.56	0.440
Body: long	2.16	0.81–5.79	0.125
Paint: short	2.55	1.03–6.33	0.043
Paint: long	1.37	0.37–5.04	0.634
Hard trim: short	1.86	0.81–4.29	0.145
Hard trim: long	0.27	0.03–2.10	0.210
	3. ASTHMA†		
(Adj rate: 0.06)‡			
Short tenure	0.56	0.12–2.61	0.460
Gender (0 = men, 1 = women)	4.33	1.93–9.70	0.001
Body: short	3.78	0.73–19.6	0.114
Hard trim: short	3.74	0.75–18.8	0.108
Chassis: short	5.09	1.05–24.6	0.043
Maintenance skilled: short	7.46	0.50–113.	0.147
	4. HEART DISEASE†		
(Adj rate: 0.18)‡			
Short tenure	1.34	0.85–2.09	0.206
Gender (0 = men, 1 = women)	0.94	0.60–1.47	0.784
Body: short	1.68	1.05–2.67	0.030
Body: long	2.17	1.29–3.67	0.004
Paint: short	1.86	1.11–3.09	0.018
Paint: long	1.50	0.79–2.87	0.217
Hard trim: short	1.59	1.00–2.51	0.048
Hard trim: long	1.35	0.76–2.39	0.305
Maintenance nonskilled: short	2.26	1.20–4.27	0.012
Maintenance nonskilled: long	1.75	0.86–3.57	0.125
Final: short	2.48	1.47–4.20	<0.001
Final: long	1.49	0.71–3.13	0.294
Other: short	1.83	0.77–4.33	0.172
	5. BACK PROBLEMS†		
(Adj rate: 1.33)‡			
Short tenure	1.78	1.32–2.40	<0.001
Body: short	1.51	1.15–1.99	0.003
Body: long	1.42	0.95–2.13	0.089

Table 18.5 (Continued)

Risk Factors	*Rate Ratio*	*95% CI**	p
	5. BACK PROBLEMS†		
Hard trim: short	1.59	1.22–2.08	<0.001
Hard trim: long	1.37	0.93–2.01	0.116
Chassis: short	1.43	1.08–1.89	0.012
Chassis: long	1.55	1.08–2.24	0.019
Other: short	1.09	0.61–1.94	0.777
6. ALL UPPER EXTREMITY CUMULATIVE TRAUMA DISORDERS†			
(Adj rate: 0.31)‡			
Short tenure	1.12	0.37–3.42	0.844
Body: short	5.34	2.13–13.4	<0.001
Body: long	3.33	1.48–7.49	0.004
Paint: short	3.72	1.43–9.70	0.007
Paint: long	2.20	0.88–5.50	0.092
Hard trim: short	5.97	2.40–14.8	<0.001
Hard trim: long	3.23	1.46–7.14	0.004
Soft trim: short	3.52	0.94–13.2	0.062
Soft trim: long	3.55	1.16–10.9	0.027
Chassis: short	4.63	1.84–11.6	0.001
Chassis: long	3.12	1.41–6.86	0.005
Maintenance skilled: short	7.72	0.96–62.2	0.055
Maintenance skilled: long	2.11	0.22–20.3	0.517
Material handling: short	1.71	0.46–6.36	0.427
Other: short	6.44	2.30–18.1	<0.001

*CI, confidence interval.

†Models adjusted for age, gender, race, and skilled trade status, unless too few cases.

‡Adjusted rate per 100 person years for unexposed (nonskilled, white men, aged 25–40 years and in assignment > 6 months; those not in any exposure category in model).

new job assignment (especially for ergonomic problems where the new job may also be stressful); most assignment changes resulted in no change in a worker's study exposure category; and (*3*) some job changes may occur for health reasons unrelated to workplace exposures; these high-risk individuals could exhibit a short-tenure effect but it should be independent of exposure category unless there are exposures contributing to or exacerbating their condition.

For each of the associations observed through surveillance, there were plausible sources for adverse health effects. Although the study was unable to draw specific conclusions regarding agents, it did point where investigation ought to follow and it allowed estimation of attributable fractions and hence population burdens.

Follow-up

Despite common concerns with painting in most auto assembly plants, there was no apparent interest on the part of the employer in using or developing further the findings from this study. Similarly, utilization of S&A based surveillance for ergonomics program implementation was not embraced. Extension of this approach to six other GM plants was recommended by a jointly appointed board of occupational health experts but has not yet been implemented (4 years later).

Conclusions

Unlike medical insurance, disability claims require a substantial threshold of severity. However, disability information is readily available and coverage is comprehensive, making it a surveillance tool of choice. It is not subject to the limitations of company medical visit reporting systems (which require a worker to seek company-provided medical care) or of workers' compensation systems (which require employer concurrence on work-relatedness). It has great potential for hypothesis testing in large populations.

REFERENCES

1. Park RM, Nelson NA, Silverstein MA, Mirer FE. Epidemiological surveillance using a Blue Cross medical claims data-base: meth-

ods development and pilot application to cumulative trauma disorders in five selected plants. Report to UAW/Chrysler National Joint Committee on Health and Safety, May 15, 1990. Unpublished.

2. Park RM, Nelson NA, Silverstein MA, Mirer FE. Use of medical insurance claims for surveillance of occupational disease. An analysis of cumulative trauma in the auto industry. *J Occup Med* 1992; 34:731–737.
3. Nelson NA, Park RM, Silverstein MA, Mirer FE. Cumulative Trauma Disorders of the hand and wrist in the auto industry. *Am J Public Health* 1992; 82:1550–1552.
4. Park RM, Krebs JM, Mirer FE. Occupational disease surveillance using disability insurance at an automotive stamping and assembly complex. *J Occup Environ Med* 1996; 38:1111–1123.
5. World Health Organization. *International Classification of Diseases. 9th Revision.* Geneva: World Health Organization,1978.
6. American Medical Association. *Current Procedural Terminology.* 4th ed. Chicago: American Medical Association, 1992.

19

Cancer Mortality Surveillance

MICHAEL A. SILVERSTEIN, NEIL A. MAIZLISH,
ROBERT M. PARK, AND FRANKLIN E. MIRER

This chapter describes union-based efforts to develop and use epidemiologic surveillance techniques as routine accessible tools in the day-to-day conduct of a health and safety program.

The United Automobile Workers International Union (UAW) represents 1.2 million workers in more than 2500 workplaces throughout the United States, Canada, and Puerto Rico. These workers face an enormous range of potential health hazards on jobs ranging from paint formulation to salt mining. Automobile manufacture, employing one-half of UAW members, is itself a collection of many distinctly different types of work.

The UAW has had an active health and safety program for many years, utilizing occupational health professionals and local union health and safety representatives to identify workplace hazards and to develop technical and political strategies for their control. Stimulated by intense membership concern with apparent excess cancer mortality in various workplaces, it became apparent that the health and safety program needed a new dimension—one which could evaluate patterns of illness, injury, and death that might not be apparent to even a skilled observer with the training to recognize known hazardous materials and conditions.

A practical system of epidemiologic triage was required so that threshold decisions about health and safety strategy could be made on firm grounds. For example, with several workplaces reporting apparent clusters of cancer deaths, a prompt choice among three courses of action is necessary: (*1*) a priority program to reduce worker exposure to known or likely hazards through engineering or other controls; (*2*) systematic research to explore suspected health effects supplemented with modest, interim protective measures; (*3*) reassurance to workers that work-related health problems have not been demonstrated and are unlikely to have occurred and that little additional action is needed. It is not reasonable to expect that any epidemiologic method can determine unequivocally which of these activities is correct for a given workplace. Moreover, many epidemiologic techniques are too slow and cumbersome to have short-term decision-making value in the workplace. However, it has been possible to adapt standard epidemiologic methods to serve as public health tools in the workplace so that quantitative data can be used in choosing among alternatives at a given workplace and in determining priorities among different locations according to relative urgency. One such method, addressing mortality, has been established in Michigan by making use of the state's computerized death registry. Three steps are involved:

- First, when a potential problem is identified, local and international union records are searched to produce a listing of names and Social Security numbers of persons at risk or known to have died. The full cohort of interest, all those who worked in the plant over a defined period, is not usually accessible or cannot be generated quickly. However, an inventory of available records (e.g., seniority lists, dues cards, application records, and sometimes death records) usually provides a fairly complete specification of those at risk. The fact that such a list might have gaps and sampling inconsistencies is not a deterrent in the triage process as long as there is reasonable certainty that major confounding and selection bias have been avoided. This can often be assured by using a subgroup for which nearly complete and unbiased ascertainment is possible, such as all those hourly employees with at least 10 years of credited pension service.

- Second, names and Social Security numbers on the list of deceased or at-risk persons are matched against computerized mortality files such as those obtained from the State of Michigan Department of Public Health. The Michigan files contain all in-state deaths since 1970 with underlying cause coded by the International Classification of Diseases (ICD) classification revision in effect at the year of death. As a useful but not essential adjunct, out-of-state deaths are identified by searches of Social Security Administration (SSA) records.
- Third, the resulting deaths identified, with underlying cause and demographic data, are used as input to the Monson program (with revisions) to generate standardized proportional mortality ratios (SPMR).[1]

As an example, we describe the course of a mortality investigation at a metal stamping plant where maintenance welders and millwrights were exposed to coal tar and welding emissions.

METHODS

Development of Study

The study site was a metal stamping plant located near Kalamazoo, Michigan. The plant, which began operations in 1966, has employed on average approximately 3000 UAW members. The plant operations have included metal stamping, spot welding, tool and die making, metal machining, and pattern making.

The Local Union became concerned in 1980 about a possible high number of cancer deaths among its members. The Local Union Health and Safety Representative began to compile a list of deceased members along with information about their causes of deaths and jobs, which he was able to abstract from information available at the plant. The UAW had not developed most of the epidemiologic tools described in this chapter. However, manual calculations of proportional mortality (see Chapter 5) were done and did not reveal excesses of cause-specific mortality or associations between mortality and specific work assignments.

By 1982, the number of known decedents was 58 and the UAW had developed the computerized capacity for PMR analysis.[1] Twenty-two cancer deaths among white men were observed, compared with eight expected based on national rates. The UAW decided to continue the investigation on a priority basis.

A site visit was conducted by International Union staff to gain insight into the nature of chemical exposures potentially associated with various jobs. It was observed that the floors in this plant consist of wood blocks that are set and protected with hot tar in an operation that closely resembles roof tarring. Further, employees reported that: (*1*) millwrights have been responsible for laying the floor tar and have been exposed to smoke and vapors from this work; (*2*) the millwrights at this plant also work closely with the maintenance welders who weld or flame cut floor-bolts at floor level where tar and wood blocks sometimes ignite and generate smoky emissions; (*3*) the wood blocks have been treated with wood preservatives, and have absorbed solvents and oil spills.

Historically, maintenance welding and floor tarring work had been done with a minimum of exhaust ventilation or respiratory protection. Routine quantitative measurements of these exposures had not been made, but in 1979, personal and area air samples taken by the employer revealed coal tar pitch volatiles in excess of 200 $\mu g/m^3$ TWA (8-hour time weighted average) with peak exposures much higher.

This additional information about the chemical environment prompted a decision to expand the mortality evaluation, and, simultaneously, to press for reduced exposure to tar emissions. The outcome of this more thorough review is presented below.

Study Group

The target population for the investigation was all deceased local union members ever employed at the stamping plant with a date of death between January 1, 1966 and December 31, 1982. Sources of data included local union lists of deceased workers, union pension records, and employer life insurance records. These sources routinely received reports of deaths or copies of death certificates of active workers and retirees. Additionally, the local union newsletter circulation file was used to identify those who left employment before vesting or left employment with vested pension rights but might have died before retirement. This file was matched to SSA records of deceased persons using Social Security number as the match key.

Ninety-eight deaths were reported from all sources, including eight uniquely ascertained from SSA records. Our judgement is that the group of 98 decedents is a virtually complete ascertainment of hourly workers who died while active or retired. A small group of deaths among workers on deferred vested status, or those terminated with less than 10 years seniority may have been missed.

Death certificates (or, in two cases, abstracted records) were obtained for 94 of the 98 deaths (96%). For 62 of the Michigan deaths, the underlying cause of death was determined by record-linkage of the death file to the computerized Michigan death certificate registry using Social Security numbers for matching. The remaining deaths, which included out-of-state deaths and those that occurred before the state computerized its files in 1970, were coded by the investigators according to the 8th Revision of the ICD.

The final study group included 91 white men, 2 African-American men, and 1 white woman.

Work Histories

Personnel records were obtained from the employer for 83 of the study group. Following site visits, discussions with the plant management and the Local Union, and a review of the available industrial hygiene reports, decedents were grouped into two exposure categories: (*1*) maintenance welders and millwrights, (*2*) all other job classifications. This classification scheme was based on the judgement that maintenance welders and millwrights are most likely to be exposed to coal tar pitch volatiles.

Preplant employment as a welder or millwright was coded on an ever–never basis.

Statistical Analyses

Standardized proportional mortality ratios, standardized for age, sex, race, and calendar year of death, and case-control studies within the decedent population were carried out. Standardized proportional mortality ratios for 54 causes of death were calculated for the 91 white men using deaths of white men from the United States as the reference population, updated to include National Center for Health Statistics (NCHS) mortality data through 1978. Standardized proportional mortality ratios were also calculated for restricted subgroups based on employment duration and prior history as a welder or millwright.

Case-control analyses were designed to examine the relationship between cancer mortality and specific jobs, which share, among other things, hot tar operations or welding or flame cutting near tarred surfaces. Cancer cases were defined by underlying cause of death and grouped according to specific ICD codes: lung, 162; digestive organs, 150–159; leukemia, 204–207; and all malignant neoplasms, 140–209. Controls were defined as all noncancer deaths. Nonmalignant respiratory disease deaths were therefore included as controls in the case-control analysis of lung cancer, a decision made to conserve statistical power despite the possibility that shared etiologic factors might result in a reduced ability to demonstrate associations. Exposed was defined as ever-maintenance welder or ever-millwright and nonexposed were all other job classifications.

Cases and controls were drawn from the 83 decedents with complete work histories: 80 white men, 2 African-American men, and 1 white woman. Tobacco smoking patterns were not known. Stratification was used to control potential confounding by age and preplant occupation.

RESULTS

The observed number of malignant neoplasms (Table 19.1) is nearly twice that expected (PMR = 28/14.82 = 1.89, 95% C.I. = 1.36, 2.62). Twofold to fivefold excess proportional mortality from cancer of the diges-

Table 19.1 Standardized Proportional Mortality, White Men, 1966–1982, by Cause of Death*

Cause of Death	*Observed*	*Expected*	*SPMR*	*95% CL*
All cancers	28	14.82	1.89	1.36–2.62
Cancer of lung	10	4.75	2.20	1.18–3.76
Cancer of digestive organs	7	3.10	2.26	1.12–4.56
Cancer of testis	2	0.41	4.85	—
Leukemia	4	0.94	4.28	1.75–10.45
All cardiovascular	22	26.79	0.82	0.59–1.13
All nonmalignant lung	0	2.96	0.00	—
All nonmalignant digestive	2	5.22	0.25	—
All external causes	37	33.28	1.11	0.90–1.38
All other	2	7.92	0.25	—
Total	91	91		

Source: Silverstein et al.[9]

*SPMR, standardized proportional mortality ratio; CL, confidence limit.

Table 19.2 Characteristics of Cases and Controls

Characteristic	*Cases* N = 27	*Controls* N = 56
Age at death, mean (SD)*	47 (11)	38 (12)
Age at death, range	22–66	20–68
Employment duration, mean years (SD)	9 (5)	7 (4)
Former welders/millwrights, *N* (%)	7 (26)	4 (7)

*SD, Standard deviation.
Source: Silverstein et al.[9]

Table 19.4 Association Between Cancer at Two Sites and Welder/Millwright Classification, Age 40+ at Death*

	Lung Cancer		*All Digestive Cancers*	
Classification	*Cases*	*Controls*	*Cases*	*Controls*
Welder/Millwright	3	1	3	1
Other	5	22	4	22
OR (95% CL)	13.2 (1.1–154.9)		16.5 (1.1–162.2)	

*OR, odds ratio; CL, confidence limit.
Source: Silverstein et al.[9]

tive organs, lung cancer, and leukemia accounts for most of the overall cancer excess. Essentially the same excesses were found in subgroups with 5 or more years seniority or with no preplant employment as a welder or millwright (data not shown).

Table 19.2 gives age and occupational characteristics of cases and controls. On average, both cancer cases and controls died at relatively young ages and short employment duration. Because cases tended to be older at death than controls and were overrepresented by former welders or millwrights, case-control analyses were stratified by age and preplant occupation.

Table 19.3 presents age-stratified odds ratios for the association between cancer mortality and employment as maintenance welders and millwrights. Odds ratios of more than 10 were found overall and in the 40+ age strata. Similarly, the odds ratios for lung cancer and digestive organ cancers were highly elevated in the 40+ strata (Table 19.4).

Table 19.5 presents cancer mortality and welder or millwright classification stratifying on prior welding or millwright occupation. Although odds ratios were elevated in both strata, the odds ratio was much greater and statistically more stable in the subgroup without prior welding or millwright occupations. Odds ratios for lung cancer or cancer of digestive organs followed a similar pattern.

Further case-control analysis simultaneously stratifying on age, employment duration, and prior occupation also revealed similar associations between cancer mortality and millwright or maintenance welder classification, but statistical power was diminished as expected with decreasing cell sizes.

DISCUSSION

A union-based epidemiologic surveillance program proved to be an effective and efficient guide to occupational health action in a metal stamping plant. Use of a mortality surveillance system designed for routine use revealed excess proportional mortality from cancer of the lung, digestive organs, and leukemia. This lent credibility to local union concerns and led the union to assign this situation very high priority for further investigation and to undertake interim efforts to control suspect chemical exposures. Subsequent case-control analysis documented associations between mortality from lung cancer and digestive cancers and work as maintenance welders or millwrights that involved probable exposure to coal tar pitch volatiles and welding emissions. This served as the basis for a further decision to seek more vigorous in-plant environmental intervention.

Following discussions of the findings, the employer took short-term source and area samples during tarring, which showed substantial levels of six specific polycyclic aromatic hydrocarbons with known carcinogenic or mutagenic properties (Table 19.6). Agreement was reached to take steps to reduce exposures of maintenance welders and millwrights to the suspect emissions. The employer purchased new, thermostatically controlled electric tar pots and agreed to obtain 20 portable ventilation units, construct several exhausted welding booths, purchase additional respirators, and initiate a search for noncoal tar floor coating substitutes. A series of educational meetings was held

Table 19.3 Association Between All Cancer Mortality and Welder/Millwright Classification*

	All Ages		*<40 Years*		*40+ Years*	
Classification	*Cases*	*Controls*	*Cases*	*Controls*	*Cases*	*Controls*
Welder/Millwright	10	3	2	2	8	1
Other	17	53	5	31	12	22
OR (95% CL)	10.4 (2.6–42.2)		6.2 (0.7–54.6)		14.7 (0.6–131.6)	

*OR, odds ratio; CL, confidence limit.
Source: Silverstein et al.[9]

Table 19.5 Association Between All Cancer Mortality and Job Classification by Prior Job Occupation*

	Former Welders or Millwrights		*Not Former Welders or Millwrights*	
Classification	*Cases*	*Controls*	*Cases*	*Controls*
Welder/Millwright	6	2	4	1
Other	1	2	16	51
OR (95% CL)	6.0 (0.3–107.0)		12.8 (1.3–122.5)	

*OR, odds ratio; CL, confidence limit.
Source: Silverstein et al.[9]

with more than 200 affected workers in the plant. At the urging of the union, the employer sent a bulletin to its other locations asking that floor tarring operations be evaluated and steps be taken either to reduce emissions or to find substitute materials. Follow-up area air sampling during tarring was conducted after the installation of the new tar pots and showed large reductions in airborne polycyclic aromatic hydrocarbons (Table 19.6).

We believe that these findings are sufficiently plausible to warrant an alert to the public health community of a probable, but previously unrecognized hazard. The observed associations are large; feasible control measures are readily available; and the findings have considerable biologic plausibility.[2–4] Exposure of roofers and coke oven workers to coal tar pitch volatiles containing polycyclic aromatic hydrocarbons has been associated with excess multiple-site cancer mortality.[5,6] The group experiencing excess mortality in this study uses similar materials under analogous conditions,[4] and exposures to specific mutagens and carcinogens have been documented (Table 19.6).

Efforts should be made to replicate the findings at other locations where similar work is done in such a manner that the combined and independent effects of coal tar and welding exposures can be evaluated. In our judgment, concurrent efforts should be made to notify representatives in potentially affected workplaces

Table 19.6 Concentration (mg/m^3) in Short-Term Air Samples of Six Polycyclic Hydrocarbons at a Stamping Plant Before and After Installation of New Tar Pots

	Vent	*Floor*	
Chemical	*Old Tar Pot*	*Old Tar Pot*	*New Tar Pot*
Phenanthrene	500	50	0.88
Anthracene	200	20	0.55
Acridine	10	1	ND*
Pyrene	100	10	0.16
Chrysene	20	1	ND
Benz(a)pyrene	1	ND	ND

*Non detectable.
Source: Silverstein et al.[9]

of the possible hazards (Right to Know) and to encourage actions to reduce worker exposures to chemical emissions during floor tarring operations as the prudent response to the surveillance findings.

Mortality surveillance enabled the union to distinguish this plant from others which, on the surface, might have appeared equally urgent. For example, in another location there were 54 cancer deaths in 260 total deaths among white men. More than 60 malignancies were expected. There were slight excesses of brain and lymphopoietic cancers but a review of the job histories revealed no clustering and did not direct attention to any specific chemical exposures. The mortality file has been updated yearly but no other intervention has been made.

Some advocates for an increased role for epidemiology in public health have argued that quantitative decision rules can be used by occupational and environmental health policy makers as virtually sufficient and complete guides to action. Dinman and Sussman, for example, have proposed, "a set of criteria for acceptance or rejection of any published study."[7] These criteria would be used to generate a summary score for studies in a given area of policy concern. The score would be used to ensure that "the public decision-making process optimally utilizes data in an organized, systematic fashion."[7] Although they concede that "scaled systems should not be considered as providing a mechanical method for arriving at judgment without thought,"[7] their single example seems to rely upon just such mechanical application. Dinman and Sussman calculate scores for five published studies of mortality among workers exposed to coal tar pitch volatiles in several industries. The average of the scores for two studies of workers exposed to emissions in the early stages of coal tar production (i.e., coke oven workers) and for three studies of workers exposed to emissions after coal tar has been further distilled to produce coal tar pitch (i.e., roofers and aluminum reduction workers). They direct attention to an information/option nonogram, a scale along which the epidemiologic scores correspond to policy options. Use of this scale directs that strong action is necessary to restrict manufacture in coke ovens and that the appropriate measures for roofers and aluminum reduction workers fall somewhere between no action and simple educational measures. Dinman and Sussman conclude that "fumes of pitch are indeed less carcinogenic than tar if, indeed, they are carcinogenic at all."[7]

Lanes and Poole have critiqued the Dinman and Sussman scheme and conclude that, with respect to their coal tar and coal pitch assessment, "It is difficult to imagine a less secure evaluative foundation for such strong and sweeping statements about causality."[8] We echo their critical judgment, sharing the belief that the fault not lies with the specific scoring system but with the very notion that public health decisions can be reduced to any set of epidemiologic rules and that the "formulation is best left to epidemiologists."[7]

Our concern with such reductionist systems is that even the most rigorous are essentially deceptive. Their apparent objectivity invariably masks a set of value judgments every bit as politically charged as those expressed by the most rhetorical of lay policy makers. The statistical concepts upon which scientific decision rules are based are inherently judgmental. For example, the choice of a statistically significant level expresses the willingness of the investigator to risk a conclusion that might be falsely positive. At a level of $p = 0.05$ the investigator is willing to conclude that a finding is significant unless there is less than a 5% chance of being wrong. This embodies a value judgment about the level of certainty necessary for action, one which is more stringently conservative than we apply to most decisions of daily living.

Although we advocate the increased input of quantitative epidemiologic science in workplace health and safety programs, we caution against the tendency to substitute numbers for balanced decision making that incorporates judgments and openly acknowledges differences in values.

The UAW has articulated its approach in this regard as follows:

> "We must work with what we have before us, not what we hope to learn after 5 more years of studies. We face today the growing likelihood that substantial numbers of metalworkers have been exposed to cancer hazards on the job for years. If only a fraction of the reports are eventually substantiated, we still face a public health problem of major dimension. If we wait for the final reports before deciding to warn workers of the possible risks, and before taking protective actions, we will lose years of opportunity . . ."
>
> "This means that in many situations we must take presumptive action. We have grown up believing 'innocent until proven guilty' is the essence of justice. But the workplace is not a court room and chemicals have no constitutional rights. Giving a carcinogen freedom to roam through the plant during its lengthy trial is far more dangerous than letting an accused burglar free on bail."[10]

ACKNOWLEDGMENTS

This work would not have been done without the efforts and determination of Jack Kelly and Roger Snell of UAW Local Union 488, Kalamazoo, Michigan. This research was supported, in part, by NIOSH Contract #210-81-5104. Some of these data were originally presented at the American Public Health Association Annual Meeting, Dallas, November 7, 1983.

A version of this chapter was previously published in the *American Journal of American Health* and has been used with permission.

REFERENCES

1. Monson R. Analysis of relative survival and proportional mortality. *Comput Biomed Res* 1974; 7:325–332.
2. Lindstedt G, Sollengerg J. Polycyclic aromatic hydrocarbons in the occupational environment. *Scand J Work Environ Health* 1982; 8:1–19.
3. Bingham E, Trosset R, Warshawsky D. Carcinogenic potential of petroleum hydrocarbons-a critical review. *J Environ Pathol Toxicol* 1980; 3:483–563.
4. Cooke M, Dennis A, Fisher D, eds. *Polyaromatic Hydrocarbons, 6th International Symposium.* Columbus, OH: Battelle Press, 1982.
5. Redmond C et al. Long term-mortality study of steelworkers: VI. Mortality from malignant neoplasms among coke oven workers. *J Occup Med* 1972; 14:53–61.
6. Hammond C et al. Inhalation of benzpyrene in man. *Ann NY Acad Sci* 1976; 271:116–124.
7. Dinman B, Sussman N. Uncertainty, risk and the role of epidemiology in public policy development. *J Occup Med* 1983; 25:511–516.
8. Lanes S, Poole C. Truth in packaging?: the unwrapping of epidemiologic research. *J Occup Med* 1984; 26:571–574.
9. Silverstein MA, Maizlish NA, Park R, Mirer FE. Mortality among workers exposed to coal tar pitch volatiles and welding fumes at a stamping plant. *Am J Public Health* 1985; 75:1283–1287.
10. Fraser D. Problems and challenges facing occupational medicine in the new decade from labor's viewpoint. Presented at American Occupational Health Conference, Detroit, MI, 4/22/1980.

20

Fatal Injury Surveillance

E. LYNN JENKINS

In the United States, an average of 16 workers die every day from injuries sustained on the job. This represents 16 workers who will not return home, 16 families who will mourn the loss of a loved one. For those of us in occupational safety and health, these deaths must be our guideposts for prevention. Information must be compiled on each of these deaths and examined both individually (in order to identify ways to prevent similar incidents in the future) and collectively (in order to identify patterns and trends of particular kinds of incidents).

Indeed, fatal injury surveillance data allow the description of the nature and magnitude of the occupational injury problem, the identification of potential risk factors, the generation of hypotheses for further research, and the setting of research and prevention priorities. Ongoing surveillance systems also enable the monitoring of trends over time and offer the potential to evaluate prevention efforts. In-depth investigations of workplace fatal injuries identified through surveillance systems allow additional analysis of the circumstances of incidents.

METHODS

Define Goals, Objectives, and Scope

For fatal occupational injuries, the goal of the surveillance system should be a complete census of all cases. That is, any fatality of a worker while engaged in work-related activities should be included in the system. Particular attention should be given to developing a system that includes everyone irrespective of the industry of employment, the size of the establishment, coverage by workers' compensation or other insurance system, or cause of death. (Motor vehicle related deaths and homicides have sometimes been regarded as nonoccupational events or inappropriate for inclusion in an occupational fatal injury surveillance system resulting in gross undercounting of deaths). A system might be focused on a single state, province, or other administrative district or on a collection of such units.

In the 1980s in the United States, the National Institute for Occupational Safety and Health (NIOSH) launched the National Traumatic Occupational Fatalities (NTOF) surveillance system. Information in the NTOF surveillance system is taken directly from death certificates; a death certificate is filed by local authorities for every death that occurs in their jurisdiction (see Data Collection below). To gather data for the system, NIOSH collects and automates death certificates from the 52 vital statistics reporting units (the 50 States, New York City, and the District of Columbia) for workers 16 years of age or older for whom an external cause of death (International Classification of Diseases, 9th Revision, codes E800–E999)[1] was noted, and for whom the certifier entered a positive response to the "Injury at Work?" item on the certificate.

In the early 1990s the U.S. Bureau of Labor Statistics (BLS) initiated the Census of Fatal Occupational Injuries (CFOI) system. The CFOI uses "diverse state and federal data sources to identify, verify, and profile fatal work injuries. Information about each workplace fatality is obtained by cross-referencing source documents, such as death certificates, workers' compensation records, and reports to federal and state agencies."[2]

Gaining Support

Because the NTOF system is based on data collected by states, NIOSH staff developed collaborative relationships with state vital statistics agencies. This includes not only staff interaction for the purpose of data collection, but also interaction with the professional association representing state vital registrars—the National Association for Public Health Statistics and Information Systems. Some states require review and approval of the NTOF methodology by an Institutional Review Board or other body; all states participate in the NTOF system. The CFOI system is based on a collaborative relationship between BLS and a designated office or staff in each state. The BLS provides training, software, and other support to state personnel who participate in the system; as with NTOF, all states participate in the CFOI system.

Multidisciplinary Team

A successful fatal injury surveillance system requires the input and expertise of a diverse group of professionals. In the case of both NTOF and CFOI, medical examiners and coroners who complete death certificates must recognize and record the work-relatedness of a case and the state must then have the ability to separate these cases from other cases of injury death. CFOI also relies on the diligence of the staff working in other administrative systems (e.g., workers' compensation) to complete and submit data. Once data have been collected, they must be appropriately coded and electronically stored, requiring the expertise of nosologists and computer programmers. The expertise of a diverse range of occupational safety and health professionals including epidemiologists, statisticians, engineers, physicians, nurses, and others is required to analyze and interpret the findings of fatal injury surveillance data in order to achieve the ultimate impact—the prevention of work-related injury deaths. These analyses must then be disseminated to workers, employers, labor unions, safety and health professionals, advocates, and others, requiring the knowledge and skills of health communication experts.

Data Collection

In the United States, the timing and other requirements relevant to the filing of death certificates by local authorities varies by state, but a death certificate must be filed on every fatality occurring in the United States, regardless of the residency status of the decedent. Although exact statutory language varies by state, a medical examiner or coroner is required to complete the death certificate in the case of an unexpected death, including both intentional and unintentional injuries. There is an item on the U.S. Standard Certificate of Death (Appendix A) that prompts the certifier to indicate whether the injury occurred at work.[3] For the NTOF system, NIOSH requests each of the 52 vital statistics units to, on an annual basis, review their mortality files for any cases that meet the three inclusion criteria (age 16 years or older, external cause of death, and "Injury at Work?" = "Yes"). NIOSH then automates and codes these data and maintains a master file that contains no personal identifiers. Per agreements with the states, the NTOF data have not been made a public use data set; any requests for case-specific information are referred back to the state agencies, and NIOSH analyzes the NTOF data in response to requests from researchers and the public, releasing data in aggregate or tabular form or both.

In the CFOI system, state CFOI personnel routinely review fatality data from a variety of sources and once a case has been verified by at least two sources, it is coded and entered into a database. The data for a given calendar year are submitted to BLS by the states by June of the subsequent year. The BLS then compiles the national dataset. A research file is released by BLS that does not include personal identifiers, location (state of occurrence), source document information, or information on alcohol or drug testing results.[4]

Protocol for Follow-up

Detailed follow-up investigation of cases identified through a surveillance system can provide quite useful information for preventing similar incidents in the future. One methodology for doing this is the NIOSH Fatality Assessment and Control Evaluation (FACE) program. FACE is a research program whose goal is to identify and investigate work situations at high risk for injury and then formulate and disseminate prevention strategies to those who can intervene in the workplace. The FACE program currently has two components:

1. The NIOSH in-house FACE program began in 1982. Participating states voluntarily notify NIOSH of traumatic occupational fatalities resulting from targeted causes of death that have included deaths in confined spaces, electrocutions, machine-related deaths, fatal falls from elevation, and fatalities in the logging industry. FACE is currently targeting investigations of deaths associated with machinery, deaths of youths under 18 years of age, and street and highway construction work zone fatalities.

2. The NIOSH state-based FACE program began in 1989. Currently, 15 state health departments have cooperative agreements with NIOSH for conducting surveillance, targeted investigations, and prevention activities at the state level using the FACE model.[5]

During on-site investigations, FACE investigators collect facts and data on: type of industry; number of employees; company safety program; the victim's age, sex, occupation; the working environment; the tasks the victim was performing; the tools or equipment the victim was using; the energy exchange resulting in fatal injury; and the role of management in controlling how these factors interact.[5] Specifically, this information is put into the context of what was happening just before, at the time of, and right after the fatal injury. This follows Haddon's matrix[6] for looking at injury events in order to identify various points for prevention action. The FACE model has also been applied to all deaths occurring in a single occupation; all line-of-duty deaths of fire fighters in the United States are currently investigated by NIOSH. Again, the goal of such follow-up investigations is to identify risk factors and develop strategies to prevent similar incidents from occurring in the future.

Code and Enter Data

The NTOF and CFOI data both contain variables useful for describing the characteristics of victims as well as injury circumstances—including demographic, employment, and cause of death variables. In addition to coded data, the NTOF system includes narrative text from the death certificate for industry, occupation, causes of death, and injury description. In addition to coded variables, CFOI maintains a detailed narrative description of the fatal injury event that can be up to 300 characters long. The value of having narrative data available for analysis of fatal occupational injuries cannot be overstated. Narrative data allow description of events at a greater level of detail than is possible with coded data alone and allows description of problems perhaps not previously recognized or well-described.[7]

Data on occupation and industry are coded in both NTOF and CFOI according to standardized coding schemes consistent with employment and other economic data that make it possible to calculate fatality rates for specific industry and occupation groups. For industry, the Standard Industrial Classification (SIC) manual[8] is used, whereas for occupation, the U.S. Bureau of the Census codes[9] are used. The NTOF uses the International Classification of Diseases, 9th Revision[1] to code cause of death. The CFOI cases are coded using the Occupational Injury and Illness Classification (OIIC) Manual,[10] which includes codes for the nature of injury (e.g., fracture), body part injured (e.g., leg), source of the injury (e.g., ground or working surface), and event or exposure (e.g., fall from ladder).

Analysis and Interpretation

Both NIOSH and BLS routinely analyze and publish data on fatal occupational injury deaths. These include annual summaries as well as analysis of: trends over time; nature and magnitude of deaths in particular occupations or industries (e.g., agriculture, construction, or truck drivers); particular causes of death or events (e.g., workplace homicides or motor vehicle crashes); and fatalities among special populations of workers (e.g., youth under age 18, women, or self-employed persons). These analyses focus on identifying risk factors, generating hypotheses for further research, and targeting prevention efforts.

Interventions

Fatal injury surveillance in the United States has identified industries and occupations at high risk and has suggested potential interventions for reducing those risks. Over the course of the decade from 1980 to 1989, fatal occupational injury rates declined 37%, with decreases seen in virtually every demographic and employment sector.[11] The reasons for these declines are not discernible from surveillance data alone, but are without a doubt multifactorial in nature including changes in workplace safety regulations, education and training efforts, as well as changes to the design of tools and equipment.[12]

Dissemination

The National Institute for Occupational Safety and Health has in recent years devoted considerable effort to disseminating information from fatal injury surveillance systems to those who can intervene in the workplace and reduce the risk of fatal occupational injuries. For example, information on the risk factors and related prevention strategies for fatal workplace injuries among youth under age 18 was disseminated to all high school principals in the United States. The information was mailed to them in the spring so they could distribute to school-age youth as they were looking for summer jobs. Another example is the targeted dissemination of information on workplace homicides to groups at high risk, including taxicab drivers, retail workers, and law enforcement professionals.

RESULTS

From 1980 to 1994, NTOF documented a total of 88,622 workers who died from work-related injuries.[13] As seen in Figure 20.1, the annual total number of

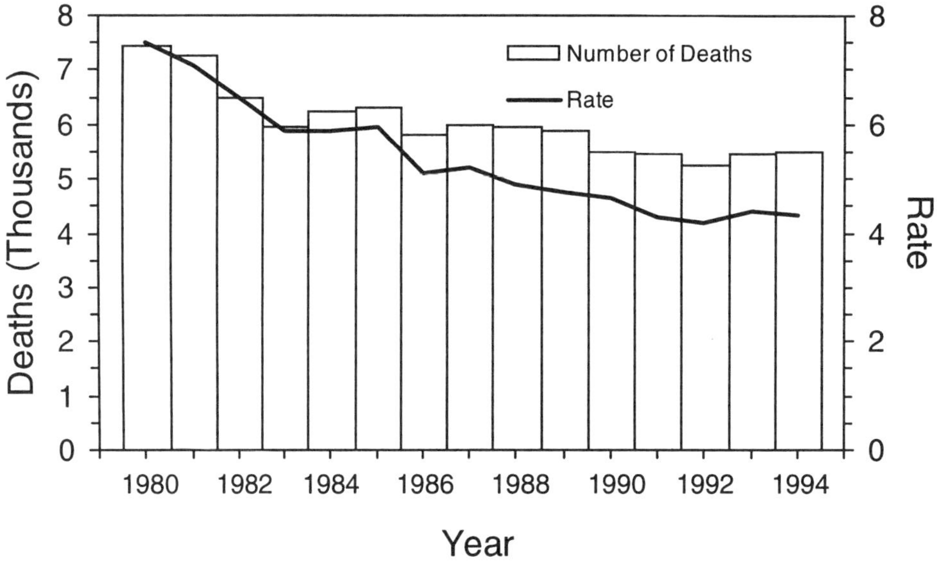

Figure 20.1 Number and rate (per 100,000 workers) of occupational injury deaths by year—United States, 1980–1994 (Centers for Disease Control).[13]

deaths and crude death rates decreased from 7405 (7.5 per 100,000 workers) in 1980 to 5406 (4.4 per 100,000 workers) in 1994.[13] Motor vehicle-related deaths were the leading cause of occupational injury death, accounting for 23% of the deaths over the 15-year period. In 1990, homicides surpassed machine-related deaths to become the second leading cause of work-related injury deaths in the United States (Fig. 20.2) Industries with the highest death rates per 100,000 workers were mining (30.5), agriculture/forestry/fishing (20.5), and construction (15.5).[13]

The CFOI data for 1998 indicate that 6026 workers died from injuries sustained in the workplace.[2] This was the lowest number of fatalities recorded since CFOI began collecting data in 1992. Work-related homicides and deaths to workers from being struck by falling objects or caught in running machinery fell in comparison to 1997, whereas fatalities in highway crashes,

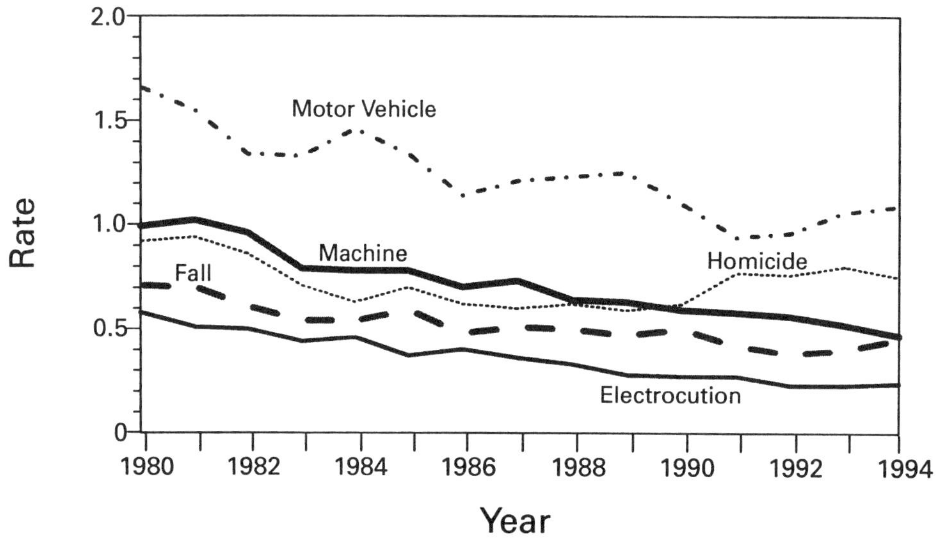

Figure 20.2 Rates (per 100,000 workers) for leading causes of occupational injury deaths, by cause and year—United States, 1980–1994. The category of motor-vehicle-related deaths includes crashes occurring on or off the road way, pedestrians struck by motor vehicles, noncollision incidences (e.g., falls from buses or cars), incidents involving off-road motor vehicles (e.g., snowmobiles and all-terrain motor vehicles) and incidents involving other road vehicles (e.g., bicycles) (Centers for Disease Control).[13]

Table 20.1 Fatal Occupational Injuries by Event or Exposure, 1993–1998

	Fatalities			
	1993–1997	*1997†*	*1998*	
*Event or Exposure**	*Average*	N	N	%
Total	6335	6238	6026	100
Transportation incidents	2611	2605	2630	44
Highway	1334	1393	1431	24
Collision between vehicles, mobile equipment	652	640	701	12
Moving in same direction	109	103	118	2
Moving in opposite directions, oncoming	234	230	271	4
Moving in intersection	132	142	142	2
Vehicle struck stationary object or equipment	249	282	306	5
Noncollision	360	387	373	6
Jackknifed or overturned—no collision	267	298	300	5
Nonhighway (farm, industrial premises)	388	377	384	6
Overturned	214	216	216	4
Aircraft	315	261	223	4
Worker struck by a vehicle	373	367	413	7
Water vehicle	106	109	112	2
Railway	83	93	60	1
Assaults and violent acts	1241	1111	960	16
Homicides	995	860	709	12
Shooting	810	708	569	9
Stabbing	75	73	61	1
Other, including bombing	110	79	79	1
Self-inflicted injuries	215	216	223	4
Contact with objects and equipment	1005	1035	941	16
Struck by object	573	579	517	9
Struck by falling object	369	384	317	5
Struck by flying object	65	54	58	1
Caught in or compressed by equipment or objects	290	320	266	4
Caught in running equipment or machinery	53	189	129	2
Caught in or crushed in collapsing materials	124	118	140	2
Falls	668	716	702	12
Fall to lower level	591	653	623	10
Fall from ladder	94	116	111	2
Fall from roof	139	154	156	3
Fall from scaffold	83	87	97	2
Fall on same level	52	44	51	1
Exposure to harmful substances or environments	586	554	572	9
Contact with electric current	320	298	334	6
Contact with overhead powerlines	128	138	153	3
Contact with temperature extremes	43	40	46	1
Exposure to caustic, noxious, or allergenic substances	120	123	104	2
Inhalation of substance	70	59	48	1
Oxygen deficiency	101	90	87	1
Drowning, submersion	80	72	75	1
Fires and explosions	199	196	205	3
Other events or exposures‡	26	21	16	—

Totals for major categories may include subcategories not shown separately. Percentages may not add to totals because of rounding. Dashes indicate less than 0.5 percent or data that are not available or that do not meet publication criteria.

*Based on the 1992 Bureau of Labor Statistics (BLS) Occupational Injury and Illness Classification Structure.[10]

†The BLS news release issued Aug. 12, 1998, reported a total of 6218 fatal work injuries for calendar year 1997.[2] Since then, an additional 20 job-related fatalities were identified, bringing the total job-related fatality count for 1997 to 6238.

‡Includes the category "Bodily reaction and exertion."

Source: Bureau of Labor Statistics.[2]

from being struck by vehicles, and from contact with overhead powerlines were at their highest levels during the 7-year period for which CFOI data exist.[2] Table 20.1 shows the distribution of fatal occupational injuries by event or exposure for the period 1993 to 1997 as well as the individual data years, 1997 and 1998; highway crashes, homicides, and falls accounted for the largest number of fatal occupational injuries.[2]

DISCUSSION AND EVALUATION

In the United States, fatal injury surveillance has improved dramatically in the last two decades with the development of the NIOSH NTOF system and the BLS CFOI system. Both systems are passive, relying on records gathered for other purposes to identify cases and provide information on the decedents and the circumstances of the workplace injury fatality.

Limitations

Despite the great progress, there remain limitations in the surveillance of fatal occupational injuries in the United States. For NTOF, which relies solely on information from death certificates, the two primary issues are: (*1*) death certificates capture only 67%–90% of all fatal occupational injuries,[14] and (*2*) medical examiners and coroners differ in their interpretation of on-the-job for the purpose of completing death certificates.[15] While CFOI overcomes these limitations to a certain extent through the use of multiple sources of data, there are likely still cases of fatal occupational injury that are not captured by the system, either because they were not recognized as work-related, were not reported through any of the administrative systems that CFOI uses to identify cases, or both.

Efforts to improve the quality of data include the development of standardized guidelines for the completion of the "Injury at Work" item on the death certificate[14] that have been published and disseminated through state vital registrars and professional organizations to medical examiners and coroners across the United States.

Future work on fatal injury surveillance in the United States will identify data gaps and explore alternative strategies for obtaining data on hard to reach populations such as migrant and seasonal workers. This may include using nontraditional sources of data as has been done in the past for particular occupational safety and health issues. For example, information on work-related violence has been gleaned from such nontraditional sources of data as criminal justice or victimization surveys when a mechanism exists to identify cases that are work-related. To the extent that all sources of injury and illness data can incorporate a designation of work-relatedness, occupational safety and health surveillance will be enhanced greatly.

ACKNOWLEDGMENTS

The author acknowledges the assistance of Suzanne Marsh and numerous other NIOSH injury surveillance staff as well as Herb Linn for their assistance in pulling together information and graphics for inclusion in this chapter.

REFERENCES

1. World Health Organization. *International Classification of Diseases: Manual on the International Statistical Classification of Diseases, Injuries, and Causes of Death, 9th* Revision. Geneva: Switzerland, 1977.
2. Bureau of Labor Statistics. *National Census of Fatal Occupational Injuries, 1998.* BLS NEWS, USDL 99-208. Washington, DC, August 4, 1999.
3. National Center for Health Statistics. *U.S. Standard Certificate of Death.* Accessed on the Internet on 11/29/99 at http://www.cdc.gov/nchs/data/std-dcrt.pdf.
4. Austin C. An evaluation of the census of fatal occupational injuries as a system for surveillance. *Compensation and Working Conditions.* Bureau of Labor Statistics, May 1995.
5. National Institute for Occupational Safety and Health. *NIOSH Fatality Assessment and Control Evaluation (FACE) Program Brochure.* Morgantown, WV: National Institute for Occupational Safety and Health, 1999.
6. Haddon W Jr. The changing approach to the epidemiology, prevention, and amelioration of trauma: The transition to approaches etiologically rather than descriptively based. *Am J Public Health* 1968; 58:1431–1438.
7. Jenkins EL, Hard DL. Implications for the Use of E-Codes of the International Classification of Diseases and Narrative Data in Identifying Tractor-Related Deaths in Agriculture, United States, 1980–1986. *Scand J Work Environ Health* 1992; 18 Suppl 2:49–50.
8. Office of Management and Budget. *Standard Industrial Classification Manual.* Washington, DC: U.S. Government Printing Office, 1987.
9. U.S. Department of Commerce, Bureau of the Census. *1990 Census of Population: Alphabetic Index of Industries and Occupations.* Publication 1990CPH-R-3.
10. Bureau of Labor Statistics. *Occupational Injury and Illness Classification Manual.* December 1992. Available on the internet at http://stats.bls.gov:80/oshoiics.htm (Accessed 11/29/99).
11. Stout NA, Jenkins EL, Pizatella TJ. Occupational injury mortality rates in the United States: changes from 1980 to 1989. *Am J Public Health* 1996; 86:73–77.
12. Centers for Disease Control. Improvements in workplace safety—United States, 1900–1999. *MMWR* 1999; 48:461–469.
13. Centers for Disease Control. Fatal occupational injuries—United States, 1980–1994. *MMWR* 1998; 47:297–302.
14. Jenkins EL, Kisner SM, Fosbroke DE et al. *Fatal Injuries to Workers in the United States, 1980–1989: A Decade of Surveillance.* National Profile. DHHS (NIOSH) Publication No. 93-108. August 1993.
15. Runyan CW, Loomis D, Butts J. Practices of county medical examiners in classifying deaths as on the job. *J Occup Environ Med* 1994; 36:36–41.

21

Exposure Surveillance for Chemical and Physical Hazards

ANTHONY D. LAMONTAGNE, A. JAMES RUTTENBER, AND DAVID H. WEGMAN

Surveillance systems can focus on hazards, health outcomes, or both. Traditionally, public health or epidemiologic surveillance has focused primarily on health outcomes, although it also includes hazard surveillance.[1–5] Hazard surveillance encompasses all health and safety hazards, including chemical, physical, ergonomic, safety, and psychosocial.[1,6–9] Hazard surveillance focuses on the source of the problem rather than the health event. Thus, being closer to the problem, it has the greatest potential for prevention. For a variety of historical, technological, and other reasons, hazard surveillance is much less developed than health surveillance.[1,10–12] Hazard surveillance is the most compelling, yet least investigated approach to surveillance. However, it is a priority area in the National Occupational Research Agenda[10] of the National Institute for Occupational Safety and Health (NIOSH), which recently included the development of exposure and hazard surveillance systems as one of its strategic goals for the year 2002.[13]

This chapter presents an overview of hazard surveillance, focusing on industrial hygiene exposure surveillance at the employer or worksite level. The first section presents the principles of exposure surveillance, and the second illustrates the application of these principles in the development and piloting of an exposure surveillance system for workers engaged in the cleanup of a former nuclear weapons site.

EXPOSURE SURVEILLANCE PRINCIPLES AND OPPORTUNITIES

Need for Improved Employer-Level Exposure Surveillance Methodologies

Thousands of industrial hygiene exposure measurements are made in U.S. workplaces each day. These include time-weighted average samples from personal breathing zones or specific work areas, and measurements made with direct-reading instruments or colorimetric tubes. In most cases, these measurements are compared with occupational exposure limits, stored for administrative or legal purposes, and never used again.[14,15] Within companies, these data could be used to manage and prioritize health and safety efforts more efficiently and to improve worker protections. Outside of these companies, these data may be used for research and policy development.[16–18] This presents a challenge to develop exposure surveillance systems at the worksite level that provide for efficient data capture; electronic storage, management, and analysis; and timely application of findings to preventive efforts.

Occupational exposure surveillance is the on-going collection, management, analysis of aggregate exposure data, and the application of findings to guide workplace prevention.[3,6,19] Exposure surveillance can be performed at many levels: within a department or section of a company (e.g., by the company itself),[20] on a companywide basis (e.g., single or multisite, national or multinational company),[21] on an industrywide basis (by a trade association, labor union, branch of military service),[22] or by broad geographic levels, such as region or nation (e.g., by a government entity).[23]

Surveillance is most useful for prevention when analyses are tailored to specific audiences. For example, company occupational health and safety (OHS) staff might examine summary measures of various exposures over time to look for trends that indicate a need for intervention. Exposure profiles for the agent of concern could then be grouped by job tasks or job titles within the company. Such analyses would provide information to directly guide exposure assessment activities (for OHS staff), exposure control efforts (for workers and OHS staff), and medical surveillance interventions (for occupational medicine providers). Feedback that is timely and specific for preventive efforts would be aided by ongoing surveillance at the plant or organizational level. This is where the connection between exposure and application of findings are the closest in both space and time.

State of Exposure Surveillance Efforts in Industry

Efficient exposure surveillance first requires that appropriate exposure data are collected, accessible in electronic databases, and analyzed. We recently performed a literature review and Internet survey of three prominent industrial hygiene E-mail lists to assess the state of exposure databases and surveillance efforts in industry.[12] Our findings suggested that relatively few organizations currently use electronic exposure database systems. The systems most commonly in use emphasize documentation, information management, and data sharing, principally for medical surveillance. Despite the continuing improvement of electronic information systems to support exposure surveillance,[24–25] our review suggests that most users of electronic systems are not likely to perform systematic aggregate analyses with feedback to primary prevention at the plant level. The need for improved capabilities for aggregate analysis and graphical presentation of data appears to be common among existing data systems.

Thus, there is a large unmet need for exposure surveillance at the workplace level. Existing exposure databases have been conceived primarily to meet the needs of regulators, policy makers, researchers, and others external to the organizations generating the majority of the exposure data.[1,8,26–30]

Recent Exposure Database and Surveillance Developments

Interest in improving the electronic accessibility and utilization of occupational exposure data has grown steadily since the late 1980's.[9,11,31–33] In 1994, the first conference devoted to occupational exposure databases reviewed the state of the art, published a comprehensive proceedings document,[14] and developed working groups to follow up recommendations.[34,35]

The Joint American Conference of Governmental Industrial Hygienists-American Industrial Hygiene Association (ACGIH-AIHA) Task Group on Occupational Exposure Databases published a 1996 report detailing the specifications of an ideal database containing 134 elements that would comprehensively describe measurements of chemical and noise exposures together with accompanying circumstances.[17] The goal was to allow various anticipated users to pick and choose relevant subsets of the 134 elements (83 were designated as key or essential elements), while preserving the possibility of pooling data sets comprised of varying, but similarly coded, sets of elements into a national data bank.

More recently, the European Working Group on Exposure Registers reviewed the scientific literature on exposure databases and surveyed the experience of its 10 members to produce a European Proposal for Core Information.[36] This group concluded that one of the most important impediments to the implementation of exposure database systems is the lack of consensus about what is termed the core information regarding exposures. This group defined core information as the minimum set of data elements needed for interpretation of the data and which should form the basis of workplace exposure databases on chemical agents. They identified 34 core elements to support efficient storage, retrieval, and transfer of data between users, as well as pooling into large data sets. Coding schemes were recommended for some of these elements, but many are narrative or free text and thus are not amenable to efficient grouped or aggregate analysis.

More recent database advances have been in developing standardized data element definitions, coding, and large database design in industrial hygiene.[14,17,33,36,37] Additional efforts are being made to improve the standardization of principles and practices of exposure assessment. This will improve general assessment, sampling strategies, and the application of exposure data to preventive efforts.[38,39]

At the same time, the broader occupational and environmental health community has taken steps to improve the theory and practice of public health surveillance, and, in particular, to move from the surveillance of disease, disability, and death to the surveillance of exposures, risk factors, and intervention efforts.[1,10,11,40,41] These recent developments provide a unique opportunity to link improvements in exposure databases, industrial hygiene practice, and public health surveillance, and to create practical and sound exposure surveillance systems that will be useful at the organizational level and above.

Merging the Strengths of Industrial Hygiene and Public Health Surveillance

Industrial hygiene, or occupational exposure assessment and control, has been described as a stepwise, cyclical process of characterizing a hazard, conducting additional evaluation as necessary, interpreting findings, and applying findings to achieve exposure control.[38,39,42,43] Both the overlap and differences between the practices of industrial hygiene and exposure surveillance are noteworthy. Most notably, the exposure assessment cycle contains the same core elements as public health surveillance.[40,44] Both consist of the repeated collection and analysis of data, with the purpose of applying findings to prevention and control efforts. The principal differences are the additional steps of electronic data entry or capture, data management and quality control, aggregate (or grouped statistical) analysis, and interpretation of aggregate analyses.

Other differences include the scale and unit of observation. Industrial hygiene exposure evaluations tend to address one defined job, group of jobs, or work process at a time. This usually includes, but is not restricted to localized worker groups with similar exposures (e.g., a worksite, or a department within a company). In contrast, surveillance has traditionally been applied to human populations at the state, regional, or other population level,[40,44] even when it is focused on a specific group such as asbestos workers. Interestingly, worksite- or company-level efforts, though prominent in the exposure assessment cycle and industrial hygiene literature, are rarely considered in the surveillance literature. Despite the similarities of strategies and goals, these two disciplines are largely separate.

From the public health surveillance perspective, the development of exposure surveillance has been overshadowed by the historical emphasis on health outcomes over risk factors, the lack of easily adaptable information infrastructures for exposure data, the incomplete understanding of exposure–disease relationships, the lack of public sources of exposure data, and the recent arrival of exposure assessment as a developed subdiscipline of epidemiology.[1,8,10,18] Worksite–based industrial hygienists continuously generate precise, documented, and interpretable exposure data required to implement exposure surveillance systems. In addition, data collected by professional industrial hygienists include the highest hazard priorities in a given worksite—another advantage of the use of industrial hygiene data in surveillance systems.

In summary, while in principle industrial hygiene and public health surveillance overlap considerably, in practice they have evolved with very different emphases. However, strengths of industrial hygiene and public health surveillance are complementary (Table 21.1). Expanded hazard surveillance at the worksite level is needed as well as improved data management and aggregate analysis in standard industrial hygiene practice. A unique opportunity exists to integrate these related fields to improve exposure databases, industrial hygiene practices, and exposure surveillance systems.

Exposure Surveillance as a Complement to Medical and Epidemiologic Surveillance

To practicing OHS professionals, medical surveillance is probably a more familiar term than exposure surveillance. Medical and epidemiologic surveillance in the workplace focus on assessing and controlling the human health effects of hazardous exposures.[2,40] However, their limitations underscore the need for including hazard or exposure surveillance. Health surveillance is by definition secondary prevention: it does not detect adverse events until after disease occurs. The development of biomarkers of exposure and new methods to detect subclinical effects of disease expand the potential of medical surveillance and its close cousin: bio-monitoring.[45,46] Nevertheless, health surveillance methods using biomarkers are currently available for only a small proportion of hazardous exposures and health effects. Even where such methods are available, diseases with long latency, such as cancers and other chronic diseases, are poorly captured through work-

Table 21.1 Complementary Characteristics of Industrial Hygiene and Public Health Surveillance

	Typical Unit of Observation	*Typical Employer*	*Electronic Data Management*	*Aggregate Data Analysis*
Industrial hygiene	Job, work process, or workplace	Company	Weak	Weak
Public health surveillance	State, regional, or larger population	Government	Strong	Strong

place surveillance programs.[47,48] Most importantly, detection of work-associated health events does not necessarily identify the exposure or exposures associated with the health outcome. In principle, detection of an occupational illness (or sentinel event) should be followed by industrial hygiene investigation and intervention, thus preventing further exposure to the affected worker and his or her coworkers.[49] Even when conscientiously practiced by occupational medicine providers, a variety of social, economic, and other factors limit the likelihood that recommended exposure control interventions occur.[50]

Hazard surveillance offers many benefits that complement and expand upon those provided by health surveillance.[7,8,51] Hazards are usually known, are easier to measure than illness and disease outcomes, and occur with higher frequency than disease events. This provides greater opportunities to detect exposures and implement control measures.[52,53]

Conclusions and Next Steps

Recent developments in industrial hygiene and public health surveillance suggest that a focus of surveillance activities at the workplace level provides new opportunities to improve worker health. Widespread implementation of exposure data systems will be more likely by meeting the needs of data generators[54] (employers, workplaces, workers) and demonstrating the utility of surveillance at the workplace level. This, in turn, will make possible broader-scale data systems for researchers, policy-makers, and other external data users. Expanded communication and collaboration among end users and developers, as well as among various occupational health subdisciplines is needed (e.g., industrial hygiene, surveillance, medicine, epidemiology, and toxicology) to achieve this goal.

DEVELOPMENT AND PILOTING OF AN EXPOSURE DATABASE AND SURVEILLANCE SYSTEM

This section provides a case study in the application of the principles and strategies outlined above to the development and piloting of an exposure surveillance system for Department of Energy (DOE) cleanup operations at the Rocky Flats Environmental Technology Site (RFETS). This work was conducted as a NIOSH-funded applied research project based on a partnership between independent occupational safety and health (OSH) researchers and practicing OSH professionals. The goal was to integrate scientific with real world perspectives to create a system that is theoretically sound and practical.

After a brief description of the project site, this section outlines the steps required in the development of an exposure surveillance system at a workplace. These are: gaining organizational support; determining the purpose and scope of the system; defining database elements and how to code them; integrating exposures to facilitate analyses; planning efficient analysis strategies; reporting capabilities; and communication strategies that promote the use of surveillance findings for prevention. We describe general background and the specific choices we made for our system. Readers can get insights for the development of similar systems in their own workplaces based on in-house solutions or commercially available industrial hygiene database software. More details are included in the references.[12,20,55]

Project Site Description

The DOE's RFETS is a former nuclear weapons plant that is now being cleaned up. From 1952–1989, RFETS produced plutonium trigger components for thermonuclear weapons, including the fabrication of beryllium and other parts. Potential exposures during cleanup include radiation, hazardous chemicals, and safety hazards.[56]

The RFETS is currently operated by one integrating contractor that directs four principal first-tier contractors as well as numerous smaller subcontractors. When the project began in 1995, we identified only one RFETS contractor that stored its industrial hygiene data in an electronic form. However, this contractor did not analyze the data, provide it to medical screening providers, nor actively use the data for other preventive applications. This is consistent with our review of practices in general industry.[12]

In 1996, we developed a partnership with a first-tier cleanup contractor at RFETS that had been previously using a hard copy industrial hygiene record keeping system. The system presented below was developed from scratch in collaboration with the industrial hygiene staff of this contractor. In brief, an integrated exposure database and surveillance system was developed and piloted over a 2-year period, as described in detail below.

Gaining Organizational Support

Organizational support is the ultimate determinant of the continuing use of any exposure database or surveillance system. As others have found,[36] the near-term needs and perspectives of those that generate exposure data must be emphasized. Support is essential from at least two organizational levels: those who authorize time and resources (usually upper management), and the OSH and related staff who are the end users. Upper management—those who authorize time and other resources—can be motivated by the need for protection of worker health, but may be more responsive to demonstrable system payback (e.g., will the system save money or reduce liabilities?).[16]

Short-term gains in record keeping efficiency, accountability, data accessibility, and quality control can be realized from the first step of implementing an electronic database system. Longer-term benefits are based on the ability to analyze and apply the data, and can result in more substantial benefits. Examples include: justifying and documenting reduced sampling—and associated expenses—for a suspected hazard, and demonstrating the effectiveness of a less costly intervention over a more expensive one in addressing a specific exposure concern. Exposure surveillance also provides a means for setting and assessing internally or externally specified performance measurements.[36] In DOE and other contracting, achieving prenegotiated OSH performance objectives is often tied directly to financial incentives.

For OSH staff, support for a system will be given if it meets their needs and improves their efficiency and effectiveness. Involvement of OSH staff is crucial to the development of sustainable systems. Convenience, simplicity, economy, and day-to-day utility must be considered. For example, a system that uses off-the-shelf software and automates required reporting (e.g., generates exposure summary reports for employees) will save OSH staff time and will help justify data entry and management efforts in the short term.

We developed our database system in collaboration with contractor OSH staff and management at RFETS. To minimize system implementation costs, we used Microsoft Access® for data entry and management, and associated Microsoft Office® applications for some analysis and reporting options.[57]

Finally, regulatory requirements can also play an important role in longer-term organizational support. Department of Energy requirements, such as the new requirement for sitewide electronic reporting of beryllium exposure data at RFETS and other sites,[58,59] are being passed down through multiple contractor levels. This improves the likelihood of broader implementation of exposure databases and surveillance systems. Such requirements may stimulate contractors to plan for and include database and surveillance costs in the bidding process without fear of decreasing their competitiveness.

Determining the Goals and Scope of the System

The broad goals of an exposure database and surveillance system for DOE cleanup operations were outlined by investigators in the proposal stage. These were to:

1. integrate occupational health research expertise with OSH practice to develop a user-friendly system that is based on sound surveillance principles and meets day-to-day OSH needs
2. emphasize the identification of exposure intervention priorities or sentinel exposure events to improve the protection of cleanup worker health
3. improve the capture and accessibility of cleanup worker exposure data to support both current and future uses

Although improvements are also needed in radiological exposure and safety hazard surveillance, we have focused the scope of our efforts on industrial hygiene exposures because this has been identified as a priority OSH area for improvement in the DOE complex.[60] Our strategy has been to work with individual contractors and other employers, believing that what is gained in terms of concrete and practical insights at the worksite level would offset a broader-based, less contact-intensive approach. We believe that the system we have developed is for the most part generalizable to other contractors and to DOE cleanup in general.

Database Elements and Coding

Working with contractor hygienists, we defined 29 core database elements that are electronically entered into our system (Table 21.2). While a greater percentage of ACGIH's 83 core elements would be desirable, the consensus between the contractor and our team was that electronic capture of this many elements would not be sustainable. Some elements can have multiple entries for a single sample (e.g., agents analyzed). In total, 38 or more elements per record are generated through automatically filled and calculated fields. To facilitate efficient data entry, analysis, and reporting, only numeric and coded elements are entered (with the exception of employee names). Coding was developed using the ACGIH-AIHA,[17] European,[37] and other guidelines. To meet RFETS needs, some variation from recommended coding was required. Review of original hard copy data sheets will be required for retrieval of narrative and other data, such as a detailed description of the work activity that was performed while the sample was collected. Although software packages for the analysis of narrative data are rapidly evolving and have been used to identify potential determinants in occupational injury surveillance systems,[61] narrative data entry and analysis are labor-intensive and require specialized training. This could be considered as a later system refinement.

Fields for industry identification (e.g., descriptive information, SIC codes) and geographic locators can be

Table 21.2 Rocky Flats Environmental Technology Site Exposure Database Elements and Coding*

Elements	*Description and Coding*
SAMPLE NUMBER GROUP (PART OF MAIN RECORD FORM)	
Entered	
Sample number	13-character numeric
Outside location	Cargo container, outside operational unit, outside (e.g., trench), trailer, valve vault, or other
Room number	Number within building, 4 character alphanumeric
Report ID	Links sets of samples to aid hygienist in generating reports, 3-character numeric
Automatically Generated	
Building number	Embedded in sample number (first three characters)
Sample date	Embedded in sample number (4th through 9th characters)
Hygienist name	Embedded in sample number as hygienist unique identifier (10th and 11th characters)
Sequence number	Sequence of sample on given date by identified hygienist (12th and 13th characters of sample number)
Survey number	Couples hygienist ID, with calendar year (from sample number), and report ID, 7-character numeric (enables generation of unique report identifier)
EMPLOYEE ID GROUP (PART OF MAIN FORM)	
Entered	
Employee ID number	Unique identifier designated by company
Social Security number	
Employee last name	Text field
Employee first name	Text field
Middle initial	Text field
Job classification	Pull-down list of generic job titles developed in consultation with contractors
Automatically Generated	
After employee ID or SS number entered once, will auto-fill all employee ID fields except Job classification (which may change) upon entry of a unique identifier	
EXPOSURE MODIFIER GROUP (PART OF MAIN FORM)	
Entered	
Type of work area	Indoor, outdoor, confined space, other, or unknown
Engineering controls	Yes or no (user enters this field or categorical field below)
Engineering controls	Charcoal drum filter, enclosure, glove box, HEPA vacuum, local exhaust, permacon
Respiratory protection	Yes or no (user enters this field or categorical field below)
Respiratory protection	None, half mask, full face mask, full face mask & airline, PAPR, supplied air with helmet or hood, supplied air garment, other
Respiratory canister	None, acid gas, charcoal, mercury, HEPA, combination HEPA and acid gas, combination HEPA, charcoal and acid gas, combination HEPA and charcoal, other
Eye/face	None, safety glasses, face shield, chemical goggles, full-face respirator, supplied air garment hood, welding helmet, welding goggles, UV lenses, laser goggles, other
Hearing	None, ear plugs, muffs, other
Hand/arm	None, impermeable gloves, permeable gloves, other
Whole body	White coveralls, blue company coveralls, smock, acid suit, PVS rain suit, Tyvek coverall, Saranex coated Tyvek coverall, supplied air garment, surgical greens, apron, other
SAMPLING GROUP (PART OF MAIN FORM)	
Entered	
Sample type	Breathing zone, area, source, blank, spike
Reason for sample	Initial characterization, periodic check, employee concern, emergency or spill, suspected high exposure, other, or unknown
Consecutive samples	One of a set of multiple partial-period samples? Yes or no
Sampling time	In minutes
Average flow rate	In liters/minute
Automatically Generated	
Measured volume	Product of sampling time and average flow rate

Table 21.2 (Continued)

Elements	*Description and Coding*
SAMPLE RESULTS SUB-FORM (≥ 1 PER SAMPLE NUMBER OR MAIN FORM)	
Entered	
Contaminant	Pull-down list based on OSHA Z Tables and previously entered contaminant names
Lab result units	Mg, mcg, or fibers/square mm
Below LOD	Yes or no, below Limit of Detection
Lab result	Results from laboratory analysis
Automatically Generated	
TWA units	Mg/cubic meter, ppm, or fibers/cc
TWA	Measured quantity divided by sample volume
8-Hour TWA	TWA normalized to 8 hours, assuming zero exposure for nonsampled time
WORK DESCRIPTOR SUB-FORM (≥ 1 PER SAMPLE NUMBER OR MAIN FORM)	
Entered	
Work package number	Unique identifier of short-term (weeks to months) specific work activity (similar to a work order number)
Work descriptor code	Two-tiered (work type and task group or task) hierarchy including 33 alpha-numerically coded selections
Task duration	Estimated percent of sampling time associated with each selected work descriptor code

*HEPA, high efficiency particulate; PAPR, powered air-purifying particulate respirator; PVS, polyvinyl synthetic; LOD, limit of detection; TWA, time-weighted average.

added to all records for a given contractor's or company's database for external data sharing or pooling across DOE sites or wider industrial groupings. In this way, system users need not be concerned with such data for day-to-day system use.

Task Data

For surveillance purposes, aggregate analyses of exposure measurements stratified by task are extremely valuable because they provide the most refined, specific problem definitions (e.g., which tasks are associated with the highest exposures), and thus can be used to direct the most targeted primary prevention efforts (e.g., reorganization of task or preventive measures). Job classifications can be useful, depending on the size of the company, the diversity of its operations, and the ease of translating administrative job titles to classifications that capture similarly exposed groups of workers.[62] For our RFETS system, we used job descriptions to collapse 280 administrative job titles for the RFETS integrating contractor plus 4 first-tier contractors into 10 job-exposure categories for surveillance analyses.

For our system, we developed and piloted a two-tier coding system comprising 33 categories of task groups (Table 21.3). The first tier contains seven categories of work type, each of which includes one or more task groups and a category for miscellaneous tasks not covered by the coding scheme. The frequency of use of miscellaneous categories guides coding revisions. This coding scheme was developed through ongoing observations and interviews with industrial hygienists, other health and safety staff, and workers at RFETS. Industrial hygienists select one or more of the 33 unique combinations of work type and task group and record the appropriate codes at the time of sample collection. An optional field is also included for estimated percent of sampling period associated with each task group. In the electronic database, a subform and drop-down pick list of the codes and definitions allow multiple entries for each record. We originally developed a scheme with a third tier for specific tasks, but it was too unwieldy for field use.

The task coding system was first applied by investigators to previously collected contractor data (review of narrative notes on hard copy datasheets). Only personal breathing zone samples were coded for task. Two investigators coded 215 datasheets independently, and agreed on initial coding of 93% percent of the datasheets. Investigators came to consensus on disparate codings, then the codings were checked by RFETS staff hygienists. One new code was added after initial retrospective testing of the coding scheme (CU17: Polymer Macro-Encapsulation). The RFETS hygienists have since coded all personal breathing zone samples at the time of sample collection.

Process and task data are likely to be the most useful within a given company. However, methods for the collection of process and task data are the least developed of all exposure determinants, the most challenging and labor-intensive to obtain and update, and the least amenable to pooling across industries, regions, nations, and other broad-based levels of analysis. Thus,

Table 21.3 Work Descriptor Coding Scheme for Rocky Flats Clean-Up Activities

Work Type	*ID*	*Task Group or Task*
Cleanup	CU1.	Use of hand tools for size reduction, disassembly, etc.
	CU2.	Use of powered tools (e.g., Sawzall, drill) for size reduction, disassembly, etc.
	CU3.	Hot cutting or welding
	CU4.	Decon: Wet methods
	CU5.	Decon: Mechanical methods (e.g., dry wiping, sweeping)
	CU6.	HEPA vacuuming
	CU7.	Abrasive methods (e.g., sanding, grinding, CO_2 blasting)
	CU8.	Draining of pipe, tank, or other container
	CU9.	Coating removal (paint, adhesives, etc.)
	CU10.	Asbestos removal and abatement (including clearances samples)
	CU11.	On-site transport of waste materials
	CU12.	Materials consolidation
	CU13.	Sorting, packaging, or repackaging waste materials
	CU14.	Demolition of buildings or other large structures
	CU15.	Environmental remediation
	CU16.	**Miscellaneous—not covered by current coding choices**
	CU17.	Polymer Macroencapsulation
Waste management	WM1.	Waste treatment (e.g., thermal desorption, vitrification)
	WM2.	Waste storage operations (draining, venting, aspirating, etc. of any type of container, including tanks, drums, pipes, etc.)
	WM3.	Handling wet combustibles (high solvent content)
	WM4.	Leak or spill response or follow-up (environmental or indoors)
	WM5.	**Miscellaneous—not covered by current coding choices**
Assessment of contamination	AC1.	Collection of samples or use of direct reading instrument (e.g., Geiger Counter, Organic Vapor Meter)
Observation	OB1.	Observation of any work type or task group
Facility Maintenance	FM1.	Housekeeping (e.g., mopping, sweeping, trash removal)
	FM2.	Ventilation system maintenance
	FM3.	General maintenance of equipment or building (e.g., building repairs, bulb replacement, minor construction)
	FM4.	**Miscellaneous—not covered by current coding choices**
Process verification	PV1.	Production, usually limited, done for purposes of verifying processes or techniques
	PV2.	**Miscellaneous—not covered by current coding choices**
Conversion	CV1.	Refurbishment of equipment
	CV2.	Refurbishment of building
	CV3.	**Miscellaneous—not covered by current coding choices**

*HEPA, high efficiency particulate.

there is an inherent tension between the analysis needs of companies versus those of external data users (such as researchers and policy makers).

Database Structure

Some of the database elements described above can have a many-to-one relationship with the sample (e.g., many tasks for one sample, or many analytes for one sample). This is accommodated through a relational database structure of one main form or table (sample information), a sample results subtable, a task subtable, and a subtable for noting that a given sample is also representative of the exposure of one or more additional workers (explained in further detail in Van Dyke).[55] In addition, several system lookup tables provide information on task ID and description, employee information, hygienist information, personal protective equipment details, and analysis information (measurement units and exposure limits).

Analysis, Interpretation, and Reporting

Pilot Data Overview

The data system contained 901 air samples from 16 different RFETS buildings collected from March 1995 through August 1998. Air samples are made up of 376 personal breathing zones, 379 areas, 142 blanks, and 3 source samples. In addition, there were 404 bulk samples in the database. Investigators entered 640 air samples retrospectively during development and refining of entry screens, coding schemes, and report generation capabilities (including samples collected before the partnership began in March 1995). The most recent 261 samples were coded and entered by contractor hygienists. The contractor now operates the system. The database contained measurements of 47 different agents. Up to 19 different agents were analyzed per sample (for a series of chlorinated hydrocarbons), yielding a total of 1504 air sample records. For breathing zone samples: (*1*) 113 unique employees are represented; (*2*) the most common agents monitored were beryllium, lead, carbon tetrachloride, and asbestos; and (*3*) 85% of all samples were below detection limits.

Development and Examples of Analysis Strategies

The most common analyses requested by database users were for single measurements or for small groups of measurements. For example, most commercial software packages for industrial hygiene data management provide a comparison of single measurements to chosen occupational exposure limits (OELs), usually as a percentage of the chosen OEL (e.g., OSHA, NIOSH, ACGIH, or internal reference values). At the request of contractor hygienists, we have incorporated this useful feature into our system and linked it to an employee notification report generator (Fig. 21.1).

At the small group level, some in-house databases and numerous stand-alone software packages provide statistical analyses of exposure group homogeneity. This is a

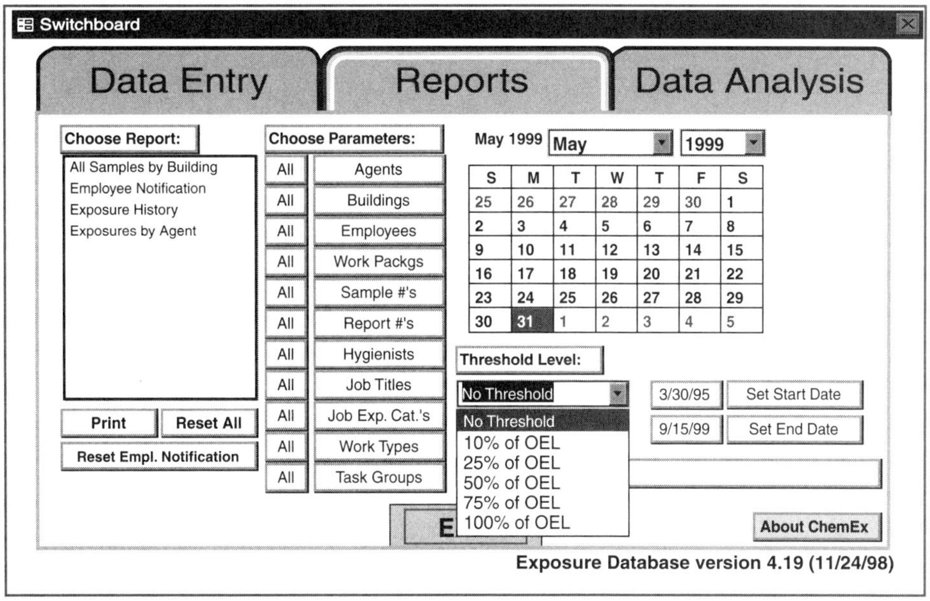

Figure 21.1 System Report Generator. Four report templates are described in the upper left corner. The user is able to choose all available choices for each of several parameters (middle), as well as the start and end dates (lower right), and a threshold level (percentage of occupational exposure limit [OEL], open drop-down menu).

Table 21.4 Exposure Surveillance Analysis Strategies

Analysis Goal and Applicability of Findings	*Analysis Procedure*	*Analysis or Report Audience*	*Recommended Frequency*
Identification of activities with higher exposure potential to enable targeted exposure control efforts	Summary measures or exposure profiles, by one or more potential exposure determinants (e.g., job title, task, location)	Health and Safety staff, workers, supervisors, managers	Monthly, bimonthly, or as needed
Detection of sentinel exposure events to enable timely exposure control interventions; assessment of Health and Safety performance goals	Filter full data set for personal or other exposure measurements above chosen administrative control level (e.g., % of a PEL* or TLV†)	Health and Safety staff, workers, supervisors, managers	Weekly, monthly, or as needed
Identification of workers in need of specific medical surveillance	Filter full data set for personal exposures above OSHA or other medical surveillance triggers	Occupational medicine providers, supervisors, workers	Weekly or monthly
Characterization of individual exposure history to determine secondary prevention needs, summarization of exposure histories for external use	Exposure profiles (e.g., scatterplot over time, distribution of exposures, median, and range)	Occupational medicine providers, individual workers (e.g., for outside medical providers, or to fill Freedom of Information Act requests)	Yearly, or by request
Periodic assessment of sitewide or specific subgroup trends over medium long term; early trend identification	Summary exposure measures over time by agent (and by one or more potential exposure determinant)	Managers, regulators, policy makers, Health and Safety staff, occupational medicine providers	Periodic: e.g., quarterly or semiannually

*PEL, permissible exposure limit.
†TLV, threshold limit value.

useful feature for production or other stable work settings where exposures are expected to be within a consistent range over time. For the DOE cleanup work environment—which is constantly changing in location, materials, and processes—the statistical process control assumptions for exposure assessment in production work environments[63] may not hold. Thus, we do not plan to incorporate exposure group homogeneity analysis into our system, and will rely on stand-alone packages.

For the DOE cleanup work environment, ongoing aggregate surveillance analyses were the most important feature. Aggregate surveillance analyses are statistical summaries of all measurements of a particular kind (e.g., same contaminant and sampling method, similar time period), grouped by various potential exposure determinants (e.g., task, work location, time period, individual worker). These analyses were simple and descriptive, but can vary widely depending on analysis goals and available data on potential exposure determinants (Table 21.4). Aggregate analysis should be specific to exposures, industries, organizational structures, and other characteristics. However, we believe that the small set of aggregate analysis strategies outlined are broadly applicable across most industries and work settings (Table 21.4). Each of these analysis strategies is illustrated below using our pilot data.

Potential Exposure Determinants

Our analysis focused on the potential exposures by task. Analyses of exposures stratified by task or task groups are poorly developed in commercially available packages and rarely appear in the published exposure surveillance literature. Yet, this type of analysis is extremely useful for guiding exposure control efforts in a timely and targeted fashion.

Our two-tier task-coding system (Table 21.3) supports exposure summary analyses by work type and by task group. Sixteen of the 33 task codes were used in the pilot period. The work type category of cleanup accounts for 85% of the task-coded samples. The most common cleanup task groups are draining of pipes, tanks, or other containers; sorting, packaging, and repackaging waste materials; and wet method decontamination. As a specific example, analysis of beryllium samples by task (202 samples over 11 different tasks) shows sorting, packaging, and repackaging to be the task with the highest airborne exposures (Fig. 21.2). These data provided a justification for focusing exposure control efforts on this task, and adjusting exposure control (e.g., measures to prevent resuspension of dusts during repackaging) and personal protective measures. It was also confirmed that respirators were being worn during all of the high measurements for this task. Details of respiratory protection and other personal protective equipment are printed with all employee notification reports (Fig. 21.1, second choice under Choose Report).

Graphs are readily generated using the built-in analysis generator of the system (Fig. 21.3), which supports stratification by up to three potential exposure determinants, or parameters (Fig. 21.2). For example, task group summaries could be generated by agent and building for the specific work type of cleanup. Thus, highly specific analysis queries can be conducted effi-

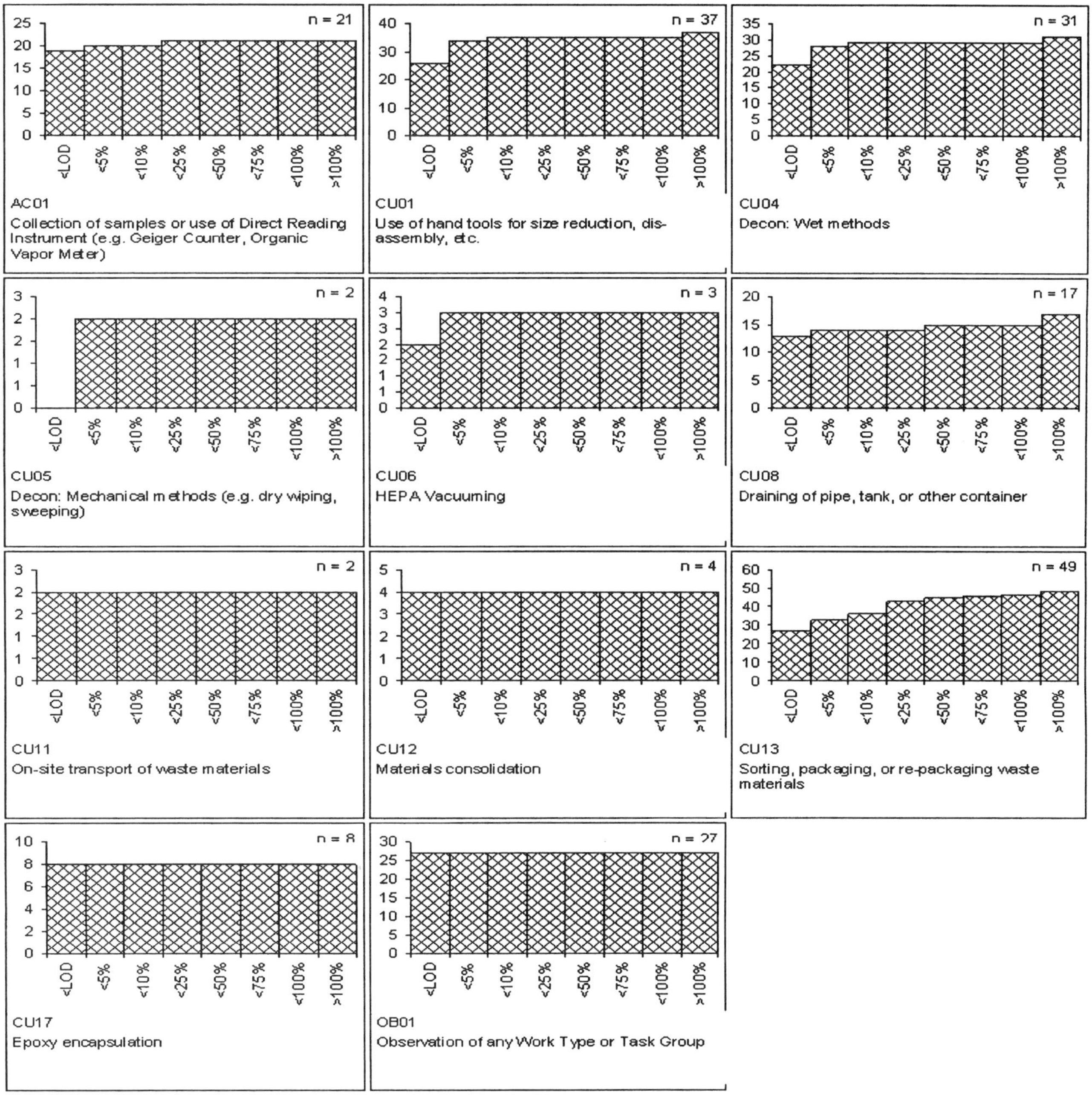

Figure 21.2 Cumulative frequency distributions of personal breathing zone beryllium exposures, split by task group. Presents time-weighted average (TWA) exposure measurements (without adjustment to 8-hour work shift) as fractions of OSHA permissible exposure limit (PEL) of 2 mcg/m^3. Output generated by system analysis generator (see Fig. 21.3).

ciently at any point in time with relative ease and minimal computer programming or statistical training. As emphasized by contractor hygienists, a short timeline between data entry and analysis is crucial for enabling application of results to on-going projects, which are sometimes only a matter of days or weeks in duration. For exposure distributions, simple visual scanning helped identify task groups with the highest exposures (greatest deviation from square), in both relative (percent of total measurements in given range) and absolute terms (total numbers of measurements).

Filtered Exposure Data

For some users, presentation or reporting of filtered data would be preferable to analyses of all available exposure data (Table 21.4, second row). For example, an overseer of a multicontractor site (as occurs at many DOE and construction sites) might want regular reporting of all ex-

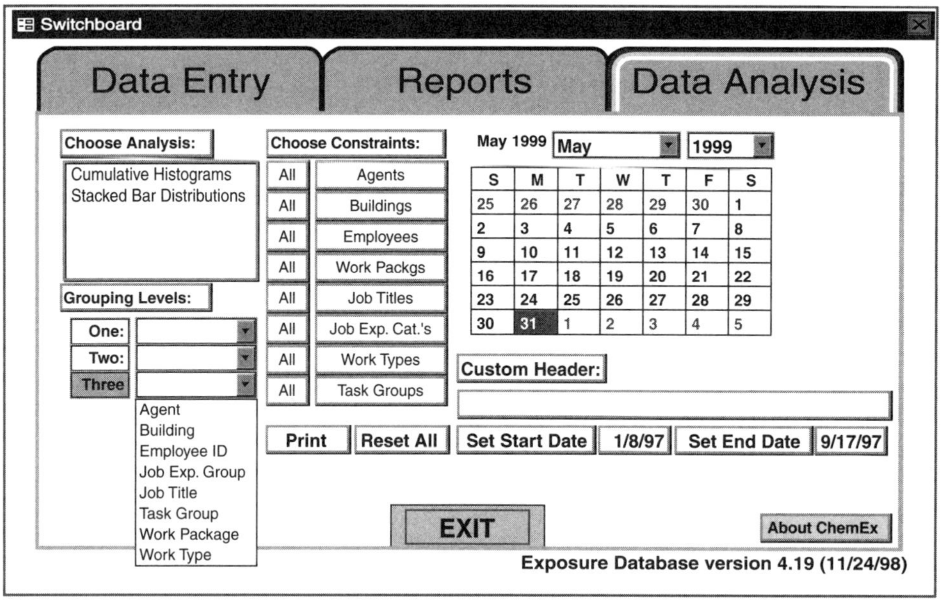

Figure 21.3 System Analysis Generator. Three analysis templates are described in the upper left corner. Users specify analysis templates, up to three grouping levels, specific constraints, start and end dates, and—if desired—a custom header. Figure 21.2 was generated as a Stacked Bar Distribution grouped by Task Group with beryllium specified as the single Agent of interest for the full calendar period (March 1995–August 1998, Start and End Dates) with a custom header.

posure events that exceed a given exposure limit (e.g., 10% of an OSHA PEL or ACGIH TLV, a performance goal recommended by the AIHA[39]). This strategy is the same as sentinel hazard or exposure event surveillance in the public health surveillance field.[49,64]

Figure 21.4 presents 3 years of exposure data for several agents exceeding a threshold of 10% of current OSHA PELs. Unadjusted time-weighted averages (TWAs) are presented in addition to TWA normalized to a full 8-hour work shift. This emphasizes the important distinction between summarizing exposure data from a compliance versus a prevention and control perspective. In DOE cleanup work, sampling periods are often shorter than 8 hours. Thus, opportuni-

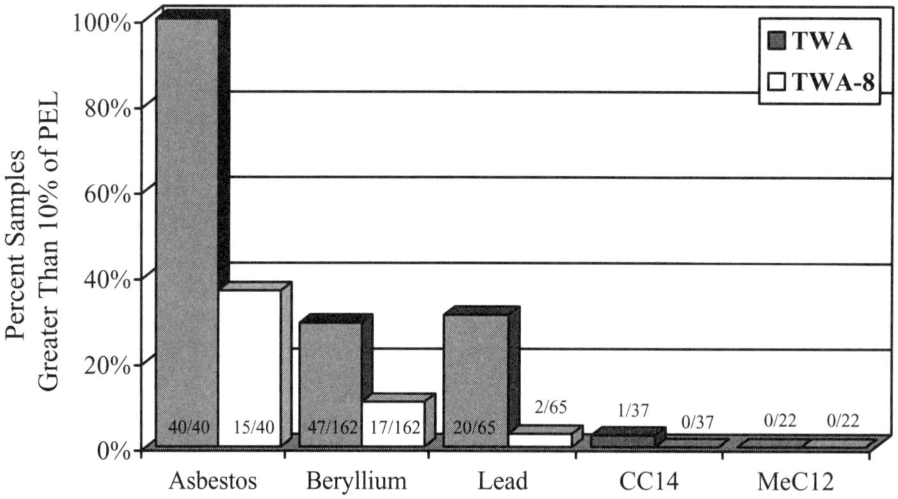

Figure 21.4 Time-weighted average (TWA) personal breathing zone samples greater than 10% of OSHA PEL, by agent, TWA normalized to sampling period versus 8 hours, 1995–1998. Numbers of samples from which percentages are derived are provided at the foot of each bar (numerator/denominator). CCl_4, carbon tetrachloride; $MeCl_2$, methylene chloride.

Table 21.5 Filtering for Medical Surveillance Requirements

Agent	*Total Pesonal Breathing Zone Samples (1995–1998)*	*TWA*-8 Medical Surveillance Criteria*	*Number of Employees Above Criteria (# of samples per employee)*
Asbestos	40	0.1 f/cc†	0
Beryllium	162	0.5 mcg/cu m‡	7 (1), 1 (2)
Lead	65	30 mcg/cu m†	1 (1)
Methylene chloride	22	12.5 ppm†	0

*TWA, time-weighted average.
†From Occupational Safety and Health Administration standards.
‡From proposed Department of Energy beryllium rule (Department of Energy[59]).

ties for exposure control might be missed by review of TWA-8 measurements (e.g., see bars for lead in Fig. 21.3). In some cases, high percentages of measurements above 10% of the PEL are expected. For instance, all asbestos work is required to be conducted under abatement conditions with Level A worker protection.

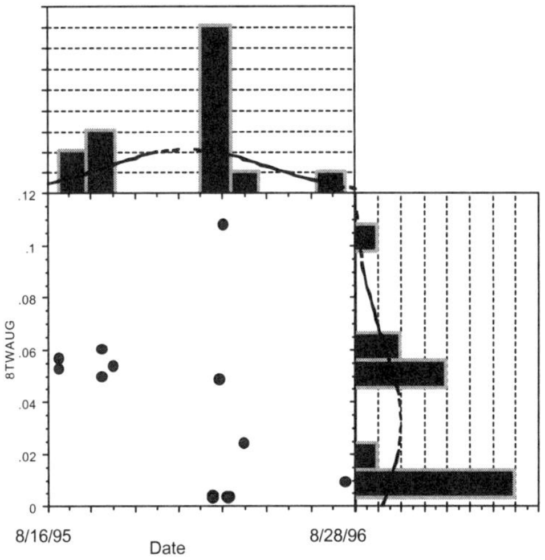

Exposure Profile for Employee 126 for Beryllium

Total # of Measurements	**15**
# > 10% of the PEL	**0**
# Below LOD	**13**
Mean	**0.032 μg/m³**
Median	**0.024 μg/m³**
Standard Deviation	**0.032 μg/m³**
Minimum	**0.003 μg/m³**
Maximum	**0.108 μg/m³**

Figure 21.5 Employee exposure profile: scatterplot of comprehensive personal breathing zone beryllium exposure history for an individual cleanup worker over a 1-year term of employment. Central panel shows TWA exposure levels normalized to sampling period (raw TWA, mcg/m^3) over calendar time. Panel above scatterplot indicates relative sampling frequency over time; panel to right of scatterplot gives graphical distribution of raw TWA levels, reflecting computed descriptive statistics in tables below. Tables present numerical frequencies of exposure measurement values and summary statistics. Output generated using Statview® (Abacus Concepts, Inc.) scatterplot with histograms command.

Other applications of filtering analyses include identification of workers in need of medical surveillance (Table 21.4, third row). Many agents with OSHA standards include TWA-8 triggers for medical surveillance. For example, Table 21.5 presents four agents with TWA-8 triggers. Sometimes these triggers are only formally activated if the TWA-8 trigger is exceeded for 30 or more working days in a given year. There are other medical surveillance triggers in OSHA standards, such as specific short-term TWA exposures or exposures during accidents. Respirator usage can also be factored into medical surveillance decisions. The summary presented in Table 21.5 provides a means of ensuring that more highly exposed workers have been provided appropriate medical surveillance.

An efficient means for identifying sentinel exposures, medical surveillance, and similar analyses is provided by an easy-to-use report generator similar to the analysis generator described above (Figure 21.1). The threshold level box allows the user to specify percentage of the OELs being used. In addition, anywhere from one to all of various parameters can be chosen ranging over any calendar period. Four standard report types have been programmed to date (upper left of Fig. 21.1).

Exposure Histories

In some circumstances, individual exposure histories are needed (Table 21.4, fourth row). For example, exposure information needed in medical surveillance varies by the toxicology of the agent in question. However, most of the information needed by agent is available from the concise profiles presented in Figure 21.5 (e.g., average and median over employment period, highest exposures with their timing and frequency). Medical surveillance providers also gain a better understanding of work and exposure histories. The system supports informed recommendations for biomonitoring, as well as information to discuss exposure prevention and health promotion with workers.

Time Trending

Time can also be incorporated into periodic analyses of summary measures. Figure 21.6 provides an example of a time series of the percentage of beryllium measurements that exceeded 10% of OSHA's current PEL.

The recommended frequency of analysis in the far right column of Table 21.4 (for time trending as well as other analyses) are rough guidelines. Appropriate timing will depend on the number of samples collected, the nature of the work being performed, the natural history of potential occupational diseases or illnesses of concern, and other factors. The more frequent the analyses, the greater the opportunity for primary versus secondary prevention.

Report and Analysis Output

We continue to improve the graphical capabilities of our system. However, some of the graphs presented in this chapter were done by export of data to other statistical, spreadsheet, or graphics packages (e.g., MS PowerPoint® for Figures 21.4 and 21.6, Statview® for Figure 21.5). Our goal is to provide graphical output with minimal programming or statistical training required for system users. Graphical and chart output is generally preferred over tabular format for its ease of interpretation and suitability for the broadest array of potential audiences.[65] Strategies being explored include the use of customized links between the exposure database and external programs, and using add-in programs (e.g., for Microsoft Office® programs).[57]

Application of Findings to Prevention

The goal of both surveillance and industrial hygiene is to complete the prevention cycle by channeling information for action.[12,38,39,40,65,66] Careful attention to the communication of this information increases the likelihood of achieving the desired action. To promote this end, surveillance reports should include only the relevant results for a specific audience and a clear message. Messages are distilled from the goals and analyses outlined in Table 21.4.[65,67] Sometimes the message will be reassuring and will not require a specific action from the recipient (e.g., worker exposures to agent X continued to decline in the most recent quarter). The desired action should be part of the message. In response to elevated exposures, a message to workers might emphasize the need to improve work practices whereas the message regarding the same situation to an administrator might justify the expense of expanded sampling and staff time devoted to improving passive exposure controls.

CONCLUSION

This chapter provides the rationale and illustrates the power of integrated exposure database and surveillance systems for prevention. In addition to the work conducted with one RFETS contractor described above, we also work with the broader RFETS OSH community. Based on the success of the system with the first-tier contractor, the integrating contractor of RFETS

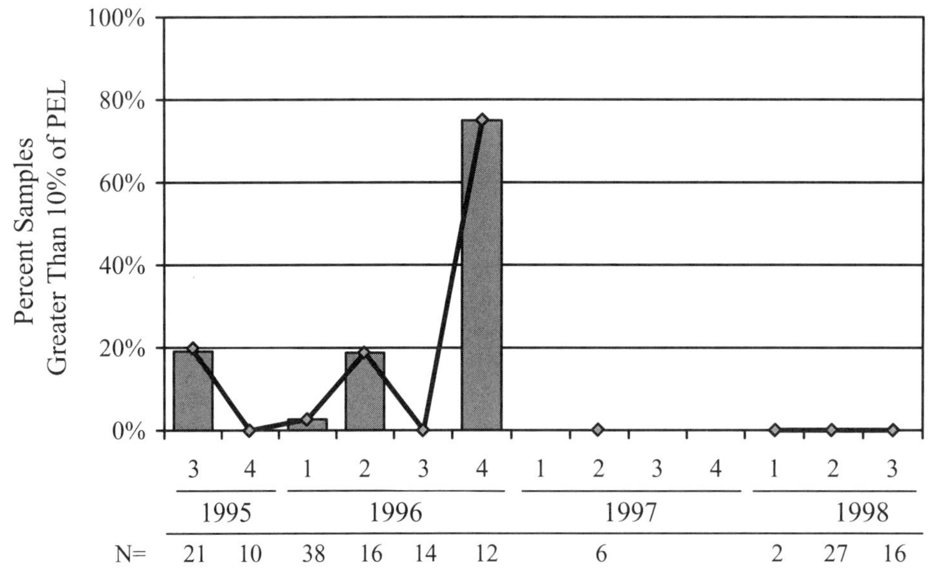

Figure 21.6 Percentage of personal breathing zone (BZ) beryllium measurements over 10% of OSHA PEL (0.2 mcg/m^3), by quarter, 1995–1998. Presents TWA-8 personal breathing zone measurements by calendar quarter (3-month periods). Graphic generated using Microsoft PowerPoint.®

adopted our system as a prototype for RFETS-wide implementation. The system described above provided the basis for design of the user interface, or front-end. It is now supported by a networked Oracle® database, or back-end. We continue to refine our sample number, task, and some other fields to improve generalizability across RFETS and the DOE complex.

While the specifics of the system were tailored to DOE cleanup work, most aspects of the system are generalizable. The integration of exposure databases and surveillance systems similar to this one will help to realize the full prevention potential of the vast amount of exposure data collected at many workplaces.

REFERENCES

1. Greife A, Halperin W, et al. Hazard Surveillance: Its Role in Primary Prevention of Occupational Disease and Injury. *Appl Occup Environ Hyg* 1995; 10: 737–742.
2. Halperin WE. The role of surveillance in the hierarchy of prevention. *Am J Ind Med* 1996; 29:321–323.
3. National Institute for Occupational Safety and Health. *National Occupational Research Agenda.* U.S. Public Health Service, Centers for Disease Control: National Institute for Occupational Safety and Health, 1996.
4. Pastides H, Mundt KA. Epidemiological Surveillance. In: DiNardi SR, ed. *The Occupational Environment—Its Evaluation and Control.* Fairfax, VA: American Industrial Hygiene Association; 1997: 92–102.
5. Buehler JW. Surveillance. In: Rothman KJ, Greenland S, eds. *Modern Epidemiology.* Philadelphia, PA, Lippincott–Raven Publishers; 1998: 435–457.
6. Sundin DS, Frazier TM. Hazard surveillance at NIOSH. *Am J Public Health* 1989; 79(Suppl):32–37.
7. Wegman D. Hazard surveillance. In: Halperin W, Baker EL, Monson RR, eds. *Public Health Surveillance.* New York: Van Nostrand Reinhold, 1992:62–75.
8. Wegman DH, Stellman SD. *Occupational Hazard Surveillance.* International Labor Organization: Encyclopaedia of Occupational Safety and Health; 1997:32.8–32.9.
9. National Institute for Occupational Safety and Health. *Exposure Assessment Methods.* National Occupational Research Agenda, U.S. Department of Health & Human Services (NIOSH) Publication No. 96–115. Cincinnati, OH: National Institute for Occupational Safety and Health, 1996.
10. Hertz-Picciotto I. Comment: toward a coordinated system for the surveillance of environmental health hazards. *Am J Public Health* 1996; 86:638–641.
11. National Institute for Occupational Safety and Health. *Surveillance Research Methods.* National Occupational Research Agenda, U.S. Department of Health & Human Services (NIOSH) Publication No. 96–115. Cincinnati, OH: National Institute for Occupational Safety and Health, 1996.
12. LaMontagne AD, Herrick RF, et al. Exposure databases and exposure surveillance: promise and practice. *AIHA Journal* (in press).
13. National Institute for Occupational Safety and Health. *National Institute for Occupational Safety & Health: Strategic Plan 1997–2002.* Washington, DC: National Institute for Occupational Safety and Health, 1998.
14. Gomez MR, Rawls G. Conference on occupational exposure databases: a report and look at the future. *Appl Occup Environ Hyg* 1995; 10:238–243.
15. Lippmann M. Henry F. Smyth, Jr. Lecture: advancing the mission: occupational and environmental hygiene in the information age. *Appl Occup Environ Hyg* 1996; 11:1287–1293.
16. Boden LI. Policy evaluations: better living through research. *Am J Ind Med* 1996; 29:346–352.
17. Joint ACGIH-AIHA Task Group. Data elements for occupational exposure databases: guidelines and recommendations for airborne hazards and noise. *Appl Occup Environ Hyg* 1996; 11:1294–1311.
18. Gomez MR. Exposure surveillance tools needed in agency GPRA plans. *AIHA J* 1998; 59:371–374.
19. Baker E. Surveillance in occupational health and safety. Challenges for the future. *Am J Public Health* 1989; 79(Suppl.):61–63.
20. LaMontagne AD, Van Dyke MV, et al. Development and piloting of an exposure database and surveillance system for DOE cleanup operations. *AIHA J* (in press).
21. Holzner CL, Hirsh RB, et al. Managing workplace exposure information. *Am Ind Hyg Assoc J* 1993; 54:15–21.
22. Morgan DA. U.S. Army Center for Health Promotion and Preventive Medicine's Electronic Information Resources. *Appl Occup Environ Hyg* 1997; 12:524–527.
23. Heikkila P, Kauppinen T. Occupational exposure to carcinogens in Finland. *Am J Ind Med* 1992; 21:467–480.
24. Whyte A. Computerizing an industrial hygiene program. In: Plog B, Niland J, Quinlan P, eds. *Fundamentals of Industrial Hygiene.* Chicago, IL: National Safety Council; 1996:759–766.
25. Stewart JH. Use of computers in occupational hygiene. In: DiNardi SR, ed. *The Occupational Environment and Its Evaluation.* Fairfax, VA: AIHA Press; 1997:1153–1166.
26. Gomez MR. A proposal to develop a national occupational exposure databank. *Appl Occup Environ Hyg* 1993; 8:768–774.
27. Burke TA, Sexton K. Integrating science and policy in a National Human Exposure Assessment Survey. *J Expo Anal Environ Epidemiol* 1995; 5:283–296.
28. Wagener DK, Selevan SG, et al. The importance of human exposure information: a need for exposure-related data bases to protect and promote public health. *Ann Rev Public Health* 1995; 16:105–121.
29. Thacker SB, Stroup DF, et al. Surveillance in environmental public health: issues, systems, and sources. *Am J Public Health* 1996; 86:633–638.
30. Gomez MR. Recommendations for optimizing the usefulness of existing exposure databases for public health applications. *AIHA Journal* 1997; 58:181–182.
31. Botkin A, Conway H. Relevance of exposure data to regulatory impact analyses: overcoming availability problems. *Appl Occup Environ Hyg* 1995; 10:383–390.
32. Fehrenbacher MC. The Environmental Protection Agency's use of occupational exposure databases for screening level assessments under the Toxic Substances Control Act. *Appl Occup Environ Hyg* 1995; 10:374–378.
33. Lippmann M. Exposure data needs in risk assessment and risk management: database information needs. *Appl Occup Environ Hyg* 1995; 10:244–250.
34. Creek K, Schinkel J. Workshop on key data needs for an occupational exposure database, session II. *Appl Occup Environ Hyg* 1995; 10:408–410.
35. Rawls GM, Haring CL. Workshop on key data needs for an occupational health database, session I. *Appl Occup Environ Hyg* 1995; 10:404–407.
36. Rajan B, Alesbury R, et al. European proposal for core information for the storage and exchange of workplace exposure mea-

surements on chemical agents. *Appl Occup Environ Hyg* 1997; 12:31–39.

37. Randolph BL, Damiano J. Workshop on serving multiple needs with exposure databases. *Appl Occup Environ Hyg* 1995; 10:415–416.
38. Hawkins NC, Norwood SK, et al., eds. *A Strategy for Occupational Exposure Assessment.* Fairfax, VA: American Industrial Hygiene Association,1991.
39. Mulhausen JR, Damiano J, eds. *A Strategy for Assessing and Managing Occupational Exposures,* Second Edition. Fairfax, VA: AIHA Press, 1998.
40. Halperin W, Baker EL, et al., eds. *Public Health Surveillance.* New York: Van Nostrand Reinhold, 1992.
41. Morabia A. Annotation: from disease surveillance to the surveillance of risk factors. *Am J Public Health* 1996; 86:625–626.
42. Leidel NA, Busch KA, et al. *Occupational Exposure Sampling Strategy Manual, DHEW (NIOSH) Publication No. 77–173.* Cincinnati, OH: National Institute for Occupational Safety and Health; 1977.
43. Rose VE. History & philosophy of industrial hygiene. In: SR DiNardi, ed. *The Occupational Environment and Its Evaluation.* Fairfax, VA: AIHA Press; 1997:3–18.
44. Teutsch S, Churchill RE, eds. *Principles and Practice of Public Health Surveillance.* New York: Oxford University Press, 1994.
45. Mendelsohn ML, Peeters JP, et al., eds. *Biomarkers and Occupational Health: Progress and Perspectives.* Washington, D.C.: Joseph Henry Press, 1995.
46. Mendelsohn, ML, Mohr LC, et al. *Biomarkers Medical and Workplace Applications.* Washington, DC: Joseph Henry Press, 1998.
47. Institute of Medicine. *Role of the Primary Care Physician in Occupational and Environmental Medicine.* Washington, DC: National Academy Press, 1988.
48. Leigh JP, Markowitz SB, et al. Occupational injury and illness in the United States. Estimates of costs, morbidity, and mortality. *Arch Int Med* 1997; 157:1557–1568.
49. Seligman PJ, Frazier TM. Surveillance: the sentinel health event approach. In: Halperin W, Baker EL, Monson RR. *Public Health Surveillance.* New York: Van Nostrand Reinhold, 1992:16–25.
50. Bracker A, Blumberg J, et al. Industrial hygiene recommendations as interventions: A collaborative model within occupational medicine. *Appl Occup Environ Hyg* 1999; 14:85–96.
51. Froines J, Wegman D, et al. Hazard surveillance in occupational disease. *Am J Public Health* 1989; 79(Suppl):26–31.
52. Gochfeld M, Favata E, et al., eds. *Hazardous Waste Workers. Occupational Medicine: State of the Art Reviews.* Philadelphia, PA: Hanley & Belfus, Inc., 1990.
53. Beall JR. Low-level exposures: some implications for the U.S. Department of Energy. *Env Health Perspectives* 1998; 106(Suppl 1):383–385.
54. Rawls G. The worlds of occupational exposure databases. *Appl Occup Environ Hyg* 1995; 10:237.
55. Van Dyke MV. Industrial hygiene databases: structure and function. *Appl Occ Env Hygiene Journal* 1999; 14:427–432.
56. Office of Technology Assessment. *Hazards Ahead: Managing Cleanup Worker Health and Safety at the Nuclear Weapons Complex, OTA-BP-O-85.* Washington, D.C., US Government Printing Office, 1993.
57. Microsoft Corporation. *Microsoft Office Professional.* Redlands WA: Microsoft Corporation, 1997.
58. Department of Energy. *Interim Chronic Beryllium Disease Prevention Program.* DOE Notice 440.1, U.S. Department of Energy, 1997.
59. Department of Energy. *Chronic Beryllium Disease Prevention Program; Proposed Rule.* Federal Register 10 CFR Part 850: 66940–66975, 1998.
60. Department of Energy. *Chemical Safety Vulnerability Working Group Report* (September 1994), Volume 1 of 3, U.S. Department of Energy, DOE/EH-0396P, 1994.
61. Sorock GS, Smith GS, et al. Three perspectives on work-related injury surveillance systems. *Am J Ind Med* 1997; 32:116–128.
62. Harber P, Miller G, et al. Work coding: beyond SIC and SOC, BOC and DOT. *J Occup Med* 1991; 33:1274–1280.
63. Hewett P. Interpretation and use of occupational exposure limits for chronic disease agents. In: Bang KM, ed. *Occupational Epidemiology.* Philadelphia, PA: Hanley & Belfus; 1996:561–590.
64. Aldrich TE, Leaverton PE. Sentinel event strategies in environmental health. *Ann Rev Public Health* 1991; 14: 205–217.
65. Goodman RA, Remington PL, et al. Communicating information for action. In: Teutsch SM, Churchill RE, eds. *Principles and Practice of Public Health Surveillance.* New York, Oxford University Press, 1994:150–157.
66. Blanc P. Linking surveillance to prevention [comment]. *Public Health Rev* 1995; 23:75–77.
67. Remington PL. Communicating epidemiologic information. In: Brownson RC, Petitti DB. *Applied Epidemiology.* New York: Oxford University Press; 1998:323–348.

22

Hospital Discharge Data

MARTHA W. STANBURY

Computerized information from hospital discharge summaries is routinely collected and coded using standard data set formats in over half of the states and nationally for all Medicare-covered patients. This administrative data set is assembled primarily for billing purposes, but it has application for public health surveillance and research because it compiles population-based diagnostic and demographic information on hospitalized patients. It is an important alternative to physician reporting as a source of surveillance data. Hospital discharge data have been used for a variety of condition-specific, case-based occupational health surveillance programs under the SENSOR model;[1] and they have been used to describe trends, geographic patterns, and costs of occupational disease. Several exploratory studies have demonstrated their potential usefulness for other occupational health surveillance activities, although the findings from these studies have not yet been applied to public health practice.

There are several important limitations to the use of hospital discharge data for occupational health surveillance. First, personal identifiers are not available in most states' data sets, making counts of unduplicated patient discharges depend on the development of computer algorithms for matching, and making case follow-back difficult or impossible. Second, in most states these data are not timely because they are not usually available to a state agency until one or more years after the close of a given calendar year due to the lengthy process of compiling data from multiple hospitals. Additionally, the data are limited by the coded diagnostic information because the International Classification of Diseases (ICD) coding system for discharge diagnoses does not identify work-related disorders, except for the codes for the pneumoconioses and some cause-of-injury E-codes. These limitations are addressed in this chapter, in regard to applying hospital discharge data to specific occupational disease and injury surveillance projects in New Jersey and elsewhere.

DESCRIPTION OF STATE HOSPITAL DISCHARGE DATA

Forty-four states collect data on all hospital discharges from acute care hospitals in their states; 34 states require reporting of hospital discharge data (HDD), and 10 states obtain the information voluntarily.[2] The data set that is reported is very large; in New Jersey, for example, there are on average approximately 1.2 million hospital discharges per year for its population of 7.7 million.

The data are reported using the Medicare Uniform Bill-92 format (UB-92, Appendix A) in 34 states, using the Uniform Hospital Discharge Data Set (UHDDS) in 4 states, and in unique data formats in 6 states.[2] These data sets collect the same kinds of information, including patient demographics, diagnostics, and billing information. The minimum data set of the UB-92, the most widely used format, includes a field to link back to the hospital medical record (usually a medical record number), patient demographics, a string of up to 9 discharge diagnoses coded in the clinical modification of ICD-9, a string of up to 8 procedures using the Current Procedural Terminology (CPT) procedure code system, a hospital identifier, a physician identifier, and insurance coverage. Until recently, very few hospital discharge systems included ICD E-codes for injury, although this is changing and as of 1999 at least 32 states require an E-code whenever there is an injury. In the ICD system, injuries can be coded with a nature of injury code, which tells the type of injury, e.g., burn, poisoning, fracture, etc., and part(s) of body affected, and with an E-code, which is the external source of the injury (e.g., accident caused by agricultural machines). Primary and secondary insurance payer fields usually include codes for the major insurance carriers, self-pay, and workers' compensation. The patient name and address are collected by very few states.[3] The UB-92 data set does not include information about the patient's employer or occupation.

The accuracy and reliability of each data element varies depending on the reason for its collection and when it was collected during the patient admission. For example, the accuracy and the length of the ICD code string has probably been influenced over time by changes in billing reimbursement practices. Insurance coverage information is usually collected at the time of admission and often not corrected after patient discharge; this field has been found to have many inaccuracies in New Jersey hospital discharge data. Additionally, as with any large data set, random error is a certainty, impacting both on sensitivity and specificity of the data for surveillance.

CASE-BASED SURVEILLANCE

Case-based surveillance requires the availability of personal identifiers to assure that preventive intervention takes place. Hospital discharge data have been used effectively by occupational health surveillance projects for case-based surveillance in several states where personal identifiers are available or can be obtained from follow-back with the discharging hospital. These projects have focused primarily on a number of work-related respiratory diseases. Hospital discharge data are not as useful for case-based surveillance and follow-up of acute diseases and injuries as they are for chronic diseases because of the long lag time between discharge and availability of the data.

Pneumoconiosis Surveillance

The ICD classification system identifies one class of important occupational diseases—the pneumoconioses (ICD 500–505). Individuals discharged with one of these diagnostic codes can be assumed to have a work-related disease. The long lag time between discharge and availability of the data set is not a major concern because these diseases are chronic and of long latency.

Silicosis

Health departments in New Jersey, Michigan, Ohio, and Illinois have developed case-based surveillance systems for silicosis (ICD 502) that are based primarily, but not exclusively, on identification of cases from HDD.[4] (Other sources of case reports have included mandatory hospital reports, mortality data, physician reports, employer reports, and workers' compensation data.) These state-based systems have used similar procedures to confirm cases and initiate intervention and control activities. Procedures for case confirmation are driven by a surveillance case definition for silicosis that has been published by the Centers for Disease Control (CDC).[5] The components of this case definition include establishing that the individuals worked in an industry where silicosis exposure was likely; and, confirming the presence of the disease by radiology or pathology report or, preferably by a reading of the chest x-ray by a NIOSH-certified B reader (see Chapter 14).

Data on individuals discharged with ICD 502 anywhere in the discharge diagnosis string are subsetted from the discharge data set. Matching on a unique identifier is then completed in order to identify repeat admissions. Finally, personal identifying information for each patient that is obtained from the data file (name, if available, medical record number or another patient identifier, birth date, discharge date) are submitted to the discharging hospital with a request for the patient's medical records. To eliminate repeat cases, the returned medical record with the patient's name can then be matched with the list of previously identified cases.

In 1995, the New Jersey Department of Health mandated hospital reporting of patients with ICD 502 in the discharge diagnosis string (as well as other selected respiratory conditions and poisonings) within 30 days of discharge, both to ensure legal access to medical records and to obtain more timely reports with patient names and addresses. By obtaining reports of hospital discharges that included the patients' names, the reports could be matched against the existing silicosis registry database to eliminate repeat cases and thereby eliminate requests for medical records of previously ascertained cases. New Jersey uses its HDD to supplement hospital reporting because, although the reports are timely, hospital compliance with the reporting regulations is only approximately 50% of actual discharges. In 1994, hospitals were required to submit the patient's name in the HDD set, eliminating the necessity of the first step of the follow-back process when using the UB-92 data set for case ascertainment.

Medical records requested from the hospital include the face page, discharge summary, and radiology reports. Chest x-rays are requested from the radiology department. (Original films, not duplicates, are requested, because duplicate films usually do not have sufficient detail for review according to the International Labor Organization's system for radiologic interpretation of pneumoconiosis.) Legal authority to access to medical records varies from state to state. In New Jersey and Michigan, regulations give the state access under hospital reporting requirements.

Medical records are screened for false positives, including coding errors (e.g., scoliosis being misread by the coder as silicosis and thus being assigned ICD 502). Available work history information is abstracted, although often it is missing from the discharge summary. In some states, x-rays are read and interpreted by a NIOSH-certified B reader. Cases not ruled out by this review are considered suspect cases. Patients, or their next-of-kin, are then interviewed to obtain a work history that will identify the source of exposure to silica. Prior to contacting the patient or next-of-kin, New Jersey notifies the attending physician identified on the discharge face page by mail, but not all other states with silicosis surveillance systems include this step in the process. Silicosis surveillance is described in detail in Chapter 14.

Asbestosis

Comprehensive case-based surveillance of asbestosis (ICD 500) has not been conducted by any state health department. The New Jersey Department of Health and Senior Services has conducted more limited surveillance-related activities because of the concern that individuals with asbestosis may need information about medical monitoring and their legal rights regarding financial compensation. The New Jersey Department of Health and Senior Services conducted a series of mailings to individuals with asbestosis who were identified by HDD. The process of identifying cases from the data set was similar to that with silicosis, although diagnostic information was not confirmed by having x-rays read by B readers. First, a survey was sent to 1079 individuals with asbestosis, who were reported by hospitals, to determine if they needed information about asbestosis.[6] When the respondents overwhelmingly indicated a desire for greater understanding of the ramifications of their disease, the Department undertook a proactive series of educational mailings to all individuals identified by hospital discharge data as having asbestosis. Medical records were reviewed to sort out false positives. The physicians of record were notified, and then patients received the educational mailing. Individuals indicated by return post card whether the materials were very helpful and informative.[7]

Coal Worker's Pneumoconiosis

No state has used HDD for case-based surveillance of coal worker's pneumoconiosis (CWP) (ICD 501) primarily because the federal government has a comprehensive, registry-based, surveillance system for CWP.

Other Pneumoconioses

New Jersey and Michigan silicosis surveillance projects review ICD 505 (pneumoconiosis other and unspecified) hospital discharges because some silicosis cases are coded ICD 505 rather than 502. There may be other important sentinel cases of work-related disease under ICD 503 and 504 codes, because these ICD codes include a number of occupational diseases (e.g., aluminosis, berylliosis, graphite fibrosis, byssinosis, and flax-dressers' disease). However, current resources and mandates in state-based programs have not supported surveillance initiatives for these conditions.

Work-Related Asthma

Case-based surveillance systems for occupational asthma have used HDD to identify potential cases. The ICD codes with potential cases include ICD 506—respiratory conditions due to fumes and vapors, and ICD 493—asthma—when linked to workers' compensation as the primary payer. Interviews with patients are necessary to rule out false positives.

Work-Related Asthma Identified Through ICD 506 (Respiratory Conditions Due to Fumes and Vapors)

International Classification of Diseases code 506 has the following subgroups: 506.0, bronchitis and pneumonitis resulting from fumes and vapors; 506.1, acute pulmonary edema resulting from fumes and vapors; 506.2, upper respiratory inflammation resulting from fumes and vapors; 506.3 other acute and subacute respiratory conditions resulting from fumes and vapors; 506.4, chronic respiratory conditions resulting from fumes and vapors; and 506.9, unspecified respiratory conditions resulting from fumes and vapors. The ICD code 506 includes patients with occupational and nonoccupational sources of exposure. The New Jersey SENSOR program evaluated the positive predictive value of ICD 506, 507 (pneumonitis due to solids and liquids), and 508 (respiratory conditions due to other and unspecified external agents) for acute work-related respiratory disease surveillance by conducting medical records reviews of cases identified by HDD with these ICD codes. This study found that in 39% of the patients discharged with ICD 506, the diagnosis was related to work exposure; however, this was true for only 2% of the discharges under ICD 507 and 508.[8] The Michigan SENSOR project subsequently investigated ICD 506 in greater detail.[9] This study confirmed the New Jersey finding that approximately one-third of

ICD 506 discharges were work-related. House fires and exposure to household cleaners were the most frequent causes of the nonwork-related discharges.

Based on these findings, the New Jersey and Michigan occupational asthma disease surveillance projects now follow-up on patient hospital discharges with ICD 506 as the primary or secondary discharge diagnosis, limiting the records reviews to those aged 18–65. The same approach for identifying silicosis cases apply: matching names against the surveillance database to identify duplicates; medical records review of new cases to screen out false positives; notification of the attending physician; followed by contact with the patient or next-of-kin to obtain information to confirm the diagnosis.[10,11]

Asthma and Workers' Compensation

The SENSOR surveillance programs in New Jersey, Michigan, and Massachusetts for occupational asthma review records and conduct follow-back with patients using the above procedures where ICD 493 is the primary discharge diagnosis and workers' compensation is the primary payer. New Jersey has found that there are a considerable number of false positives, mostly due to coding errors in the primary payer field. For example, one large hospital was coding all its employees who were hospitalized with asthma as having workers' compensation as the primary payer, even though the asthma was not occupationally related. In New Jersey, although hospital reporting of ICD 493 is not mandatory under the state's hospital reporting regulations, physician reporting of occupational asthma is, and hospitals release records to the state under the physician reporting regulation.

Other Potential Uses of Hospital Discharge Data for Case-Based Surveillance

There have been a number of feasibility studies for other case-based, condition-specific surveillance systems, although these have not yet been established because of a lack of resources in state health departments.

Sorock et al.[12] interviewed a series of patients identified from HDD with several types of injuries to determine their work-relatedness. They sent letters to 809 individuals with discharge ICD codes for selected injuries (finger and thumb amputations, lower limb crush injury, toxic effects of heavy metals, and eye burns) inviting them to be in the study; 61% of those who completed the interview said their injury was work-related. There was a high correlation between self-reported work-related injury and workers' compensation as the primary payer.

Table 22.1 is a list of poisonings that are included in New Jersey's regulations for mandatory reporting by hospitals. These ICD codes capture patients with occupational exposure, with nonoccupational exposure and with intentional exposure—suicide or homicide. Exploratory studies of medical records similar to those that have been done for ICD 506 have been conducted for ICD 989—pesticides—and 987—toxic effects of other gases, fumes, or vapors—in New Jersey. No cases of work-related pesticide toxicity were found on that medical records review. Approximately 38% of the discharges where ICD 987 was the primary discharge diagnosis were work-related, of which 50% were related to fires (unpublished data). Evaluation of all of the ICD codes on the list in Table 22.1 would be useful.

Balmes et al.[13] reviewed medical records and conducted interviews of patients discharged with lung cancer, bladder cancer, and toxic hepatitis, three conditions considered to be Sentinel Health Events/Occupational.[14] They concluded that the work-relatedness of these conditions can be determined if adequate occupation and industry (O/I) information is available. However, the accuracy and completeness of O/I in hospital charts was relatively low.[13] The National Research Council has noted that inclusion of occupation and industry information on hospital discharge abstracts would make HDD more useful for ongoing occupational disease surveillance activities.[15]

In New Jersey, a medical records review has also been conducted for patients with ICD 495—extrinsic allergic alveolitis. A medical records review of 47 cases identified from New Jersey hospital discharge data with this discharge diagnosis found that 27% met clinical crite-

Table 22.1 Poisonings Reportable by Hospitals in New Jersey*

ICD 9th Revision	*ICD-9 Code*
Toxic effect of alcohol	ICD 980; E860 (E860.0–.9)
Toxic effect of petroleum products	ICD 981; E862 (E862.0–.9)
Toxic effect of solvents other than petroleum based	ICD 982; E862 (E862.0–.9)
Toxic effect of corrosive aromatics, acids, and caustic alkalis	ICD 983; E864 (864.0–.4)
Toxic effect of lead and its compounds	ICD 984; E866 (E866.0)
Toxic effect of other metals	ICD 985; E866 (E866.1–.4)
Toxic effect of carbon monoxide	ICD 986; E867, E868 (E868.0–.9)
Toxic effect of other gases, fumes, or vapors	ICD 987; E869 (E869.0–.9)
Toxic effect of other substances Chiefly nonmedicinal as to source	ICD 989;E861 (E861.0–.9), E863 (E863.0–.9) E866 (E866.0–.9)

*ICD, International Classification of Diseases.

ria for this disease, and that 52% were due to coding errors rather than misdiagnosis.[16] States with larger farming populations than New Jersey may have more valid data on this condition, and this evaluation deserves to be repeated elsewhere.

All disease and injury discharges with workers' compensation as the primary payer logically should be work-related, bearing in mind that the diseases identified in this way are much more likely to be acute, as is the case in state-based workers' compensation data sets, than chronic or multifactorial in etiology. Suspected coding errors have limited the exploration of this approach to identifying cases in New Jersey, although it is used for occupational asthma surveillance. New Jersey has approximately 20,000 hospital records annually (not deduplicated—includes repeat admissions) where workers' compensation is the primary payer. Twenty percent of the discharges are suspected of being false positives because they are for children or for conditions such as childbirth that are not likely to be work-related. Approximately 33% of the discharges of adults are for diseases of the musculoskeletal system and approximately 35% are for injury and poisoning (unpublished data). Michigan's hospital discharge data have similar findings (Table 22.2).[17] Additional studies are needed to determine the usefulness of this surveillance strategy. Follow-back to hospitals where nonrandom coding and classification errors in the payer field are identified could greatly improve the usefulness of HDD for the identification of work-related acute disease and injury.

As noted above, the current long lag time between discharge and data availability has meant that HDD are not very useful in case-based surveillance and follow-up interventions for acute diseases and injuries. Even though E-codes are now mandated by 32 states' hospital discharge systems, most of the case-based occupational injury surveillance systems that have evolved in states have been based on other sources of data (e.g., active reporting from hospital burn centers and trauma centers, from workers' compensation systems, and from physician reports.) In the near future, lag time is less likely to be an issue because of the rapid evolution of electronic reporting systems. In New Jersey, for example, the state is planning to receive HDD electronically within 30 days of discharge by 2001. Timely case-based poisoning and injury surveillance systems can have significant public health impact.

Table 22.2 Primary Diagnosis of Workers' Compensation Hospitalizations in Michigan 1992–1997*

	1992–1993		*1994–1995*		*1996–1997*	
Primary Diagnosis	*Mean*†	%	*Mean*	%	*Mean*	%
Infectious and parasitic diseases (001–139)	21	0.3	43	0.6	58	1.0
Neoplasms (140–239)	30	0.4	15	0.2	15	0.2
Endocrine, nutritional, metabolic diseases and immunity disorders (240–279)	31	0.4	26	0.4	15	0.2
Diseases of the blood and blood forming organs (280–289)	7	0.1	5	0.1	7	0.1
Mental disorders (290–319)	124	1.6	97	1.4	61	1.0
Diseases of the nervous system and sense organs (320–389)	220	2.9	185	2.6	111	1.8
Diseases of the circulatory system (390–459)	215	2.8	185	2.6	173	2.8
Diseases of the respiratory system (460–519)	103	1.3	78	1.1	68	1.1
Diseases of the digestive system (520–579)	167	2.2	139	2.0	116	1.9
Diseases of the genitourinary system (580–629)	68	0.9	45	0.6	40	0.7
Complications of pregnancy, childbirth, and the purpureum (630–676)	65	0.9	25	0.4	37	0.6
Diseases of the skin and subcutaneous tissue (680–709)	199	2.6	249	3.6	210	3.4
Diseases of the musculoskeletal system and connective tissue (710–739)	3251	42.5	2866	41.0	2499	40.9
Congenital anomalies (740–759)	37	0.5	24	0.3	17	0.3
Conditions originating in the perinatal period (760–779)	1	< 0.1	1	< 0.1	1	< 0.1
Symptoms, signs, and ill-defined conditions (780–799)	100	1.3	108	1.5	105	1.7
Injury and poisoning (800–999)	2750	35.6	2719	38.9	2435	39.9
V codes	286	3.7	183	2.6	139	2.3
Total	7675	100	6993	100	6107	100

*Principal diagnosis was unknown for 14 cases in 1992–1993, 17 cases in 1994–1995 and 14 cases 1996–1997.

†Number of cases per year averaged over the 2 years.

From: Summary of Occupational Disease Reports to the Michigan Department of Consumer and Industry Services: 1998. Michigan State University.

HOSPITAL DISCHARGE DATA FOR POPULATION-BASED SUMMARIES: TRENDS, MAGNITUDE, GEOGRAPHIC DISTRIBUTION, AND COSTS

National, population-based trend data on pneumoconioses have been published by NIOSH in a series of reports using Medicare data and data from the National Hospital Discharge Survey that is conducted annually by the National Center for Health Statistics. Numbers, rates, and geographic distributions nationally of these diseases are presented.[18–21] State-specific data are included. Methods and results are described in detail in these reports. Table 22.3 illustrates trend data by state for silicosis from Medicare hospitalization data.

Trend analyses using HDD must address the problem of repeat admissions if the data set does not include patient name. Algorithms that can effectively eliminate repeat admissions by applying matching procedures to selected available variables (e.g., age, other demographic information, and hospital) have been developed.[22] New Jersey has analyzed hospital discharge data for the geographic distribution of pneumoconiosis cases[23] and their temporal trends[24,25] using matching algorithms. New Jersey publishes annual summary reports of occupational disease surveillance data that include cases identified from HDD (Table 22.4).

Hospital discharge data can be used to critique other sources of occupational health surveillance data. Windau et al.[26] published a study comparing the number of hospital discharges for pneumoconiosis and selected acute lung diseases (ICD 493 and 506) in four states to the number of cases that were reported in the annual survey of occupational injuries and illnesses conducted by the federal Bureau of Labor Statistics (BLS) for the same period. Approximately twice as many reports of pneumoconiosis were identified in the four states' HDD than in the BLS survey for the entire United States. Markowitz et al.[27] compared pneumoconiosis in New York State HDD to data in the state's workers' compensation system, and found six times more cases in HDD than in workers' compensation. Hospital discharge data have been used to study the costs of occupational disease. A study of hospital discharges for pneumoconiosis (1987–1990) in New Jersey found that workers' compensation covered an average of only about 2% of the annual costs for the approximately $7 to $8 million annual costs of these hospital stays.[24] A cost analysis of New Jersey hospitalizations for pneumoconiosis using a different methodology estimated that these hospitalizations in 1998 cost almost $6 million dollars.[28] Hospital discharge data were used in estimate costs in Pennsylvania, with a total estimated cost of $797 million in medical care for occupational diseases and injuries in 1988.[29]

RELATED RESEARCH

Hospital discharge data have been used for some studies that estimate the burden and scope of occupational disease.

A survey was conducted of 762 physicians who were identified by hospital discharge records of patients with pneumoconiosis. The names and addresses of the discharging physicians were determined by matching medical license number in the HDD with the list of licensed physicians maintained by the State of New Jersey. The survey showed that these physicians were seeing three to four times as many patients with work-related lung disease in their outpatient practices as were being hospitalized.[30]

Hospital discharge data from Michigan were used to examine potential associations between pneumoconioses and several other diseases including lung cancer that may be caused by exposure to the same mineral dusts, using a Standard Incidence Ratio analysis methodology. The data suggested that the association between lung cancer and coal worker's pneumoconiosis was secondary to misdiagnosis. Pneumoconiosis was found to be associated with cor pulmonale and obstructive lung disease.[31] The Michigan study was modeled on a study from Ontario Canada that had similar findings.[32]

Table 22.3 Medicare Hospitalizations with Any Mention of Silicosis, by State, from 1984 to 1989*

	Year of Hospitalization					
State	*1984*	*1985*	*1986*	*1987*	*1988*	*1989*
Alabama	34	40	59	42	58	48
Alaska	4	10	8	7	2	1
Arizona	88	45	63	58	33	42
Arkansas	17	10	17	19	13	15
California	151	152	107	141	120	113
Colorado	35	57	76	52	38	57
Connecticut	28	25	22	26	12	15

Table 22.3 (Continued)

State	Year of Hospitalization					
	1984	*1985*	*1986*	*1987*	*1988*	*1989*
Delaware	—†	1	—	—	6	4
District of Columbia	4	—	4	10	3	6
Florida	76	62	83	80	95	62
Georgia	60	73	97	68	61	36
Hawaii	2	6	—	—	—	—
Idaho	22	14	4	18	16	18
Illinois	94	92	129	95	87	70
Indiana	69	78	35	31	30	22
Iowa	12	12	15	14	13	12
Kansas	14	15	6	15	7	8
Kentucky	42	24	29	50	72	50
Louisiana	50	49	48	36	32	37
Maine	13	9	13	17	7	—
Maryland	8	22	36	29	25	24
Massachusetts	14	42	47	44	27	21
Michigan	81	136	96	128	88	89
Minnesota	35	33	34	44	42	44
Mississippi	13	19	10	12	4	14
Missouri	60	95	80	55	77	89
Montana	9	12	30	22	10	17
Nebraska	9	1	—	1	3	6
Nevada	22	9	15	24	10	13
New Hampshire	12	8	2	5	25	4
New Jersey	64	50	101	88	88	64
New Mexico	16	41	27	14	16	16
New York	54	91	121	115	135	103
North Carolina	62	90	75	86	77	69
North Dakota	5	—	1	—	—	3
Ohio	197	195	228	270	220	191
Oklahoma	11	13	18	28	16	16
Oregon	12	18	21	12	8	12
Pennsylvania	422	432	375	325	310	345
Rhode Island	9	11	21	1	2	3
South Carolina	34	17	9	11	21	19
South Dakota	19	7	4	7	5	7
Tennessee	46	70	39	63	35	36
Texas	97	79	73	88	90	69
Utah	30	52	49	13	17	54
Vermont	20	11	12	26	12	10
Virginia	87	52	74	61	60	58
Washington	38	51	54	41	44	38
West Virginia	42	45	42	33	37	44
Wisconsin	76	91	90	77	90	54
Wyoming	6	4	5	4	4	4
Total	2425	2573	2600	2506	2303	2152

Silicosis = ICD-9CM code 502.

*Table reprinted from: NIOSH. Work-Related Lung Disease Surveillance Report. DHSS (NIOSH) Publication No. 91-113. Morgantown, WV: National Institute for Occupational Safety and Health; 1991.

†—, quantity zero. Empty space indicates information not available.

Source: Medicare Provider Analysis and Review (MEDPAR), Office of Statistics and Data Management, Bureau of Data Management and Strategy, Health Care Financing Administration.

Table 22.4 Number of New Cases Reported by the New Jersey Department of Health and Senior Services Occupational Disease Reporting that Includes Hospital Discharge Data

	From beginning of reporting through:										
*Condition**	*1988*	*1989*	*1990*	*1991*	*1992*	*1993*	*1994*	*1995*	*1996*	*1997*	*Cumulative Total*
Occupational†	32	46	65	66	47	70	41	57	39	72	529
Silicosis‡	691	53	66	74	46	46	26	25	15	21	1100
Other§	1883	801	760	609	676	624	474	655	611	498	7591
Acute lung§	271	154	115	76	65	75	57	68	82	59	1022
Chemical poisonings§	894	257	248	293	217	207	141	216	150	129	2752

*Includes confirmed and unconfirmed cases.
†Data sources: hospital reports, physicians. Reporting began in 1988.
‡Data sources: hospital reports, physician reports, death certificates. Reporting began in 1979.
§Data source: hospital reports. Reporting began in 1985.

ETHICAL ISSUES

Hospital discharge data have been used by states to conduct a variety of surveillance projects that include accessing medical data on named individuals without their consent. The critical importance of the data for public health interventions is demonstrated in other chapters. Currently there are no national standards for access and protection of the privacy of medical records, and state statutes and regulations vary considerably. States with mandatory hospital reporting requirements may have easier access than states without such regulations. Researchers will need to go to their Institutional Review Boards in order to use state HDD for studies that access personal identifying information.

Although protection of patient privacy and proper use of patient medical records under research conditions is safeguarded by federal regulations, public health surveillance is considered to be exempt from these requirements.[33] Public health ethics may conflict with standards for privacy of medical records in that public health generally assumes that individual's rights may be ethically superseded for the good of the greater public. Even where state statute or regulation provides for access to medical records for the benefit of public health, generally accepted principles of ethics that have been developed for epidemiologists should apply.[34] Confidentiality guidelines for public health surveillance have been developed and these guidelines should be observed when using hospital discharge data.[34]

CONCLUSION

In spite of its limitations, HDD have been of critical importance for case-based surveillance and the development of intervention programs in several states. Several pilot studies suggest that they potentially have more applications than those currently underway; however, additional resources would be needed for the labor-intensive records reviews and required patient contacts. Their use in population-based surveillance activities have not been as extensive because of difficulties in defining denominators and the problems of disease definitions for multifactorial diseases.

ACKNOWLEDGMENTS

The author thanks her colleagues in the Occupational Health Service, New Jersey Department of Health and Senior Services, who have contributed in so many ways to the development of the surveillance systems described here.

REFERENCES

1. Baker EL. Sentinel Event Notification System for Occupational Risks (SENSOR): the concept. *Am J Public Health* 1989; 79(suppl):18–20.
2. National Association of Health Data Organizations. *1998 State Data Availability Report.* Church Falls, VA: National Association of Health Data Organizations, 1999.
3. National Association of Health Data Organizations. Personal Communication, 1999.
4. Centers for Disease Control. Surveillance for silicosis, 1993—Illinois, Michigan, New Jersey, North Carolina, Ohio, Texas, and Wisconsin. *MMWR* 1997; 46 (No. SS-1):13–28.
5. Centers for Disease Control. Silicosis; Cluster in sandblasters—Texas, and occupational surveillance for silicosis. *MMWR* 1990; 39:433-7.
6. Stanbury M, Tepper A, Ramaprasad R. Solice-Sample G. Asbestosis in New Jersey. *New Jersey Medicine* 1991; 88:195–199.
7. Stanbury M, Solice-Sample G, Pescatore J. Asbestosis disease risk communication conducted by the New Jersey Department of Health. *Am J Ind Med* 1993; 23:97–104.
8. Kipen H, Gelperin K, Tepper A, Stanbury MJ. Acute occupational respiratory diseases in hospital discharge data. *Am J Ind Med* 1991; 19:637–642.
9. Reilly MJ, Rosenman KD. Use of hospital discharge data for surveillance of chemical-related respiratory disease. *Arch Environ Health* 1995; 50:26–30.
10. Reilly MJ, Rosenman KD, Watt FC, et al. Surveillance for occupational asthma—Michigan and New Jersey, 1988–1992. *MMWR* 1994; 43(No. SS-1):9–17.

11. Jajosky RA, Harrison R, Reinisch F, et al. Surveillance of work-related asthma in selected U.S. states using surveillance guidelines for state health departments—California, Massachusetts, Michigan, and New Jersey, 1993–1995. *MMWR* 1999; 48 (No. SS-3):1–20.
12. Sorock GS, Smith E, Hall N. An evaluation of New Jersey's hospital discharge database for surveillance of severe occupational injuries. *Am J Ind Med* 1993; 23:427–437.
13. Balmes J, Rempel D, Alexander M, Reiter R, Harrison R, Bernard B, Benner D, Cone J. Hospital records as a data source for occupational disease surveillance: A feasibility study. *Am J Ind Med* 1992; 21:341–351.
14. Rutstein DD, Mullan RJ, Frazier T, Halperin W, Melius J, Sestito J. Sentinel health events (occupational): A basis for physician recognition and public health surveillance. *Am J Public Health* 1983; 73:1054–1059.
15. Pollack ES, Keimig DG. Counting Injuries and Illnesses in the Workplace: Proposals for a Better System. Washington DC: National Academy Press; 1987: 93.
16. Kipen H, Tepper A, Rosenman KD, Weinrib D. Limitations of hospital discharge diagnoses for surveillance of extrinsic allergic alveolitis. *Am J Ind Med* 1990; 17:701–709.
17. Hall JM, Reilly MJ, Rosenman KD, Kalinowski DJ. *Summary of 1998 Occupational Disease Reports to the Michigan Department of Consumer & Industry Services. Joint Report of Michigan State University and the Michigan Department of Consumer & Industry Services.* Lansing, MI; April 20, 1999.
18. National Institute for Occupational Safety and Health. *Work-Related Lung Disease Surveillance Report.* DHSS (NIOSH) Publication No. 91-113. Morgantown, WV: National Institute for Occupational Safety and Health, 1991.
19. National Institute for Occupational Safety and Health. *Work-Related Lung Disease Surveillance Report Supplement, 1992.* DHSS (NIOSH) Publication No. 91-113S. Morgantown, WV: National Institute for Occupational Safety and Health, 1992.
20. National Institute for Occupational Safety and Health. *Work-Related Lung Disease Surveillance Report, 1994.* DHSS (NIOSH) Publication No. 94-120. Morgantown, WV: National Institute for Occupational Safety and Health, 1994.
21. National Institute for Occupational Safety and Health. *Work-Related Lung Disease Surveillance Report, 1996.* DHSS (NIOSH) Publication No. 94-134. Morgantown, WV: National Institute for Occupational Safety and Health, 1996.
22. Keller JE, Howe HL, Noak JR. An algorithm for matching anonymous hospital discharge records used in occupational disease surveillance: Anonymous record matching algorithm. *Am J Ind Med* 1991; 20:657–661.
23. Rosenman KD. Use of hospital discharge data in the surveillance of occupational disease. *Am J Ind Med* 1988; 13:281–289.
24. Henneberger P, Stanbury MJ. Patterns of asbestosis in New Jersey: 1979–1986. *Am J Ind Med* 1992; 21:689–697.
25. Ramaprasad R. *Trends in Hospitalizations for Occupational Disease in New Jersey.* Presented at the annual meeting of the American Public health Association, November 1992.
26. Windau J, Rosenman K, Anderson H, Hanrahan L, Rudolph L, Stanbury M, Stark A. The identification of occupational lung disease from hospital discharge data. *J Occup Med* 1991; 33:1060–1066.
27. Markowitz S, Fisher E, Fahs M, Shapiro J, Landrigan P. Occupational disease in New York State: A comprehensive examination. *Am J Ind Med* 1989; 16:417–435.
28. Markowitz S, Landrigan P. *Occupational Disease in New Jersey: Report to the New Jersey Department of Health,* December 1989.
29. Bresnitz EA. *Occupational Disease and Injury in Pennsylvania: Report to the Pennsylvania Department of Health,* June 1990.
30. Rosenman KD, Trimbath L, Stanbury M. Surveillance of occupational lung disease: Comparison of hospital discharge data to physician reporting. *Am J Public Health* 1990; 80:1257–1258.
31. Rosenman KD, Zhu Z. Pneumoconiosis and associated medical conditions. *Am J Ind Med* 1995; 27:107–113.
32. Kasiak R, Liss GM, Gailitis MM. Cor pulmonale and pneumoconiotic lung disease: An investigation using hospital discharge data. *Am J Ind Med* 1993; 23:161–173.
33. Centers for Disease Control/Agency for Toxic Substances and Disease Registry. *Decision Making about Human Subjects Review Requirements: A Guide for CDC/ATSDR Scientists.* U.S. Department of Health and Human Services, Public Health Service, July 1994.
34. Hahn RA. Ethical Issues. In: Teutsch SM, Churchill RE, eds. *Principles and Practice of Public Health Surveillance.* New York: Oxford University Press, 1994:175–189.

23

Poison Control Centers

PAUL D. BLANC

In the United States, poison control centers (PCC) comprise a national network of consulting services to promote the prevention and treatment of poisoning and drug overdose. Similar centers exist worldwide, functioning in both industrialized nations, and, to a lesser extent, in countries with developing economies.

Since their founding in the mid-1950s, PCCs have evolved from small-scale and ad hoc emergency consultative services focused primarily on unintentional pediatric ingestions of toxins into highly structured, database-dependent full-service resources. Originally, the centers were local, typically serving one urban area. Currently, however, the U.S. American Association of Poison Control Centers is comprised of Regional Poison Control Centers that must meet a series of standard criteria to participate in the network.[1,2]

The key characteristics of poison control service are summarized in Table 23.1. Poison control centers represent a unique mechanism to capture a limited number of variables that are consistently collected on a broad range of cases.

Advantages of Poison Control Centers for Surveillance

The most important aspect of PCC case identification in the United States is its direct public access. Although health care providers are an important source of initial telephone contacts, especially for the most severely ill cases, most calls come directly from either the exposed person or a family member. Internationally, PCCs vary in this regard, with some accessible to health care professionals only. In practice, this broad access means that U.S. PCC data are not dependent on health care access nor are consultations impacted by insurance eligibility. This latter aspect is particularly relevant to exposures that may be occupationally related because no eligibility screen precludes poison control case reporting, for example, self-employed status or nonsalaried employment. Moreover, there is no minimum severity cut-off: neither lost work time duration or any other definition of severity limits case identification if exposure has taken place. Poison control center reporting does handle informational calls somewhat differently, but these are defined as telephone queries where no exposure has taken place.

Incoming telephone consultations are initially handled by staff with a wide range of training and expertise. Although there is a certification process for poison control specialists, many of whom hold advanced degree training (especially at the Doctor of Pharmacy [Parm. D.] level), paraprofessionals are also used widely.[2] Despite these differences in staffing, physician back-up and quality assurance oversight is integral to the system, insuring a fairly consistent level of service nationwide. A key element of consistency is built into the structure of data collection, which is standardized.[1]

The data collection structure is directly relevant to any potential application of case reporting to occupational disease surveillance. This structure builds in two critical data fields that can identify occupationally related events: one field classifies type of case, with occupational as one of multiple options (alternate choices include intentional-abuse, environmental, and general); and a second field identifies the location of exposure (home being the predominant entry).

Another strength is the consistent emphasis given to exposure identification. In the occupational arena this

Table 23.1 Key Characteristics of Regional Poison Control Center Services in the United States

STRENGTHS

- Direct telephone access to both the general public and to health care professionals
- No link to general insurance or dependence on workers' compensation criteria
- Varying levels of expertise of initial telephone consultant, but physician back-up at all times
- Structured data collection into a computerized format
- Coding of site of exposure with workplace
- Coding of exposure type with occupational
- Aggressive identification of exposure, at least at the level generic descriptors
- Case fatalities studied in detail

LIMITATIONS

- Potential case detection (selection) biases related to awareness and severity
- No classification of occupation or industry even if occupationally related
- Demographic data are limited and inconsistent
- Symptom assessment targeted and not structured
- Outcome severity broadly defined as mild, moderate, severe
- Follow-up contact information voluntary on part of caller
- Follow-up limited to more severe, acute cases

can be limited to a generic exposure classification only, depending on the information available. This is particularly true of commercial products, for example sealant, paint, or detergent. Industrial chemicals are far more likely to be specified both by a generic classification that codes at a material-specific level (epoxy or trichloroethylene rather than glue or solvent) and, additionally, by chemical specific code number (CAS) as well. Poison control center data also include a route of exposure field that includes options for dermal and ocular exposure as well as toxin inhalation, ingestion, or envenomation.

American Association of Poison Control Centers policies put additional emphasis on supplemental data collection and reporting for all cases with fatal outcomes. This includes detailed information in a narrative format drawing on medical records and coroner case investigations when available. Selected narratives are summarized in annual reporting.[1]

Limitations of Poison Control Center Data

Case detection is passive. It depends on factors such as awareness and satisfaction of both the general public and health care providers. The data are population-based, but do not reflect systematic outreach and sampling. For these reasons, case reporting biases can impact the data in important ways. First is that more severe cases are more likely to be reported. This became evident, for example, when cases identified through an active surveillance system, such as the Drug Awareness Warning Network (DAWN) were checked against PCC consultations.[3] Secondly, more exotic or combinations of toxins are more likely to lead to consultation, for example a medication or drug new on the market or poly-drug overdose compared to a familiar material, whether legal or illegal.

There is a more specific limitation in occupational disease surveillance: the lack of routine and systematic collection of occupation (job) or industry of employment. Although such data may sometimes be imbedded within the narrative text of a case consultation, it is difficult to extract and inconsistent when present. Demographic data are routinely collected, but with less severe intoxications, age is not always specified (the notation of adult is common). Gender is typically available and reliable. Another limitation is that prominent symptoms are elicited and coded, but systematic symptom reviews are not carried out. The majority of case referrals have either no symptoms or minimal symptoms, the latter classified as a minor effect. Symptoms can also be classified as moderate or major using guidelines promulgated by the American Association of Poison Control Centers.[1] Nonetheless, these are fairly broad and overlapping categories, thus limiting interpretation. The principal effort in follow-up is appropriately directed to the moderate-major cases. In those cases, the call has typically been initiated by a health care provider, insuring call-back access. Calls into the PCC that do not originate from health care centers often cannot be returned for follow-up because a call-back number has either not been requested or has not been provided by the caller. Also, there is no fixed or standardized period for PCC follow-up telephone calls. For these reasons it is not possible to estimate from routine PCC data morbidity measures such as restricted activities days or lost workdays. In contrast, variables such as hospitalization (yes or no) or mortality are more readily interpretable from the data.

Incidence Data

Poison control centers commonly consult in occupational cases. Table 23.2 summarizes incidence data from a series of reports of occupational illness derived from poison control center data.[4–10] The consistency across the United States and worldwide is impressive. The choice of denominator used has a large impact on the incidence and proportion of cases specific to age groups. Poison control centers receive relatively few reports of occupational exposures among children. In the large U.S. series, only 1.2% of 25,368 occupational

Table 23.2 Poison Control Center Reporting of Occupational Illness

		% Occupational		
Poison Center Location	*Total Cases*	*All Cases*	*Adult Cases*	*Ref. No.*
United States national data	1,368,748	1.8	5.5*	4
Philadelphia region	7760	NA†	4.8	5
San Francisco region	10,277	1.8	NA	6
Cincinnati	32,000	1.9	NA	7
Taiwan	23,436	5.5	7.2	8
Netherlands	6856	NA	4.4*	9
Switzerland	4830	3.2	NA	10

*Adult defined in these studies as age ≥ 13 years.
†NA, not available.

cases were reported to be among those younger than 13 years of age;[4] in a series from Taiwan the proportion among those 18 years or younger was 2.2% of 1293.[8] A comparison between these two studies also underscores the variation in overall case mix and how it can impact these estimates. In the United States, approximately 65% of cases were under age 13, whereas in the Taiwan data set, only 21% fell into this age range. Because varying proportions of pediatric cases will dilute the estimate of the proportion of occupational cases, expressing the incidence in terms of adult cases may allow more standard comparisons across centers. Nonetheless, even a small number of cases in the pediatric age group may be of interest because other data sources for detecting occupational illness among adolescents are so fragmentary. This would identify a need for surveillance that would be unlikely to be met by workers' compensation data, and where even limited numbers of PCC cases could provide important insights.

Another way in which raw PCC incidence can be compared is on the basis of symptomatic (minor effect or greater severity) compared to asymptomatic (no effect) cases. As noted previously, asymptomatic cases form an important contribution to overall PCC incidence, disproportionately so among younger age groups. This trend is further amplified by disproportionate severity among occupational cases. In the large U.S. series, 71% of the occupational cases were symptomatic compared to 27% of all others (excluding environmental cases).[4] In a follow-up study based on a second series of San Francisco Bay Area Regional Poison Control Center data (not shown in Table 23.2) limited to symptomatic cases, the occupationally related cases comprised 456 of 5849 (7.8%) consultations over the 6-month study period.[11] Age, occupation, and symptoms appear to be interrelated. This suggests that the proportions cited in Table 23.2 would rise even higher if they were restricted to symptomatic adult cases. It is reasonable to summarize the data among all adult cases. Thus, approximately 4%–5% of adult PCC cases are occupational.

Descriptive Data by Route of Exposure

Routinely collected PCC data also provide a basis for comparing route of exposure in different groups and surveillance systems. Exposure by route of inhalation or dermal (skin) contact has been reported more frequently among occupational cases compared to other cases for which ingestion is the predominant route. For example, in the United States, 44% of the occupational cases were by inhalation and 26% by skin contact compared to only 4% and 10%, respectively, among more than a million nonoccupational, nonenvironmental cases.[4] Overall, 13% of all inhalation or dermal cases were occupational. In the Netherlands, 81% of the occupational cases reported inhalation or dermal contamination as the primary exposure route;[9] in Taiwan, the combined proportion was greater than 90%.[8]

Another important exposure route among occupational cases is ocular contact, reported by 22% of occupational compared to less than 6% of all others in the United States.[4] Expressed proportionally among ocular cases alone, 8% of cases with this route of exposure category were occupational. In the San Francisco Bay Area Regional Poison Control Center, 42 (11%) of all 368 symptomatic ocular exposure cases over 5 years of age were occupational.[12]

These data indicate that the proportion of occupationally related cases may be high enough to impact the overall frequencies of descriptive variables (demographics, exposure types, case severity). Furthermore, they suggest that subcategories of subjects can be identified, independent of the case type field (where the occupational designation is one option), where an enriched proportion of occupational cases can be expected, for example, adult, symptomatic, inhalation exposures. This enrichment could be used to facilitate interpretation of surveillance data.

Because the exposure routes differ between occupational and nonoccupational cases, this could lead to reporting biases if there are systematic differences in PCC referrals driven by this factor. This would be possible, for example, to the extent that public or health care provider awareness of poison control relevance to inhalations or skin exposure might be less than public awareness of the availability of poison control intervention for ingested toxins. One study assessing whether toxic exposures treated in an emergency department resulted in a PCC consultation, observed that although 31% of all cases were indeed referred, this proportion fell to only 14% among inhalation cases.[13]

Even relatively uncommon routes of exposure may be particularly relevant to targeted surveillance questions. Within the occupational context, for example, high pressure injection injuries comprise an infrequent but important group of PCC case referrals. These exposures, due to misfiring of paint spray guns, for example, can lead to significant morbidity. For such events, the appropriate classification in the PCC schema for route of exposure would be parenteral. Although this is the least frequent exposure category reported for occupational cases (0.5% nationally) it is more common than among all others (0.3%).[4] Another example of PCC data used to target a relatively uncommon route of exposure would be the category of bite/sting (also less than 1% of occupational cases), particularly if the focus were on occupations of anticipated risk of such events, such as agricultural workers or laboratory animal handlers.

Exposure Frequencies

The level of detail is often variable for specific exposures obtained through routine PCC consultation. Across broadly defined groups of chemicals, it is easier to interpret for surveillance purposes. Pesticides are one such example, accounting for 8% of U.S. occupational cases;[4] 21% in the Netherlands;[9] and 61% in Taiwan.[8] In the urban San Francisco (U.S.) regional center, only 3% of occupational cases had pesticide exposures.[6]

Comparing the frequency of cases by exposure category can also be a useful alternative approach to case detection. For example, in cases of pesticides, a significant number of these exposures would be anticipated to arise from occupational causes, but this can vary widely. In the United States, the proportion is less than 5% and in a Minnesota study it is even lower (4%), largely because asymptomatic household exposures to low toxicity pesticides are major contributors to incidence.[4,14] In contrast, in a poison control series of 1274 pesticide exposure cases from Costa Rica, 34% were occupational.[15] The State of California, as an adjunct to its pesticide illness reporting system, has used PCC data as supplementary case-finding sources for both occupational and nonoccupational cases.[16]

For specific chemicals, PCC data are particularly well-suited to surveillance because the identification of exposure is fairly specific and reliable. Examples include carbon monoxide, cyanide, and methylene chloride. In addition, acute toxic syndromes due to exotic or novel chemicals are also likely to be reported to PCCs. This is most relevant to the surveillance goal of identifying sentinel health events. Case detection at PCCs has indeed been pivotal in a number of toxic chemical illness outbreaks.

Special Categories of Exposure

Case detection has particular advantages for certain categories of exposure and disadvantages for others. One prominent class of exposures that results in fairly frequent PCC consultations is potential reproductive hazards. Although the bulk of these are prescription and nonprescription pharmaceuticals, occupationally related exposures are common. In one series of 335 reproductive exposure case consultations over a 3-month period to the Washington State Regional Poison Control Center, 38 (11%) were occupational.[17] The occupational reproductive health consultations were slightly less than one call per thousand total calls to the center, underscoring their frequency.

Exposures classified as environmental present a distinct disadvantage in the interpretation of PCC data. The intent of this category is to identify exposure scenarios such as ambient or bystander contamination or ingestion of materials contaminating food or beverages. Exposures that may occur on the job are commonly classified as environmental if not arising out of routine work activities of the person exposed. This could include inhalation exposure to cleaning fumes or paint vapors in an office being cleaned or under maintenance or contaminated air due to malfunction of high volume air cleaning (HVAC) equipment. Environmental cases are one-third as frequent as those classified as occupational in national data.[4] Nonetheless, they probably do lead to undercounting when occupational cases are defined narrowly. For example, in a study of 323 inhalation exposure cases reported to a poison control center, 96 (30%) were initially coded as occupational.[18] Based on detailed systematic follow-up interviews, 6 of these were found to be coded incorrectly as occupational, while 32 were found to have been miscoded predominantly as environmental, for a total occupational increase of 27%.

Time Trends

One important use of surveillance data is to track time trends. U.S. PCC data from 1983 through 1988 were analyzed in this regard. Because the number of PCCs participating in the national data collection system has shifted over time, the denominator has not been stable. Expressed as a rate per million population served by the poison centers each year, occupational case reporting however, demonstrated an increase from 57 to 163 per million over 5 years.[4] Moreover, the increase showed a strong linear trend from year to year. The nearly threefold rise compared with a less than twofold rise for environmental cases over the same period. By 1996, the rate of occupational cases (based on 47,033 reports) was 202 per million, a further increase of 23% during a period when overall poison center reporting increased by approximately 12%.[1] Time trends in reporting can reflect two forces at work: a true increase in incidence, and an increased utilization rate of poison control services in the catchment population. Poison control centers refer to this as penetrance, reflecting, in part, public awareness of and access to the services offered. International time trends have not been reported.

Comparative Case Detection

Another critical issue in any surveillance data base is its potential overlap with other existing case detection systems. Because of the advantages listed in Table 23.1, particularly its independence from workers' compensation, poison control incidence would appear to be an ideal data set for novel case detection. Multiple investigators have indeed found this to be the case.[5,6,9–11] Major studies examining this question are summarized in Table 23.3.

The best studied overlap has been the comparison between surveillance through the California State Doctor's First Report (DFR) program and PCC case detection. Because the DFR is a physician-mandated reporting program independent of workers' compensation or U.S. Occupational Safety and Health Administration (OSHA) data, that program is considered to be a near gold standard against which other surveillance approaches can be measured. In two separate analyses, the first using broad matching criteria across cases and the second through direct manual review, fewer than one-quarter of PCC cases were captured by the DFR.[6,11] Part of this was accounted for by ineligibility: the PCC consultations included cases that were not physician-treated or were for self-employed persons for whom a DFR need not be filed. But even among hospitalized cases, capture was poor.

Table 23.3 Poison Control Detection: Case Overlap With Other Surveillance Systems

Comparison System	*Percent Case Overlap*	*Ref. No.*
California Doctor's First Report	16	6
California Doctor's First Report		11
All cases	22	11
Hospitalized cases	29	11
OSHA* log	23	11
Workers' Compensation	7	5
Dutch Directorate General of Labor	3	9
Swiss Occupation Insurance Fund		10
All cases	66	10
Worksites < 15 employees	28	10

*OSHA, Occupational Safety and Health Administration.

Other studies, although limited, suggest that surveillance based on OSHA logs or workers' compensation data are likely to miss at least as many cases captured though PCC surveillance.[5,11] Despite the potential richness of PCC data as a surveillance tool, relatively few studies of overlap have been made, especially in terms of workers' compensation data. The estimate of 7% workers' compensation overlap (Table 23.3) is based on 5 of 73 cases that reported having sick leave covered by compensation insurance.[5] In the earlier California study, although claims data were not available, only 17% of the cases reported at least 2 lost workdays, a typical cut-off for workers' compensation reporting.[11] Internationally, the picture is very much the same. Even the Swiss Occupational Insurance Fund, which has a 66% overlap with poison center cases overall, falls off sharply to 28% when smaller sites of employment are considered separately.[10] Formal capture–recapture modeling (Chapter 13) estimating case overlap with poison control data has not been reported.

Poison Control Case Follow-up Studies

Because routine PCC data collection has limitations, investigators have exploited the initial case detection in order to carry out more detailed follow-up investigations. In the simplest model, poison control consultations are considered as index cases. For example, four cases over 4 years of severe methylene chloride toxicity reported to the Rocky Mountain Poison and Drug Center occurring in small-scale furniture-stripping shops, prompted a systematic survey of 21 shops in the poison center's catchment area.[19] Targeted case follow-up has also been used to gather information on factors influencing patient referral and follow-up in green tobacco sickness, a form of nicotine poisoning in agricultural tobacco workers.[20]

Detailed follow-up interviews of PCC cases have allowed analysis of a variety of symptom and treatment-related questions that cannot be easily studied otherwise. Of particular surveillance interest are data addressing the circumstances of exposure. In a California study, 19% of all exposures occurred via a spill, splash, or spray.[11] Researchers in Switzerland estimated 22% with this exposure scenario.[10] In contrast, siphoning exposures occurred in 4% of the former and only 1% of the latter series. The two studies can also be compared in terms of recent similar coworker exposures (separate from the event in question) that were reported by 17% of the California series[11] and 19% of the Swiss series.[11] Worker awareness of Right-to-Know legislation has also been ascertained in at least two separate studies. The study cited previously estimated such awareness among 43% of those surveyed (California),[11] whereas a second study estimated a lower proportion of 27% (Delaware Valley).[5] Follow-up studies have also been used to assess risk factors and outcomes in inhalational and ocular poison control cases.[12,18,21,22]

Health Services Research

To a limited extent, PCCs have been the focus of research addressing health services as they relate to occupational health. A 1989 survey of 49 PCCs found that only 8% had occupational health specialists within their center and less than half had ongoing access to such a specialist outside the center.[23] Ten years later, a survey of 33 regional poison control centers found that most purported to have high levels of occupationally related services, but when some of these centers participated in a blinded role-playing exercise, the consultation services actually offered fell short, with only 2 of 19 centers actually recommending that the employee in the simulated case actually report the illness as work-related.[24]

Other health services studies have addressed theoretical models of PCC services or training needs to address occupational disease.[7,25] Of greater relevance to surveillance, one study systematically analyzed why both physician and nonphysician care providers contacted the PCC for consultations following occupational exposures.[2] For the nonphysician case contacts, less than half were aware that the PCC specifically dealt with occupational exposures, whereas three-quarters of the physicians were not only aware, but had actually consulted the PCC in such cases previously.[26] Only 11% of the nonphysician cases consulted poison control in order to identify the exposure, whereas this was the motivating factor for 21% of the physician calls. In contrast, the proportion seeking risk assessment was similar in the two groups (41% compared to 38%). Earlier analysis of the same data found that the specialty of the physician-treated occupational cases referred to the PCC was occupational or preventive medicine in only 2% of the cases.[11]

CASE STUDY

Details of the methods and outcomes of one PCC study illustrates the strengths and weaknesses of this approach to surveillance.[11]

Define Goals, Objectives, and Scope

The primary goal was to use PCC data to identify previously uncaptured incidence of occupational cases. Preliminary analyses showed that occupational case reports were fairly frequent and were weighted to types of illnesses less common in standard surveillance. By identifying new cases, more accurate estimates of underreporting by established surveillance schemes could be made.

The geographic scope was limited to cases reported to the regional PCC of the San Francisco Bay Area, which is predominantly urban. This made the surveillance less likely to capture certain groups of exposures, for example, agricultural chemicals or exposures encountered in primary metal manufacturing. The nature of PCC reporting also made it less relevant for occupational illnesses such as asbestosis or silicosis, or to most occupational trauma, whether acute or chronic.

The scope of the project was influenced strongly by earlier experience with an analysis of occupational cases in PCC data.[6] From the analyses it was apparent that a study confined to the information in the basic case PCC log (Fig. 23.1) would seriously limit the scope of the project in such key areas as occupation, lost work time, and even personal identifiers that could be used to match cases to other surveillance systems. The key element to the expanded scope of this surveillance project was the use of structured follow-up interviews. A second element was the intention to manually review data from one surveillance system—the California Doctor's First Report (DFR)—and to obtain copies of a limited number of OSHA injury logs (Appendix A).

Based on the previous studies, it was estimated that up to 1000 symptomatic cases might be reported to the PCC over a 1-year period. Given the labor intensive nature of the proposed follow-up, including multiple interviews and manual records review, a sample of 300 cases was targeted. Because the occupations in the catchment area of the PCC were not seasonal, the project began on July 1 and ended on December 31 of a single calendar year.

Assemble a Multidisciplinary Team

Most PCCs function in an interdisciplinary environment with both physician and nonphysician poison specialists. This was reflected in the study team assembled for this project. Another key aspect was the integration of staff from the state health department's occupational health program. This included epidemiologic expertise.

Gain Support

A critical aspect of support was that the principal investigator had clinical duties with the PCC, but was

```
CENTER     Friday  07/23/99     11:00        Page 1 of 10
Date:07/23/99     Reviewer# 999      Time:    :    #FU    #FU-SPI#    Case #:4108712
Substance 1:
 Contents 1:                                              Mg-1:
 Exposure 1:             Generic 1:
Substance 2:
 Contents 2:                                              Mg-2:
 Exposure 2:             Generic 2:

 History Entry
 History: Memo



Patient Name:                              Age:  -      Time  -
         Zip:                 Patient phone: (   )      -     Lbs:     Kg:
 Caller Name:                                           Relation:
Hospital:                                               Pt ID#
    City:                     Caller# (   )    -        ER#(   )    -
    QFI?F    Consult?F     Consultant          Hazmat/911->          2ndary PCC?F
```

```
Call & Caller Type - Sex - Age Entry
Month:   7 Day: 23  Year:99 DOW: FRIDAY      Time:   0          Case #:4108712
   Mg/Kg calculations                                         Victim Type
 Substance 1 Component         Mg/Kg:                       Patient:     Multiple
                                                            1.) Human   0.) Single
 Substance 2 Component         Mg/Kg:                       2.) Animal  1.) Multiple

                                                              Sex
 Call Type        Acute/Chronic                                   Sex:
 0.) Exposure     1.) Acute    2.) Acute-on-Chronic               1.) Male
 1.) Drug Info    3.) Chronic 4.) Unknown                         2.) Female
 2.) Drug ID                                                      3.) Unknown
 3.) Environment  Duration:                                       4.) Pregnant
 4.) Medical      1.) >8hrs   <=24hrs                            Weeks pregnant
 5.) Occupation   2.) >24hrs <=1Wk                            (Code 99 for unknown)
 6.) Poison       3.) >1Wk    <=1Mo
 7.) Prev/Safety  4.) >1Mo   <=3Mo    Age Entry
 8.) Teratogen    5.) >3Mo           Age:    Age Type:  (1=yr/2=mo/3=day)
 9.) Other        6.) Unknown        Unknown Age:   Enter for lookup Table
```

```
AAPCC Substance Entry - Route of Exposure
Product Codes/Generic Codes                                 Case Number:    4108712
Substance 1:
   AAPCC#->                     Generic#->                     Location:
Substance 2:                                                       (Zip Code)
   AAPCC#->                     Generic#->                        State: 05
Total Substances Involved:      Reverse Priority                  (Ca.-05)
** From 3 - 9 Substances **     -Enter 1 to Reverse-              Center: 14

         Exposure Route
      Ingestion                      Animal Species
      Inhaled/Nasal                   Species:
      Aspiration                      1.) Cat      6.) Horse
      Ocular                          2.) Dog      7.) Rodent/LM
      Dermal                          3.) Bird     8.) Sheep/Goat
      Bite/Sting                      4.) Aquatic 9.) Other
      Parenteral                      5.) Cow
      Unknown
```

Figure 23.1 Selected data entry screens of poison control center automated log.

also an independent occupational health researcher with an academic base. The principal investigator served as a bridge between the state health department and the PCC. A key aspect of buy-in was the willingness of the PCC telephone specialists to go out of their way to note personal identifiers for call-back in some cases that might otherwise not have been recontacted as part of routine PCC activities. During peak times, even a few extra moments on the telephone can be a burden to the staff. The PCC alliance was critical in

```
Patient Flow
Patient Flow                                            Case Number:     4108712
   1.) Managed on site (non-HCF)
   2.) Patient was in (or enroute to ) HCF when PCC called *(Code)

Hospital Flow -----------------------------------------------------------------
 1.) Treated/evaluated and released       4.) Admitted to psychiatric facility
 2.) Admitted to critical care unit       5.) Patient Lost to FU/Left AMA
 3.) Admitted to noncritical care areas

   3.) Patient was referred to PCC to a HCF
   Referral: ------------------------------------------------------------------
 1.) Treated/evaluated and released       4.) Admitted to psychiatric facility
 2.) Admitted to critical care unit       5.) Patient refused referral/no show
 3.) Admitted to noncritical care unit    6.) Patient lost to FU/left AMA

   4.) Other *(Code)    Initial HCF                  Referred HCF
   5.) Unknown            Initial HCF:                 Referral HCF:
                        Enter 6 digit HCF Code       Enter 6 digit HCF Code
```

```
Therapy Provided
Therapy Provided:                        Medical Outcome        Case No: 4108712
1.) No therapy necessary              Followed to known outcome-----------------
2.) Observation only                  0.) No effect
3.) Patient refused any help          1.) Minor effect      Duration of Effect
4.) Unknown if Tx provided            2.) Moderate effect   Enter for Look-up
                                      3.) Major effect
Decontamination                       4.) Death
Ipecac                                Not Followed to Known Outcome-------------
Charcoal (Single)                     5.) Judged as nontoxic-effect no effect
Lavage (MDAC)                         6.) Minimal clinical effects possible
Cathartic                             7.) Unable to follow-potentially toxic exp
Whole Bowel Irrigation              Exposure probably not responsible for effect
Other emetic                          8.) Unrelated-probably not responsible
Dilute/Irrigate/Wash                  9.) Confirmed non exposure
Fresh air                                                               OVERRIDE
Food/Snack                                  Use to override data QA =>Override F
```

```
Symptoms Coding
Symptoms Coding - Hematologic/Neurologic/Ocular
Case No: 4108712                     Neurologic
1=Related  2=unrelated         Agitated/irritable         Muscle Rigidity
3=Unknown if related           Ataxia                     Muscle Weakness
Hematological                  Coma                       Paralysis
AST, ALT >100 <=1000           Confusion                  Peripheral Neuropathy
AST, ALT >1000                 CVA                        Sz (single)
Bilirubin                      Dizziness/vertigo          Sz (Mult./discrete)
Cytopenia                      Drowsiness/lethargy        Sz (status)
DIC                            Dystonia                   Slurred speech
Hemolysis                      Fasiculations              Syncope
PT prolongation                Hallucin./Delusions        Tinnitus
Other Coagulopathy             Headache                   Tremor
Other LFT                      Intracranial bleed

Ocular Effects
Blurred Vision           Irritation/pain    Mydriasis     Pupil(s) nonreactive
Burns                    Lacrimation        Nystagmus     Visual defect
Corneal Abrasions        Miosis             Papilledema
```

Source: San Francisco Bay Area Poison Control Center, 1999

Figure 23.1 (Continued)

that health care providers contacted as part of a PCC-based study were more likely to cooperate in being interviewed and in helping locate the cases for call-back (i.e., pulling emergency department records for review), because of a positive view of PCC services based on pervious personal experience. This also promoted participation by the cases once they were contacted for interview. Compliance would likely have been less successful had the follow-up been carried out outside the PCC structure. Another key aspect of support was the leverage of the state health department, which provided legal access to DFRs and pesticide illness reports held by other state agencies, and OSHA logs held by employers.

Case Definition and Data Collection

Eligible PCC cases were defined as follows:

1. the case originated in California, and
2. the case was coded according to the American Association of PCC criteria as:
   a. occupational
   b. symptomatic
   c. the symptoms were assessed by the PCC as related or potentially related to the presumed exposure

Because the log data were not computerized at the time of the study and data were manually extracted, the minimum data set included case demographics, exposure, case type, physician treatment, and outcome of case.

This study used data from the PCC log (Fig. 23.1) and a follow-up questionnaire administered by telephone. Because the initial PCC contact could have been the exposed person, a health care provider or a third party (i.e., family member or coworker), three separate structured interviews were used: (*1*) a brief interview for the health care provider, (*2*) a brief interview for a third party, and (*3*) a longer interview for the exposed person.

The interview for the health care provider focused on case mix and practice setting, familiarity with PCC services, and the reason for referral. The third-party interview covered the nature of the referral and familiarity with the PCC. The in-depth interview with the exposed person assessed the circumstances of exposure, duration and severity of symptoms, health care utilization, and details of employment. Most questionnaire items were close-ended, but items on exposure circumstances were open-ended and coded later into categories: spill, spray, or splash; lack of process or product familiarity, work in a closed space; siphoning, leak from an otherwise closed system; other equipment malfunction; exposure arising from routine operations; and not otherwise classified.

Interviews of exposed persons took about 20–30 minutes, and those for health care providers were 5–10 minutes.

This study compared PCC cases with those identified through three separate California surveillance systems: Doctor's First Reports (Department of Industrial Relations), Pesticide Illness Reports (California Department of Pesticide Regulation), and OSHA 200 logs. Because of concerns with confidentiality at small worksites, OSHA logs were requested only for workplaces with 10 or more employees. Many callers still declined to specifically identify their workplaces. By ascertaining lost workdays in the follow-up questionnaire, it was possible to determine if the cases were eligible for workers' compensation.

Mechanism for Reporting

The basic mechanism for reporting was telephone calls to the PCC. Fax transmission is increasing in importance to exchange follow-up information and even emergency department charts between health care providers and the PCC. However, at the time of this study this was not available.

Selecting, Recruiting, and Training Reporters

The reporters include health care professionals and the general public, which are a self-selected group with access to a telephone. The PCC staff itself is highly trained in poison management, although occupational events comprise only a small fraction of their case load.

Protocols for Follow-up

The case definition was designed to screen out calls that were informational by requiring symptoms to be noted in the initial PCC log. Thus, cases that become symptomatic after the initial PCC contact were screened out, as well as cases that did not report their symptoms in the initial contact with PCC staff. An important limitation is that only cases noted as occupational were followed-up. Many cases miscoded as environmental may have been occupational.

Analysis and Interpretation

There were 461 cases on the PCC logs that met the eligibility criteria for being symptomatic occupational cases. Of these, 135 (29%) could not be contacted. All but 10 were due to insufficient contact information, since providing such data is voluntary; only 2% of the eligible subjects declined to participate when contacted. There was an important difference between those contacted and those lost to follow-up. Of the 301 cases that were interviewed, 60% were referred by health care professionals. Of the 161 not interviewed, 33% were referred by health care professionals. There was no statistical difference in the pattern of exposures either by type or route, and, despite the difference in referral source, the proportion classified by the PCC as having moderate to severe symptoms was similar (18% versus 20%). The distribution of broad occupational categories was also similar between the cases from the two referral sources.

Key findings for the overlap of cases reported in the other California surveillance systems are presented in Table 23.3. Because 26% of the cases were not treated by physicians, they were not eligible for reporting in the physician-based surveillance systems. Even after taking this into account, the actual detection of cases through the DFR was much lower—in the range of 15%–30%. If the DFR appeared to miss four out of five cases of acute occupational illnesses, it is likely that detection of chronic disease would be even poorer. A conservative estimate of the true annual incidence of occupational illness in California could be as high as 185,000 cases, based on the 35,000 to 40,000 DFRs reported annually. Since California represents approximately 10% of the work force, the national estimate may be near 2 million cases per year.

Feedback and Dissemination of Results

The results of the study were disseminated largely through peer-reviewed publications. In those publications, priority was given to general medical publications more likely to be read by physicians in general practice.[11,26] In addition, the data were presented in detailed reports circulated by the state health department.

CONCLUSION

Poison control center case detection of occupationally related illness presents a rich source of data that can be exploited for surveillance. The cases are frequent, approximating 50,000 per year in the United states. The proportion of general PCC referrals that are occupational is 4%–5% of all adult case consultations and of even greater relative frequency among certain broadly defined types of cases, such as inhalational or ocular exposures. The greatest advantage of PCC case detection is the broad surveillance net it throws out by providing direct access to the general public as well as to health care providers. Of particular importance, PCC reporting is completely independent of workers' compensation. For this reason, most PCC cases do not appear to be captured by other surveillance mechanisms. The limitations of PCC surveillance result from the nature of the basic data collection, geared to acute management questions. This shortcoming can be addressed by structured follow-up studies where additional data can be gathered by questionnaire, medical record review, or even worksite visits.

REFERENCES

1. Litovitz TL, Smilkstein M, Felberg L, Klein-Schwartz W, Berlin R, Morgan JL. 1996 annual report of the American Association of Poison Control Centers Toxic Exposure Surveillance System. *Am J Emerg Med* 1997; 15:447–500.
2. Geller RJ, Fisher JG, Leeper JD, Rangathan S. American poison control centers: still not all the same. *Ann Emerg* Med 1988; 17:599–603.
3. Blanc PD, Jones MR, Olson KR. Surveillance of poisoning and drug overdose through hospital discharge coding, poison control center reporting, and the Drug Abuse Warning Network. *Am J Emerg Med* 1993; 11:14–19.
4. Litovitz T, Oderda G, White JD, Sheridan MJ. Occupational and environmental exposures reported to poison centers. *Am J Public Health* 1993; 83:739–743.
5. Bresnitz EA. Poison control center follow-up of occupational disease. *Am J Public Health* 1990; 80:711–712.
6. Blanc PD, Olson KR. Occupationally related illness reported to a regional poison control center. *Am J Public Health* 1986; 76:1303–1307.
7. Bonfiglio JF, Clark CS, Sigell LT, Subet V, Rice CH, Radike MJ, Hayes KM. Poison centers: a resource for occupational health services. *Vet Hum Toxicol* 1988; 30:569–572.
8. Yang CC, Wu JF, Ong HC, Hung SC, Kuo YP, Sa CH, Chen SS, Deng JF. Taiwan National Poison Center: epidemiologic data 1985-1993. *Clin Toxicol* 1996; 34:651–663.
9. Lam de Cort W, Sangster B. Acute intoxications during work. *Vet Hum Toxicol* 1988; 30:9–11.
10. Hinnen U, Hotz P, Gossweiler B, Gutzwiller F, Meier PJ. Surveillance of occupational illness through a national poison control center: an approach to reach small scale enterprises? *Int Arch Occup Environ Health* 1994; 66:117–123.
11. Blanc PD, Rempel D, Maizlish N, Hiatt O, Olson KR. Occupational illness: case detection by poison control surveillance. *Ann Int Med* 1989; 111:238–244.
12. Saunders SK, Kempainen R, Blanc PD. Outcomes of ocular exposures reported to a regional poison control center. *J Toxicol Cut Ocular Toxicol* 1996; 15:249–259.
13. Clark RF, Harchelroad F, Dean B, Krenzelok E. Treated vs. reported toxic exposures: discrepancies between a poison control center and a member hospital.(Abstract). *Vet Hum Toxicol* 1989;31:330.
14. Olson DK, Sax L, Gunderson P, Sioris L. Pesticide poisoning surveillance through regional poison control centers. *Am J Public Health* 1991; 81:750–753.
15. Leveridge YR. Pesticide reporting in Costa Rica during 1996. *Vet Hum Toxicol* 1998; 40:42–44.
16. Richmond D. *Pesticide Exposure and Information Calls Handled by the Los Angeles County Medical Association Regional Poison Information Center June, 1986.* HS-1395. Sacramento, California: California Department of Food and Agriculture, Division of Pesticide Management Branch, 1987.
17. Luderer U, Burgess JL, Polifka JE, Robertson WO. Calls on reproductive and developmental toxicants to a regional poison control center. *Vet Hum Toxicol* 1999; 41:42–46.
18. Blanc PD, Galbo M, Hiatt P, Olson KR. Morbidity following acute irritant inhalation in a population-based study. *JAMA* 1991; 266:664–669.
19. Hall AH, Rumack BH. Methylene chloride exposure in furniture-stripping shops: ventilation and respirator use practices. *J Occup Med* 1990; 32:33–37.
20. McKnight RH, Dawson SK, Westneat SC, Rodgers GC, Ross MP. Delay among the general public in telephoning a poison center. *Vet Hum Toxicol* 1996; 38:92–95.

21. Blanc PD, Galbo MS, Balmes JR, Olson KR. Occupational factors in work-related inhalations: inferences for prevention strategy. *Am J Ind Med* 1994; 25:783–791.
22. Blanc PD, Galbo M, Hiatt P, Olson KR, Balmes JR. Symptoms, lung function and airway responsiveness following irritant inhalation. *Chest* 1993; 103:1699–1705.
23. Grbcich PA, Pepper LB, Brooks D, Woolf AD. Provision of occupational health services: report of a survey of poison centers. (Abstract) *Vet Hum Toxicol* 1989; 31:366.
24. Bresnitz EA, Gittleman JL, Shic F, Temple B. A national survey of regional poison control centers' management of occupational exposure calls. *J Occup Environ Med* 1999; 41:93–99.
25. Bresnitz EA. A model system for occupational disease surveillance activities applying Centers for Disease Control guidelines to poison control centers. *J Occup Med* 1990; 32:255–259.
26. Blanc PD, Maizlish N, Hiatt P, Olson KR, Rempel D. Occupational illness and the poison control center: referral patterns and service needs. *West J Med* 1990; 152:181–184.

24

Workers' Compensation Information Systems

NEIL A. MAIZLISH AND LINDA A. RUDOLPH

The Division of Workers' Compensation (DWC) is the state agency in the California Department of Industrial Relations (DIR) that oversees the administration of workers' compensation benefits to the nearly 1.5 million injured workers each year.[1] Approximately $8 billion annually is spent; benefits include medical care, wage replacement income, vocational rehabilitation, and death benefits. Workers' compensation claims are administered by over 500 insurance companies, third party administrators, or self-insured and self-administered businesses.

The lack of credible information was a common theme during the 1990–1993 workers' compensation crisis in California. The workers' compensation system was marked with escalating costs from medical treatment and forensic medical evaluations, fraud, and delayed resolution of cases.[2,3] With the severest economic recession since the Great Depression as a backdrop, the inhospitable workers' compensation environment was singled out as a leading cause of business flight. Throughout the debate about proposed reform measures, policy makers and state agencies confronted gaps in basic information and statistics regarding injury incidence, costs, timeliness of benefit delivery, adequacy of benefits, satisfaction with services, and other outcomes.

California and over 25 other states have completed a pilot of electronic transmission of First Reports of Injury (FROI) (See Appendix A), demonstrating the feasibility of using standardized data elements and file specifications and electronic data transmission. A few states (Texas, Florida, Wisconsin) already routinely accept electronic FROIs. Automation of claims handling by workers' compensation insurers is rapidly becoming commonplace, as is automation of medical billing, and, at a slightly lesser pace, computerization of medical records.

This chapter describes the design and development of the California Workers' Compensation Information System (WCIS), which builds on these current trends in the medical and workers' compensation marketplaces.

Goals, Objectives, and Scope

The goals and scope were guided by a mandate from the California legislature (Labor Code §138.6) that directed DWC to develop an information system to:

- manage the workers' compensation system in an effective and efficient manner
- facilitate the evaluation of the efficiency and effectiveness of the benefit delivery system
- measure how adequately the system indemnifies injured workers and their dependents
- provide statistical data for research into specific aspects of the workers' compensation system
- be compatible with national standards for electronic commerce being developed by the International Association of Industrial Accidents Boards and Commissions (IAIABC)[4–6]

Gaining Support

Workers' compensation is a contentious issue among the stakeholders, who include government agencies such as DWC and the state's Department of Insurance, labor unions, injured workers support groups, commercial insurers, self-insured employers, third-party claims administrators (TPAs), medical and chiropractic associations, rehabilitation professionals, defense and applicants attorneys, medical bill review companies, private research institutes, and health maintenance organizations. Changes in law usually create a realignment of the economic fortunes of the participants.

The stakeholders participated directly in the design process. The concerns of the stakeholders were:

- how was the information going to be used by DWC?
- how was confidentiality going to be guarded?
- how was reporting to multiple government agencies going to be simplified?

The Division of Worker's Compensation recruited high profile leaders among all the different stakeholders to participate in an advisory committee. The tasks were to jointly develop policy recommendations for how the data collected from the information system was going to be used and how its confidentiality protected. Each subcommittee included policy makers, (who were the chairpersons), business officials, and technical staff from insurance and government stakeholders, including DWC. The recommendations were used by DWC technical staff who ultimately were responsible for the design of the information system.

The DWC's administrative director was an advocate of the concept of the information system. DWC held leadership positions on the steering committee and technical committees of the IAIABC, which developed national standards for electronic data interchange (EDI) between claims administrators and state workers' compensation agencies.[4–6]

Inventory of Data

The DWC staff made an assessment of existing data related to occupational injury and illness incidence, costs, timeliness and adequacy of benefits, and outcomes.

Incidence of Injuries and Illnesses, and Claims

Under California's labor code, employers and physicians report the occurrence of injuries and illnesses on prescribed forms, Doctor and Employer FROI. These reports are usually the first notification that a work injury or illness has occurred. These forms are sent by employers and physicians via the workers' compensation carrier or the claims administrator to DIR, which receives nearly two million one-page reports annually. The employer and physician reports contain similar information that encompasses approximately 75 mostly text fields that include the names and addresses of the worker, employer, claims administrator, industry type, occupation, description of the injury or illness, date of injury or onset, diagnosis, etc. Historically, these reports were coded for industry,[7] occupation,[8] body part, nature of injury, type of injury, and agent;[9] key-entered, and tabulated. Since 1992, they have not been key entered nor analyzed.

The DIR does produce annual reports on injury incidence based on a federally funded statistical sample of OSHA 200 logs. These logs provide less detail on nature, cause, and body part than is required on the employers' or doctors' FROIs.

The California Workers' Compensation Insurance Rating Bureau (WCIRB) collects information on the roughly two-thirds of claims that are covered by commercial insurers. Detailed information on individual claims is collected only for claims that exceed $5000.[10] The WCIRB uses insurance industry code lists to categorize injuries and illnesses.[11] No data on nature or cause of injury is reported for the one-third of the claims that are covered by self-insured employers.[12]

Cost Data

Cost data are reported entirely differently for claims covered by insured and self-insured employers. For insured employers, indemnity and medical costs are available on open and closed claims at the individual claim level; whereas for self-insured employers, this information is reported to the state's Self-Insurance Program (SIP) for only open claims and aggregated for closed claims. The WCIRB collects data relating to costs of forensic medical evaluations, but this is not available for self-insured claims.

Medical Data

Medical data such as final medical diagnosis or information on the utilization of medical services linked to claims are lacking in any currently publicly available system.

Timeliness of Benefit Delivery

California law requires claims administrators to send letters (notices) explaining the nature of benefits to injured workers. Before 1992, DWC received mailed-in report forms based on these notices that contained date information that permitted DWC to assess the timeliness of benefit delivery. The volume of reports—up to 2 million per year based on an estimated 2–5 notices per 400,000 beneficiaries—was so overwhelming that DWC suspended collecting these data in 1992. Neither the WCIRB nor SIP databases contain the first or last date associated with individual benefit payments.

Adequacy of Benefits, Satisfaction with Services, Consequence of Work Injuries

Information regarding adequacy of benefits, satisfaction with services (claims handling, legal, adjudicative, medical), reasons for disputes, or short and long-term consequences of work injuries is not captured by existing data systems. The extent to which injured workers utilize personal income and resources (out-of-pocket, home care by family members), public assistance programs (e.g., food stamps, welfare, Medi-Cal, State or Social Security Disability), and private health and disability insurance for work injuries is also unknown.

In sum, existing data systems are fragmented and limited, and cannot provide the data required to assess key questions about the California workers' compensation system.

Defining the Data Set and Mechanisms for Reporting

The methodology to define the data needed was based on posing questions that the information system should answer. The questions were asked in plain language by the WCIS advisory committee (Table 24.1) based on a template jointly developed by the University of California and DWC. Once key questions were agreed upon, measures addressing each question were expressed as outcomes, benchmarks, or performance indicators. Data elements necessary to calculate each measure were then identified, including data elements required for stratification or use as covariates.

Each data element was assessed for possible data sources, and compatibility with collection in a standard electronic format. Where possible, data elements were drawn from those contained in employers FROI, physician FROI, standard benefit notices, standard medical bills for doctors and hospitals (HCFA 1500 and UB92) (Appendix A), and their electronic equivalents.[13]

The final list of required data elements was mapped to EDI transaction sets of the IAIABC. IAIABC has released EDI standards for first and subsequent report of injury (benefits), proof of coverage, and the payment of medical bills.[4–6] The focus for standardizing electronic business transactions in the United States is the American National Standards Institute,[13] which identifies business requirements, data elements and their definitions, code lists, file specifications, and communication protocols. State workers' compensation agencies

Table 24.1 Key Questions, Benchmarks, and Data Elements

Key Question	*Performance Measure or Benchmark*	*Data Elements or Data Source*
	Incidence of Injuries, Illnesses, Fatalities	
How many injuries, illnesses, and deaths occur in the workplace in California?	Number and incidence rate of injuries, illnesses, and deaths officially and unofficially reported	Unreported morbidity and mortality will require special surveys.
How many *reported* injuries, illnesses, and deaths occur in the workplace?	Number and incidence rate of injuries, illnesses, and deaths officially reported; baseline year 1998 when electronic reporting is mandatory	Claim number and date of injury. Denominator for incidence rate is the arithmetic average of monthly state employment censuses taken by California's employment development/ security agency.
What are the characteristics of injured workers?		Social Security Number and see stratification variables (Table 24.2)
	Benefits and Costs to Employers	
What benefits are received?	Benefit (dollars) paid to injured workers Median amount per claim	Payment start and stop dates and codes for indemnity type and vocational rehabilitation amounts; settlement amounts and awards of a sample of adjudicated cases at DWC Workers' Compensation Appeals Boards
	Benefit dollars paid to other participants	Paid medical amounts for providers services and hospital services; payment start and stop dates and indemnity type, vocational, med-legal, defense attorney fees; future medical and applicant lawyers fees from a sample of adjudicated cases at DWC Workers' Compensation Appeals Boards
Who pays and receives how much of the workers' compensation dollar?	Insurers general costs (dollars)	Insurer survey for acquisition costs, allocated loss adjustment expenses, taxes, and profits

(Continues on next page)

Table 24.1 (Continued)

Key Question	*Performance Measure or Benchmark*	*Data Elements or Data Source*
	Benefits and Costs to Employers	
	Employer costs (premium dollars)	Above survey and survey of employer liability and productivity losses due to work injuries
When are benefits delivered?	Number and percentage of first payments made after statutory timelines (generally 14 days after eligibility begins for each benefit type)	Stop–start dates for benefit types
	Adequacy of Benefits	
Medical Treatment		
What services are injured workers receiving and is there adequate access to services?	Days from injury to treatment Days from first treatment to maximum medical improvement (permanent and stationary) Days from first to last treatment	Date of injury or illness, medical service codes and their dates
Are patient satisfied with the medical treatment they receive?	Patient satisfaction measures	Routine survey
Are lifetime medical benefits adequate?	Percentage of total medical bills paid by workers' compensation	Special survey of nonworkers' comp participants (government health payers, group health plans, self-pay)
Level of Indemnity		
Is the temporary disability benefit adequate?	Percentage of preinjury wages and earnings provided by workers' compensation benefits	Wage at time of injury, and special survey or record linkage to wage earnings in unemployment insurance system, or both
Is the benefit adequate for permanent disability, vocational rehabilitation, and death? and what are the long-term economic and noneconomic consequences of a work injury or claim for the workers and their families?		Special survey of preinjury employer-provided benefits, long-term disability, public-provided benefits, (SDI, SSDI, UI); family or self-subsidy; nonwage financial loses; postinjury wages for control group; quality of life changes; PD rating and method of settlement (prenegotiated, trial decision)
What are the return-to-work outcomes of the injury?	Percentage returning at time intervals (or disability days) from injury date to return-to-work; percentage returning at time intervals (or disability days) from injury date to return-to-work without reinjury in a prescribed time period (sustained return-to-work)	Date of injury or illness; code for release to return to work; special survey for actual return to work date, type of release (e.g., regular work, modified), same or different job; same or different employer; structure and process of employer incentives for RTW
Claim Resolution		
How promptly are claims resolved?	For nondisputed claims: time distribution (number and percentage at a given point in time) and median time from injury or illness date to last benefit payment	Claim number, date of injury or illness, stop date of benefit payment, and payment adjustment reason codes
	For disputed indemnity claims: time distribution (number and percentage at a given point in time) and median time from date of injury or illness to date of approval of negotiated settlement or judge's decision to award or deny benefits	Division of Workers' Compensation case number, date of declaration of readiness to proceed to date DWC approves prenegotiated settlements (stipulation, compromise, and release) or judge issues decision (finding and awards)
What are the issues in dispute?		Survey of DWC's adjudicated cases; initiating party
How promptly are disability ratings done?	Number and percent of requests completed within statutory time period of 20 days	Disability case number, date of request, date of rating
How consistent are ratings between raters?		Special survey
How promptly are vocational rehabilitation plans approved?	Number and percent of requests completed within statutory time period of 20 days	Division of Workers' Compensation rehabilitation case number, date of request, date of approval

*DWC, Division of Workers' Compensation; PD, Permanent Disability; SDI, State Disability Insurance; SSDI, Social Security Disability Insurance; UI, unemployment insurance; RTW, return-to-work.

Source: Maizlish et al.[19]

participate through IAIABC, a nonprofit professional and educational association of state workers' compensation executives. Data elements not present in any IAIABC EDI transaction list were identified as candidates for collection via survey, database linkage, or other collection methods (e.g., claims file sample).

The agency carried out pilot projects with actual data transmissions among volunteer insurers, and general public education to the workers' compensation community.

RESULTS

The most significant and frequently asked questions about the workers' compensation system, proposed measures, and the data elements needed to answer them are summarized in Table 24.1. Tables 24.2 to 24.4 show approximately 75 data elements that would allow assessment of these measures. Three mechanisms for data collection were identified: (*1*) rapid EDI for a minimum number of data elements currently found in FROIs and benefit notices for *all* claims, (*2*) electronic collection of data on medical bills for a sample of claims, and (*3*) surveys of persons and claims files (Fig. 24.1).

The DWC proposed that all EDI data be composited from employer and physician FROIs, medical bills, benefit notices and other source documents, and sent from claims administrators and medical bill review companies to a state-sponsored data repository. The data repository will distribute data to other government agencies to satisfy existing, mandated reporting requirements of insurers, claims administrators, employers, and physicians. The data repository will edit and reduce the information into statistical work files, carry out analyses, generate reports, and create public use files without individual identifiers.

Standard Industrial Classification code[7] and annual average employment by SIC code will be captured through linkage with Federal Employer Identification Number (FEIN) or unemployment insurance code to databases of California's state employment development agency. The DWC proposes to code occupation description using a combination of automated methods analyzing text strings[14] and manual coders.

Criteria for sampling for medical services data and survey administration will be determined by DWC in conjunction with a technical advisory committee. The DWC will provide claims administrators with lists of cases comprising the sample. Telephone and mail surveys will be conducted on a sample of approximately 2000 cases, following development of survey instruments that assess adequacy of benefits, return to work outcomes, satisfaction with services, and other outcomes.

Data Quality

Data reporting will incorporate an electronic acknowledgement with receipt date, and an error-checking program that analyzes logical date sequences, valid codes and ranges, and completeness of mandatory fields. Following development of data quality standards (in conjunction with the advisory committee), a data quality assurance program will use both computer and field audits to document accuracy and validity of data. A program of technical assistance and education for data providers will include an orientation to EDI and the IAIABC implementation guides, train the trainer sessions, and a help desk function for ongoing assistance. The WCIS will be phased in over a period of several years. For each phase, a year-long voluntary testing program will precede mandatory reporting.

Confidentiality

Individual identifier information on both injured workers and employers, and claims administrators, will be protected to the extent feasible under workers' compensation law, which mandates access to specified individual records in litigated cases. Publicly available data files will be stripped of all individual identifier information, and DWC reports will include only aggregate data. Legitimate researchers will be able to access data with assurances that adequate protection of human subjects has been reviewed and approved by formal institutional review boards.

DISCUSSION

Many technical and organizational challenges were encountered and remain in the implementation of the information system. However, the direct involvement of policy makers—the users—in developing outcome measures and defining the data needs was a crucial passage. Several data elements not normally integrated into insurance databases may be key to the success of the WCIS, including, for example, standard entity identifiers for key parties, medical diagnosis by physician, paid medical amounts, and type of health care arrangement. One approach to overcoming this barrier is to phase in data collection, starting with only those data elements that are more universally available, and providing a long lead time before mandatory collection of data elements not currently integrated into insurers systems. Data quality remains another major challenge.

California and 29 other states have already initiated or completed EDI pilots. In California, six workers' compensation carriers accounting for approximately 25% of the annual claim volume transmitted approx-

Table 24.2 Selected Variables for Stratification and Subgrouping*

Variable	*Code List*
INCIDENCE OF INJURY, ILLNESS, AND FATALITIES	
Date of injury	
Nature of injury code	IAIABC
Part of body code	IAIABC
Cause of injury code	IAIABC
Claim type: temporary partial (±wage continuation), temporary total, permanent partial, permanent total, vocational rehabilitation, death	IAIABC
Diagnosis	ICD9
Date of birth	
Gender code	IAIABC
Employment status	IAIABC
Industry, via record linkage on Employer FEIN or UI code	SIC
Occupation (description)	BOC
Geographic area (employer zip code)	USPS
BENEFITS	
Indemnity benefit type	IAIABC
Medical provider specialty	HCFA
Hospital	HCFA
Provider gatekeeper code (primary treating physician)	IAIABC
Health care arrangement (PPO, HMO, fee schedule)	IAIABC
Security arrangement (deductible, group or individual, self-administered, TPA, legally uninsured, carve out)	IAIABC (partial)
OUTCOMES	
Diagnosis and injury or illness severity (additional diagnoses)	ICD9
Worker demographics (age, sex, occupation)	IAIABC
Employer demographics (SIC, size); record linkage (FEIN/UI)	IAIABC
Health care arrangement (PPO, HMO, fee schedule)	IAIABC
CLAIM RESOLUTION	
Claim type	IAIABC
Diagnosis	ICD9
Claims administrator (FEIN)	IAIABC
Represented or nonrepresented	DWC†
Claim adjusting location	DWC†
DWC district office	DWC†
DWC judge	DWC†
DWC disability rater	DWC†
DWC vocational rehabilitation consultant	DWC†
Law firm	DWC†
Settlement type (prenegotiated; judge decision after trial)	DWC†

*BOC, Bureau of the Census; DWC, Division of Workers' Compensation; FEIN, Federal Employer Identification Number; HCFA, Health Care Financing Agency; HMO, health maintenance organization; IAIABC, International Association of Industrial Accidents Boards and Commissions; ICD, International Classification of Diseases, 9th Revision; PPO, Preferred Provider Organization; SIC, Standard Industrial Classification; TPA, third-party claims administration; UI, unemployment insurance; USPS, United States Postal Service

†non-IAIABC codes specific to DWC

Source: Maizlish et al.[19]

imately 27,000 employer FROIs from the claims administrator to DWC. The pilot demonstrated the feasibility of using IAIABC standards for specifications of files and data elements, the use of an electronic mailbox for claims administrators to send American Standard Code for Information Interchange (ASCII) files, and development of applications to acknowledge receipt of the transactions and provide an error report.

Evaluation of managed care presents many conceptual and analytic challenges. Most workers' compen-

Table 24.3 Data Elements Required to be Submitted Electronically on All Claims to California Workers' Compensation Information System*

Data Element Name
INSURER
FEIN
Name
CLAIMS ADMINISTRATOR
FEIN
Name
Address line 1
Address line 2
City
State
Postal code
Claim number
EMPLOYER
Employer FEIN
Insured name
Employer name
Address line 1
Address line 2
City
State
Postal code
INJURY OR ILLNESS
Date of injury or illness
Nature of injury code
Part of body injured code
Cause of injury code
Accident description
Date reported to employer
EMPLOYEE
Last name
First name
Middle initial
Address line 1
Address line 2
City
State Postal code
Telephone
Social Security Number
Date of birth
Gender code
Date disability began
Date of death
Employment status code
Occupation description
Wage
Wage period
MAINTENANCE REASON AND PAYMENT ADJUSTMENT CODES
First payment code, temporary disability
Last payment code, temporary disability
Payment adjustment code, temporary disability
Delay temporary disability payment
First permanent disability payment
Last permanent disability payment
Delay permanent disability payment
First VRMA
Last VRMA
Vocational rehabilitation, evaluation
Vocational rehabilitation, training
First death benefit payment
Last death benefit payment
Delay in death benefits
Medical-legal costs-applicant
Medical-legal costs-defense
Penalties
Incurred versus paid qualifier
INDEMNITY PAYMENT AMOUNTS
Dollar amount of payment
PAYMENT START/END DATES
Date of payment

*FEIN, Federal Employer Identification Number; VRMA, Vocational Rehabilitation Maintenance Allowance.
Source: Maizlish et al.[19]

sation claims systems lack a methodology to allocate prepaid medical care of a population of enrollees to individual claims. Without service level detail, costs or cost equivalents may not be calculable.

The use of survey research to supplement administrative data has many precedents, but in the design of WCIS, surveys are not an add-on, but an integral means of capturing data to answer key questions when administrative databases fall short. The database on all claims will serve as a sample frame, and, through record linkage, claims information will be available on cases selected into survey samples. The DWC has already developed and field tested a survey of patient satisfaction with workers' compensation medical care that will serve as a prototype.[15]

Reducing the costs of claims handling and mandatory reporting to state agencies is an impetus to automating claims administration.[16] Costs for manual processing FROIs are not widely published. Based on estimates from advisory committee members, costs range from $5 to $20 per FROI, taking into account transmission costs incurred by mail, fax, and telephone, key-entry and rekey-entry costs between employers, insurers, claims administrators, and state agencies. One advisory committee member reported that EDI saved

Table 24.4 Data Elements Required to be Submitted Electronically on a Sample of Medical Bills to California Workers' Compensation Information System*

DATA ELEMENT NAME
Service date range
Hospital admission date
Hospital discharge date
Treatment code, CPT
Diagnosis codes, ICD9
Provider gatekeeper indicator (PTP)
Provider credential code
Provider specialty code
Place of service
Amount paid, professional services
Amount paid, hospital services
Health care arrangement
(Provider Agreement Code: PPO, HMO, fee schedule, etc.)

*CPT, current procedural terminology; ICD9, International Classification of Diseases, 9th Revision; PTP, Primary Treating Physician; PPO, Preferred Provider Organization; HMO, health maintenance organization.

Source: Maizlish et al.[19]

79 cents per FROI in transmission costs and up to $45 per claim in labor and overhead incurred for state-mandated reporting of benefit notice detail. Of course, the move to EDI will also require investments in technology. Systemwide estimates of these costs are not available. The potential indirect savings associated with the impact of improved information on claims management is unknown, but many observers expect it to be greater than the direct benefits of automating the claims administration process.[17] Finally, state workers' compensation agencies will save considerable costs of key entry of FROIs and can electronically recycle name, address, and other case make-up information, if parties to a dispute later request DWC's services.

The choice of specific data standards, what state agencies will do with the data, financing of the data repository, costs to data providers, control and access to information, and confidentiality were candidly discussed by the advisory committee. The move to EDI requires the adoption of standards. However, no individual or group of players in California's decentralized workers' compensation market wields enough clout to dictate a standard. Multistate carriers are particularly interested in national standards so they can reduce the costs associated with maintaining idiosyncratic reporting systems for each of 50 states.

A major recurrent issue in development of the WCIS was ownership of the data. Some participants encouraged privatization of the data repository and standards and the sale of data products. Some insurer participants voiced concern that DWC might use benefit notice data as the basis for levying fines against insurers. Some worker advocates expressed fear that the increased access to information afforded by the WCIS might give employers a tool to blacklist injured workers, or provide a source for lawyers and providers to solicit injured workers. Limitation of data collection to those data elements required to answering key administrative and policy questions about the workers' compensation

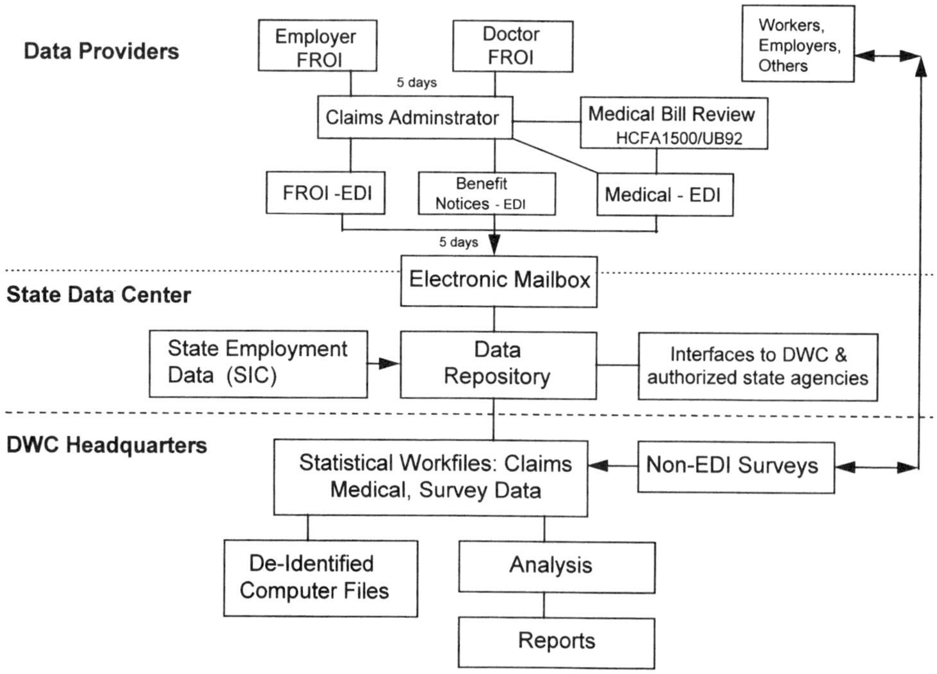

Figure 24.1 Data flow in California's workers' compensation information system (Maizlish et al.[19]).

system has helped to dispel some of these concerns. It is crucial that confidentiality of individual identifier information and access to WCIS data be explicitly addressed to assure that information in the WCIS will not be used against individuals. DWC has adopted confidentiality and access regulations.

It was acknowledged that the use of electronic commerce to administer claims will save millions of dollars annually. Consequently there was stronger support for the EDI claims component than the medical data and surveys. Some participants suggested that part of the potential cost savings be used to finance the state repository. Employers were generally skeptical of paying for another government program. Predictably, DWC's avowed use of WCIS data to carry out electronic screening of timeliness to direct its auditors to claim adjusting locations with a high likelihood of problems was well received by labor advocates and not welcomed by others. DWC's current practice of auditing a 1.5% random sample of claims[18] is often criticized for its small impact and low specificity because claims adjusting locations with few violations are frequently selected.

The proposed WCIS will provide information to improve the performance and to increase the accountability of all the participants in California's workers' compensation system. More importantly, it will provide information that will allow improved quality in the provision of mandated benefits to injured workers. This, in turn, may decrease disputes in the system. The WCIS will provide information for monitoring trends in the workers' compensation system, and will allow both administrators and policy makers to take action before problems reach crisis proportions. In this sense, the WCIS may truly mark the dawn of a new era in California's workers' compensation system.

ACKNOWLEDGMENTS

Thanks are due to Casey Young, former Administrative Director of DWC and the members of the Workers' Compensation Information System Advisory Committee for their time, energy, and interest. The authors also gratefully acknowledge the contributions of Glenn Shor, Walter Sensing, and other DWC staff; the technical assistance of Henry Brady, John Wiley, and Frank Neuhauser, University of California Data Archive and Technical Assistance, Berkeley; and Richard Brand, University of California.

Portions of this chapter were published previously in the *American Journal of Industrial Medicine* and have been used with permission.

REFERENCES

1. Division of Labor Statistics and Research. *Work Injuries and Illnesses, California, 1991.* San Francisco: California Department of Industrial Relations, 1992.
2. Barth P, Telles C. *Workers' Compensation in California: Administrative Inventory.* WC-92-8. Cambridge, MA: Workers' Compensation Research Institute, 1992.
3. Aubry L. *Meaningful Reform of Workers' Compensation in California.* San Francisco: Department of Industrial Relations, 1995.
4. International Association of Industrial Accidents Boards and Commissions (IAIABC). *First Report of Injury, Subsequent Report, Release 1.* Kansas City: Electronic Data Interchange Development Committee, International Association of Industrial Accidents Boards and Commissions, 1995. (Those wishing to obtain copies of the technical documentation should contact IAIABC at http://www.iaiabc.org.)
5. International Association of Industrial Accidents Boards and Commissions (IAIABC). *Proof of Coverage.* Release 1. Kansas City: Electronic Data Interchange Development Committee, International Association of Industrial Accidents Boards and Commissions, 1996.
6. International Association of Industrial Accidents Boards and Commissions (IAIABC). *Medical Bill Payment Report.* Release 1. Kansas City: Electronic Data Interchange Development Committee, International Association of Industrial Accidents Boards and Commissions, 1996.
7. Office of Management and Budget. *Standard Industrial Classification Manual, 1987.* Washington, DC: U.S. Government Printing Office, 1989.
8. Bureau of the Census. *Classified Index of Industries and Occupations. The 1990 Census of the Population.* Washington, DC: U.S. Government Printing Office, 1992.
9. American National Standards Institute Z16.2 Subcommittee. *Method of Recording Basic Facts Relating to the Nature and Occurrence of Work Injuries, ANSI Z16.2-1962 (R1969).* American National Standard for Information Management for Occupational Safety and Health. 3rd Draft, March 1995.
10. Workers' Compensation Insurance Rating Bureau. *California Workers' Compensation Uniform Statistical Reporting Plan, 1995.* San Francisco: Workers' Compensation Insurance Rating Bureau, 1996.
11. National Council on Compensation Insurance. *Classification Codes and Statistical Codes for Workers Compensation and Employers Liability Insurance.* Boca Raton: National Council on Compensation Insurance, 1995.
12. Office of Self-Insurance. *Reports.* Sacramento: Department of Industrial Relations, Office of Self-Insurance, 1996.
13. American National Standards Institute. *Electronic Data Interchange Standards.* Draft Version 4 Release 1. Alexandria VA: Data Interchange Standards Association. Accredited Subcommittee X12. Transaction sets 148 (First Report of Injury); 837 (Health Care Claim), 1997.
14. National Institute for Occupational Safety and Health. *The SOIC System User's Manual," Version 1.3.* Morgantown: Division of Safety Research, National Institute for Occupational Safety and Health, 1998.
15. Rudolph L, Wiley J, Dervin K, Garrett K, Maizlish N, Chang YT. *What Do Injured Workers Think About Their Medical Care?* San Francisco: California Division of Workers' Compensation, 1998.
16. Woodward E. *Electronic Data Interchange: Forum VII.* Sponsored by the International Workers' Compensation Foundation. Newport News, May 23, 1995.
17. Akabas SH, Gates LB, Galvin DE. *Disability Management: A Complete System to Reduce Costs, Increase Productivity, Meet Employee Needs, and Ensure Legal Compliance.* New York: AMACOM, American Management Association, 1992.
18. Audit Unit. *Report to the California Legislature on Claims Handling Practices of Workers' Compensation Administrators. 1995 Audits.* San Francisco: Department of Industrial Relations, 1996.
19. Maizlish NA, Rudolph LA, Young C. Design of a state-based workers' compensation information system. *Am J Ind Med* 1999; 35:564–573.

25

Closing the Loop: Impact of a Lead Poisoning Prevention Project

JIM BELLOWS, LINDA A. RUDOLPH, NEIL A. MAIZLISH, AND KATHY A. DERVIN

During the 1990's, state-based occupational health surveillance was revitalized in the United States.[1,2] State public health agencies started playing a stronger and complementary role to that of the Bureau of Labor Statistics[3] and the Occupational Safety and Health Administration for surveillance and enforcement.

New initiatives launched by the National Institute for Occupational Safety and Health (NIOSH) stimulated the reporting of sentinel occupational illnesses,[2] the follow-up of occupational fatalities,[4,5] and the inclusion of occupational health topics into national health surveys.[6] NIOSH's Sentinel Events Notification System for Occupational Risks (SENSOR) supported state public health agencies to experiment with different data sources and surveillance techniques. Some states improved existing passive surveillance systems to generate information on the extent of the problem, to identify high-risk groups, and to monitor trends.[7] In this approach, the feedback was statistical information without direct links to specific worksites. Other states linked case reporting of occupational sentinel events at specific worksites so that enforcement agencies, universities, consultants, or personnel from the surveillance system could provide prevention services to those worksites. This approach, in its most simple application, proceeds worksite-by-worksite. By combining approaches, other surveillance systems evolved into comprehensive disease control programs with an industrywide or geographic focus.

This chapter describes the evolution of a disease control model by the California Department of Health Services (CDHS) for occupational lead poisoning. This occurred in successive stages in which surveillance influenced the intervention strategy, and the intervention impacted the surveillance system—closing the loop.

DEVELOPMENT OF THE MODEL

The successive stages in developing the surveillance-intervention model were:

- measure the extent of the problem with a statewide prevalence survey
- establish a case registry that links laboratory reporting of elevated blood lead to follow-up at specific worksites; and, target a high-risk group for intervention based on statistical data from the prevalence survey and blood lead registry
- carry out an intervention aimed at primary prevention in the targeted risk group and channel newly identified cases to the surveillance system (lead registry)

Prevalence Survey

By the mid 1980s, several states (New York, New Jersey, and Texas) had established lead registries compiled from mandatory reports of private analytical laboratories.[8,9] Before a similar occupational lead registry was established in California in 1987, questions were raised regarding the usefulness and validity of case-based registries as public health prevention tools. The proportion of true cases likely to be reported (sensitivity) was

Table 25.1 Estimated Number of Employees Who Are Receiving Routine Biological Monitoring in Selected Standard Industrial Classifications, California, 1986

*SIC Code**	*Industry*	*Employees potentially exposed to lead*	*Employees receiving routine biological monitoring*	
			N	*% of exposed*
1711	Plumbing, heating, and air conditioning	22,742	0	0.99
3341	Secondary lead smelting nonferrous metals	393	132	33.59
3691	Storage battery manufacture	1850	1762	95.25
3731	Shipbuilding and repair	1089	477	43.79
7538	Automotive repair	6561	1	0.02
7539	Radiator repair	903	70	7.95
7692	Welding repair	312	0	0.00
All	Total	229,434	5919	2.58

*SIC, Standard Industrial Classification.
Source: Rudolph et al.[10]

unknown and their representativeness suspect. Cases most likely to be reported might be limited to severe cases that bypassed worksite medical services and low-risk cases among workers in medical monitoring programs of large lead employers.

To put the results of the future case registry in context, a statewide survey was administered to a stratified cluster sample of California worksites.[10] The survey estimated nearly 230,000 lead-exposed workers, of whom only 2.6% (~5919) had routine blood lead testing (Table 25.1).

Case-Based Lead Registry

The prediction of low sensitivity and bias was borne out (Chapter 11).[11] By 1990, only about 4000 different individuals entered the lead registry. A disproportionate number of highly exposed workers were referred by their family physicians. The registry also received a large number of reports on workers with relatively low blood lead levels who were employed by a few large companies in battery manufacturing and secondary lead smelting. These employers conducted supervised, periodic blood lead screening as suggested in the prevalence survey.

Despite these limitations, the lead registry was a safety net for a large number of workers with highly elevated blood lead levels (≥60 μg/dl). Intervention was limited to telephone follow-up with the case, attending physician, and the employer, and referrals to other agencies. This exemplifies a one-on-one, worksite-by-worksite sentinel event model focusing on medical treatment of already overexposed workers, their medical removal, and blood lead retesting (Fig. 25.1). The futility of this approach for hundreds of cases of elevated blood lead made it necessary to search for a comprehensive model that reoriented the registry to broader interventions emphasizing primary prevention and increasing workers' access to occupational health services (Fig. 25.2).

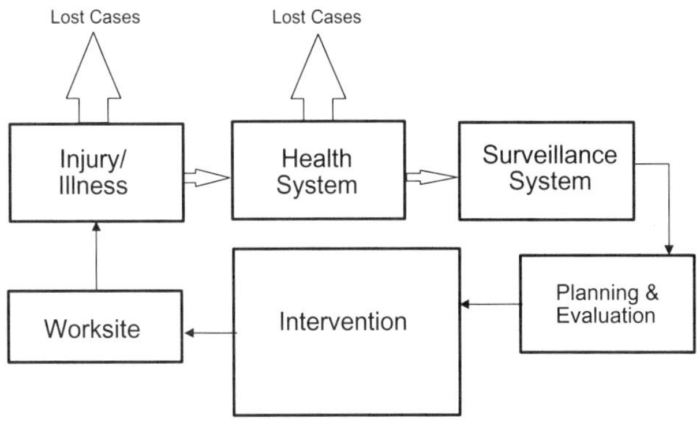

Figure 25.1 Sentinel events model that takes a case-by-case approach and does not target interventions to stem the loss of cases from worksites and the health care system.

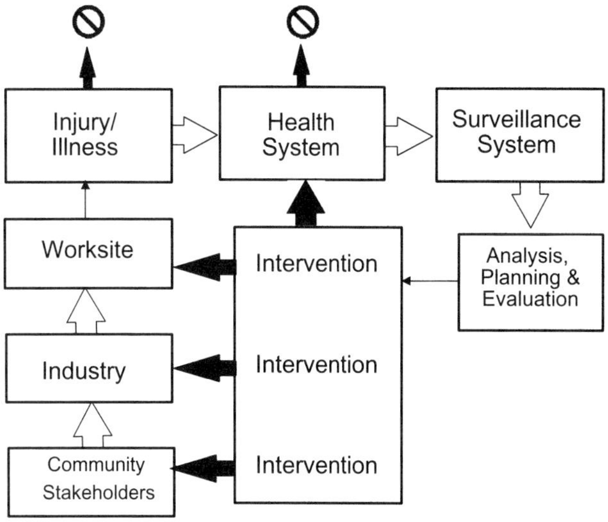

Figure 25.2 Sentinel events model that closes the loop by funneling cases into the health care system and coordinates primary and secondary prevention for individuals, workplaces, and an entire industry.

Selecting and Targeting the Intervention

The first steps at reaching some of these untested workers was a community-based intervention targeting all Los Angeles and San Bernardino County radiator repair shops.[12] Radiator repair workers were selected because they have well-documented lead hazards, were seriously underreported in the lead registry, and represented a disproportionate number of emergency cases that were reported. Targeting Los Angeles and San Bernardino counties was a strategic decision to focus limited resources and capitalize on local interest.[13]

Community-based means a broad range of stakeholders and their constituencies of employers and employees, labor and industry associations, medical providers, and others in the same geographic area. Organizing coordinated, collective action was directed at stakeholders in the community, the radiator repair industry, and specific workplaces. The role of CDHS was one of convener and coalition builder. The members of the coalition were active participants in the intervention.

METHODS

The intervention program focused on three areas: identifying companies, developing and marketing resources to facilitate employers' own lead-poisoning prevention activities, and maintaining regular contact with individual companies to stimulate and monitor their progress.

The project's strategy was to get companies started with the relatively simple step of blood lead testing. Occupational Safety and Health Administration (OSHA) regulations imply that air monitoring should be the initial means of hazard evaluation, but blood lead offers several advantages over air monitoring. Blood lead reflects ingestion as well as inhalation exposures[14] and has less daily variability than air monitoring. It is also less expensive, allowing companies to save limited funds for exposure control. Blood lead testing also provided a key link between the companies and the lead registry at CDHS. Mechanisms were already in place to follow-up individuals with highly elevated blood lead levels (Chapter 11). Perhaps most important, documented high blood lead levels could provide strong motivation for employers to reduce workplace exposures.

A key aspect in gaining companies' cooperation was presenting a step-by-step approach by which they could achieve compliance with the principal OSHA regulations. This approach encouraged employers to work first on measures that were likely to be the most cost-effective in reducing exposures.

Company Identification

Four hundred fifty-nine Los Angeles County and San Bernardino County radiator industry companies were identified from local telephone directories and local environmental health agencies. A baseline telephone survey of these companies was conducted during July and August 1990. Of the 495 surveyed, 275 were apparently engaged in radiator repair or manufacturer and were enrolled into the intervention. Those excluded included 76 companies that were apparently out of business, 94 that were engaged in wholesale or retail sales only. Fourteen did not respond.

Resource Development

A local ad hoc advisory committee was convened to enhance the project's sensitivity to the needs of the industry, to encourage the use of newly developed resources, and to establish a foundation for sustainability of prevention by local participants. The advisory committee's 26 members represented the occupational health program in CDHS; local, state, and national radiator industry trade groups; a national lead industries' association; workers' compensation insurance companies (including the state fund); occupational health faculty and labor occupational health educators from the University of California; maternal and child health and occupational health programs from county health departments; county hazardous waste and environmental health divisions; radiator trade press; immigrant workers association; legal aid foundation; Cal/OSHA Consultation Services; an environmentalist organization; applicants attorneys association; occupational medical association; and labor health and safety advocates (committee on occupational safety and health).

The state health department provided no direct professional services, such as blood lead testing or air monitoring. Instead, existing providers were urged to tailor their services to the needs of the participating companies. These resources were publicized by project staff and cosponsoring organizations, many of whom had links to the advisory committee.

The resources that resulted from the project included:

- A comprehensive 140-page manual[15] produced by CDHS (*Prevent Lead Poisoning—Before It Poisons Your Business*) to guide companies step-by-step in creating a lead poisoning prevention program
- A low-cost blood lead screening program sponsored by the National Automotive Radiator Service Association and the Western Occupational Medicine Association
- A model contract for use by employers and physicians establishing medical surveillance programs

- Seminars for participating employers, sponsored by the CDHS
- Worker health and safety training in English and Spanish, sponsored by the Los Angeles City College
- A bilingual motivational video (*He's Not the Man I Married . . . Could It Be Lead?*) for workers and their employers, produced by CDHS with funding from the California State Compensation Insurance fund (the workers' compensation insurer covering the vast majority of radiator repair shops)
- Continuing medical education courses sponsored by local medical groups
- Marketing of low-cost ventilation systems developed by private local vendors specifically for use in radiator repair
- Testing of lead-free solders for radiator repair, sponsored by the Copper Development Association

Tracking of Companies' Progress

Companies were first notified of the intervention in October 1990. They were informed that active participation in the project was voluntary but that compliance with OSHA regulations was mandatory. Failure to cooperate might result in a referral to Cal/OSHA for enforcement. The companies were encouraged to initiate lead-poisoning prevention activities by conducting blood lead testing or air monitoring. They were asked to submit their test results on standardized progress report forms (Figs. 25.3, 25.4, 25.5). Employers that provided no evidence of testing were sent a friendly reminder letter 5 weeks after the initial contact, followed 3 weeks later by a bluntly worded letter warning that they might soon be identified to Cal/OSHA. A final warning was sent by certified mail. Companies without hired employees were not sent warnings because they are exempt from OSHA. During this period, project staff responded to many telephone requests for information. Intensive case follow-up (similar to that for other cases reported in the lead registry) was conducted for individuals with reported blood lead levels of 60 μg/dL or higher.

Data Collection and Analysis

A database was created that held information from the baseline survey about companies business activities and any previous blood lead testing or air monitoring. In-

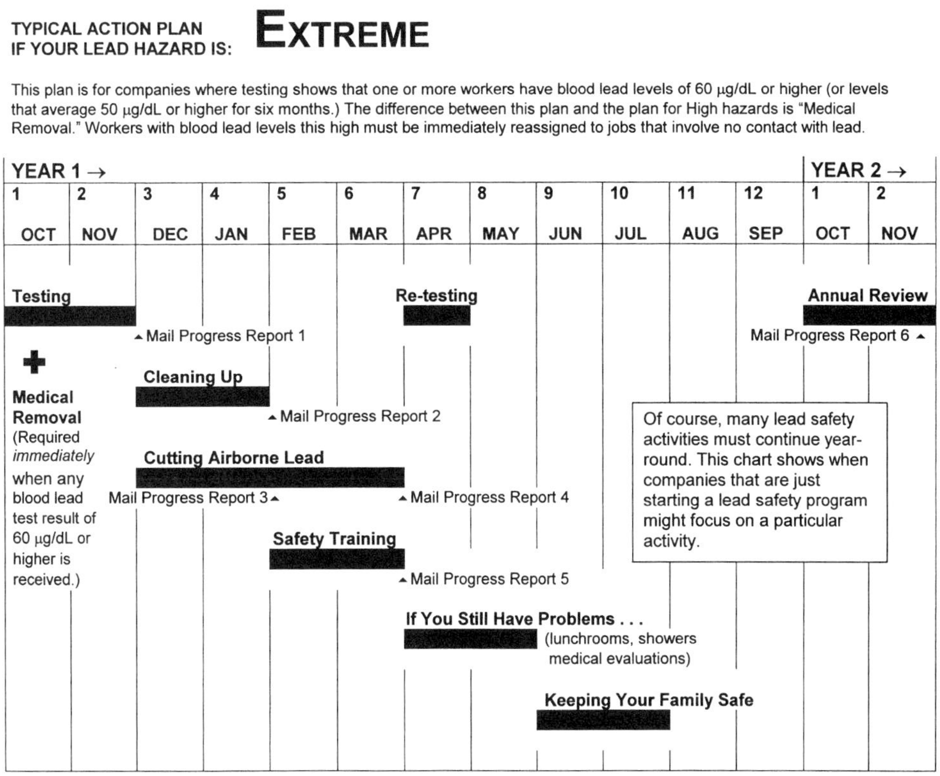

Figure 25.3 Action plan for employers with workers who had a blood lead test of 60 μg/dL or greater. (California Occupational Health Program[15])

PROGRESS REPORT 1: TESTING

COMPANY:

NAME ____________________

STREET ____________________

CITY ____________ ZIP ______

REPORT PREPARED BY:

NAME ____________________

POSITION ____________________

Date: __/__/__

INSTRUCTIONS *Complete all sections, on both sides of the page. For items that refer to "workers," include yourself (or other owners, managers, etc.) IF you work in areas that may have lead dust or fumes.*

A. Blood-Lead Testing

1. This company has done blood-lead testing.
   ☐ Yes ☐ No
2. The medical doctor in charge is:

   NAME ____________________

   STREET ____________________

   CITY ____________ STATE ______ ZIP ______
3. We used COHP's "Model Contract for a Lead Medical Program."
   ☐ Yes ☐ No
4. Blood-lead testing has been provided as follows: *(Fill in a number in each space below.)*
   a. ____ workers had blood-lead tests.
   b. ____ workers declined to have their blood-lead levels tested free-of-charge.
   c. ____ workers were not offered blood-lead tests because they have no possible contact with lead-containing dusts or fumes.
5. Write the results of each worker's most recent blood-lead test on the back of this report.

B. Air Sampling

1. This company has done air sampling.
   ☐ Yes ☐ No
2. The industrial hygienist in charge is:

   NAME ____________________

   STREET ____________________

   CITY ____________ STATE ______ ZIP ______
3. This industrial hygienist is employed by:
   ☐ Cal/OSHA Consultation Service
   ☐ an insurance company: ____________
   ☐ a consulting firm: ____________
   ☐ this company.
4. We used COHP's "Model Contract for Air Sampling." ☐ Yes ☐ No
5. Air sampling has been done on: *(Fill in a number in each space below.)*
   a. ____ work days,
   b. ____ workers (one or more days each)
6. Write the results for each worker tested on the back of this page and attach a copy of the industrial hygienist's report.

C. Follow-up Actions

1. The results of the testing described above show that:
   ☐ No further testing or lead-control measures are required at this time.
   ☐ Too much airborne lead is present and/or workers' blood-lead levels are too high. (Be sure to follow the steps described in the manual's *Chapter 5: Cutting Airborne Lead* and *Chapter 7: If You Still Have Problems...*)

   (If you are unsure what the testing results show, review the manual's Chapter 3: Blood Testing and Air Sampling, or talk to the medical doctor or industrial hygienist who did the testing.)
2. I authorize the California Occupational Health Program, California Department of Health Services, to contact the medical doctor and/or industrial hygienist listed above and to obtain information about the services provided.

SIGNATURE ____________________ DATE ________

CALIFORNIA OCCUPATIONAL HEALTH PROGRAM
(415) 540-2115

2151 BERKELEY WAY, ANNEX 11
BERKELEY, CA 94704

DECEMBER 1990

Figure 25.4 The first step of the action plan is blood lead testing or air monitoring. The results are indicated on the progress report that the employer sends to the state health department. (California Occupational Health Program[15])

D. Testing results Please list all employees below. Fill in their testing results or explain why they were not tested. If your employees do not all fit on this page, use additional copies.

Employees who had blood-lead testing and/or air sampling. (For tests not done, write "none" under Result.)

Name	Job	Date Hired	Date of Birth	Blood-lead testing Date	Blood-lead testing Result	Air Sampling Date	Air Sampling Result (circle units)
		/ /	/ /	/ /		/ /	µg/m3 mg/m3
		/ /	/ /	/ /		/ /	µg/m3 mg/m3
		/ /	/ /	/ /		/ /	µg/m3 mg/m3
		/ /	/ /	/ /		/ /	µg/m3 mg/m3
		/ /	/ /	/ /		/ /	µg/m3 mg/m3
		/ /	/ /	/ /		/ /	µg/m3 mg/m3
		/ /	/ /	/ /		/ /	µg/m3 mg/m3
		/ /	/ /	/ /		/ /	µg/m3 mg/m3
		/ /	/ /	/ /		/ /	µg/m3 mg/m3
		/ /	/ /	/ /		/ /	µg/m3 mg/m3

Employees who did not have blood-lead testing or air sampling.

Name	Job	Date Hired	Reason not tested (check one)
		/ /	☐ no contact with lead ☐ refused to participate
		/ /	☐ no contact with lead ☐ refused to participate
		/ /	☐ no contact with lead ☐ refused to participate
		/ /	☐ no contact with lead ☐ refused to participate

Figure 25.5 Testing results form for recording the names and blood lead levels of employees tested. These data were checked against the results of the lead registry. (California Occupational Health Program[15])

formation about new blood lead testing and air monitoring was taken from the companies' progress reports. Data in the lead registry provided a basis for validating information on the progress reports.

Simple descriptive statistics were generated to examine the frequency of blood lead testing pre-/postintervention. In describing companies blood lead levels, peak levels were used rather than means or medians because a company was considered to have a lead exposure problem if any worker had a high blood lead level.

RESULTS

Study Group

Of the 275 companies enrolled in the intervention, 23 were dropped because they went out of business or because they repaired fewer than 10 radiators per week. Of the 252 active companies, 148 (58%) had employees and 104 (42%) were owner-operated. Companies with employees had on average 6 employees per shop, of which 2 were engaged in radiator repair work. Two-hundred forty-seven companies repaired used radiators and five manufactured new radiators or cores.

Progress reports submitted by 171 companies listed 495 individuals who participated in blood lead testing. Three hundred eighty-six were employees and 109 were owners or managers. Over half of the companies used the trade association's low-cost screening program. Twenty-four individuals declined blood lead testing, and 141 were considered unexposed by their employer. Most individuals tested were radiator repair workers (50%) or owners or managers (22%). Participants averaged 36 years of age and had been at their current companies for a mean of 3.2 years. Sixty percent had Hispanic surnames. Eight (1.6%) were female.

Blood Lead Testing

Blood lead testing increased sharply during the study period among both employers (9%–95%) and owner-operators (1%–29%). Nearly half (47%) of the companies initiated blood lead testing only after the first

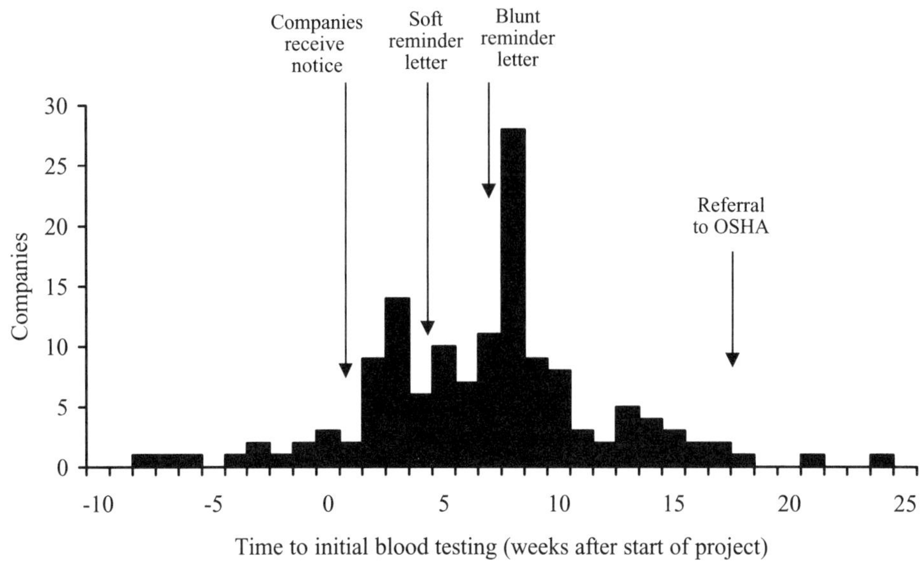

Figure 25.6 Relationship between time of project activities and initiation of company sponsored blood lead testing at 171 companies. (Bellows et al.[12])

strong warning of referral to Cal/OSHA if they failed to conduct testing (Fig. 25.6). By January 1991, only seven employers (<3%) had failed to provide evidence that the required blood lead testing or air monitoring had been conducted. Enforcement inspections were initiated by Cal/OSHA at each of the seven.

Blood lead levels of 40 μg/dL or higher were reported for 69 individuals (14%), including 54 radiator repair workers (22% of those tested). More than 25% of the companies had at least one worker with a level of 40 μg/dL or higher (Table 25.2). Of the 218 individuals listed with blood lead levels of 25 μg/dL or more on progress reports, 162 (74%) were also reported by laboratories to the lead registry. The reported values were identical in 93% of pairs and minor discrepancies accounted for the remainder. For only one company were blood lead levels exceeding 40 μg/dL reported in the registry but not on a corresponding progress report.

Air Monitoring

Six companies conducted air monitoring. Each also conducted blood lead testing. Data provided by these companies showed maximum airborne lead exposures of 9–97 $\mu g/m^3$ with a median of 21 $\mu g/m^3$.

DISCUSSION

The enormous increase in blood lead testing activity resulting from this project indicates that companies that have been largely out of compliance with required worker protection can successfully be urged to begin taking action on lead-poisoning prevention. The increase in testing generated a similar increase in registry reporting from 5 companies where blood lead levels exceeded 40 μg/dL during 1989 to 49 such companies during the project's first 5 months. Companies with

Table 25.2 Individual's Blood Lead Levels and Companies' Maximum Blood Lead Levels

Group	*N*	*% ≥ 25 μg/dL*	*% ≥ 40 μg/dL*	*% ≥ 60 μg/dL*	*% ≥ 80 μg/dL*
Individuals	495	44	14	4	1
Radiator repair workers	246	60	22	6	1
Owners and managers	109	38	12	5	1
Employees in other jobs	140	21	1	0	0
Companies	171	70	29	10	3
Employers	141	71	31	11	4
Owner-operators	30	63	17	7	0

Source: Bellows et al.[12]

levels of 60 μg/dL were followed up in the CDHS lead registry and employers were referred to free consultation services from Cal/OSHA that they probably would not have otherwise sought.

Most public monies spent on occupational illness and injury prevention have gone into the development and enforcement of regulations. Most observers concur that in the case of lead, the results of this command and control approach have fallen short of the goals of the original OSHA regulations.[16] Existing enforcement programs have been particularly ineffective at changing the practices of very small business, such as those targeted in this project. The need for locally based, industry focused outreach programs has already been recognized, and has been addressed in at least one location with a series of on-site surveys.[17]

This project fills a need for occupational health intervention models that spread limited resources over a substantial number of companies, yet are still able to demonstrate real impact in those companies. The number of companies in this project was far larger than the number that could have been affected by on-site consultation at individual workplaces. The project was able to amplify its impact by adopting a community-based approach, drawing on the resources of existing organizations such as trade associations, insurance companies, medical associations, and suppliers of safety-related goods and services.

The project's success cannot be attributed to any single factor. There is a general consensus that lead causes illness, a strong OSHA standard, a biologic exposure (blood lead) that has a built in severity scale, preexisting blood lead reporting by a limited number of laboratories subject to quality control, a surveillance system that actively followed up cases of elevated blood lead, and well-developed control technologies.

The coalition of stakeholders generated substantial interest and awareness at the level of individual worksites. Although coordinated by the state health department, many tasks were delegated via enlightened self-interest to various constituent groups. For example, the clinical services for blood lead testing was organized by a medical association that negotiated price discounts with laboratories. A low-cost ventilation blueprint for radiator repair shops was developed so that local sheet metal contractors could install new ventilation systems. An industry development association offered radiator shop owners lead-free solder as an inducement to rid the workplace altogether of new sources of lead. Training was offered at local technical high schools, and a Spanish-English educational video for workers was developed by the health department and underwritten by the state's largest workers' compensation carrier.

Overall coordination was facilitated by a step-by-step manual for employers written by the state health department. The manual included a written, scheduled timeline for blood lead-testing and follow-up activities for training employees and implementing industrial hygiene controls. Targeting a cohort of geographically defined businesses all at the same time probably eliminated the temptation of some companies to gain a competitive advantage by not participating. Moreover, not participating was not an option. There was an agreement from OSHA to grant a temporary grace period followed by vigorous enforcement of nonparticipating employers.

The success of the initial phase warrants the extension of the model to other lead-using industries and other locations. The model also could well be applied to prevention of other types of occupational injury and illness.

ACKNOWLEDGMENTS

This project was supported in part by the California Department of Health Services (Contract 89-97661), the National Institute for Occupational Safety and Health (Cooperative Agreement U60-CCU-029990-03), and the California Department of Industrial Relations.

The authors acknowledge the many contributions of the project staff: Elizabeth Abello, Robin Dewey, David Harrington, Lucia Mireles, Kate Nichol, Sarah Royce, Glenn Shor, Joan Sprinson, and Pat Young. The authors also acknowledge the guidance and feedback of the ad hoc advisory committee. The project would not have been possible without the cooperation and contributions of the California Division of Occupational Safety and Health (Cal/OSHA).

Portions of this chapter were published previously in the *American Journal of Public Health* and have been used with permission.

REFERENCES

1. Millar D. Testimony before a subcommittee of the Committee on Governmental Operations. U.S. House of Representatives, June 20, 1984, 98th Congr. Second Session.
2. Baker EL. Sentinel event notification system for occupational risks (SENSOR): The concept. *Am J Public Health* 1989; 79(suppl): 18–20.
3. Bureau of Labor Statistics. *Survey of Occupational Injuries and Illnesses in 1997.* Washington, DC: U.S. Department of Labor, 1998.
4. National Institute for Occupational Safety and Health. *Fatal Accident Circumstances and Epidemiology (FACE).* Morgantown, WV: Division of Safety Research, 1989.
5. National Institute for Occupational Safety and Health. *National Traumatic Occupational Fatalities: 1980–1985.* Division of Safety Research. DHHS (NIOSH) Publ. No. 89-116. Washington, DC: U.S. Government Printing Office; 1989.
6. Behrens V, Seligman P, Cameron L, Mathias CGT, Fine L. The prevalence of back pain, hand discomfort, and dermatitis in the US working population. *Am J Public Health* 1994; 84:1780–1785.
7. Hanrahan LP, Higgins D, Anderson H, Haskins L, Tai S. Project SENSOR: Wisconsin surveillance of occupational carpal tunnel syndrome. *Wisconsin Med J* 1991; 90:80–83.

8. Baser ME, Marion D. A statewide case registry for surveillance of occupational heavy metals absorption. *Am J Public Health* 1990; 80:162–164.
9. Tepper A. Surveillance of occupational lead exposure in New Jersey: 1986 to 1989. *Am J Public Health* 1992; 82:275–277.
10. Rudolph L, Sharp DS, Samuels S, Perkins C, Rosenberg J. Environmental and biological monitoring for lead exposure in California workplaces. *Am J Public Health* 1990; 80:921–925.
11. Maizlish NA, Rudolph LA. California adults with elevated blood lead levels, 1987 through 1990. *Am J Public Health* 1993; 83: 402–405.
12. Bellows J, Rudolph L. Initial impact of a workplace lead-poisoning prevention project: expanded blood-lead testing improves surveillance and focus follow-up effort. *Am J Public Health* 1993; 83:406–410.
13. Papenek PJ, Ward CE, Gilbert KM, Frangos SA. Occupational lead exposure in Los Angeles county: An occupational risk surveillance strategy. *Am J Ind Med* 1992; 21:199–208.
14. American Conference of Governmental Industrial Hygienists. *Documentation of the Threshold Limit Values and Biological Exposure Indices.* 5th Ed. Cincinnati, OH: American Conference of Governmental Industrial Hygienists, Inc., 1986.
15. California Occupational Health Program. *Prevent Lead Poisoning—Before It Poisons Your Business.* Berkeley, CA: California Department of Health Services, 1991.
16. Silbergeld EK, Landrigan PJ, Froines JR, Pfeffer RM. The occupational lead standard: a goal unachieved, a process in need of repair. *New Solutions* 1991; (Spring):20–30.
17. Tuskes PM, Key MM. Potential hazards in small business—a gap in OSHA protection. *Appl Ind Hyg* 1988; 3:55–57.

26

Frontiers of Occupational Health Surveillance

LINDA A. RUDOLPH AND NEIL A. MAIZLISH

This book focuses on ways surveillance can be used for primary prevention. This approach emphasizes the causes rather than the consequences of illness and injury. However, for the large numbers of workers who do become ill or injured from work, the prevention of disability is a major goal. Over the last decade, interest in factors that influence disability[1–3] has grown steadily as well as concerns with the effectiveness and quality of occupational health services.[4] These are emerging concerns in which surveillance can play a role.

DISABILITY SURVEILLANCE

Disability can be defined as not being able to work due to an occupational injury or illness. Disability is measured by days away from work, or days in which work is restricted by a physician's orders. Disability arises when there is loss of physical or mental function that interferes with the demands of the employee's usual job or other jobs that are available and appropriate. For example, any person with a severe scrape on the knee will have a limited range of motion in his or her leg and will experience difficulty walking and bending down. Accountants, however, can still perform most of their jobs because walking and bending down are not part of the sedentary work of an accountant at a computer station or desk. The same severe scrape on the knee for a fire fighter makes it impossible to climb a ladder quickly or to drag a heavy hose. The accountant may have pain and discomfort that interferes with productivity but is not disabled. However, the fire fighter is disabled by the same, equally severe injury.

The general objectives of surveillance apply to disability outcomes: estimating the magnitude of the problem, identifying high-risk groups, identifying trends, and linking case reporting to active follow-up. Individual case follow-up may reveal difficulties that can be addressed by changes in the medical treatment plan, rehabilitation, evaluation of work restrictions, changes in an alternative work program, modifications to the work station, or a change in the hours of work.

Health care professionals and employers play key roles in preventing disability. Physicians determine the work restrictions as a part of releasing a patient to return to work. During the recovery period, employers can offer alternative work or make other types of accommodations. Some larger employers have started disability management programs in which a coordinator works with supervisors, injured workers, the treating physician, claims administrators, or case managers in workers' compensation managed care organizations.

Data Collection

Many of the data elements that are outcomes and risk factors for disability are found in employer work absence records and existing workers' compensation databases. These include the beginning and ending dates of spells of disability, the date released to work by the attending physician, the type of release (with or without restrictions), the date of actual return-to-work, the nature and date of injury, the age, gender and occupation of the injured or ill employee, the geographic location and industry of the company. With linkage to medical billing databases, it is possible to expand the number of data elements to include the type, intensity, duration, and timing of medical treatments and the type of health services organization. Linkage to state employment databases may capture standard industrial classification (SIC) code and employer size. Chapter 24 describes efforts to standardize states' workers' compensation databases and make data publicly accessible.

Measures of Frequency

Return to work after an injury or illness is a key outcome. Rather than a healthy population, the return-to-work population starts off injured or ill. Return-to-work typically has a curve similar to Figure 26.1. For most lost time injuries, the medical condition stabilizes quickly, and the workers recuperate without loss of function and return to work without medical restrictions. This is reflected in the initial steep rise during the first 30 days after an injury in Figure 26.1. There is a gradual plateauing between 60 and 90 days, and after 90 days a small percentage of workers have an extended period to return-to-work. This small percentage or tail of the curve can account for a significant percentage of lost workdays.

To calculate return-to-work, first, the population is defined as injuries and illnesses that occurred within a specified time (e.g., between two calendar dates). Then, for each case, return-to-work is put on a common scale, such as days after the date of injury or onset of illness. It is customary to follow-up each case for a preset minimum amount of time after the injury or illness such as 30, 60, or 90 days. For example, for return-to-work 90 days after injuries that occurred in a calendar year (January through December), the year-end cases from October 1 to December 31 must be followed up into the next calendar year until March 31 so there will be a full 90 days of follow-up for each case. Thus, to analyze a group of injuries or illnesses that occur between two dates, it is necessary to specify a third date through which follow-up occurs.

As in measures of incidence, return-to-work can be measured in three ways: a single point in time, repeated censuses, and as a continuous disability-time (rather than person-time).

Single Point in Time

The bottom part of Figure 26.2 shows the percent of return-to-work of 10 workers on each day after the date of injury. The 10 workers can be incident cases that occurred during a specified time period (e.g., cases with a date of injury or illness between January 1 and June 30, 2000). Return-to-work at a point in time is expressed as the number or percent that have returned to work from the initially injured or ill population by a specified time after the injury or onset of illness. For example, return-to-work 90 days after an injury is defined as:

$$\text{Percent Return-to-Work}_{90\text{Days}} = \frac{\begin{array}{c}\text{Number of workers with injuries and}\\ \text{illness occurring within a specified time}\\ \text{period who are back at work by 90}\\ \text{days after the date of injury or illness}\end{array}}{\begin{array}{c}\text{Number of injured or ill workers with}\\ \text{injuries and illness occurring in}\\ \text{specified time period}\end{array}} \times 100$$

This percent includes workers who returned to work in fewer than than 90 days and remained working

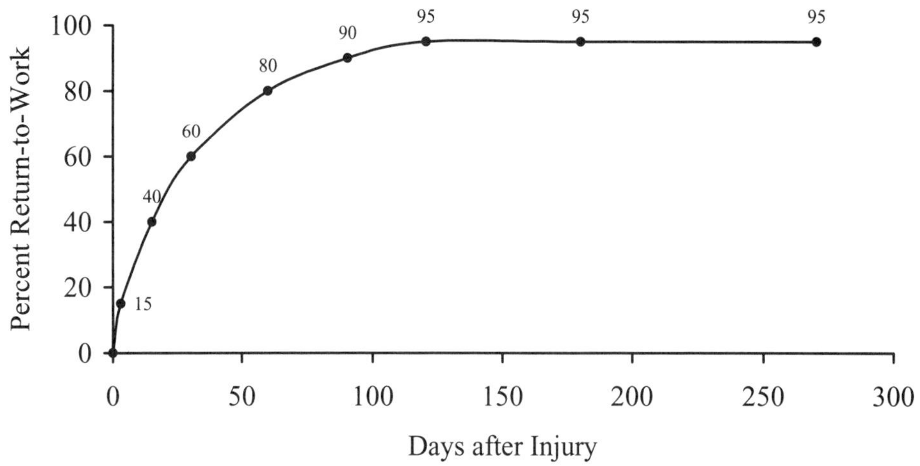

Figure 26.1 Typical plot of percent return-to-work at specified days after the date of injury.

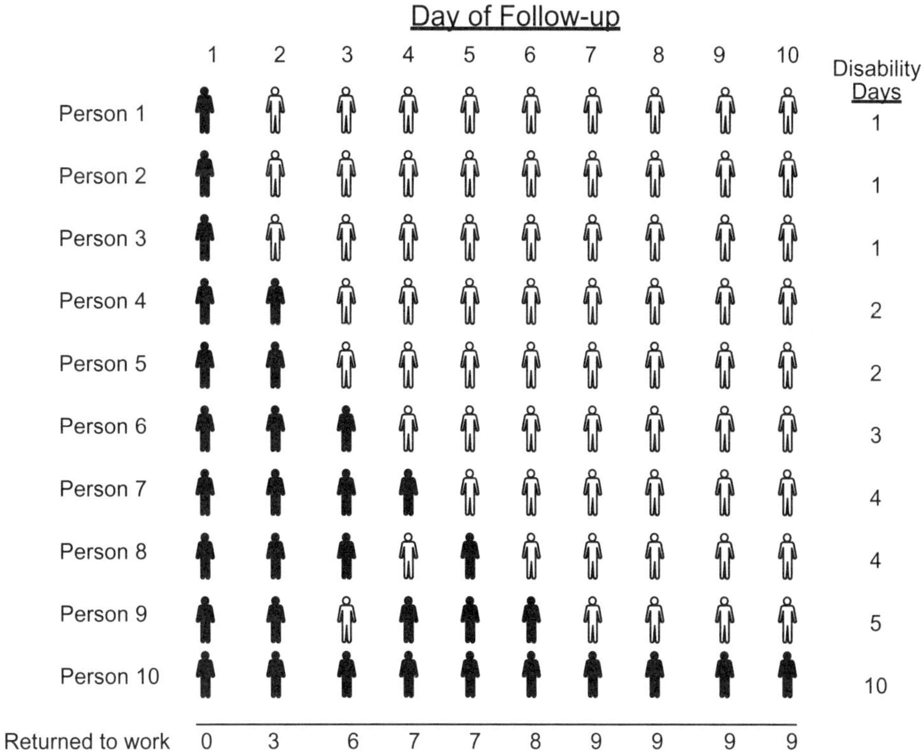

Figure 26.2 Return-to-work at specified days after the date of injury and cumulative disability days. Note that Person 8 accumulates 4 disability days over 5 calendar days.

through 90 days after the date of injury or illness. It is cumulative over time and sometimes stated as the cumulative percent return-to-work.

Repeated Censuses

For repeated census measurements, one examines the profile of percentages of return-to-work at several time intervals after the date of injury. This is shown in the first three columns of Table 26.1 and the bottom of Figure 26.2. Figure 26.3 plots the percent returned-to-work on days after the injury.

Cumulative Disability Days

Some workers experience difficulties staying on the job after an initial return to work, and have repeated episodes of return-to-work, each of which generates disability days. This pattern occurs in about 20% of occupational back injuries.[5] Examining the distribution of cumulative disability days allows each day off work to be counted. The distribution of cumulative disability days answers the question "What percentage of workers lost up to 1 day, 2 days, 3 days, etc?" For example, the right most columns in Table 26.1 tally dis-

Table 26.1 Return-to-Work and Disability Days in a Cohort of Injured Workers*

Day After Injury	*Number RTW*	*% RTW*	*Days of Disability*	*Workers*	*Cumulative No. of Workers*	*Cumulative %*
1	0	0	1	3	3	30
2	3	30	2	2	5	50
3	6	60	3	1	6	60
4	7	70	4	2	8	80
5	7	70	5	1	9	90
6	8	80	6	0	9	90
7	9	90	7	0	9	90
8	9	90	8	0	9	90
9	9	90	9	0	9	90
10	9	90	10	1	10	100

*RTW, return-to-work.

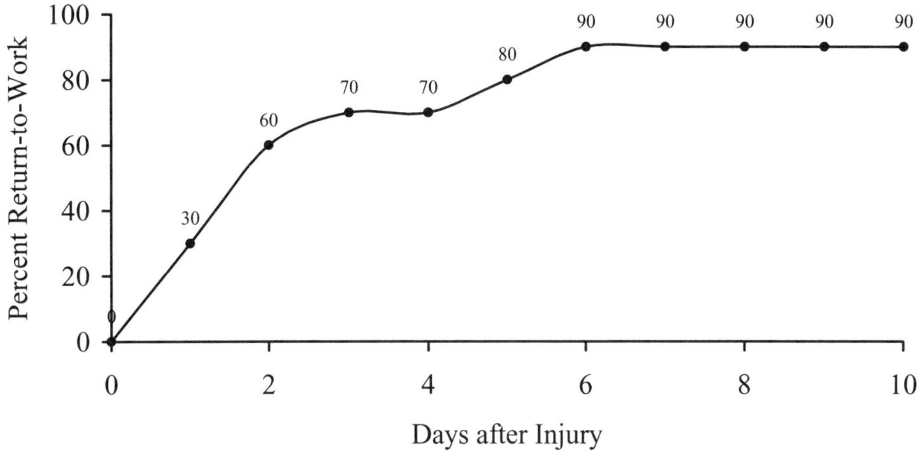

Figure 26.3 Return-to-work at specified days after the date of injury. This is an example of censuses taken each day after the day of injury in Figure 26.2.

ability days for each worker. Three of 10 (30%) workers each lost 1 day, 2 workers (20%) lost 2 days, 1 (10%) worker lost 1 day, etc. These percentages of workers are added as a cumulative tally as well. The plot of cumulative disability days is shown in Figure 26.4 for data on the right side columns of Table 26.1.

Analysis and Interpretation

In theory, the analysis of disability data for the purpose of surveillance is similar to other types of outcomes. The general objectives of the analysis are to estimate the magnitude of the problem, identify high-risk groups (for slow return-to-work), track trends in time or geographic area, and link case reporting to active follow-up. For active case follow-up, the criteria for follow-up can use the diagnosis, the actual or projected duration of the disability, the treatment setting (e.g., hospitalized cases, surgical cases), the clustering of cases, and epidemiologic measures such as rates of return-to-work.

The analysis can be considered rate-based because a denominator is defined. Using a single-point-in-time measure, a univariate analysis would examine how return-to-work at a specific point in time after injury or illness varies one variable at a time (e.g., diagnosis, age, sex, occupation, industry, geographic area). For individual employers, the specific departments or supervisory units may be included among the possible risk factors. Using repeated census or disability days, return-to-work curves can be plotted for each category of a risk factor (Fig. 26.5). Bivariate analyses can examine these relationships in more detail. Several advanced techniques under the heading of survival analysis have been used to analyze return-to-work.[6]

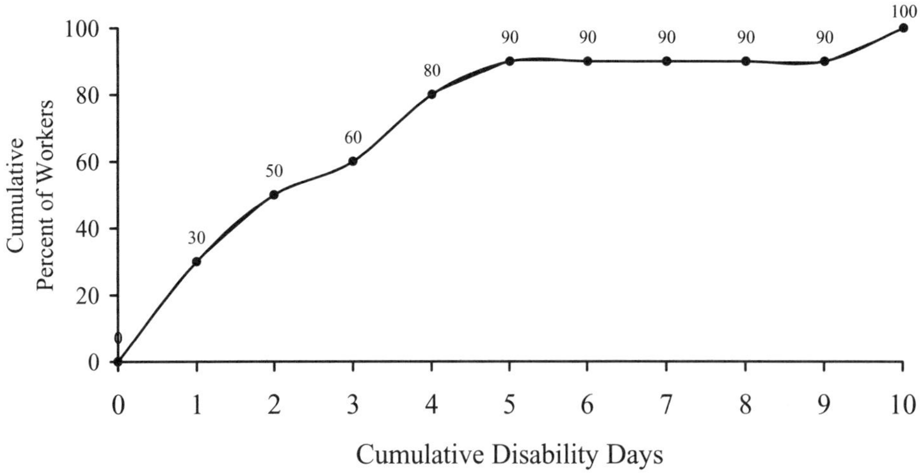

Figure 26.4 The graph describes the distribution of workers who lost up to the specified number of disability days. Thirty percent of the workers lost 1 day, 50% lost up to 2 days, 60% lost up to 3 days, etc.

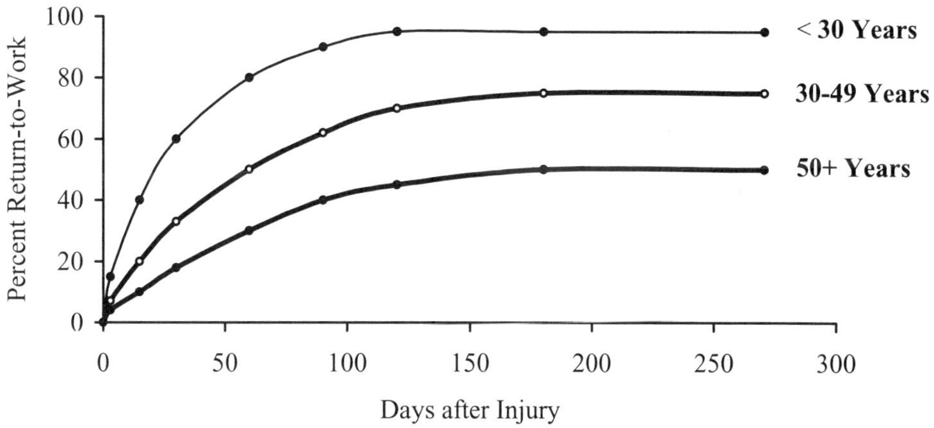

Figure 26.5 Univariate analysis of return to work by age. The graph illustrates that at any given point after the date of injury, the percent of returning older workers is less than younger workers.

The analysis of return-to-work at an individual employer has advantages and limitations. An employer large enough to have several different supervisors or department heads can analyze return-to-work by supervisor or department, changes before and after the implementation of disability policy, and other types of very specific issues not addressed in other databases. However, certain types of questions require external comparison groups. Injured workers at a single employer may be seen by only one medical group or have workers' compensation claims handled by a single administrator during a policy period. This will not allow an employer-specific analysis to examine how disability varies with these factors.

Data involving multiple employers, health care organizations, and claims administrators pose opportunities and many challenges for analysis and interpretation. There are significant issues regarding data quality, comparability of coding of variables, and confounding, which makes comparisons difficult to interpret. For example, small employers and other employers who cannot get workers' compensation insurance in the commercial market are often assigned to a state fund as their insurer. This may make it difficult to separate the effects of employer size and claims administrator. Many risk factors may be interrelated involving employers, the types of diagnoses (case-mix), work force demographics and size, health care providers, managed care arrangements, return-to-work policies and programs, and workers' compensation claims administrator.

Interpretation also depends on the operational definition of return-to-work or disability. A standard definition has yet to be adopted. An initial estimated date of return-to-work may be given by the treating physician. Released to return-to-work is based on physician's judgement that an injured worker is well enough to resume work with or without medical restrictions. Actual return-to-work is when a worker physically returns to the worksite. Sustained return-to-work is actual return without losing a set number of workdays due to relapses or reinjury. Depending on the definition, the percentage of return-to-work and disability duration can vary significantly.[5,7]

Feedback

Disability surveillance also involves information for action. Workers, employers, health care personnel, managed care organizations, rehabilitation and disability management professionals, claims administrators, workers' compensation administrative agencies, and lawmakers are among those with a need to know. Each has a sphere of influence, and a surveillance organization can develop messages, target the message to specific audiences, select appropriate channels for dissemination, market the message, and evaluate the impact. Feedback can also involve investigations into the causes of prolonged disability and basic research.

IMPROVING THE QUALITY AND EFFECTIVENESS OF OCCUPATIONAL HEALTH SERVICES

Surveillance can play a role in improving the quality and effectiveness of health services. The following is a brief overview of basic concepts of quality of health care and approaches to assessing and improving the quality of occupational health care through the use of indicators or performance measures. Some of these indicators may be suitable for surveillance.

The use of managed care in occupational medicine is increasing rapidly, in large part due to the desire of employers and insurers to better control workers' compensation costs. However, there is increasing recognition that indiscriminate cost cutting may have an adverse impact on the quality of care.[8] Increasingly, large purchasers—including the federal government—are turning their focus to the concept of health care value, where Value = Quality/Cost.

Value-based purchasing requires a mechanism to measure both cost and quality. On the cost side of the equation, employers and insurers can monitor their own dollar and productivity costs associated with health benefits, workers' compensation premiums, absence days, etc. But measuring the quality of health care is extremely challenging.

The interest in assessing quality of care is not limited to purchasers and consumers. Medicine is evolving rapidly toward a focus on medical effectiveness and outcomes and evidence-based care.[9] Numerous studies suggest the persistence of wide variations in medical practice, some of which raise questions about the quality of care.[10] Health care providers and managed care organizations are struggling to identify the parameters of quality care, and are striving to improve performance in the face of increasing financial and time constraints.

Defining Quality

The Institute of Medicine defines quality of care as the degree to which health services for individuals and populations increase the likelihood of desired health outcomes and are consistent with professional knowledge.[11] Poor quality of care may increase morbidity and mortality, decrease ability to function after an injury, and fail to improve the public health. Aspects of poor quality of care include:

- Shortcomings in interpersonal care. The nature of interactions between the physician, health care personnel, and the patient influences the development of patient trust in the physician, the extent of patient understanding, and the willingness of the patient to follow instructions or return for follow-up care. In occupational health, shortcomings in interpersonal care additionally may impact the patient's trust in the appropriateness of return-to-work recommendations, the understanding of work restrictions, and the likelihood of litigation.
- Shortcomings in the technical aspects of care. Overuse of ineffective therapeutic modalities, use of inappropriate treatments, or under-use of effective treatments all contribute to poor outcomes. Several studies suggest that overuse may be a problem in workers' compensation medical care, particularly in the care of common musculoskeletal problems such as low back pain.[12–14] Overuse may increase complications and iatrogenic poor outcomes,[15] or may simply drive up costs of care. Although managed care organizations (MCOs) tend to focus on identification of over-utilization, several recent studies in the group health arena suggest that under-use is also a significant problem;[16] further studies in occupational medicine are warranted. Deficiencies in skill and judgment of individual providers also lead to poor quality of care. There is considerable evidence that, at least in the performance of coronary artery by-pass grafts (CABG), high volume is associated with lower mortality.[17] Studies of the association between volume and, for example, outcome after low back surgery, are lacking, as are assessments of the appropriateness of selected procedures.
- Shortcomings in the organizational aspects of care. The health care delivery system influences access to care (both initial and access to specialty care), continuity of care, and coordination of care. The traditional workers' compensation fee-for-service system, in which the injured worker, claims examiner, or attorney has often managed care, has been characterized by fragmented, uncoordinated care.

In assessing the quality of care, experts have focused on three aspects of care: structure, process, and outcomes.[18] Structure includes the organization of the health care delivery system, the nature of the provider network, the facilities that are available—in other words, the overall physical and organizational context in which health care providers actually provide care. Process refers to everything that happens between the provider and the patient: communications, medical decision-making, and diagnosis and treatment choices. Outcomes reflect changes in health status that occur subsequent to the delivery of care, and can be attributed to the health care that was provided.

In order to evaluate or monitor the quality of care, there must be both a standard of care to use as a benchmark, and a standardized method for evaluation. Performance measures, or quality indicators, provide a tool to monitor the extent to which the health care providers meet a standard of care; they are signs that can point to problems, indicate changes in complex systems, or compare different areas or groups.[19] Although it is beyond the scope of this chapter to discuss specific occupational medicine performance measures in depth, several examples are provided below.

Properly developed and used, performance measures and quality indicators can be used by health care providers, managed care organizations, purchasers, consumers, and health care regulators. Such measures can provide insight into the strengths and weaknesses of care delivery systems, providing useful information for quality improvement efforts and for selection of health care.[20–22]

In the group health arena, several organizations have devoted considerable resources to the development of performance measures, including the National Council on Quality Assurance, the Joint Commission for the Accreditation of Healthcare Organizations, and the Foundation for Accountability.[23–24] These performance measures, for the most part, focus on diagnoses and services that have high impacts on cost and outcome (e.g., postoperative CABG mortality, mammography and immunization rates, screening for complications of diabetes, and hospitalization for asthma). They provide little help in the evaluation of the quality of occupational medical care, because, with few exceptions, they are not relevant to the practice of occupational medicine.

The first step in developing performance measures is determining what one wishes to assess and in what population. Clearly, performance measures for occupational medical care should address work-related illnesses and injuries. High-frequency diagnoses in occupational medicine include low back pain, fractures, dermatitis, upper extremity complaints and cumulative trauma of the upper extremities, and eye injury; less frequent events may, however, have particularly serious consequences (e.g., occupational cancer) or may be particularly amenable to quality improvement efforts (e.g., treatment of occupational asthma).

Performance measures are most reliable when used to assess outcomes in specific populations. Understanding the population of interest thus provides additional important information for the development of performance measures.[25] Knowledge of population characteristics is also important in identifying risk adjusters, which may be critical in the analysis of data used for performance measurement. Generally, the occupational medicine patient population is between the ages of 16 and 65, and sufficiently healthy (at least preinjury) to be working; it is a population characterized by ethnic, linguistic, and literacy diversity. The usual patterns of care for this population vary tremendously—ranging from rich group health benefits to no usual health care.

Occupational medicine encompasses a wide scope of activities, including primary prevention, clinical diagnosis and treatment, and disability prevention and management. Performance measures should address the breadth of occupational medical practice, and may pertain to the structure, process, or outcomes of health care.

Ideally, the quality of the structure and process will contribute to the nature of the outcomes; however, this is not always the case. In selecting performance measures, it is important to assess the extent to which a particular structure or process is really associated with an outcome of interest. There is good evidence, for example, that immunizations really do prevent polio; therefore, immunization rates of children are a reasonable indicator of quality of pediatric care, as a proxy for measuring polio case rates. Surgery utilization rates, however, are not a reasonable proxy for measuring outcomes after back surgery.

When using outcome measures, it is very important to consider key contributors to the outcome that may lie outside the health care provider's domain. Teen pregnancy rates, for example, certainly reflect factors other than the quality of counseling by pediatricians. Return-to-work outcomes similarly reflect workplace conditions and employer policies that are beyond the control of the individual physician. Thus, although the physician may play an important role in the return to work process, good return-to-work outcomes also require employer policies and behaviors conducive to return-to-work.

The following discusses examples of the types of performance measures that might be used to assess the quality of occupational medicine services, and some of the problems in using performance measures. These examples are not meant to be exhaustive, but rather illustrative of the range of issues that warrant examination if we are committed to developing performance measures and using them to improve the quality of occupational medical care.

Access

Simple measures of access include time from injury to first doctor's visit (which can be obtained from medical bill data), or standard patient satisfaction survey questions regarding geographical convenience and waiting time in doctors' offices.[26] However, assessing access in occupational medicine should also include a measure of the extent to which workers with occupational illness have access to the workers' compensation system. This poses a larger measurement problem because we have no ability to routinely and systematically identify occupational illnesses treated outside of the workers' compensation system.

Clinical Diagnosis and Treatment

Process quality indicators for clinical diagnosis and treatment, including provision of clinical preventive services, must be carefully derived from professionally developed and accepted clinical guidelines of care. Medical services utilization rates may be difficult to use as

Table 26.2 Performance Measures for Clinical Care in Occupational Medicine: Examples*

Condition	*Examples of Performance Measures*
CARPAL TUNNEL RELEASE SURGERY	
1. Was there an adequate trial of conservative care prior to surgery?	
a. Percentage of patients with appropriate activity restrictions for at least 1 month prior to surgery	
b. Percentage of patients with night splint prior to surgery	
c. Percentage of patients with localized injection of lidocaine or corticosteroid prior to surgery	
2. Was there appropriate NCV testing done prior to surgery?	
a. Percentage of patients with documented decreased NCV	
3. Is there documented counseling regarding outcomes, risks, and benefits prior to surgery?	
a. Percentage of patients with counseling documented in chart	
ACUTE LOW BACK PROBLEMS	
1. Were appropriate assessment techniques used?	
a. Percentage of medical records with documentation of screening for serious underlying condition	
b. Percentage of patients with plain x-rays of lumbar spine in absence of red flag	
c. Percentage of patients with CT or MRI in first month in absence of red flag	
2. Was appropriate conservative care provided?	
a. Percentage of patients with chart documentation of patient education/counseling	
b. Percentage of patients with appropriate analgesic prescribed (acetaminophen, NSAIDs, aspirin)	
c. Percentage of patients with bed rest longer than 4 days	
d. Percentage of patients with oral steroids prescribed	
e. Percentage of patients receiving TENS	
f. Percentage of patients receiving trigger point or ligamentous injections	
3. If performed, was surgery appropriate?	
a. Percentage of patients with chart documentation of discussion of treatment options	
b. Percentage of patients with documented persistent severe sciatica	
c. Percentage of patients with documented clinical evidence of nerve root compromise	

*NCV, nerve conduction velocity; CT, computed tomography; MRI, magnetic resonance imaging; NSAID, non-steroidal antiinflammatory drug; TENS, transcutaneous electrical nerve stimulation.

Source: Rudolph.[36]

quality indicators, unless there is reasonable evidence regarding what constitutes an appropriate rate of services, or there is clear-cut evidence of services that should or should not be provided in particular patient groups. Clinical indicators must be carefully defined.[27] Examples of possible clinical performance measures are provided in Table 26.2, based in large part on clinical standards of care presented in the American College of Occupational and Environmental Medicine (ACOEM) Treatment Guidelines.[28]

Prevention

Occupational medicine is a preventive medicine specialty, and high quality occupational medical services should play a role in the prevention of occupational injury and illness.[29] Components of the process of care may be important indicators of the quality of preventive services. Failure to take a good occupational history makes it difficult to identify hazardous exposures that warrant intervention. However, taking a good history is not sufficient, and may not lead to primary prevention interventions. Thus, examining the occupational physician's records to assess the frequency with which an occupational history is taken may also not be a good measure of the quality of prevention services.

A better measure for occupational medicine prevention may be the record of communicating recommendations for primary prevention to the employers of injured workers, or the number of times a provider has visited a worksite in the prior year. The Association of Occupational and Environmental Clinics (AOEC) asks applicants for membership to describe a primary prevention intervention in which the clinic has been involved.[30] Employer surveys could be another source of information about primary prevention efforts by an occupational medicine provider.

Other measures of preventive services include: the proportion of high-risk health workers who receive necessary immunizations (e.g., Hepatitis B); the proportion of exposed individuals who receive appropriate biological monitoring (e.g., blood lead testing); the proportion of exposed individuals who receive appropriate medical screening for early disease detection (e.g., audiometry, pulmonary function testing); or the proportion of cumulative trauma cases in which appropriate work restrictions or modifications are prescribed.

Outcomes

Outcome measures provide the only indicator of the extent to which health care actually impacts health status. A number of outcomes are of considerable interest. These include easily measured clinical outcomes of both preventive and treatment interventions (e.g., decrease in blood lead levels after intervention to reduce lead exposure; improved nerve conduction velocity after carpal tunnel release surgery).

Patient-perceived outcomes such as frequency and severity of pain or functional impacts of injury at work and at home are clearly extremely important outcomes, requiring surveys of injured workers. Patient satisfaction with medical care is another important outcome that in the workers' compensation arena, may impact not only patient compliance with treatment, but also employer control over medical care, litigation, and disability outcomes.[31] Measures of employer satisfaction (e.g., with adequacy of communications regarding appropriate work restrictions) may also provide insight into occupational medicine quality.

The use of outcome measures requires careful attention to other factors, which may also impact outcome. In the analysis of hospital mortality rates, for example, intensive effort has gone into developing methods for risk adjustment that consider patient demographics, severity, and case mix, in order to allow more confidence in using these rates to compare the quality of care among hospitals.[32] Different risk adjustment methods, however, may yield different results when comparing hospital mortality experience.

This should give us pause when considering the use of some outcome measures of great interest in occupational medicine, particularly given the complexity of the workers' compensation system.

Rates of injury and illness, for example, are the outcome most reflective of the success of prevention efforts, and could certainly be used to assess the quality of preventive services. However, it is the employer, not the physician, who has the lion's share of responsibility and the ability to maintain a safe workplace free of hazards; claims rates may also reflect aspects of labor-management relationships. Injury rates may thus not be a fair indicator of the physician's performance with regard to prevention. Indeed, using injury rates as a performance measure for the health care provider organization could create perverse incentives to provide services only to those employers with good safety programs.[33]

Some purchasers and managed care organizations view return-to-work outcomes as a paramount measure of occupational medicine quality—even proposing that physician reimbursements be tied to return-to-work outcomes. Yet even the best disability management skills on the part of a provider may not result in a good return-to-work outcome if the supervisor is unwilling to cooperate. Without a method for risk adjustment that takes into account the nature and severity of injury or complaint, the specific job and characteristics thereof, and the willingness of the employer to implement appropriate work modifications or restriction, return-to-work is a very fuzzy measure of occupational medicine performance.

Performance measures may be extremely useful in improving the quality of care and facilitating the health care choices of consumers and purchasers. However, to be useful, information derived from performance measurement must be both understandable and meaningful.[34] For workers, this means there must be considerable attention to worker concerns, literacy levels, and presentation formats.[35] For physicians and health care organizations, this requires a level of buy-in that may be facilitated by an inclusive measures development process by a credible organization, and a nonpunitive approach to the discussion of performance measurement results.

The use of quality indicators is a new phenomenon in health care. In occupational medicine, developing meaningful and valid performance measures will require a concerted effort involving health care providers, employers, labor representatives, and public health experts. Embarking on that effort will provide the information we need to improve the quality of preventive and treatment services for workers.

ACKNOWLEDGMENTS

Portions of this chapter on the quality and effectiveness of occupational health services were published previously in *Occupational Medicine* and have been used with permission.

REFERENCES

1. Cheadle A, Franklin G, Wolfhagen C, Savarino J, Liu PY, Salley C, Weaver M. Factors influencing the duration of work-related disability: a population-based study of Washington State workers' compensation. *Am J Public Health* 1994; 84:190–196.
2. Kraus N, Dasinger LK, Wigand A. *Does Modified Work Facilitate Return to Work for Temporarily or Permanently Disabled Workers? Review of the Literature and Annotated Bibliography.* Berkeley: University of California; 1997.
3. McGrail MP Jr, Tsai SP, Bernacki E. A comprehensive initiative to manage the incidence and cost of occupational injury and illness. Report of an outcomes analysis. *J Occup Environ Med* 1995; 37:1263–1268.2.
4. Rudolph L. A call for quality (editorial). *J Occ Med.* 1996; 38:343–344.
5. Krause N, Dasinger LK, Deegan L, Brand R, Rudolph L. Alternative approaches for measuring duration of work disability after low back injury based on workers' compensation data. *Am J Ind Med* 1999; 35:604–618.
6. Selvin S. *Statistical Analysis of Epidemiologic Data.* New York: Oxford University Press, 1991.
7. Dasinger LK, Krause N, Deegan LJ, Brand RJ, Rudolph L. Duration of work disability after low back injury: a comparison of administrative and self-reported outcomes. *Am J Ind Med* 1999; 35:619–631.

8. Chelimsky E. The political debate about health care: are we losing sight of quality. *Science* 1993; 262:525–528.
9. Ellwood P. Shattuck Lecture—Outcomes Management: A Technology of Patient Experience. *New Engl J Med* 1988; 318(23): 1549–1556.
10. Welch WP, Miller ME, Welch HG, Fisher ES, Wennburg JE. Geographic variation in expenditures for physicians' services in the United States. *New Engl J Med* 1993; 328:621–627.
11. Institute of Medicine. *America's Health in Transition: Protecting and Improving Quality*. Washington, DC: National Academy Press; 1994.
12. Zaidman B. *Industrial Strength Medicine: Report to the Minnesota Legislature*. Minnesota Department of Labor and Industry. 1990.
13. Johnson WG, Baldwin ML, Burton JF Jr. Why is the treatment of work-related injuries so costly? New evidence from California. *Inquiry* 1996; 33:53–65.
14. Mardon R, Mitchell G. *The Impact of Florida's Low-Back Practice Guideline on Treatment of New Workers' Compensation Injuries*. State Center for Health Statistics, Agency for Health Care Administration, 1997.
15. Franklin G, Haug J, Heyer N, McKeefrey S, Picciano J. Outcome of lumbar fusion in Washington State workers' compensation. *Spine* 1994; 19:1897–1904.
16. Chassin M. Assessing strategies for quality improvement. Health Affairs 1997; 16:151–161.
17. Grumbach K, et al. Regionalization of cardiac surgery in the U.S. and Canada: Geographic access, choice, and outcomes. *JAMA* 1995; 274:1282–1288.
18. Donabedian A. *The Methods and Findings of Quality Assessment and Monitoring: An Illustrated Analysis*. Ann Arbor, Michigan: Health Administration Press, 1985.
19. Institute of Medicine. *Access to Health Care in America*. Washington, DC: National Academy Press, 1993.
20. Corrigan J. How do purchasers develop and use performance measures. *Medical Care* 1995; 33(1)Suppl:JS25–JS30.
21. Karpatkin R, Shearer G. A short-term consumer agenda for health care reform. *Am J Public Health* 1995; 85:1352–1355.
22. O'Leary D. Performance Measures: How are they developed, validated, and used? *Medical Care* 1995; 33(1)Suppl:JS13–JS17.
23. NCQA. *Medicaid HEDIS*. Washington, DC: National Committee for Quality Assurance, 1996.
24. Nadzam D, Turpin R, Hanold L, White R. Data-driven performance improvement in health care: the Joint Commission's Indicator Measurement System (IMSystem). *Jt Comm J Qual Improv* 1993; 19:492–500.
25. Palmer RH. *Understanding and Choosing Clinical Performance Measures: Development of a Typology*. U.S. Department of Health and Human Services. Agency for Health Care Policy and Research. AHCPR Publ. No. 95-N001, 95-N002.
26. Agency for Health Care Policy and Research. *Consumer Assessment of Health Plans Survey*. Baltimore, MD: U.S. Department of Health and Human Services, 1997.
27. NCQA. *Health Plan Employer Data and Information Set*, version 3.0. Washington, DC: National Committee for Quality Assurance, 1997.
28. American College of Occupational and Environmental Medicine. *Acute Medical Problems in Working Adults: A Clinician's Guide to Assessment and Treatment*. Arlington Heights, IL: ACOEM, 1997.
29. ACOEM Committee on Ethical Practice in Occupational Medicine. Committee report: Commentaries on the code of ethical conduct. *J Occup Med* 1995; 37:201–206.
30. Association of Occupational and Environmental Clinics. *Application Standards*. Washington, DC: Association of Occupational and Environmental Clinics, 1993.
31. Rudolph L, Wiley J, Dervin K, Garrett K, Maizlish N, Chang YT. *What Do Injured Workers Think About Their Medical Care?* San Francisco: California Division of Workers' Compensation, 1998.
32. Iezzoni L. *Risk Adjustment for Measuring Health Outcomes*. Ann Arbor: Health Administration Press, 1994.
33. Schauffler H, Rodriguez T. Exercising Purchasing Power for Prevention. In: Wilkerson J, Given R, ed. *Competitive Managed Care: The Emerging Health Care System*. San Francisco: Jossey-Bass, 1997.
34. Office of Technology Assessment. *Health Care Reform: Report Cards Are Useful but Significant Issues Need to Be Addressed*. Washington, DC: U.S. GAO, 1994.
35. Sum J. *What Workers Know About the Workers' Compensation System*. San Francisco: California Commission on Workers' Compensation and Health and Safety, 1997.
36. Rudolph LA. Performance measures in occupational medicine: A tool to manage quality. *Occup Med* 1998; 13:747–753.

Appendix A

Standardized Forms Used in Occupational Health Surveillance

NEIL A. MAIZLISH

The OSHA 200 summary page (Fig. A.1) is divided into injuries (*left*) and seven categories of illness (*right*). Each case has to be logged within 6 days of becoming aware of its occurrence. At least once a year employers count the number of cases and the lost days away from work and workdays of restricted work activity. Cases are defined as fatalities and nonfatal injuries or illnesses, including those that cause a loss in consciousness, a work restriction, transfer to another job, or medical treatment other than first aid.

Employer's Report of Occupational Injury or Illness (Fig. A.2) is used by California employers to report each case of job injury or illness to their insurance carrier within 5 days of its occurrence. Insurance carriers use the form to help establish a workers' compensation claim, and then forward the report to the state's Division of Labor Statistics and Research.

California is one of 28 states that requires physicians to report cases of suspected occupational injury and illness. The form used is the Doctor's First Report of Occupational Injury or Illness (Fig. A.3). Approximately 40,000 Doctor's First Reports are received each year for occupational illness.

The standard billing form for doctors and other health professionals in the United States is called a health insurance claim form (Fig. A.4). The form, known as the HCFA-1500, or its electronic equivalent (837) is submitted to insurance companies and to the federal government. It is for reimbursement of professional services rendered by doctors and other health care professionals in fee-for-service types of medical care. It lists several fields for a coded diagnosis linked to coded treatments, dates of service delivery, and costs. However, occupation of the patient is not included on the form.

The standard billing form for hospitals and health care facilities is shown in Figure A.5. It is known as the UB-92 or HCFA-1450 form. The form or its electronic equivalent (837) are also submitted to insurance companies and the federal government. It is for reimbursement of costs of facilities (hospital bed, food, supplies, operating rooms, etc.) in fee-for-service types of medical care. It lists several fields for a coded diagnosis linked to coded treatments. Occupation is not included on the form.

The standard death certificate used in the United States is shown in Figure A.6. A death certificate must be filled out by a physician before a body can be buried. The top part of the form about the personal background of the decedent, including usual occupation and industry worked, is usually filled in by a funeral director or house staff of a hospital.

U.S. Department of Labor

For Calendar Year ___________ Page: _____ of _____

Company Name	Form Approved
Establishment Name	O.M.B. No. 1218-0176
Establishment Address	See OMB Disclosure
	Statement on reverse.

Extent of and Outcome of Injury						Type, Extent of, and Outcome of Illness												
Fatalities	Nonfatal Injuries					Type of Illness							Fatalities	Nonfatal Illnesses				
Injury Related	Injuries with Lost Workdays				Injuries Without Lost Workdays	CHECK Only One Column for Each Illness (See other side of form for terminations or permanent transfers)							Illness Related	Illnesses with Lost Workdays				Illnesses without Lost Workdays
Enter Date of death. mm/dd/yy	Enter a Check if injury involves DAYS away from work or restricted work activity or both.	Enter a Check if injury involves DAYS away from work.	Enter number of DAYS away from work	Enter number of DAYS of restricted work activity	Enter a Check if no entry was made in column 1 or 2 but the injury is recordable as defined above.	Occupational Skin Disorder or Disease	Dust Disease of the lungs	Respiratory Conditions due to toxic agents	Poisoning (systemic effects of toxic materials)	Disorders due to physical agents	Disorders associated with repeated trauma	All other occupational illnesses	Enter DATE of death, mm/dd/yy	Enter a CHECK if Illness involves DAYS away from work, or DAYS of restricted work activity or both.	Enter a CHECK if Illness involves DAYS away from work.	Enter number of DAYS away from work.	Enter number of DAYS of restricted work activity	Enter a CHECK if no entry was made in columns 8 or 9
						(7)												
(1)	(2)	(3)	(4)	(5)	(6)	(a)	(b)	(c)	(d)	(e)	(f)	(g)	(8)	(9)	(10)	(11)	(12)	(13)

Certification of Annual Summary Totals by: ____________________ Title: ____________________ Date: __________

OSHA 200

POST ONLY THIS PORTION OF THE LAST PAGE NO LATER THAN FEBRUARY 1

Figure A.1 OSHA 200 Form.

Log and Summary of Occupational Injuries and illnesses

NOTE: This form is required by Public Law 91-596 and must be kept in the establishment for 5 years. Failure to maintain and post can result in issuance of citations and assessment of penalties. (*See posting requirements on the other side of form*)

RECORDABLE CASES: You are required to record information about every occupational death; every nonfatal occupational illness; and those nonfatal occupational injuries which involve one or more of the following: loss of conciousness, restriction of work or motion, transfer to another job, or medical treatment (other than first aid) (*See definitions on the other side of form*)

Case or File Number	Date of Injury or Onset of Illness	Employee's Name	Occupation	Department	Description of Injury or Illness
Enter a nonduplicating number which will facilitate comparisons with supplementary records.	Enter Mo/Day	Enter first name or initial, middle initial, last name	Enter regular job title, not activity employee was performing when injury occurred or at onset of illness. In the absence of a formal title, enter a brief description of the employee's duties.	Enter department in which the employee is regularly employed or a description of normal workplace to which employee is assigned, even though temporarily working in another department at the time of injury or illness.	Enter a brief description of the injury or illness and indicate the part or parts of the body affected. Typical entries for this column might be: Amputation of 1st joint right forefinger; Strain of lower back; Contact dermatitis on both hands; Electrocution - body.
(A)	(B)	(C)	(D)	(E)	(F)
					PREVIOUS PAGE TOTALS ⇒
					TOTALS (Instructions on other side of form) ⇒
OSHA No. 200					

Figure A.1 (Continued)

State of California

EMPLOYER'S REPORT OF OCCUPATIONAL INJURY OR ILLNESS

Please complete in triplicate (type, if possible) Mail two copies to:

OSHA
Case No.

☐ Fatality

Any person who makes or causes to be made any knowingly false or fraudulent material statement of material representation for the purpose of obtaining or denying workers' compensation benefits or payments is guilty of a felony

NOTICE: California law requires employers to report within **five days** of knowledge every occupational injury or illness which results in lost time beyond the date of the incident **OR** requires medical treatment beyond first aid. If an employee subsequently dies as a result of a previously reported injury or illness, the employer must file within **five days** of knowledge an amended report indicating death. In addition, every serious injury/illness, or death must be reported **immediately** by telephone or telegraph to the nearest office of the California Division of Occupational Safety and Health.

EMPLOYER

1. FIRST NAME — 1A. POLICY NUMBER

2. MAILING ADDRESS (Number and Street, City Code) — 2A. PHONE NUMBER

3. LOCATION, IF DIFFIRENT FROM MAILING (Number and Street, City, Zip) — 3A LOCATION CODE

4. NATURE OF BUSINESS, e.g., painting contractor, wholesale grocer, sawmill, hotel, etc. — 5. STATE UNMPLOYMENT INSURANCE ACCT. NO.

6. TYPE OF EMPLOYER ☐ ☐STATE CITY COUNTY SCHOOL DISTRICT ☐

EMPLOYEE

EMPLOYEE NAME — 8. SOCIAL SECURITY NUMBER — 9. DATE OF BIRTH (mm/dd/yy)

10. HOME ADRESS (Number and Street, City, Zip) — 10A. Phone Number

11. SEX ☐MALE ☐FEMALE — 12. OCCUPATION (Regular job title) – No initial, abbreviations or numbers — 13. DATE OF HIRE (mm/dd/yy)

14. EMPLOYEE USUALLY WORKS ____ hours per day ____ days per week ____ total weekly hours — 14A. EMPLOYEMENT STATUS (State applicable status at time of injury) ___ Regular Full Time ____ Part Time ______ temporary ____ seasonal — 14B. Under what class code of your policy were wages assigned?

15. GROSS WAGES/SALARY $_____ PER _____________ — 16. OTHER PAYMENTS NOT REPORTED AS WAGES/SALARY (e.g., tips, meals, lodging, overtime, bonuses, etc)? ☐ YES, $______________ Per __________ ☐ NO

INJURY OR ILLNESS

17. DATE OF INJURY OR ONSET OF ILLNESS (mm/dd/yy) — 18. TIME INURY/ILLNESS OCCURRED ______A.M. ______P.M. — 19. TIME EMPLOYEE BEGAN WORK ______A.M. ______P.M. — 20. IF EMPLOYEE DIED, DATE OF DEATH (MM/DD/YY)

21. unable to work for at least one full day after date of injury ☐ yes ☐no — 22. DATE LAST WORKED (mm/dd/yy) — 23. DATE RETURNED TO WORK (mm/dd/yy) — 24. IF STILL OFF WORK CHECK THIS BOX. ☐

25. PAID FULL WAGES FOR DAY OF INJURY OR LAST DAY WORKED? ☐YES ☐NO — 26. SALARY BEING CONTINUED ☐YES ☐NO — 27. DATE OF EMPLOYER'S KNOWLEDGE/NOTICE OF INJURY/ILLNESS (MM/DD/YY) — 28. DATE EMPLOYEE WAS PROVIDED EMPLOYEE CLAIM FORM (MM/DD/YY)

29. SPECIFIC INJURY/ILLNESS AND PART OF BODY AFFECTED, MEDICAL DIAGNOSIS, if available e.g., second degree burns on right arm, tendentious of left elbow, lead poisoning.

30. LOCATION WHERE EVENT OR EXOSURE OCCURRED (Number, Street, City) — 30A. County — 30B. ON EMPLOYER'S PREMISES? ☐YES ☐NO

31. DEPARTMENT WHERE EVENT OR EXPLOSURE OCCURRED, e.g., Shipping department, machine shop. — 32. OTHER WORKERS INJURED/ILL IN THIS EVENT? ☐YES ☐NO

33. EQUIPMENT, MATERIALS AND CHEMICALS THE EMPLOYEE WAS USING WHEN THE EVENT OR EXPOSURE OCCURRED, e.g., acetylene, welding torch, farm tractor, scaffold.

33. SPECIFIC ACTIVITY THE EMPLOYEE WAS PERFORMING WHEN EVENT OF EXPOSURE OCCURRED e.g., welding seams of metal forms, loading boxes onto truck.

35. HOW INJURY/ILLNESS OCCURRED. DESCRIBE SEQUENCE OF EVENTS. SPECIFY OBJECT OR EXPOSURE WHICH DIRECTLY PRODUCED THE INJURY/ILLNESS, e.g., worker stepped back to inspect work and slipped on scrap material. As he fell, he brushed against fresh weld, and burned right hand, USE SEPARATE SHEET IF NECESSARY.

36. NAME AND ADRESS OF PHYSICIAN (Number and Street, City, Zip — 36A. PHONE NUMBER

37. IF HOSPITALIZED AS AN INPATIENT, NAME AND ADDRESS OF HOSPITAL (Number and Street, City, zip) — 37A. PHONE NUMBER

Completed by (Type or Print) — Signature — Title — Date

DO NOT USE THIS COLUMN: Case NO; Ownership; Industry; Occupation; Sex; AGE; Daily hours; Days per week; Weekly hours; Weekly Wage; County; Nature of injury; Part of Body; Source; Event; Sec. Source; Extent of injury

FORM 5020 (REV. 6)

FILING OF THIS REPORT IS NOT ADMISSION OF LIABILITY

Figure A.2 Employer's First Report of Injury and Illness (6th Rev, 1993), California.

STATE OF CALIFORNIA

DOCTOR'S FIRST REPORT OF OCCUPATIONAL INJURY OR ILLNESS

Within 5 days of your initial examination, for every occupational injury or illness, send tow copies of this report to the employer's workers' compensation insurance carrier or the insured employer. Failure to file a timely doctor's report may result in assessment of a civil penalty. In the case of diagnosed or suspected pesticide poisoning, send a copy of the report to Division of Labor Statistics and Research, P.O. Box 420603, San Francisco, CA 94142-0603, and notify your local health officer by telephone within 24 hours.

			PLEASE DO NOT USE THIS COLUMN
1. INSURER NAME AND ADDRESS			
2. EMPLOYER NAME			Case No.
3. Address No. and Street City Zip			Industry
4. Nature of business (e.g., food manufacturing, building construction, retailer of women's clothes.)			County
5. PATIENT NAME (first name, middle initial, last name)	6. Sex ☐ Male ☐ Female	7. Date of Birth Mo. Day Yr.	Age
8. Address: No. and Street City Zip		9. Telephone number ( )	Hazard
10. Occupation (Specific job title)		11. Social Security Number - -	Disease
12. Injured at: No. and Street City County			Hospitalization
13. Date and hour of injury or onset of illness Mo. Day Yr. Hour ______ a.m. ______ p.m.		14. Date last worked Mo. Day Yr.	Occupation
15. Date and hour of first examination or treatment Mo. Day Yr. Hour ______ a.m. ______ p.m.		16. Have you (or your office) previously treated patient? ☐ Yes ☐ No	Return Date/Code

Patient please complete this portion, if able to do so. Otherwise, doctor please complete immediately, inability or failure of a patient to complete this portion shall not affect his/her rights to workers' compensation under the California Labor Code.

17. **DESCRIBE HOW THE ACCIDENT OR EXPOSURE HAPPENED.** (Give specific object, machinery or chemical. Use reverse side if more space is required.)

18. **SUBJECTIVE COMPLAINTS** (Describe fully. Use reverse side if more space is required.)

19. **OBJECTIVE FINDINGS** (Use reverse side if more space is required.)
A. Physical examination

B. X-ray and laboratory results (State if non or pending.)

20. **DIAGNOSIS** (if occupational illness specify etiologic agent and duration of exposure.) Chemical or toxic compounds involved? ☐ Yes ☐ No
ICD-9 Code ___ ___ ___ - ___ ___

21. Are your findings and diagnosis consistent with patient's account of injury or onset of illness? ☐ Yes ☐ No If "no", please explain.

22. Is there any other current condition that will impede or delay patient's recovery? ☐ Yes ☐ No If "yes", please explain.

23. **TREATMENT RENDERED** (Use reverse side if more space is required.)

24. If further treatment required, specify treatment plan/estimated duration.

25. If hospitalized as inpatient, give hospital name and location Date admitted Mo. Day Yr. Estimated stay

26. WORK STATUS -- Is patient able to perform usual work? ☐ Yes ☐ No
If "no", date when patient can return to: Regular work ___/___/___
Modified work ___/___/___ Specify restrictions ________

Doctor's Signature ________ CA License Number ________

Doctor Name and Degree (please type) ________ IRS Number ________

Address ________ Telephone Number (____)________

FORM 5021 (Rev. 4)
1992

Any person who makes or causes to be made any knowingly false or fraudulent material statement or material representation for the purpose of obtaining or denying workers' compensation benefits or payments is guilty of a felony.

Figure A.3 Doctor's First Report of Injury and Illness (4th Rev., 1992), California.

PLEASE DO NOT STAPLE IN THIS AREA

APPROVED OMB-0938-0008

CARRIER

PICA

HEALTH INSURANCE CLAIM FORM

PICA

1. MEDICARE (Medicare #) MEDICAID (Medicaid #) CHAMPUS (Sponsor's SSN) CHAMPVA (VA File #) GROUP HEALTH PLAN (SSN or ID) FECA BLK LUNG (SSN) OTHER (ID)

1a. INSURED'S I.D. NUMBER (FOR PROGRAM IN ITEM 1)

2. PATIENT'S NAME (Last Name, First Name, Middle Initial)

3. PATIENT'S BIRTH DATE MM DD YY SEX M F

4. INSURED'S NAME (Last Name, First Name, Middle Initial)

5. PATIENT'S ADDRESS (No., Street)

6. PATIENT RELATIONSHIP TO INSURED Self Spouse Child Other

7. INSURED'S ADDRESS (No., Street)

CITY STATE

8. PATIENT STATUS Single Married Other

CITY STATE

ZIP CODE TELEPHONE (Include Area Code) ( )

Employed Full-Time Student Part-Time Student

ZIP CODE TELEPHONE (INCLUDE AREA CODE) ( )

9. OTHER INSURED'S NAME (Last Name, First Name, Middle Initial)

10. IS PATIENT'S CONDITION RELATED TO:

11. INSURED'S POLICY GROUP OR FECA NUMBER

a. OTHER INSURED'S POLICY OR GROUP NUMBER

a. EMPLOYMENT? (CURRENT OR PREVIOUS) YES NO

a. INSURED'S DATE OF BIRTH MM DD YY SEX M F

b. OTHER INSURED'S DATE OF BIRTH MM DD YY SEX M F

b. AUTO ACCIDENT? PLACE (State) YES NO

b. EMPLOYER'S NAME OR SCHOOL NAME

c. EMPLOYER'S NAME OR SCHOOL NAME

c. OTHER ACCIDENT? YES NO

c. INSURANCE PLAN NAME OR PROGRAM NAME

d. INSURANCE PLAN NAME OR PROGRAM NAME

10d. RESERVED FOR LOCAL USE

d. IS THERE ANOTHER HEALTH BENEFIT PLAN? YES NO *If yes*, return to and complete item 9 a-d.

READ BACK OF FORM BEFORE COMPLETING & SIGNING THIS FORM.

12. PATIENT'S OR AUTHORIZED PERSON'S SIGNATURE I authorize the release of any medical or other information necessary to process this claim. I also request payment of government benefits either to myself or to the party who accepts assignment below.

SIGNED ______ DATE ______

13. INSURED'S OR AUTHORIZED PERSON'S SIGNATURE I authorize payment of medical benefits to the undersigned physician or supplier for services described below.

SIGNED ______

PATIENT AND INSURED INFORMATION

14. DATE OF CURRENT: MM DD YY ILLNESS (First symptom) OR INJURY (Accident) OR PREGNANCY(LMP)

15. IF PATIENT HAS HAD SAME OR SIMILAR ILLNESS. GIVE FIRST DATE MM DD YY

16. DATES PATIENT UNABLE TO WORK IN CURRENT OCCUPATION FROM MM DD YY TO MM DD YY

17. NAME OF REFERRING PHYSICIAN OR OTHER SOURCE

17a. I.D. NUMBER OF REFERRING PHYSICIAN

18. HOSPITALIZATION DATES RELATED TO CURRENT SERVICES FROM MM DD YY TO MM DD YY

19. RESERVED FOR LOCAL USE

20. OUTSIDE LAB? YES NO $ CHARGES

21. DIAGNOSIS OR NATURE OF ILLNESS OR INJURY. (RELATE ITEMS 1,2,3 OR 4 TO ITEM 24E BY LINE)

1. ___ . ___

2. ___ . ___

3. ___ . ___

4. ___ . ___

22. MEDICAID RESUBMISSION CODE ORIGINAL REF. NO.

23. PRIOR AUTHORIZATION NUMBER

24. A DATE(S) OF SERVICE From MM DD YY To MM DD YY	B Place of Service	C Type of Service	D PROCEDURES, SERVICES, OR SUPPLIES (Explain Unusual Circumstances) CPT/HCPCS MODIFIER	E DIAGNOSIS CODE	F $ CHARGES	G DAYS OR UNITS	H EPSDT Family Plan	I EMG	J COB	K RESERVED FOR LOCAL USE
1										
2										
3										
4										
5										
6										

25. FEDERAL TAX I.D. NUMBER SSN EIN

26. PATIENT'S ACCOUNT NO.

27. ACCEPT ASSIGNMENT? (For govt. claims, see back) YES NO

28. TOTAL CHARGE $

29. AMOUNT PAID $

30. BALANCE DUE $

31. SIGNATURE OF PHYSICIAN OR SUPPLIER INCLUDING DEGREES OR CREDENTIALS (I certify that the statements on the reverse apply to this bill and are made a part thereof.)

SIGNED DATE

32. NAME AND ADDRESS OF FACILITY WHERE SERVICES WERE RENDERED (If other than home or office)

33. PHYSICIAN'S, SUPPLIER'S BILLING NAME, ADDRESS, ZIP CODE & PHONE #

PIN# GRP#

PHYSICIAN OR SUPPLIER INFORMATION

(APPROVED BY AMA COUNCIL ON MEDICAL SERVICE 8/88) ***PLEASE PRINT OR TYPE*** FORM HCFA-1500 (12-90), FORM RRB-1500, FORM OWCP-1500

Figure A.4 Health Insurance Claim Form (HCFA-1500).

APPROVED OMB NO. 0938-0279

ST11843 1PLY UB-92

1

2

3 PATIENT CONTROL NO.

4 TYPE OF BILL

5 FED. TAX NO. | 6 STATEMENT COVERS PERIOD FROM THROUGH | 7 COV D. | 8 N-C D. | 9 C-I D. | 10 L-R D. | 11

12 PATIENT NAME | 13 PATIENT ADDRESS

14 BIRTHDATE | 15 SEX | 16 MS | ADMISSION 17 DATE 18 HR 19 TYPE 20 SRC | 21 D HR | 22 STAT | 23 MEDICAL RECORD NO. | CONDITION CODES 24 25 26 27 28 29 30 | 31

32 OCCURRENCE CODE DATE | 33 OCCURRENCE CODE DATE | 34 OCCURRENCE CODE DATE | 35 OCCURRENCE CODE DATE | 36 OCCURRENCE SPAN CODE FROM THROUGH | 37 A B C

a
b

38

39 VALUE CODES CODE AMOUNT | 40 VALUE CODES CODE AMOUNT | 41 VALUE CODES CODE AMOUNT

a b c d

42 REV. CD.	43 DESCRIPTION	44 HCPCS / RATES	45 SERV. DATE	46 SERV. UNITS	47 TOTAL CHARGES	48 NON-COVERED CHARGES	49

1 2 3 4 5 6 7 8 9 10 11 12 13 14 15 16 17 18 19 20 21 22 23

50 PAYER | 51 PROVIDER NO. | 52 REL INFO | 53 ASG BEN | 54 PRIOR PAYMENTS | 55 EST. AMOUNT DUE | 56

A B C

57

DUE FROM PATIENT ▶

58 INSURED'S NAME | 59 P. REL | 60 CERT. - SSN - HIC. - ID NO. | 61 GROUP NAME | 62 INSURANCE GROUP NO.

A B C

63 TREATMENT AUTHORIZATION CODES | 64 ESC | 65 EMPLOYER NAME | 66 EMPLOYER LOCATION

A B C

67 PRIN. DIAG. CD. | OTHER DIAG. CODES 68 CODE 69 CODE 70 CODE 71 CODE 72 CODE 73 CODE 74 CODE 75 CODE | 76 ADM. DIAG. CD. | 77 E-CODE | 78

79 P.C. | 80 PRINCIPAL PROCEDURE CODE DATE | 81 OTHER PROCEDURE CODE DATE A | OTHER PROCEDURE CODE DATE B | 82 ATTENDING PHYS. ID

OTHER PROCEDURE CODE DATE C | OTHER PROCEDURE CODE DATE D | OTHER PROCEDURE CODE DATE E

83 OTHER PHYS. ID A a b

OTHER PHYS. ID B a b

84 REMARKS a b c d

85 PROVIDER REPRESENTATIVE X | 86 DATE

UB-92 HCFA-1450 OCR/ORIGINAL I CERTIFY THE CERTIFICATIONS ON THE REVERSE APPLY TO THIS BILL AND ARE MADE A PART HEREOF.

Figure A.5 Hospital Billing Form (UB-92).

TYPE/PRINT IN PERMANENT BLACK INK FOR INSTRUCTIONS SEE OTHER SIDE AND HANDBOOK

U.S. STANDARD
CERTIFICATE OF DEATH

LOCAL FILE NUMBER | STATE FILE NUMBER

DECEDENT

1. DECEDENT'S NAME (*First, Middle, Last*) | 2. SEX | 3. DATE OF DEATH (*Month, Day, Year*)

4. SOCIAL SECURITY NUMBER | 5a. AGE—Last Birthday (*Years*) | 5b. UNDER 1 YEAR Months, Days | 5c. UNDER 1 DAY Hours, Minutes | 6. DATE OF BIRTH (*Month, Day, Year*) | 7. BIRTHPLACE (*City and State or Foreign Country*)

8. WAS DECEDENT EVER IN U.S. ARMED FORCES? (*Yes or no*)

9a. PLACE OF DEATH (*Check only one; see instructions on other side*)
HOSPITAL: ☐ Inpatient ☐ ER/Outpatient ☐ DOA
OTHER: ☐ Nursing Home ☐ Residence ☐ Other (*Specify*)

9b. FACILITY NAME (*If not institution, give street and number*) | 9c. CITY, TOWN, OR LOCATION OF DEATH | 9d. COUNTY OF DEATH

SEE INSTRUCTIONS ON OTHER SIDE →

10. MARITAL STATUS—Married, Never Married, Widowed, Divorced (*Specify*) | 11. SURVIVING SPOUSE (*If wife, give maiden name*) | 12a. DECEDENT'S USUAL OCCUPATION (*Give kind of work done during most of working life. Do not use retired.*) | 12b. KIND OF BUSINESS/INDUSTRY

13a. RESIDENCE—STATE | 13b. COUNTY | 13c. CITY, TOWN, OR LOCATION | 13d. STREET AND NUMBER

13e. INSIDE CITY LIMITS: (*Yes or no*) | 13f. ZIP CODE | 14. WAS DECEDENT OF HISPANIC ORIGIN? (Specify No or Yes—If yes, specify Cuban, Mexican, Puerto Rican, etc.) ☐ No ☐ Yes *Specify:* | 15. RACE—American Indian, Black, White, etc. (*Specify*) | 16. DECEDENT'S EDUCATION (*Specify only highest grade completed*) Elementary/Secondary (0-12) College (1-4 or 5+)

PARENTS

17. FATHER'S NAME (*First, Middle, Last*) | 18. MOTHER'S NAME (*First, Middle, Maiden Surname*)

INFORMANT

19a. INFORMANT'S NAME (*Type/Print*) | 19b. MAILING ADDRESS (*Street and Number or Rural Route Number, City or Town, State, Zip Code*)

DISPOSITION

20a. METHOD OF DISPOSITION
☐ Burial ☐ Cremation ☐ Removal from State
☐ Donation ☐ Other (*Specify*) ____________
| 20b. PLACE OF DISPOSITION (*Name of cemetery, crematory, or other place*) | 20c. LOCATION—City or Town, State

SEE DEFINITION ON OTHER SIDE

21a. SIGNATURE OF FUNERAL SERVICE LICENSEE OR PERSON ACTING AS SUCH | 21b. LICENSE NUMBER (*of Licensee*) | 22. NAME AND ADDRESS OF FACILITY

PRONOUNCING PHYSICIAN ONLY

Complete items 23a-c only when certifying physician is not available at time of death to certify cause of death. | 23a. **To the best of my knowledge, death occurred at the time, date, and place stated.** *Signature and Title* | 23b. LICENSE NUMBER | 23c. DATE SIGNED (*Month, Day, Year*)

ITEMS 24-26 MUST BE COMPLETED BY PERSON WHO PRONOUNCES DEATH →

24. TIME OF DEATH M | 25. DATE PRONOUNCED DEAD (*Month, Day, Year*) | 26. WAS CASE REFERRED TO MEDICAL EXAMINER/CORONER? (*Yes or no*)

CAUSE OF DEATH

SEE INSTRUCTIONS ON OTHER SIDE

27. PART I. Enter the diseases, injuries, or complications that caused the death. Do not enter the mode of dying, such as cardiac or respiratory arrest, shock, or heart failure. List only one cause on each line. | Approximate Interval Between Onset and Death

IMMEDIATE CAUSE (Final disease or condition → resulting in death) a. ____________
DUE TO (OR AS A CONSEQUENCE OF):
b. ____________
DUE TO (OR AS A CONSEQUENCE OF):
c. ____________
DUE TO (OR AS A CONSEQUENCE OF):
d. ____________

Sequentially list conditions, if any, leading to immediate cause. Enter **UNDERLYING CAUSE** (Disease or injury that initiated events resulting in death) **LAST**

PART II. Other significant conditions contributing to death but not resulting in the underlying cause given in Part I. | 28a. WAS AN AUTOPSY PERFORMED? (*Yes or no*) | 28b. WERE AUTOPSY FINDINGS AVAILABLE PRIOR TO COMPLETION OF CAUSE OF DEATH? (*Yes or no*)

29. MANNER OF DEATH
☐ Natural ☐ Pending Investigation
☐ Accident
☐ Suicide ☐ Could not be Determined
☐ Homicide
| 30a. DATE OF INJURY (*Month, Day, Year*) | 30b. TIME OF INJURY M | 30c. INJURY AT WORK? (*Yes or no*) | 30d. DESCRIBE HOW INJURY OCCURRED

30e. PLACE OF INJURY—At home, farm, street, factory, office building, etc. (*Specify*) | 30f. LOCATION (Street and Number or Rural Route Number, City or Town, State)

CERTIFIER

SEE DEFINITION ON OTHER SIDE

31a. CERTIFIER (*Check only one*)
☐ CERTIFYING PHYSICIAN (*Physician certifying cause of death when another physician has pronounced death and completed Item 23*)
To the best of my knowledge, death occurred due to the cause(s) and manner as stated.
☐ PRONOUNCING AND CERTIFYING PHYSICIAN (*Physician both pronouncing death and certifying to cause of death*)
To the best of my knowledge, death occurred at the time, date, and place, and due to the cause(s) and manner as stated.
☐ MEDICAL EXAMINER/CORONER
On the basis of examination and/or investigation, in my opinion, death occurred at the time, date, and place, and due to the cause(s) and manner as stated.

31b. SIGNATURE AND TITLE OF CERTIFIER | 31c. LICENSE NUMBER | 31d. DATE SIGNED (*Month, Day, Year*)

32. NAME AND ADDRESS OF PERSON WHO COMPLETED CAUSE OF DEATH (ITEM 27) (*Type/Print*)

REGISTRAR

33. REGISTRAR'S SIGNATURE | 34. DATE FILED (*Month, Day, Year*)

PHS-T-003
REV. 1/89

NAME OF DECEDENT: ____________ For use by physician or institution

DEPARTMENT OF HEALTH AND HUMAN SERVICES—PUBLIC HEALTH SERVICE—NATIONAL CENTER FOR HEALTH STATISTICS—1989 REVISION

Figure A.6 U.S. Standard Certificate of Death.

Appendix B

Questionnaires for Active Surveillance of Cumulative Trauma Disorders

A. Active risk factor surveillance

General assessment questionnaire

Please answer the questions listed below regarding your health and your work.
We want to know how you have felt this **past month** including today.
Do **not** put your name on this questionnaire, but be sure to indicate your job title and department at the bottom.
No one will know how you answered these questions.
This information will help us improve your working conditions.

Thank you.

Please circle the number that indicates how often you have experienced each of the following in the last month.

	Never	Sometimes	Often	Always
1. You had headaches	1	2	3	4
2. Your hands or fingers got numb	1	2	3	4
3. You had a cold or sore throat	1	2	3	4
4. You had back pain	1	2	3	4
5. Your wrists or hands hurt	1	2	3	4
6. You woke up at night with hand pain	1	2	3	4
7. You felt nervous or irritable	1	2	3	4
8. Your arm hurt or felt numb	1	2	3	4
9. You felt very tired at work	1	2	3	4
10. You had pain in your neck or shoulder	1	2	3	4
11. You felt pressured to work faster	1	2	3	4
12. You felt you were in control of your job	1	2	3	4
13. You had chest pains	1	2	3	4
14. You liked your job	1	2	3	4
15. Your legs hurt	1	2	3	4
16. Your lower back hurt	1	2	3	4

Please fill in your job title, employee study ID# (if appropriate), and department below. Thank you for your help.

______________	______________	______________	__/__/__
Job title	Employee study ID#	Department	Date

B. Discomfort Survey. An example of a tool to evaluate the effectiveness of workplace/job interventions.

DISCOMFORT SURVEY

Last Name ______________________ First Name ______________________

Date ______________________ Time ______________________ am pm

Department Name ______________________ Job Title ______________________

Shift ______________________

Think about how you feel RIGHT NOW

1. Shade in all the areas of discomfort on the figure.

2. Rate the discomfort for each left and right side of the body part named in the box below. Rate the discomfort using the scale below in which 0 = no discomfort at all and 10 = worst imaginable discomfort. Write the score in the box.

SCALE

No discomfort at all — Worst imaginable discomfort

0 1 2 3 4 5 6 7 8 9 10

DISCOMFORT AREA	RATING SCORE	
	RIGHT	LEFT
Neck		
Shoulder		
Chest		
Elbow		
Hand / wrist		
Hip / thigh		
Knee		
Lower leg		
Ankle / foot		
Other		

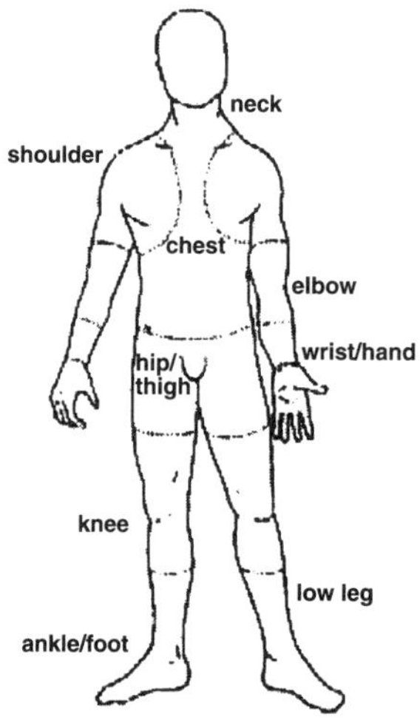

FRONT

SCALE

No discomfort at all										Worst imaginable discomfort
0	**1**	**2**	**3**	**4**	**5**	**6**	**7**	**8**	**9**	**10**

Think about how you feel RIGHT NOW

DISCOMFORT AREA	**RATING SCORE**	
	RIGHT	**LEFT**
Neck		
Shoulder		
Chest		
Elbow		
Hand / wrist		
Hip / thigh		
Knee		
Lower leg		
Ankle / foot		
Other		

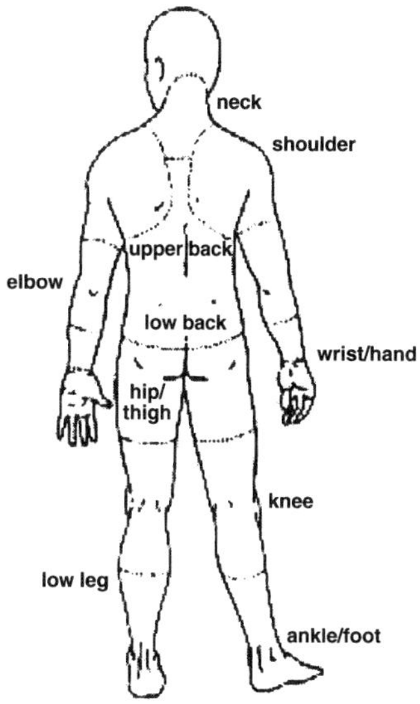

BACK

WHOLE BODY: Overall Discomfort Rating (use the same scale)	

Source: Silverstrein B. Health and risk factor surveillance for work related musculoskeletal disorders. In Kuorinka I, Forcier L, eds. Work Related Musculoskeletal Disorders (WMSDS): A Reference Book for Prevention. London: Taylor & Francis; 1995: 213–245. (Reprinted with permission)

Appendix C

Statistics for Describing Distributions

NEIL A. MAIZLISH

Any characteristic that is measured on a scale that has no gaps, like age, noise level in decibels, or blood lead level can be made into categories. Other characteristics occur in a limited number of categories like gender (male, female), job classification (welder, assembler, doctor, machine operator, supervisor, etc.), industry, or department. For example, in a group of 10 workers with blood lead levels we can create five categories such as <20 μg/dL, 20–29.9 μg/dL, 30–39.9 μg/dL, 40–49.9 μg/dL, and 50 μg/dL and above. The individual values and categories are shown in Table C.1.

The number and percent in each category describe the distribution. Graphing the distribution also helps us see the pattern (Fig. C.1). Some distributions are symmetrical, that is, they have the same, but mirrored shape to the left and right of the midpoint. We can use various points along the distribution to describe the group. The minimum (smallest) and maximum (largest) give the range (19.2–52.3). The mean is the arithmetic average, which is the sum of the values divided by the number of values:

$$\text{Average} = \frac{19.2 + 24.3 + 27.8 + 32.1 + 35.4 + 36.5 + 39.9 + 46.9 + 47.5 + 52.3}{10}$$

$$= \frac{361.9}{10} = 36.2$$

Another point that helps describe the distribution is the median. When all the points are put in ascending or descending order, the median is the value that has an equal number of points above and below. For a distribution with 11 points, point number 6 has 5 values above and 5 values below. For distributions that have an even number of points, we usually take the arithmetic average of the two middle points and call that the median. When the population is very large we generally have enough data to make many fine categories that appear continuous. This approximates the smooth curve in the Figure C.1. Many characteristics in human populations have a distribution that looks like this bell-shaped curve. This distribution is also called the normal distribution.

A statistic that describes whether the data points vary a little or a lot around the average is called the standard deviation. It is calculated by taking the difference between the average and each point. This difference, or deviation from the average, is multiplied by itself (squared). The squared differences are then summed up and divided by the number of points, minus 1. This is an average of the sum of squared deviations, and is called the variance of a mean. Finally, the square root of this term is taken, and is called the standard deviation. For the example,

Standard Deviation =

$$\sqrt{\frac{(19.2 - 36.2)^2 + (24.3 - 36.2)^2 + (27.8 - (36.2)^2 + (32.1 - 36.2)^2 + (35.4 - 36.2)^2 + (36.5 - 36.2)^2 + (39.9 - 36.2)^2 + (46.9 - 36.2)^2 + (47.5 - 36.2)^2 + (52.3 - 36.2)^2}{9}} = 10.8$$

Some distributions are not symmetrical and look lopsided, as if the hump in the normal distribution had been pushed left or right. An example of a skewed distribution comes from another plant (Table C.2) where blood lead values were taken (Fig. C.2).

In this example, the hump in the normal curve was pushed to the left because a greater proportion of the 10 points are in the lower blood lead categories. We also see that when the curve is symmetrical, the median and the mean are the same. When the distribution is not symmetrical the mean and the median can have a pronounced separation.

Table C.1 Distribution of Blood Lead Levels at Plant 1

Median = $$\frac{35.4 + 36.5}{2} = 35.9$$

Plant 1 Individuals	*Blood Lead µg/dL*	*Categories µg/dL*	N	%
Worker 1	19.2	Less than 20	1	10
Worker 2	24.3			
Worker 3	27.8	20–29.9	2	20
Worker 4	32.1			
Worker 5	35.4	30–39.9	4	40
Worker 6	36.5			
Worker 7	39.9	40–49.9	2	20
Worker 8	46.9			
Worker 9	47.5	50 or more	1	10
Worker 10	52.3	Total	10	100

Range	19.2–52.3
Average	36.2
Median	35.9
Standard deviation	10.7

If we only compared means and medians we might think that the profile of blood leads at the second plant was better because the mean and median at plant 2 (mean = 34.9; median = 28.5) are lower than at plant 1 (mean = 36.2; median = 35.9).

While means and medians are useful, they may hide important features of a distribution. In surveillance activities, we frequently use cut points along the distribution to trigger preventive actions. For blood lead, one such trigger occurs at 40 µg/dL. At plant 1, 30% of the population meets or exceeds this level, but only 20% at plant 2 do. This suggests that plant 1 may have a more widespread problem than plant 2. However, a closer look at plant 2 shows that even though moderately elevated blood lead values (40–55 µg/dL) are not as widespread, an extremely elevated level occurred with one case at 89 µg/dL. Under OSHA regulations, worker 10 must be removed immediately

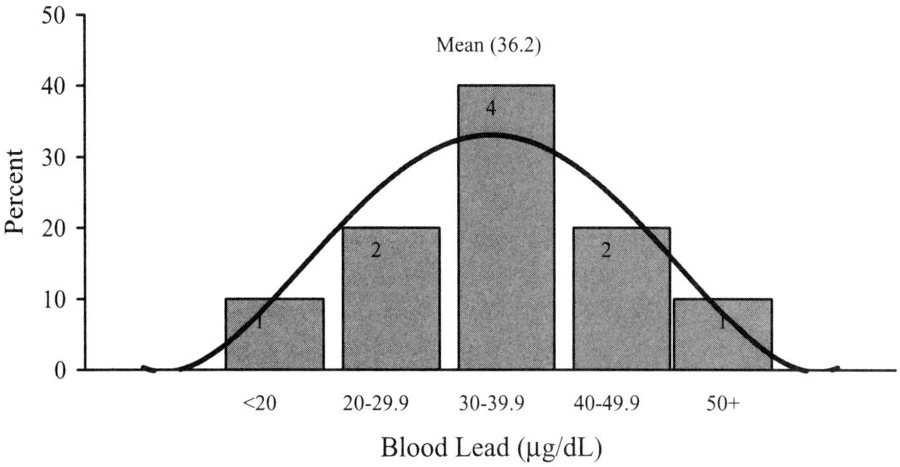

Figure C.1 Blood lead levels with a symmetrical distribution and descriptive statistics at plant 1.

Table C.2 Distribution of Blood Lead Levels at Plant 2

Plant 2 Individuals	*Blood Lead µg/dL*	*Categories µg/dL*	*Number*	*Percent*
Worker 1	19.4	Less than 20	1	10
Worker 2	20.1	20–29.9	5	50
Worker 3	22.5	30–39.9	2	20
Worker 4	24.3	40–49.9	1	10
Worker 5	27.8	50 or more	1	10
Worker 6	29.2	Total	10	100
Worker 7	34.3			
Worker 8	34.7			
Worker 9	47.6			
Worker 10	89.1			
		Range	19.4–89.1	
		Average	34.9	
		Median	28.5	
		Standard deviation	20.8	

Median = $\frac{27.8 + 29.2}{2} = 28.5$

from the lead-exposing job and be provided with medical follow-up. It is possible to miss the importance of high values by lumping together all values greater than a particular cut point, or by just looking at an average. This underscores the importance of examining the entire distribution as well as summary statistics, such as the mean, median, and standard deviation.

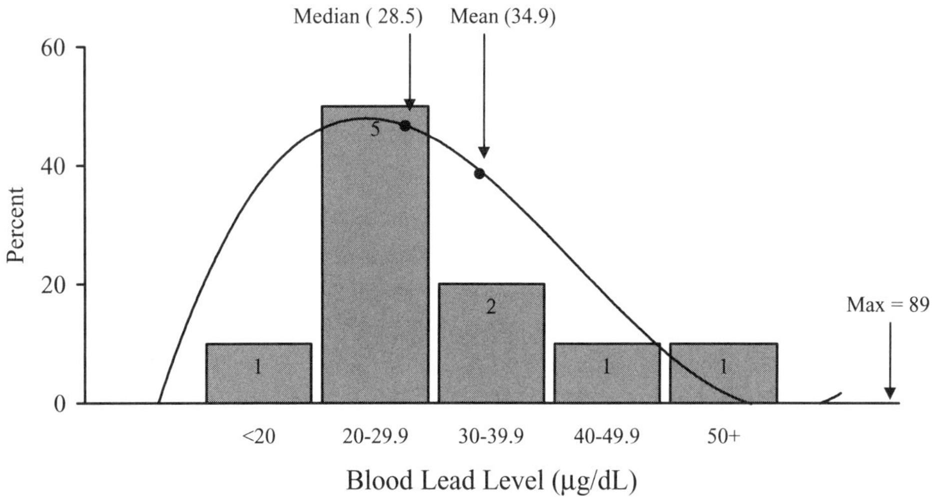

Figure C.2 Blood lead levels with a lop-sided distribution and descriptive statistics at plant 2.

Appendix D

Analysis and Annual Report for an Individual Workplace

NEIL A. MAIZLISH

The following is an example of analysis and interpretation of rate-based injury and illness data that many employers collect. It is a univariate analysis of injury and illness by nature of injury, external cause, department, occupation, and month of injury or illness. The format is a 2–3 page summary followed by about a dozen tables oriented to a technical person on a surveillance team or health and safety committee. For a general audience, the findings are more effectively communicated with graphs and less text.

Even though the data are made up, the analysis and tables were generated with public domain software[1,2] from an example database.

INCIDENCE OF OCCUPATIONAL INJURY AND ILLNESS, FOOD PRODUCTS FACTORY, 1999

Nature of Injury and External Cause

In 1999, of 3000 employees, 378 workers experienced 191 new, work-related injuries and 187 illnesses, which accounted for 34,836 lost workdays (Tables D.1 and D.2). The incidence rate of all injuries and illness combined was 12.6 per 100 full-time equivalents (FTE), an increase of 10% from 1998. The incidence rate of cases with lost workdays (LWD) did not change between years (4.0 per 100 FTEs). In contrast, the lost workday incidence rate decreased 10% to 1161 LWD per 100 FTE from 1277 per 100 FTEs in 1998.

The most common diagnoses (Table D.1) were musculoskeletal disorders (MSDs) (~25%) and sprains and strains (~25%). There were 133 cases of MSDs of the back (Table D.3), which accumulated 13,759 LWDs, 39% of all lost workdays. These diagnoses were followed in frequency by open wounds, diseases of the nervous systems, poisoning, and fractures, which with MSDs and sprains accounted for 70% of cases and lost workdays. Among injuries, motor vehicle injuries (84 cases, 42% of lost workdays due to injuries) was the leading cause followed by injuries due open flames, environment, and poisoning (Table D.2).

The monthly injury and illness rate varied between 9.6 and 18.4 per 100 FTEs with peaks in January, June, and December (Table D.4).

Departments and Occupations

The department with the highest incidence rate for injury and illness combined was **Line 1**, which at 22 cases per 100 FTE was 3.4 times higher than **Shipping and Receiving** (S&R) (Table D.5). If the other production departments could achieve the same rate as **Shipping and Receiving**, 183 cases and 18,629 LWDs could be avoided. Using the ballpark figure of $5000 per case (direct and indirect costs) from the Risk Management Department, this represents nearly $1 million per year in potentially avoidable costs if the injury and illness rate observed in **S&R** could be reached by other departments. The principal impact would be seen in **Line 1** and **Line 2** with 137 excess cases and 13,062 excess LWDs. Among occupations (Table D.6), **Machine Operators** had the highest injury and illness rate combined—22.1 cases per 100 FTEs, which was 3.1 times higher than **Mechanics**, the occupation with the lowest rate. In each department and occupation the leading diagnosis was musculoskeletal disorder or sprains. In each department and occupation diagnoses that achieved 10% or more of cases or lost workdays included open wounds, poisoning, diseases of the nervous system, and circulatory diseases. Disease-specific illness or injury with 10% or more of cases included circulatory disease in **S&R**, and internal organ injury among **fork lift operators** (tables not shown). In **Inspection**, poisoning, machinery accidents, and objects penetrating the eyes were the cause of 10% or more of the cases. Injuries due to being struck by objects and collisions are leading causes in **Maintenance**. Among injuries, motor vehicles were the major cause in each department and occupation. Poisoning was 10% or more of the external causes in each occupation, except **mechanics**, where injuries due to fire and confined space were leading causes.

Return-to-Work

Of the incident cases in 1999, approximately one-third (119) had not returned to work by December 31. There was little variation in the return-to-work rates by department (Table D.7) or occupation (Table D.8).

Case Follow-up

Forty-seven cases were selected for follow-up that consisted of interviews and investigations of the work stations (Table D.9). By 12/31/99, of these, 4 cases were closed and 43 were still open. Thirty-four of the open cases missed their deadlines (1 month from injury to finish of the injury investigation). Based on investigations finished in 1999, a total of 124 recommendations were made: 14 for changes in workstation design, 32 for training or retraining, 45 for changes in work practices, and 33 for the use of personal protective equipment. Of these recommendations, 68 were implemented immediately, 8 were approved but not implemented, 23 were deferred for feasibility analysis, and 25 were rejected for lack of feasibility.

Interpretation and Recommendations

Incidence and Severity

The main finding is that although the number and rate of injuries and illnesses increased from 1998 to 1999, the severity decreased resulting in 2355 fewer days lost in 1999. The overall injury and illness rate at 12.6 per 100 FTEs is slightly lower than our industry rate (spaghetti and macaroni production, SIC 2098; 14.4 cases per 100 FTE).[3] The decrease in LWD incidence was observed across diagnosis, external causes, departments, and occupations. Because hours worked were practically the same in 1999 and 1998, the increase in the number of cases is due to an increase in the rate. The pattern of increased case incidence and decreased LWD incidence is consistent with the early reporting of milder cases. This is a predicted effect of the plantwide safety training in February 1999, in which each worker received 2 hours of general training about job safety that emphasized the early reporting of cases. If the entire difference in workdays lost (2255 fewer days) is attributed to the safety training, it produced a net benefit of $225,500.

Groups at High Risk and Recommendations

Disabling back injuries remain a significant and persistent problem impacting **Line 1** and **Line 2**, where the majority of cases occurred. We are waiting for the results a ergonomic analysis and a new engineering design that will substantially reduce lifting. Preventive actions should be directed to the following areas:

Area of the plant	Recommendation or Action
• All areas	Motor vehicle injuries are a leading cause of injuries for which a control program already exists. We will review the existing safety procedures to identify weaknesses and lack of compliance immediately.
• Line 1 and 2	1. Machine operators in Line 1 and 2 are a high-risk group for back injuries. An ergonomic assessment should be undertaken to determine what preventive steps can be taken until Lines 1 and 2 are redesigned. 2. Fire safety and confined space injuries were also identified in Line 1.
• Inspection	Eye safety and safe handling practices for solvents should be reinforced.
• Shipping & receiving	Forklift safety should be reinforced
• Mechanics	1. Fire safety 2. Confined space 3. Lock-out procedures to prevent struck and trapped by injuries
• Operators	Safe handling of solvents

New findings in 1999 include the appearance of nervous system disorders in **Inspection** and cardiovascular disease in **Shipping & Receiving**, each disease consisting of 10% of all cases of these departments. Because of the recognized solvent exposures and poisoning cases, we recommend including a neurological exam in the year 2000 annual medical exams.

Return to Work and Disability Management

A high percentage of injured workers (31%) did not return to work rapidly (by 90 days from injury date). This did not vary by department or occupation. A key recommendation is to develop a plantwide program that will coordinate return to work between the injured worker, human resources, the medical group, and supervisors. We are working with the medical group to identify appropriate alternative work.

Case Follow-up

There is significant slippage in deadlines to complete injury and illness investigations within our goal of 30 days. We will work with the Information Services Department to determine if new document assembly software can help us speed up the report writing part of the investigation, which has been a long-standing bottleneck.

REFERENCES

1. Dean AG, Dean JA, Coulombier D, et al. *Epi Info, Version 6: A Word Processing, Database, and Statistics Program for Epidemiology on Microcomputers.* Atlanta, GA: Centers for Disease Control and Prevention, 1994.
2. Maizlish N. Designing prevention-oriented software for workplace health and safety. *Am J Ind Med* 1997; 31:64–74.
3. Bureau of Labor Statistics. *Survey of Occupational Injuries and Illnesses, 1993.* Summary 95-5. Washington, DC: U.S. Department of Labor, February 1995.

Table D.1a Screen by Nature of Injury or Illness 01/01/1999–12/31/1999

*ICD 9**	*Nature of Injury or Illness*	N	%	*Rate†*
710–739	Musculoskeletal diseases	98	26	3.3
840–848	Sprains and strains	90	24	3.0
999–999	Other illnesses and injuries	36	10	1.2
320–389	Diseases of the nervous system	22	6	0.7
870–904	Open wounds	19	5	0.6
960–989	Poisoning	19	5	0.6
800–829	Fracture	18	5	0.6
910–924	Superficial wounds	13	3	0.4
950–959	Injuries to the spinal cord and nerves	11	3	0.4
860–869	Internal organ injuries	8	2	0.3
001–139	Infectious diseases	7	2	0.2
830–839	Dislocations	6	2	0.2
940–949	Burns	6	2	0.2
390–459	Diseases of the circulatory system	5	1	0.2
140–239	Cancer	4	1	0.1
460–519	Respiratory diseases	4	1	0.1
850–854	Intracranial injury and concussion	4	1	0.1
520–579	Digestive organ diseases	3	< 1	< 0.1
680–709	Skin diseases	2	< 1	< 0.1
780–799	Symptoms and ill-defined conditions	2	< 1	< 0.1
580–589	Diseases of the genitourinary system	1	< 1	< 0.1
001–999	Total	378	100	12.6

*International Classification of Diseases, 9th Revision.
†Cases per 100 full-time equivalents per year.

Table D.1b Lost Workdays* by Nature of Injury, 01/01/1999–12/31/1999

ICD 9†	*Nature of Injury or Illness*	N	%	*Rate‡*
840–848	Sprains and strains	9394	27	313.1
710–739	Musculoskeletal diseases	8859	25	295.3
999–999	Other illnesses and injuries	2609	7	87.0
870–904	Open wounds	1682	5	56.1
960–989	Poisonings	1603	5	53.4
320–389	Disease of the nervous system	1320	4	44.0
800–829	Fractures	1254	4	41.8
910–924	Superficial wounds	1203	3	40.1
950–959	Injuries to the spinal cord and nerves	1145	3	38.2
830–839	Dislocations	734	2	24.5
860–869	Internal organ injury	712	2	23.7
390–459	Diseases of the circulatory system	697	2	23.2
001–139	Infectious diseases	651	2	21.7
460–519	Respiratory diseases	603	2	20.1
940–949	Burns	575	2	19.2
520–579	Diseases of the digestive system	484	1	16.1
140–239	Cancer	430	1	14.3
850–854	Intracranial injury and concussion	410	1	13.7
680–709	Skin disease	311	1	10.4
780–799	Symptoms and ill-defined conditions	105	<1	3.5
580–589	Diseases of the genitourinary system	55	<1	1.8
001–999	Total	34836	100	1161.2

*Lost workdays for cases with missing return-to-work date are calculated from date of injury or illness to 12/31/1999.
†International Classification of Diseases, 9th Revision.
‡Lost Workdays per 100 full-time equivalents per year.

Table D.2a Injuries by External Cause, 01/01/1999–12/31/1999

*ICD 9**	*External Cause of Injury*	N	%	*Rate†*
	Other traffic injuries	56	29	1.9
810–825	Motor vehicle injuries	28	15	0.9
	Other injuries	21	11	0.7
900–909	Environmental factors	17	9	0.6
890–899	Injuries caused by fires and flames	13	7	0.4
866–869	Poisoning by other solids, liquids, or gases	12	6	0.4
860–862	Poisoning by solvents and disinfectants	8	4	0.3
916–918	Struck by, caught by, hit by persons or objects	7	4	0.2
882–884	Fall from one level to another	5	3	0.2
910–912	Drowning and submersion	4	2	0.1
865	Poisoning by plants	3	2	0.1
919	Injury by machinery	3	2	0.1
885–886	Fall on same level	2	1	0.1
913	Suffocation (confined space)	2	1	0.1
914	Foreign objects in the eye	2	1	0.1
927	Overexertion	2	1	0.1
846	Injury due to forklift	1	<1	0.1
863	Poisoning by pesticides	1	<1	0.1
864	Poisoning by corrosives and caustics	1	<1	0.1
880	Fall from or on ladders or steps	1	<1	0.1
887–888	Other fall	1	<1	0.1
920	Injuries due to hand tools	1	<1	0.1
800–999	Total	191	100	6.3

*International Classification of Diseases, 9th Rev., external cause "E" Code.
†Cases per 100 full-time equivalents per year.

Table D.2b Lost Work Days* by External Cause, 01/01/1999–12/31/1999

ICD 9†	*External Cause of Injury*	N	%	*Rate‡*
	Other traffic injuries	5055	28	168.5
810–825	Motor vehicle injuries	2454	14	81.8
	Other injuries	1875	10	62.5
900–909	Environmental factors	1677	9	55.9
860–862	Poisoning by solvents and disinfectants	1155	6	38.5
890–899	Injuries caused by fires and flames	910	5	30.3
866–869	Poisoning by other solids, liquids, or gases	767	4	25.6
916–918	Struck by, caught by, hit by persons or objects	675	4	22.5
913	Suffocation (confined space)	544	3	18.1
919	Injury by machinery	480	3	16.0
910–912	Drowning and submersion	458	3	15.3
914	Foreign body in eyes	336	2	11.2
882–884	Fall from one level to another	272	2	9.1
865	Poisoning by plants	246	1	8.2
846	Injury due to forklift	239	1	8.0
885–886	Fall on same level	210	1	7.0
920	Injuries due to hand tools	199	1	6.6
927	Overexertion	137	1	4.6
880	Fall from or on ladders or steps	76	<1	2.5
887–888	Other falls	71	<1	2.4
863	Poisoning by pesticides	70	<1	2.3
864	Poisoning by corrosives and caustics	27	<1	0.9
800–999	Total	17933	100	597.8

*Lost workdays for cases with missing return-to-work date are calculated from date of injury or illness to 12/31/1999
†International Classification of Diseases, 9th Rev., external cause "E" Code.
‡Lost Workdays per 100 full-time equivalents per year.

Table D.3a Screen of Musculoskeletal Disorders, 01/01/1999–12/31/1999

Body Part	N	%	*Rate**
Back	133	70	4.4
Hand-wrist-arm	28	15	0.9
Neck	21	11	0.7
Shoulder	8	4	0.3
Total Musculoskeletal Disorders	190	100	6.3

Selection of Musculoskeletal Disorders

Nature of the Musculoskeletal Disorder	N	%	*Rate*
Bursitis of occupational origin	3	2	0.1
Ganglion	2	1	0.1
Thoracic outlet syndrome	12	6	0.4
Raynaud's disease	1	1	0.0
Carpal tunnel syndrome	9	5	0.3
Flexor tendinitis	4	2	0.1
Bicipital tenosinovitis	4	2	0.1

*Cases per 100 Full-Time Equivalents per Year.

Table D.3b Screen of Musculoskeletal Disorders, 01/01/1999–12/31/1999 Lost Workday* Rate × 100 Full-Time Equivalents per Year

Body Part	N	%	*Rate†*
Back	13759	78	458.6
Hand-wrist-arm	1816	10	60.5
Neck	1579	9	52.6
Shoulder	517	3	17.2
Total Musculoskeletal Disorders	17671	100	588.9

Selection of Musculoskeletal Disorders:

Nature of the Musculoskeletal Disorder	N	%	*Rate†*
Carpal tunnel syndrome	793	4	26.4
Thoracic outlet syndrome	491	3	16.4
Bicipital tenosinovitis	352	2	11.7
Bursitis of occupational origin	204	1	6.8
Ganglion	174	1	5.8
Flexor tendinitis	165	1	5.5
Raynaud's disease	61	0	2.0

*Lost workdays for cases with missing return-to-work date are calculated from date of injury or illness to 12/31/1999.

†Lost Workdays per 100 Full-Time Equivalents per Year.

Body Part	ICD Codes
Back	721.2,721.3,721.40–721.49,722.10–722.19, 722.50–722.59,722.72,722.73,722.92,722.93, 724.0–724.99,846.0–846.99,847.2–847.4,847.9.
Neck	721.0,721.1,722.0,722.4,722.71,722.91,847.0, 723–723.9.
Shoulder	726.1,726.12,726.2.
Hand-wrist-arm	353.0,354.0–354.9,443.0,726.31,726.32,726.90, 726.91, 727.02–727.05,727.09,727.2,727.40–727.49.

Table D.4 Monthly Injury and Illness Rate, 01/01/1999–12/31/1999

Month	N	%	*Rate**
01	39	10	15.6
02	25	7	10.0
03	38	10	10.0
04	24	6	9.6
05	25	6	9.6
06	39	10	15.6
07	29	8	11.6
08	25	7	9.6
09	24	6	9.6
10	32	9	12.8
11	32	9	12.8
12	46	12	18.4
Total	378	100	12.6

*Cases per 100 full-time equivalents.

Table D.5a Incidence Rate by Department, 01/01/1999–12/31/1999

Department	*Cases*	*Person-Years*	*Rate**	*Rate Ratio*	*Excess Cases†*	*Excess Costs‡*
Line 1	99	450	22.0	3.4	70	350,000
Line 2	109	650	16.8	2.6	67	335,000
Inspection	69	600	11.5	1.8	30	150,000
Maintenance	65	750	8.7	1.3	16	80,000
Shipping and receiving	36	550	6.5	1.0	0	0
Total	378	3000	12.6		183	915,000

*Cases per 100 full-time equivalents per year.
†Excess cases = (Rate − lowest $\text{rate}_{S\&R}$) × Department Person-Years.
‡Estimated costs/case = $5000; Excess costs = cost/case × excess cases.

Table D.5b Lost Workday Rate by Department, 01/01/1999–12/31/1999

Department	*Lost Workdays*	*Person-Years*	*Rate**	*Rate Ratio*	*Excess Days†*
Line 1	9347	450	2007.1	3.8	6916
Line 2	9658	650	1485.8	2.8	6146
Inspection	6955	600	1159.2	2.1	3714
Maintenance	5905	750	787.3	1.5	1853
Shipping and receiving	2971	550	540.2	1.0	0
Total	34,836	3000	1161.2		18,629

*Lost Workdays per 100 full-time equivalents.
†Excess days = (Rate − lowest $\text{rate}_{S\&R}$) × Department Person-Years.

Table D.6a Incidence Rate by Occupation, 01/01/1999–12/31/1999

Occupation	*Cases*	*Person-Years*	*Rate**	*Rate Ratio*	*Excess Days†*
Machine operators	166	750	22.1	3.1	113
Material handlers	75	500	15.0	2.1	40
Inspectors	66	750	8.8	1.2	13
Mechanics	71	1000	7.1	1.0	0
Total	378	3000	12.6		166

*Cases per 100 full-time equivalents per year.
†Excess cases = (Rate − reference $\text{rate}_{\text{Mechanics}}$) × Department Person-Years.

Table D.6b Lost Workday Incidence Rate by Occupation, 01/01/1999–12/31/1999

Department	*Lost Workdays*	*Person-Years*	*Rate**	*Rate Ratio*	*Excess Days†*
Machine operators	16,752	750	2233.6	3.5	12,023
Material handlers	6489	500	1297.8	2.1	3337
Inspectors	5290	750	705.3	1.1	561
Mechanics	6305	1000	630.5	1.0	0
Total	34,836	3000	1161.2		15,921

*Lost Workdays per 100 full-time equivalents.

†Excess days = (Rate − lowest $rate_{Mechaniscs}$) × Department Person-Years.

Table D.7 Rate of No Return-to-Work by Department, 01/01/1999–12/31/1999

Department	*Cases Not RTW**	*Cases*	*Rate†*	*Rate Ratio*	*Excess Cases‡*
Inspection	25	69	36.2	1.3	6
Shipping and receiving	12	36	33.3	1.2	2
Maintenance	21	65	32.3	1.2	3
Line 2	34	109	31.2	1.1	4
Line 1	27	99	27.3	1.0	0
Total	119	378	31.5		15

*RTW, return-to-work.

†Cases not RTW per 100 injured workers per year.

‡Excess cases = (Rate − lowest $rate_{Line\ 1}$) × Cases.

Table D.8 Rate of No Return-to-Work by Occupation, 01/01/1999–12/31/1999

Occupation	*Cases Not RTW**	*Cases*	*Rate*	*Rate Ratio*	*Excess Cases†*
Mechanics	25	71	35.2	1.6	9
Machine operators	57	166	34.3	1.5	19
Material handlers	22	75	29.3	1.3	5
Inspectors	15	66	22.7	1.0	0
Total	119	378	31.5		33

*RTW, return-to-work.

†Excess cases = (Rate − lowest $rate_{Inspectors}$) × Cases.

Table D.9 Follow-up Status of Incident Cases, 01/01/1999–12/31/1999

Cases Followed-up	N	%
No	315	87
Yes	47	13

Case Status	N	%
Open—pending	4	9
Open—missed deadline	34	72
Closed	9	19

Appendix E

Example of a Rate-Based Analysis at an Individual Workplace

NEIL A. MAIZLISH

You are responsible for health and safety at an automobile parts factory that employs 193 workers in 4 different departments: fabrication, assembly, maintenance, and shipping & receiving. An epidemic of work-related musculoskeletal disorders (MSDs) might be occurring in the plant based on a causal review of the log of first-time medical visits. Musculoskeletal disorders appear to be related to the repetitive use of the hands but affect body parts from the shoulder to the fingers.

Workers in the early stages of illness have pain, swelling, and inflammation of the tendons. It seems that nerves such as the median and ulnar of the arm and wrist are affected because the reported symptoms follow the distribution of these nerves. Some of the patients also complain of numbness (paresthesia), cramping, loss of touch in the hands, and a radiating pain toward the forearm.

You would like to answer these questions:

- What is the rate of MSDs in 1998?
- Which is the department most affected by MSDs?
- Which is the department least affected by MSDs?
- Assuming the MSDs are all work-related, if it were possible to eliminate the risk factors, how many cases of MSD could be prevented per year?

You would like to see management fix the problem without hesitating, but that does not seem likely. Every little safety improvement is now subject to a cost-benefit analysis. A few cases of MSDs have already resulted in significant permanent disability, and the costs could be as much as $75,000 per case. You've talked to the plant manufacturing engineer about making changes to some of the work stations that seem to be problematic, and the engineering department has made some estimates of the costs to change workstations in each of the four production departments. A preliminary cost-effectiveness or cost-benefit analysis based on available data may help argue in favor of changes.

As inputs, you will need the following materials:

- Overview of the steps needed to carry out the analysis (Table E.1)
- Medical department log for 1998 (Table E.2)
- Hours-worked for each of the four departments in 1998 (Table E.3)
- Lost workdays due to MSDs for each of the four departments for 1998 and 1999 (Table E.3)
- Summary data tables or spreadsheets to consolidate information on hours worked, number of cases and workdays lost, incidence rates, attributable risk, and excess cases and lost workdays (Table E.4 and E.5)

The following will be needed for a cost-benefit analysis (Appendix F):

- Cost estimates per case of MSDs or the costs of an hour (or day) of production, or both
- Cost estimates for engineering changes to workstations for each department

Although appearing straight forward, this example is difficult to carry out because there are numerous steps, ambiguities, and very limited data—a not uncommon real-world situation. We do not have access to precise medical information, and, we must make many assumptions to create a case definition. How does one define a case of MSD? What body parts should be included or excluded in the definition? What symptoms, signs, or diagnoses are included or excluded? Are the conditions all work-related? Depending on the assumptions, there may be several correct answers to this example. However, only through careful documentation of the assumptions and process can one reproduce and defend the result.

This example can be carried out using pencil and paper, manual counting, and a calculator. One can be effective with these tools and even semiautomate the cal-

Table E.1 Overview of Steps for a Rate-Based Analysis of Surveillance Data of Musculoskeletal Disorders at an Auto Parts Factory*

Step A	Construct a written case definition of work-related musculoskeletal disorders of the upper extremities	
Step B	Define the time period of analysis and the eligible population	
Step C	Calculate the annual number of hours worked for all departments combined and each department separately	
Step D	Compare the written case definition of an MSD of the upper extremity to each entry in the medical log and decide whether it meets the case definition	
Steps E–K	There are two parallel tracks for MSD a) case incidence and b) lost workday incidence:	
	a. Case incidence	b. Lost Workday Incidence
Step E	Count the number of MSD cases for each of the four departments and for all departments combined	Count the number of lost workdays for MSDs for each of the four departments and for all departments combined
Step F	Calculate the incidence rates for MSD cases	Calculate the incidence rates for lost workdays due to MSDs
Step G	Calculate the rate ratio for MSD cases	Calculate the rate ratio for lost workdays due to MSDs
Step H	Calculate the attributable risk for MSDs cases	Calculate attributable risk for lost workdays due to MSDs
Step I	Calculate the number of excess cases for each department and sum up all excess cases for the entire plant	Calculate the number of excess workdays lost for each department and sum up all excess lost workdays for the entire plant
Step J	Identify the high-risk and low-risk departments based on number of cases, relative risks, and excess cases, and interpret the findings	Identify the high-risk and low-risk departments based on number of lost workdays, relative risks, and excess lost workdays, and interpret the the findings
Follow-up Steps	• Prioritization of follow-up by department • Selection of intervention and its implementation • Evaluation of the impact on reducing MSD frequency, severity, and costs	

*MSD, musculoskeletal disorder.

Table E.2 Medical Department Log of Visits, Auto Parts Factory, 1998, by Department*

Visit No.	*Date*	*Department*	*Reason for Visit*†
1	1/3/98	S	Finger caught in parts tray
2	1/9/98	F	Pain in shoulder
3	1/14/98	A	Pain in elbow, tendinitis
4	1/15/98	M	Lost sense of touch in fingers
5	1/19/98	S	Sprained right wrist
6	1/25/98	A	Dislocated left wrist
7	1/28/98	M	First degree burn right thumb
8	1/31/98	S	Open fracture, right thumb
9	2/2/98	A	Hematoma at base of right thumb
10	2/3/98	A	Deep cuts, right index finger
11	2/7/98	S	Backache
12	2/8/98	F	Open wound scalp
13	2/15/98	S	Fracture, right forearm
14	2/19/98	S	Fracture, right elbow
15	3/1/98	A	Swelling, right wrist
16	3/4/98	A	Cut on right pinky finger
17	3/5/98	S	Dislocation, right thumb
18	3/11/98	A	Hematoma, right palm
19	3/17/98	S	Carpal tunnel syndrome
20	3/18/98	M	Cut on right hand
21	3/20/98	S	Contusion, right hand
22	3/23/98	S	Contusion, right thumb
23	3/27/98	S	Dislocated right index finger
24	3/30/98	A	Cramp in right hand
25	4/2/98	S	Pain in right shoulder
26	4/6/98	M	Hit right hand fingers by part
27	4/11/98	F	Radiating pain, right forearm
28	4/12/98	M	Debris in right eye
29	4/15/98	S	Sprained right elbow
30	4/20/98	M	Part fell on right hand
31	4/22/98	A	Loss of feeling in fingers of right hand
32	4/29/98	S	Open fracture in right palm area
33	5/2/98	A	Tendinitis of muscle flexors in right hand
34	5/5/98	S	Ganglion, right wrist
35	5/9/98	F	Edema in left wrist
36	5/14/98	M	Blister, right index finger
37	5/23/98	A	Pain in wrist
38	5/26/98	F	Tendinitis in right thumb flexor
39	5/28/98	S	Tendinitis in right thumb flexor
40	6/1/98	S	Complex fracture, right hand
41	6/6/98	A	Conjunctivitis, noninfectious
42	6/7/98	M	Difficulty breathing
43	6/8/98	S	Sprained left shoulder
44	6/10/98	S	Tendinitis muscle abductors, left arm
45	6/13/98	S	Carpal tunnel syndrome, left hand
46	6/21/98	A	Pain in elbow with swelling
47	6/24/98	S	Acute bronchitis
48	6/28/98	M	Foreign object in eye
49	6/29/98	A	Contact dermatitis, hands
50	7/2/98	M	Hurt back while lifting part
51	7/4/98	F	Tendinitis, right wrist
52	7/9/98	S	Allergic rhinitis

Table E.2 (Continued)

Visit No.	*Date*	*Department*	*Reason for Visit*†
53	7/19/98	A	Chemical conjunctivitis
54	7/21/98	M	Twisted ankle
55	7/22/98	S	Acute bronchitis
56	7/28/98	F	Inflammation of left wrist
57	8/1/98	S	Muscle spasm, low back
58	8/4/98	A	Hurt back while braking fall
59	8/9/98	S	Dermatitis, abdominal region
60	8/11/98	S	Fractured right humerus
61	8/15/98	S	Deep cuts in deltoid region
62	8/22/98	A	Pain in right elbow
63	8/23/98	A	Chemical conjunctivitis, right eye
64	8/29/98	S	Bronchial asthma crisis
65	9/3/98	F	Bumped back of head in fall
66	9/4/98	S	Contusion, right index finger
67	9/10/98	M	Pain in wrist from repetitive use
68	9/13/98	A	Inflammation, right wrist
69	9/17/98	S	Allergic rhinitis
70	9/18/98	S	Sprained joint in left wrist
71	9/22/98	A	Dislocated joint in left wrist
72	9/24/98	F	Open fracture, left ring finger
73	9/27/98	S	Abraded fingers, right hand
74	9/30/98	A	Fracture in left forearm
75	10/2/98	M	Felt dizzy
76	10/6/98	S	Contusion of right middle finger
77	10/11/98	A	Sprained right hand and wrist
78	10/14/98	S	Dislocation, 1/3 distal right thumb
79	10/18/98	F	Contusion in left hand
80	10/22/98	M	Twisted knee while lifting box
81	10/23/98	S	Constant pain in left shoulder
82	10/27/98	S	Loss of touch, fingers right hand
83	10/27/98	A	Stiff right index finger
84	10/27/98	S	Pain in hand from repetitive use
85	11/3/98	M	Pain in right elbow
86	11/5/98	A	Dislocated left elbow
87	11/11/98	F	Tendinitis in right wrist
88	11/14/98	S	Complex fracture, right hand
89	11/22/98	A	Radiating pain through forearm
90	11/25/98	S	Bilateral chemical conjunctivitis
91	11/29/98	A	Allergic dermatitis
92	11/30/98	F	Contusion of right index finger
93	12/2/98	S	Acute bronchitis
94	12/3/98	M	Constant pain in right shoulder
95	12/15/98	S	Chronic obstructive lung disease
96	12/18/98	A	Mycosis in nails of fingers of right hand
97	12/19/98	F	Contusion of left hand
98	12/20/98	A	Contusion of left index finger
99	12/22/98	F	Dislocated joint, left wrist
100	12/22/98	S	Amputation of fingers of right hand
101	12/23/98	M	Sprained back after fall
102	12/29/98	F	Fractured left middle finger

*S, Shipping and Receiving; F, Fabrication; A, Assembly; M, Maintenance.

†MSDs = Visit No. 2, 3, 4, 15, 19, 24, 25, 27, 31, 33, 34, 35, 37, 38, 39, 44, 45, 46, 51, 56, 62, 67, 68, 81, 82, 83, 84, 85, 87, 89, 94

Table E.3 Hours Worked and Incident Cases of Musculoskeletal Disorders in 1998, and Lost Workdays, 1998–1999

A *Department*	B *Hours Worked 1998*	C *No. of Cases, 1998*	D *Lost Workdays, 1998–1999*
Assembly	189,413	11	115
Fabrication	114,114	7	84
Shipping and receiving	64,286	9	117
Maintenance	19,048	4	56
Total	386,861	31	372

culations by entering summary data into commercial spreadsheet programs. However, there are obvious advantages of automating this process (see Chapter 10). Unfortunately, at many workplaces, data that draw from medical departments, personnel, accounting, payroll, and risk management are not integrated. Even when they are, a custom software application must be written to perform the following calculations because commercial off-the-shelf software usually lacks an epidemiologic orientation. The steps for carrying out this example are presented in overview in Table E.1, and follow below.

A. CONSTRUCT A WRITTEN CASE DEFINITION OF WORK-RELATED MUSCULOSKELETAL DISORDERS OF THE UPPER EXTREMITIES

Ideally one would like to define cases in terms of laboratory results such as nerve conduction tests, x-rays, physical findings, and other hard data. After reading just a few medical log entries, it becomes clear that the reason for the medical visit is a hodge-podge of signs, symptoms, diagnoses, and the external cause of the injury or illness. Making matters worse, the reason for the visit is a brief text narrative rather than a standard numeric or alphanumeric code that a computer can process easily.

To make an operational definition, one can construct a checklist of key words and synonyms that are consistent with symptoms, signs, and diagnoses of MSDs. Some entries in the log are so ambiguous that this may seem like a leap of faith, but let us assume this is the only source of data available.

Because work history is not on the log, it is not apparent how one can tell if the injury involves the repetitive use of the hands or even if the condition is work-related. However, it is not unreasonable to infer that medical conditions such as fractures, burns, contusions, and cuts are traumatic rather than repetitive. This still leaves sprains and strains, which may or may not be the result of repetitive use. One must make a decision, and for this example, sprains and strains will be excluded from case definition. This increases the specificity of the definition, that is, noncases are more likely to be excluded. However, this will decrease sensitivity because some true MSD cases called sprains or strains will probably be excluded. (See Chapter 3, Scientific Classification Systems for a discussion of sensitivity and specificity.) Work-relatedness is also an assumption. One can argue that if none of the conditions is work-related or exacerbated by work, the MSDs will be distributed with equal probability across departments (rate ratio of 1 for each department). This assumes that distributions of age and gender that might influence the MSDs are similar across the departments, but this can be tested, too.

A simple case definition and eligibility may be stated as follows:

- Visit with upper extremity body part affected: hand, wrist, elbow, shoulder, neck, AND
- Visit with mention of pain, cramping, loss of sense of touch, or swelling *or* a diagnosis of tendinitis, carpal tunnel syndrome, or other recognized MSD of the upper extremity listed in a reference guide[1,2]
- Exclude mention of sprain or strain of upper or lower extremity
- Assume all visits are on the log are work-related

Table E.4 Incident Cases, Rates, Rate Ratios, and Excess Cases of Injuries and Illnesses, Auto Parts Plant, 1998*

A *Department*	B *Hours Worked*	C *Cases of MSDs*	D *MSD Incidence Rate × 100*	E *Rate Ratio*	F *Attributable Risk Rate × 100*	G *Excess Cases*
Assembly	189,413	11	11.6	1.0	0.0	0.0
Fabrication	114,114	7	12.2	1.1	0.6	0.3
Shipping and receiving	64,286	9	28.0	2.4	16.4	5.3
Maintenance	19,048	4	42.0	3.6	30.4	2.9
Total	386,861	31	16.0	—	—	8.5

*MSD, musculoskeletal disorder.

Table E.5 Lost Workdays Incidence Rates, Rate Ratios, and Excess Cases of Injuries and Illnesses, Auto Parts Plant, Incident Cases in 1998*

A	B	C	D	E	F	G
Department	*Hours Worked*	*Workdays Lost from MSDs*	*MSD LDW Incidence Rate × 100*	*Rate Ratio*	*Attributable Risk Rate × 100*	*Excess Days*
Assembly	189,413	115	121.4	1.0	0.0	0.0
Fabrication	114,114	84	147.2	1.2	25.8	14.7
Shipping and receiving	64,286	117	364.0	3.0	242.6	78.0
Maintenance	19,048	56	588.0	4.8	466.6	44.4
Total	386,861	372	192.3	—	—	137.1

*MSD, musculoskeletal disorders; LWD, lost workday.

B. DEFINE THE TIME PERIOD OF ANALYSIS AND THE ELIGIBLE POPULATION

The log does not state whether the date of visit is the date of onset or diagnosis. In this example the period of observation is 1 year, beginning January 1 and ending December 31. However, it is not clear that calendar dates of the hours-worked of the population (Table E.3) will match the calendar dates of the diagnoses of new cases. It is preferable to use the date of diagnosis or onset rather than the date of visit or the date of report. In this example we must make an assumption that the date of visit is sufficiently close in time to the date of diagnosis that the results will not be skewed.

Comparability between the numerator (cases) and denominator (population) also applies to what type of worker is eligible to be counted as a case and whose hours-worked are included. Will just production workers be included, or will management, supervisory, and administrative workers be included? This exercise does not include data on this question, so we will assume that only hourly production workers are included.

We now need to revise our case definition as follows:

Case Definition:

- Visit with upper extremity body part affected: hand, wrist, elbow, shoulder, neck, *and*
- Visit with mention of pain, cramping, loss of sense of touch, or swelling *or* diagnosis of tendinitis or carpal tunnel syndrome
- Exclude sprain or strain of upper or lower extremity

Eligibility:

- Exclude cases with date of visit before January 1, 1998 or after December 31, 1998
- Restrict the analysis to production workers in the four departments

Assumptions:

- Assume that the date of visit is the same or nearly the same as the date of diagnosis
- Assume all cases are work-related or are exacerbated by work

C. CALCULATE THE ANNUAL NUMBER OF HOURS WORKED FOR EACH DEPARTMENT

Table E.3 gives the hours-worked for 1998 for each department and for the entire eligible population. This table is sometimes built up from 12 monthly tallies (not shown). To keep this example simple, only an annual analysis will be shown. Record the hours worked from Column B in Table E.3 into Column B of Table E.4.

D. COMPARE THE WRITTEN CASE DEFINITION OF A MUSCULOSKELETAL DISORDER TO EACH ENTRY IN THE MEDICAL LOG

One should pilot the case definition before accepting it as final. A medical log from the previous year may be used to test and debug the definition.

Given that the medical history is not available, it is not possible to tell whether the case is new or occurred in 1997 or earlier. We must make an assumption that these are new cases and not follow-up visits. To record your decision, manually add an extra column in the medical visit log (Table E.2) so that a Yes or No note can be placed in the same row:

Visit No.	Date	Department*	Reason for Visit	Case?
1	1/3/98	S	Finger caught in parts tray	N
2	1/9/98	F	Pain in shoulder	Y
3	1/14/98	A	Pain in elbow, tendinitis	Y
4	1/15/98	M	Lost sense of touch in fingers	Y
5	1/19/98	S	Sprained right wrist	N
6	1/25/98	A	Dislocated left wrist	N

*S, Shipping and Receiving; F, Fabrication; A, Assembly; M, Maintenance.

The reader is now encouraged to try this on their own, starting at Visit No. 7 and ending at Visit 102. How many cases of MSDs do you count?

E. COUNT THE NUMBER OF MUSCULOSKELETAL DISORDERS FOR EACH DEPARTMENT

Case Incidence

For 1998, count the total number incident cases of MSDs in Table E.2 for each department and record each and the total in column C of Table E.3, and column C of Table E.4.

Lost Workday Incidence

These data come from a source other than the medical log. In this example they are provided in Table E.3. To make an accurate tally of lost workdays (LWD), the sum of lost workdays for each case in 1998 should include lost workdays in 1998 and 1999, or an estimate. If the analysis is done late in 1999 or 2000, lost workdays after the year of case incidence may already be available. Otherwise, the sum will be based either on 1998 data alone (which will lead to an underestimate), or projections such as the estimated date for first return-to-work (which also usually leads to an underestimate). Record the five entries in column C in Table E.4.

F. CALCULATE THE INCIDENCE RATES FOR MUSCULOSKELETAL DISORDERS

Case Incidence

The case incidence rates for 1998 are recorded in column D of Table E.4. Multiply the number of cases (column C) by the conversion factor of 200,000 hours worked/100 FTEs and divide by the hours actually worked (column B) for each department and overall. For example, the case incidence rate for the four departments combined is:

$$\text{Incidence Rate}_{\text{All Depts.}} = \frac{200{,}000 \times 31 \text{ cases}}{386{,}861 \text{ hours}}$$
$$= 16.0 \text{ cases per 100 FTEs}$$

LOST WORKDAY INCIDENCE

The lost workday incidence rates for 1998 are recorded in column D of Table E.5. Multiply the lost workdays (column C) by the conversion factor of 200,000 hours/100 FTEs and divide by the hours actually worked (column B) for each department and overall. For example, the lost workday incidence rate for the four departments combined is:

$$\text{LWD Incidence Rate}_{\text{All Depts.}} = \frac{200{,}000 \times 372 \text{ days}}{386{,}861 \text{ hours}}$$
$$= 192.3 \text{ days per 100 FTEs}$$

It is important to examine variation in incidence rates by time period. Depending on the amount of data available, monthly or quarterly variation for both case incidence and lost workday rates should be plotted. Figure E.1 is a plot of monthly incidence rates. It was plotted from tables (not shown) that had hours worked and cases broken down by month and department.

G. CALCULATE THE RATE RATIO FOR EACH DEPARTMENT

Case Incidence

Identify the department with the lowest MSD case incidence rate. It is Assembly with a rate of 11.6 cases per 100 FTEs. The rate ratio for the reference department (Assembly) is 1. Using this rate as the denominator for the rate ratio, calculate the rate ratios for the other three departments. Put the results in column E of Table E.4. For the Fabrication department, the Rate Ratio is:

$$\text{Rate Ratio}_{\text{Fabrication}} = \frac{\text{Incidence Rate}_{\text{Fabrication}}}{\text{Incidence Rate}_{\text{Assembly}}}$$
$$= \frac{12.2}{11.6} = 1.1$$

Lost Workday Incidence

Identify the department with the lowest incidence rate of lost workdays. This department does not have to be the same as the department with the lowest case incidence. It is possible that some departments have a high frequency of mild cases with rapid return-to-work and other departments with a fewer, but more severe cases or a few catastrophic cases that take weeks or months to return to work. In this example, Assembly is also the department with the lowest incidence rate of lost workdays at 121.4 days per 100 FTEs. The LWD rate ratio for this reference department is 1. Using this rate as the denominator, calculate the rate ratios for the other three departments. Put the results in column E of Table E.5. For the Fabrication, the Rate Ratio is:

$$\text{LWD Rate Ratio}_{\text{Fabrication}} = \frac{\text{Incidence Rate}_{\text{Fabrication}}}{\text{Incidence Rate}_{\text{Assembly}}}$$
$$= \frac{147.2}{121.4} = 1.2$$

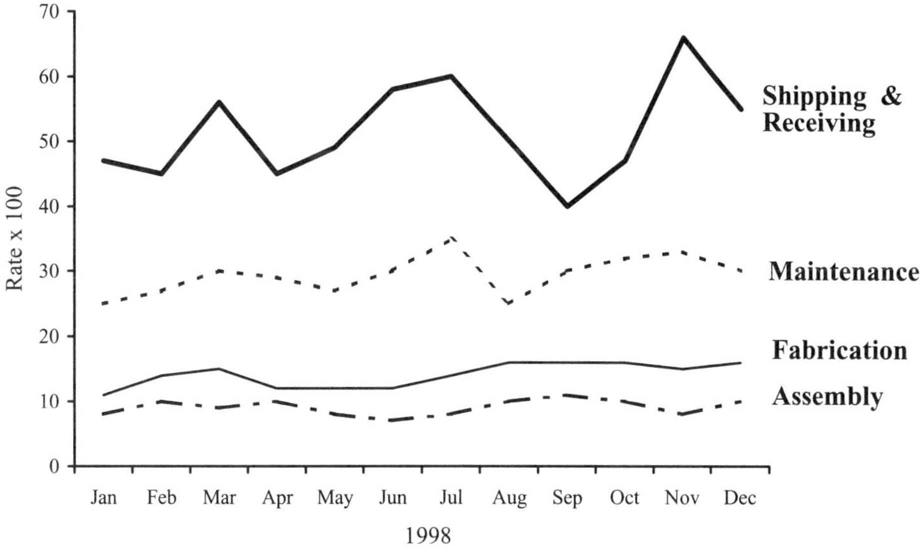

Figure E.1 Case incidence rates at an automobile parts plant by department and month, 1998.

H. CALCULATE THE ATTRIBUTABLE RISK FOR MUSCULOSKELETAL DISORDERS FOR EACH DEPARTMENT

Case Incidence

Using the same reference rate as the previous step (Assembly), subtract the reference rate from each of the other department's incidence rates. Put the results in column F of Table E.4.

$$\text{Attributable Risk}_{\text{Fabrication}} = \text{Incidence Rate}_{\text{Fabrication}} - \text{Incidence Rate}_{\text{Assembly}} = 12.2 - 11.6 = 0.6$$

Lost Workday Incidence

Using the same reference rate for lost workdays as step G (Assembly), subtract the reference rate from each of the other department's LWD incidence rates. This is repeated three times. Put the results in column F of Table E.4.

$$\text{Attributable Risk}_{\text{Fabrication}} = \text{Incidence Rate}_{\text{Fabrication}} - \text{Incidence Rate}_{\text{Assembly}} = 147.2 - 121.4 = 25.8$$

I. CALCULATE THE NUMBER OF EXCESS CASES FOR EACH DEPARTMENT

Case Incidence

Multiply the attributable risk (column F in Table E.4) for the first nonreference department by the hours-worked (column B) in that same department and divide by 200,000 to express the results as cases. In Fabrication,

$$\text{Excess Cases}_{\text{Fabrication}} = \frac{\text{Attributable Risk}_{\text{Fabrication}} \times \text{Hours Worked}_{\text{Fabrication}}}{200{,}000} = \frac{0.6 \times 114{,}114}{200{,}000} = 0.3 \text{ cases}$$

Fractional cases are not an error. Repeat for the other two departments and put the results in column G. Sum the number of excess cases for the three nonreference departments for a plantwide total.

Lost Workday Incidence

Multiply the attributable risk (column F in Table E.5) for the first nonreference department by the hours-worked (column B) in that same department and divide by 200,000 to express the results as days. For Fabrication,

$$\text{Excess Workdays Lost}_{\text{Fabrication}} = \frac{\text{Attributable Risk}_{\text{Fabrication}} \times \text{Hours Worked}_{\text{Fabrication}}}{200{,}000} = \frac{25.8 \times 114{,}114}{200{,}000} = 14.7 \text{ days}$$

Repeat for the other two departments and put the results in column G. Sum the number of excess lost workdays for the three nonreference departments for a plantwide total.

J. IDENTIFY THE HIGH-RISK AND LOW-RISK DEPARTMENTS BASED ON NUMBER OF CASES, RATE RATIOS, AND ATTRIBUTABLE CASES AND INTERPRET THE FINDINGS

Which department has the most number of cases? Does this reflect a low incidence rate in a large department? Which department has the highest incidence rate and rate ratio? Does this department also have the largest number of excess cases or lost workdays? Thus, there are several ways of defining the departments most and least affected by MSDs.

While Assembly has the greatest number of cases and lost workdays, Assembly has the lowest MSD rate for both case incidence and lost workdays. Does it make sense to follow-up first where the rates are already the lowest, or is it better to focus on the highest rates first, say in Maintenance or Shipping and Receiving? Even though Assembly has the lowest rate in the auto parts plant, perhaps it is much higher than comparable plants within the same company or industry as a whole. Should we also analyze the data using a different reference rate?

Do we need to know more specifically what are the problematic occupations, work tasks, or workstations in the high-risk departments? To follow-up, we should repeat the analysis but specifically aimed at jobs within the Maintenance or Shipping and Receiving. This would be a bivariate analysis of MSD rates by department and occupation. If these departments are small, there may be too few cases to carry out further statistical analysis. The analyses should now help guide an investigation that examines jobs in the high- and low-risk departments to determine the possible causes of the MSDs.

Are there unaccounted factors, related or unrelated to work, that occur in the high-risk or low-risk departments? For example, the frequency of some MSDs is usually higher in women than in men. Perhaps the employment patterns at this plant make it more (or less) likely that women predominate in Maintenance and Shipping and Receiving. Should we look at the gender distribution of the departments to see if proportionately more women work in the two high-risk departments? Should we now carryout separate analyses (bivariate), one for men another for women?

Are we confident enough in our data that we have not missed cases, or classified them improperly? We also need to go back over the assumptions and test each one. We may need to validate the data by looking at other data sources that confirm our operational case definition and perhaps include cases that may have escaped the medical log.

This example illustrates that there are several ways rate-based analysis can help establish priorities, and that follow-up needs to balance taking immediate action with additional data collection, analysis, and investigation.

REFERENCES

1. Putz-Anderson V. *Cumulative Trauma Disorders: A Manual for Musculoskeletal Diseases of the Upper Limbs.* New York: Taylor & Francis, 1988.
2. Park RM, Krebs JM, Mirer F. Occupational disease surveillance using disability insurance at an automotive stamping and assembly complex. *J Occup Environ Med* 1996; 38:1111–1123.

Appendix F

Economic Analysis and Employer-Based Surveillance

NEIL A. MAIZLISH

At every workplace, the selection of the solution for controlling or eliminating job exposures undergoes some kind of analysis. The analysis may be a gut reaction, or a formal economic analysis that has a business plan like the rest of the employer's operations. At workplaces where resources are limited it is legitimate to ask, given a specific prevention goal, which among the potential solutions is the most cost-effective.

Surveillance plays several roles. First, it may be the mechanism that first identified the problem and its magnitude. Second, surveillance data are inputs to economic analysis by providing information on potential benefits or cost avoidance. Third, the routine functioning of the surveillance system helps document whether the anticipated benefits were actually achieved.

There is an extensive literature on economic analysis. Some of the basic concepts are presented below with links to surveillance data and occupational health and safety. Several text books review this area.[1,2]

TYPES OF ECONOMIC ANALYSIS

There are three major approaches to economic analysis: cost-benefit analysis, cost-effectiveness analysis, and cost-utility analysis. The term *cost-benefit analysis* has taken on a generic meaning. Formally, it is a technique of expressing both the costs and benefits of the intervention on a single economic scale, usually dollars. Although it is easy to express costs in dollars, it is not easy to express benefits like the value of a human life, pain, or suffering in dollars. The cost-benefit equation usually takes one of two formats.

$$\text{Net Benefit (\$)} = \sum \text{Benefits (\$)} - \sum \text{Costs (\$)}$$

This says the sum of the benefits minus the sum of the costs is equal to the net benefit. Despite the widespread use of the term *cost-benefit ratio,* expressing the costs and the benefits as a ratio does not communicate the absolute impact. A ratio of 2 can be observed for benefits of \$200 and costs of \$100, or for benefits of \$200,000 and costs of \$100,000. However, a net benefit of \$100 may be trivial compared to \$100,000.

There is an important variant used in the business world. If the business invests in a health and safety solution now, how long will it take to recoup the costs in terms of benefits? This is known as the payback period. The costs of the intervention are assigned to a single budget year and benefits as an annual average:

$$\text{Pay Back Time} = \frac{\sum \text{Costs}}{\text{Benefits per year}}$$

From a business owner's perspective, an investment in health and safety that pays for itself in a short time period is a lot more palatable than one that takes a long time.

Cost-effectiveness analysis is a different approach that does not attempt to assign a dollar amount to the benefits, but rather uses a health outcome prevented as a unit of analysis. Cost-effectiveness is often expressed as the ratio of costs per prevented case.

$$\text{Cost Effectiveness} = \frac{\sum \text{Costs}}{\text{Number of cases prevented}}$$

Cases prevented can be the difference between the number of cases pre- and postintervention. For planning purposes, an estimate of cases prevented can be based on the number of attributable cases, or excess cases from surveillance data.

An advantage is that cost-effectiveness analysis does not have to make the difficult value judgments such as "how much does a human life cost?" A disadvantage is that a separate analysis has to be carried out for each type of health outcome. It is difficult to make direct comparisons. For example, it is not readily apparent how one compares the cost per fracture prevented with the cost per case of low back pain prevented.

Cost-utility analysis is a variant of cost-effectiveness analysis and uses a common health outcome scale for all the different types of health events, including death and disability. The common scale is usually quality-adjusted life years where both the length of life and the quality of life are considered. For fatal injuries and illnesses, the length of life is readily measurable in years of potential life lost. Deaths before the age of 65 are regarded as premature, and the years of life between age 65 and the age at death are those potentially lost. However, the quality of life still requires some kind of scale that gives weights to disability, limitations, pain, and suffering during the years lived.

In economic analysis the costs are broken down into two components: the cost of the intervention program and the cost savings brought about by the intervention program. The cost savings are costs avoided by reducing or eliminating the risk factors that contribute to the injuries and illness. The cost savings is considered a benefit. This can include both medical and indemnity costs. The intervention may also have another benefit beyond avoiding costs. The intervention may increase productivity by changing the production process or work practices. Productivity is usually expressed in terms of output per person-hour worked. The resistance to cost-benefit analysis is linked to the implications of productivity increases. One can increase productivity by maintaining the same level of output but with less hours, i.e., fewer workers and layoffs. Or, one can keep the same number of workers but achieve a new higher level of output. This second option saves jobs, and retrains or reassigns workers to other productive tasks within a workplace. Workers react to the implications of economic analyses, and their input should be taken into account.

Many economic analyses are based on assumptions and incomplete data that can create uncertainty in interpreting the results. Nonetheless, economic analysis can help improve the information available for decision-making.

ECONOMIC ANALYSIS IN OCCUPATIONAL HEALTH

Economic analysis varies depending on whether the focus is decision-making at a specific workplace or the society at large. The approach here is a specific workplace.

Two different models for economic analysis are frequently used in occupational health: the insurance model and the productivity model. The insurance model states that job injuries and illnesses are an insured cost. To spread the economic risk, employers are grouped according to the types of industries and occupations that have similar economic risks. They pay a premium according to this economic risk group or class. Sometimes insurance premiums are priced for an individual employer taking into account the average payouts (medical, indemnity, medical-legal) by their class, and their own recent injury experience. The definition of costs in the insurance model then become the costs of workers' compensation benefits and its administration.

Many costs of injuries and illness fall outside of workers' compensation insurance. Some medical costs of job injuries are paid out-of-pocket by injured workers themselves, by general health insurance of employers who offer their employees health benefits, by public hospitals who provide uncompensated medical care, by publicly financed medical programs such as Medicare for chronic job-related diseases in retired workers, and by publicly financed disability programs such as Social Security or state-disability programs.

There is substantial evidence that the costs of injuries and illnesses far exceed what employers pay in workers' compensation insurance. Productivity models suggest that the hidden or indirect costs of job injuries and illnesses can range from 0.5 to 20 times the wage cost.[3] What gets excluded from the insurance model are the following costs of lost productivity:

- structural overstaffing
- overtime due to job injuries
- lost production time
- training
- employee turnover
- substitution of goods and services for lost output
- reduced quality of services and goods

If 10% of the work force is absent on any given day due to job injuries and illnesses, an employer has two options: hire 10% more workers than is really necessary to maintain the expected level of output, or change the expected level of production to reflect the 90% attendance. The first option is called structural overstaffing and is a common response. Lowering production standards because of job injuries and illness neither solves the job-related health problem or gets production back to expected levels. Employers may try to increase the work rate, but this is not a long-lived solution and may itself increase job injuries.

For short-term injuries and illness, the absent worker can be temporarily replaced by a worker from another shift with the same skills. This is a source of overtime costs. Overtime itself may be a risk factor for job injuries. Thus, begins an spiral of job injuries, overtime, more job injuries, more overtime, etc.

If the injury or illness appears to be long-term, the employer may need to replace the worker. This involves internal promotions and transfers, or an external job search. In either event, training will be required for the new employee. Depending on the time it takes to get the new employee up to speed, the productivity of the replacement will be less than that of the experienced injured worker. Some jobs have long learning curves, which represent months of lost productivity.

Work injuries and illnesses can become an overriding aspect of working conditions and quality of work life. If conditions do not improve, workers may just leave. While not all job turnover is related to work injuries and illnesses, they may play an important part. Turnover increases training costs and productivity losses. As one mentally and physically prepares to leave employment, motivation and productivity often drops. Time is spent on nonproduction activities such as filing out personnel forms, training a new employee, or securing and shutting down equipment.

At some point, structural overstaffing, overtime, and other responses cannot compensate for reduced work hours, and production falls or shows signs of reduced quality. If the product or service cannot be delivered on time, employers lose their contracts or buy the same goods from a competitor to resell to their client. Reselling can be a costly solution. Reduced quality may be a decisive factor in a client abandoning the company. Ultimately, if clients question a company's reliability, or its product is not competitive in price and quality, the company will lose market share, potentially abandon product lines, or even go out of business. One or all of these consequences of job injuries and illnesses operate at a given business, and none are covered by workers' compensation insurance.

APPLYING THE PRODUCTIVITY MODEL

How does one carry out cost-benefit analysis using the productivity model, and what are its links to surveillance data? Figure F.1 shows the overview of the process. The cost-benefit equation is shown in an expanded form that states that the total benefits are made up of costs avoided and possible productivity increases. This version of the model does not take into account nontangible benefits like pain and suffering, but it could be adapted to do so.

At many workplaces structural overstaffing is a principal source of avoidable costs, and it can be estimated from the lost workdays due to job injuries and illness. If an intervention is successful it will reduce work hours lost. This represents a cost savings or benefit. Because the intervention may not be 100% effective at reducing the exposures that caused the lost work hours, we need to make a correction. Finally, the direct and indirect cost of a person-hour of production needs to be estimated. Avoided costs because of structural overstaffing are the product of three components: the effectiveness of the intervention, the number of excess work hours

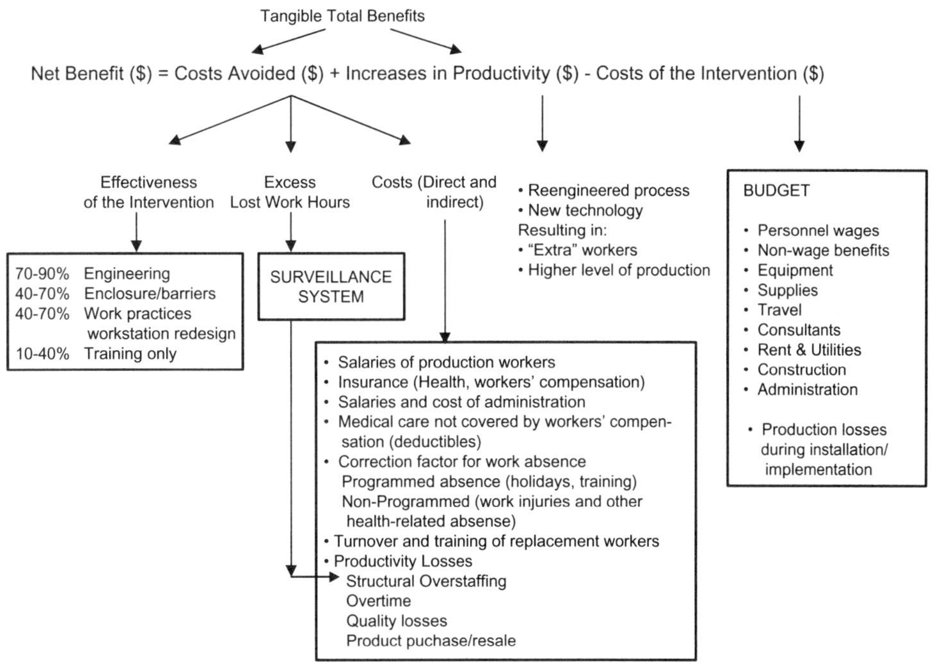

Figure F.1 Overview of cost-benefit analysis using the productivity model.

(or days) lost due to job-related injuries and illness, and the cost of a person-hour of production.

$$\text{Avoided Costs} = \text{Intervention effectiveness} \times \text{Excess lost work hours} \times \text{Cost per hour of production}$$

The effectiveness of the intervention should be based on the experience of similar companies under field conditions, and the judgment of experts, when available. Effectiveness can be judged in terms of reduction in either exposure or injury and illness rates. There is rarely precise data for effectiveness. Oxenburgh[2] has suggested broad bands for effectiveness: engineering (70%–90%), enclosure (40%–70%), change in work practices or workstation redesign (40%–70%), and training (10%–40%). Engineering changes are preferred because of their high degree of effectiveness, and because they do not require each individual to assume the responsibility of the intervention.

The excess lost work hours is generated by a surveillance system that captures lost work time. Excess lost work hours can be estimated from:

- the attributable risk using lost workday incidence rates (multiplied by 8 hours per lost workday) in the work area in which the intervention is planned minus the rate in a baseline area
- the hours worked in the area where the intervention is planned

$$\text{Excess Work Hours Lost} = (\text{LWD Rate}_{\text{Intervention}} - \text{LWD Rate}_{\text{Baseline}}) \times \frac{8\ \text{hours}}{\text{day}} \times \text{Hours Worked}_{\text{Intervention}}$$

An important assumption is that if an intervention is 100% effective by totally eliminating the exposure, the injury and illness rate will fall to the baseline level (rather than 0). For example, back strains due to occasional light lifting may occur at a low rate throughout all production areas of a plant. Work areas with only light lifting might be considered for the baseline rate of back sprains. An intervention that semiautomates constant heavy lifting in a material handling operation may eliminate back sprains because of heavy lifting, but not address back sprains because of occasional light lifting on other job tasks in the same work area. Although injury and illness rates of zero are possible, it is probably better not to overstate the potential benefits.

The cost of a productive hour has several components. Many details depend on the cost accounting methods of specific businesses. For example, some costs at a given workplace may be taken on by a corporate parent. In general, the main cost components are:

- wages of the production workers
- nonwage benefits (health, disability, pension, etc.)
- workers' compensation premium, and for policies with deductibles, direct costs under the deductible
- costs of on-site medical services, if applicable
- salaries and costs of administration of the workplace

Hours paid versus hours actually worked in most workplaces is quite different. The true cost per productive hour should be based on the time actually spent in production activities. The sources of the difference between paid time and actual hours worked include both programmed work absence and nonprogrammed events:

- paid vacation, holidays, and other paid leave (maternity, education)
- study days, job training away from workstation, health and safety training
- unscheduled work absence due to job injuries and general sick leave

In addition to the cost savings due to structural overstaffing, productivity losses because of employee turnover, training, overtime, reduction in quality, and product purchase and resale need to be estimated separately and added to the model. This requires detailed records from production, attendance, and training programs and criteria that helps identify whether a job injury or illness led to the productivity loss. Not all overtime, turnover, product rejects, and missed deadlines are caused by work injuries and illnesses. If large volumes of attendance and production data are generated daily, taking representative samples of records may help determine the proportion of the productivity loss that is because of job injuries and illness. Likewise, exit interviews of employees who quit may reveal how job exposures and injuries influenced their decision to leave. The proportion that cite job health and safety concerns as a significant reason for leaving can be multiplied by costs for general recruitment and training at the workplace.

As mentioned earlier, intervention for health and safety may have the broader consequence of increasing productivity by introducing a new technology or work practice. It may be possible to do the same work as before but with fewer workers. These are considered benefits that are added to the cost-benefit equation.

Lastly, the cost of the intervention itself must be evaluated. Most organizations have a standard budget breakdown that covers personnel, nonwage benefits, equipment, supplies, rent, utilities, communications, construction, consultants, and overhead and administrative costs.

Both the effectiveness and costs are specific to each type of intervention. Usually several alternatives are considered, and given an *equal* goal of exposure reduction, the least costly intervention program is selected. Because many interventions require time to be phased in, the cost of lost work time because of disruptions in production while the intervention is being implemented should also be included. For example, the downtime as a result of installing new equipment, or time spent on new job training should be included as part of the intervention.

Like measures of incidence, cost-benefit analysis requires a period of time to be specified. This is called the time horizon for the analysis.[1] Interventions are not expected to last forever, and must be maintained and replaced as they lose their effectiveness, or as new technologies are introduced. United States businesses typically have horizons for return on investment of 1 to 3 years.

There are several common pitfalls to carrying out economic analysis. These include:

- imprecise thinking in attributing costs and benefits
- not accounting for all the costs and all the benefits
- inaccurate estimates of the effectiveness and staying power of the interventions
- claiming credit for benefits or costs not related to the intervention, but to other factors beyond the analysis
- double counting costs or benefits
- using biased samples to estimate costs or benefits

An example is shown in Table F.1 based on the productivity model of Oxenburgh.[2] In this analysis, the benefit of the intervention is the costs avoided by reducing lost work time and structural overstaffing because of job injuries. The workplace is a hypothetical food products plant employing 3000 hourly workers (Appendix D). The factory is organized into five main departments (Line 1, Line 2, Maintenance, Shipping and Receiving, and Inspection) and four main occupations (machine operators, inspectors, material handlers, and mechanics). The time horizon for the analysis is 1 year. Data on annual costs for plant operations are meant to be illustrative rather than realistic. These are data that would be obtained from business operations and accounting, and are expressed in terms of percent of wage payroll.

The average monthly wage per worker is $3000 and the annual hourly payroll is $108 million. On top of wages, an amount equal to 4% of payroll pays for the annual group health insurance premium, and 10% of payroll pays the annual workers' compensation premium. Production workers usually get an annual 3% bonus. The plant has its own in-plant medical services staffed with a physician consultant and 2 nurses that costs $160,000 per year. Annual administrative costs are 40% of payroll and include the entire salary and operating budgets of administration. The above direct and indirect costs are $169,720,000 per year.

The annual average nominal hours worked is 1790 hours per worker. *Nominal* is not actual hours worked because during a normal work year the average worker gets paid time for vacation, sick leave, training days, etc. The nominal cost of an hour worked at this workplace is $31.60 ($169.7 million/[1790 hours/worker × 3000 workers]). After subtracting out paid time at nonproduction activities (e.g., vacation and all other paid absence) from the 1790 nominal average, the cost of an actual hour of production climbs to $36.34.

Workers are experiencing back injuries due to lifting. Workers in Line 1 have the highest rate ratio (RR) in the plant (RR = 3.4) compared to Shipping and Receiving. In the previous year, workers in Line 1 had 6916 excess lost workdays compared to Inspection. Assuming full 8-hour workdays, this is 55,328 hours lost that could be avoided if any intervention is 100% effective. Among several interventions considered, redesigning individual workstations was the most effective intervention. It is expected to reduce excess lost work time by 75%. Given the actual cost per hour is $36.34, the cost of the hours saved by the intervention is over $1.508 million per year (55,328 hours × 0.75 × $36.34/hr).

The intervention is a redesigned workstation for 250 workers in Line 1 at a cost of $2000 per station. The installation is an extra 10% of the cost per work station. Additional costs are retraining, downtime during installation, and administration. The overall costs of the intervention are $1.121 million.

In this example there is a net benefit of $386,715 ($1.508 million − $1.121 million). It is customary to assign the costs of the intervention to the first budget year, and express the benefits per year for the duration of the time horizon. After 9 months, the cost of the hours saved by avoiding injuries will pay back the investment of $1.12 million on the intervention program.

This example greatly simplifies cost-benefit analysis. In every economic analysis there are many assumptions and uncertainties. Nonetheless, this type of analysis increases the amount of information available for deci-

Table F.1 Cost-Benefit Analysis of Reengineering Line 1 to Reduce Lifting Injuries Among 250 Machine Operators at a Food Products Factory, 1999

Costs and Benefits	*Amount*
A. Annual direct* and indirect† costs of production	$169,720,000
B. Annual hours engaged in production (3000 wage employees)‡	4,671,000
• Cost per productive hour (A/B)‡	$36.34
C. Avoidable costs of lost work time because of job injuries§	$1,507,965 per year
D. Cost of the intervention program¶	$1,121,250
• Net benefit (C − D)	$386,715
• Payback period (D/C)	9 months (0.74 years)

*Direct costs, annual sum of:

Wages for 3000 production workers	$108,000,000
Bonuses for meeting production goals	$3,240,000
Workers' compensation premium	$10,800,000
Group health benefits	$4,320,000
In-plant medical services	$160,000
Total	$126,520,000

†Indirect costs (Administration)	$43,200,000
Sum of direct and indirect costs	$169,720,000

‡Cost per productive hour:

Annual sum of paid hours (PH) for 3000 production workers 1790 hours per worker per year standard × 3000 workers	5,370,000
Annual sum of hours absent (HA) from work because of work injuries, sick leave, maternity leave, training, etc.	429,000
Annual sum of vacation hours (VH)	270,000
Annual hours engaged in production (PH − HA − VH)	4,671,000
Cost per paid hour $= \left(\dfrac{\text{Direct and indirect costs}}{\text{Annual paid hours}}\right)$	$31.60
Cost per productive hour $= \left(\dfrac{\text{Direct and indirect costs}}{\text{Annual hours engaged in production}}\right)$	$36.34

§Avoidable costs of lost work time because of job injuries:

Annual excess lost workdays (LWD) from surveillance system comparing rates in area of intervention (Line 1) with that of baseline department (Shipping and receiving)	6916
$(\text{LWD incidence rate}_{\text{Line1}} - \text{LWD incidence rate}_{\text{S\&R}}) \times \dfrac{\text{Hours Worked}_{\text{Line1}}}{200{,}000}$	Appendix D, Table D.5b
$(2077.1 - 540.2) \times \dfrac{900{,}000}{200{,}000} = 6916 \text{ workdays} = 55{,}328 \text{ work hours}$	
900,000 hours = 450 FTEs × 2000 hours/year	
Annual excess lost work hours (excess lost workdays × 8 hours per workday)	55,328
Effectiveness of intervention (based on consultants' opinion)	75%
Avoidable costs = Excess hours × effectiveness × cost per productive hour‡ (55,328 hours × .75 × $36.34)	$1,507,965

¶Cost of the intervention program:

Workstation redesign (250 workstations × $2000 per workstation)	$500,000
Installation of new workstations	$375,000
Training of workers on new station	$50,000
Idle production during training period	$50,000
Project administration and overhead	$146,250
Total	$1,121,250

sion-making and may spark interest for more detailed analyses.

ACKNOWLEDGMENTS

Dr. Glenn Shor, California Division of Workers' Compensation, is gratefully acknowledged for his insight and review of this appendix.

REFERENCES

1. Haddix AC, Teusch SM, Shaffer PA, Duñet D. *Prevention Effectiveness.* New York: Oxford University Press, 1996.
2. Oxenburgh M. *Increasing Productivity and Profit through Health and Safety.* Chicago: Commerce Clearing House, 1991.
3. Andreoni D. *The Cost of Occupational Accidents and Diseases.* Geneva: International Labour Office, 1986.

Appendix G

Questionnaires for the Follow-up of Elevated Blood Lead

Staff of the California Occupational Health Program,
California Department of Health Services

EMPLOYEE QUESTIONNAIRE

CALIFORNIA LEAD REGISTRY (Adults)

Priority Cases, > 60 μg Pb/dl

Interviewer: Hello, my name is ______________________________. |__|__|__|
first last ID

I am with the California Department of Health Services—the State health department. Since January 1987, medical laboratories have been required to report the results of blood tests for lead in California residents, whenever the test shows an increased blood lead level. We recently received a notice of your test.

We are making follow-up phone calls to all people with high lead results. The purpose of this call is to provide information and other assistance regarding possible workplace exposures to lead. If your blood test was part of a company-sponsored medical program, your employer may have already received a copy of your test results.

I would like to ask you a few questions about your work and exposure to lead. The answers to these questions are confidential medical information and no information identifying you individually will be made available to your employer. The information will help make sure that your blood tests for lead are getting the proper attention and follow-up, which may lead to improving your health and workplace conditions.

1. Would you agree to a 15-minute interview now? ___Yes 1 ___No 2 ___Index case 3 already interviewed

   If NO to Question 1,

   Would you mind just telling us, your occupation and industry of employment?

2. Occupation |__|__|__|__|__|__|__|__|__|__|__|__|__|__|__|__|__|__|__|

3. Industry |__|__|__|__|__|__|__|__|__|__|__|__|__|__|__|__|__|__|__|

California Lead Registry Rev. 11/88

Patient No. ____________________ Employee Questionnaire

Interviewer: If you want information later or wish to contact us, ask for Dr. ___________, California Occupational Health Program Lead Registry, Berkeley, CA 94704. Tel. (xxx) xxx-xxxx.

4. Today's date: __ __/__ __/__ __ (Dy Mo Yr) 5. Time __ __:__ __ (hr min) AM/PM (circle)

I. Patient Demographics

Where are you residing?

1. Street |__|__|__|__|__|__|__|__|__|__|__|__|__|__|__|__|__|__|__|
2. City |__|__|__|__|__|__|__|__|__|__|__|__|__|
3. State |__|__| 4. Zip |__|__|__|__|__|
5. Telephone at home (__|__|__) |__|__|__| -|__|__|__|__|
6. Telephone for message (__|__|__) |__|__|__| -|__|__|__|__|
7. Sex: M___ (1) F___ (2) 8. What is your date of birth?__ __/__ __/__ __ (Mo Dy Yr)
9. What is the highest grade of school you completed?

   0 1 2 3 4 5 6 7 8 (Grade School) 9 10 11 12 (High School) 13 14 15 16 (College)

10. What is your race or ethnicity?

   ___White (1) __Black (2) ___Hispanic (3) ___Asian (4) ___Other (5)

11. What is the language you speak most at home?___English (1) ___Spanish (2) ___Other (3)
12. From the youngest to oldest, list the ages of all persons who live with you at the address above?

   __ __ (1) __ __ (2) __ __ (3) __ __ (4) __ __ (5) __ __ (6) __ __ (7) __ __ (8)

13. Are you, or anyone living with you, pregnant or nursing an infant?

   a. Pregnant ___Yes (1) ___No (2) b. Nursing ___Yes (1) ___No (2)

14. Have you had any of the following hobbies or nonwork activities in the last 12 months in which you have been exposed to lead, including house painting, ceramics, shot making?

   ___ none (1) ___ target practice (4) ___ stained glass making (6)

Patient No. ___________________ Employee Questionnaire

___ house painting ___ shot making ___ folk remedies
2 5 7

___ pottery/ceramics ___ serving or cooking ___ other_______________
3 8 food in dishes 9
or bowls made from glazed pottery

II. Medical Care for Current Blood Test

Interviewer: "I'd like to ask you a few questions about medical care concerning your recent blood test for lead."

1. Have you been informed of the results of this test prior to this call? ___Yes (1) ___No (2)

Interviewer: if NO, "Medical authorities believe that blood lead levels over 80 are immediately injurious, and may cause serious and lasting damage to your health. At levels above 60, most employers are legally obligated to transfer you to a job with less exposure to lead. If you are a construction worker your employer is not legally obligated to do this, but we recommend removal to a less exposed job. We will be sending you information on how to reduce your exposures to lead, your employer's responsibilities, and your rights under OSHA regulations."

2. Were you hospitalized for the high blood lead level? ___Yes (1) ___No (2)

3. Did you experience any of the following symptoms:

	Yes	No		Yes	No
a. joint or muscle pain	___ 1	___ 2	d. extreme fatigue	___ 1	___ 2
b. nausea	___ 1	___ 2	e. constipation	___ 1	___ 2
c. headaches	___ 1	___ 2	f. other _______________	___ 1	___ 2

4. Was the blood test part of a company screening program ___ (1) or did you go to a private doctor ___ (2) ?

5. Are you currently seeing a doctor for your blood lead? ___Yes (1) ___No (2)

6. IF YES, what is the physician's name and address:

Dr. First Name |__|__|__|__|__|__|__|__|__|__| M.I. |__|

Last Name |__|__|__|__|__|__|__|__|__|__|__|__|__|__|__|__|__|__|__|__|

Org. |__|__|__|__|__|__|__|__|__|__|__|__|__|__|__|__|__|__|__|__|

Street |__|__|__|__|__|__|__|__|__|__|__|__|__|__|__|__|__|__|__|__|

City|__|__|__|__|__|__|__|__|__|__|__|__|__|__|__|__|__|__|__|__|

State |__|__|__|__|__|__|__| Zip |__|__|__|__|__|

Patient No. ____________________ Employee Questionnaire

7. Is this individual your:
 __ personal physician (1) ___ company physician (2) ___ or other health provider? (3) ______________________

If NO, "We recommend that you contact your personal physician. If you do not have a personal physician or you would like your doctor to contact an occupational health physician familiar with lead-related health problems, we can recommend:" (see attached)

III. Occupational History

Interviewer: "I'd like to ask you a few questions about your work history."

1. Who is your current employer?

 Employer |__|__|__|__|__|__|__|__|__|__|__|__|__|__|__|__|__|__|__|__|

 Street|__|__|__|__|__|__|__|__|__|__|__|__|__|__|__|__|__|__|__|__|

 City |__|__|__|__|__|__|__|__|__|__|__|__|__|__|__|__|

 State |__|__| Zip |__|__|__|__|__|

 Industry |__|__|__|__|__|__|__|__|__|__|__|__|__|__|__|__| |__|__|__|__| SIC

 Occupation |__|__|__|__|__|__|__|__|__|__|__|__|__|__| |__|__|__|__| SOC

2. Who was your employer when the blood test was taken?

 Employer |__|__|__|__|__|__|__|__|__|__|__|__|__|__|__|__|__|__|__|__|

 Street|__|__|__|__|__|__|__|__|__|__|__|__|__|__|__|__|__|__|__|__|

 City |__|__|__|__|__|__|__|__|__|__|__|__|__|__|__|__|

 State |__|__| Zip |__|__|__|__|__| |__|__|__|__| SOC

 Industry |__|__|__|__|__|__|__|__|__|__|__|__|__|__|__|__| |__|__|__|__| SIC

 What job did you have when the blood test was taken?

Job Title/Occupation	Dept/Bldg/Section	Dates Worked MM/YY - MM/YY	No. of Co-workers in work area

 Description of worksite and adjacent work area(s), if any.

 Description of materials used:

Patient No. ____________________ Employee Questionnaire

____

Description of process:

____

3. Have you been transferred or removed from this job since the time the blood test was taken? ___Yes (1) ___No (2)

   IF YES, are you still getting paid the same rate as before you got transferred? ___Yes (1) ___No (2)

Interviewer: If blood lead is >60, "You may be covered by the OSHA lead standard. If so, your employer is required to remove you from your job when your blood lead is 60 μg/dl or greater. Under the OSHA law you keep your same pay rate and seniority until you are ready to go back to that job again. You may also be entitled to medical monitoring. Even if you are not covered by OSHA, removal from the source of exposure is a recommendation to prevent serious harm from lead over-exposure. We will be sending you information on medical monitoring for lead in blood."

4. What type of respirators did you use, if any?

   ___none (1) ___disposable (2) ___1/2 mask-cartridge (3)
   ___full face (4) ___ air supplied (5) ___other: ______________________ (6)

5. Is there any ventilation to remove lead fumes or dusts from the workplace? ___Yes (1) ___No (2)

6. How many other blood lead tests have you had on this job? ___ ___

7. While on this job, have you usually changed into a different set of clothes before leaving the worksite? ___Yes (1) ___No (2)

8. While on this job, was there a shower at the worksite? ___Yes (1) ___No (2)

   If YES, did you take a shower at the end of each work shift? ___Yes (1) ___No (2)

9. While on this job, did you smoke cigarettes at work, if at all?
   ___ not a smoker (1) ___ smoker, but not at work (2) ___ smoked anywhere at work (3)

10. While on this job, where did you eat at work?

    ___ never ate at work (1) ___ ate at work, location(s):__________________ (2)

11. How many hours of training, if any, have you received regarding the health effects of lead, protective clothing, or the lead standard? ___ ___

Patient No. ____________________ Employee Questionnaire

12. Is there a union that represents you at this workplace ___Yes ___No
                                                                1   2

    If YES, name unions(s)/local(s) ______________________________________

    ____
    Street City Zip Phone

Contact person/title:____

Did you have another job before this at the same or other employer in the last 12 months?

If YES, go to next page, otherwise go to Section IV.

13. Where did you work immediately before the job you just described. Start with your current employer and work backwards in time and include each separate job and transfer at each employer.

    Employer |__|__|__|__|__|__|__|__|__|__|__|__|__|__|__|__|__|__|__|__|

    Street|__|__|__|__|__|__|__|__|__|__|__|__|__|__|__|__|__|__|__|__|

    City |__|__|__|__|__|__|__|__|__|__|__|__|__|__|__|__|

    State |__|__| Zip |__|__|__|__|__| |__|__|__|__|
    SOC

    Industry |__|__|__|__|__|__|__|__|__|__|__|__|__|__|__|__| |__|__|__|__|
    SIC

    What job did you have when the blood test was taken?

Job Title/Occupation	Dept/Bldg/Section	MM/YY - MM/YY	No. of Co-workers in work area

    Description of worksite and adjacent work area(s), if any.

    ____

    Description of materials used:

    ____

    Description of process:

    ____

14. What type of respirators did you use, if any?

    ___none (1) ___disposable (2) ___1/2 mask-cartridge (3)
    ___full face (4) ___ air supplied (5) ___other: ______________________ (6)

Patient No. ____________________ Employee Questionnaire

15. Was there any ventilation to remove lead fumes or dusts from the workplace? ___Yes ___No
1 2

16. How many other blood lead tests did you have on this job? ___ ___

17. While on this job, did you usually change into a different set of clothes before leaving the worksite? ___Yes ___No
1 2

18. While on this job, was there a shower at the worksite? ___Yes ___No
1 2

If YES, did you take a shower at the end of each work shift? ___Yes ___No
1 2

19. How many hours of training, if any, have you received regarding the health effects of lead, protective clothing, or the lead standard? ___ ___

20. Was there a union that represented you at this this workplace? ___Yes ___No
1 2
If YES, name unions(s)/local(s) ______________________________________

____
Street City Zip Phone

Contact person/title:____

IV. Worker Notification and Follow-up

Employer Follow-up. We would like to talk to your employer about lead exposures at your worksite. This is important to determine whether there are measures in place to protect other current workers and future workers from toxic exposures. We also need to do this to determine whether your employer has a complete program for dealing with lead exposures, including medical testing, respirators, showers, clothing, and other industrial hygiene controls. We will do this without mentioning your name.

1. Do you object to our contacting your employer without mentioning your name? ___Yes ___No
1 2

Interviewer: for cases in manufacturing industries:

OSHA Lead Standard. There is a federal law called the "OSHA Lead Standard" that was written to protect the health of workers exposed to lead in nonconstruction industries. In this law, employers are required to provide training, limit exposures, provide showers and clean rest areas for their employees who are exposed to lead. Parts of this law require employers to hire a doctor to give free medical check-ups and blood tests for the effects of lead exposure. If the doctor finds that your blood lead is too high to keep working at your regular job, this law requires your employer to place you at a job with low- or no-lead exposure and at full pay, seniority, and benefits. Only after your blood lead level drops to a safer level are you allowed to return to your regular job.

Patient No. ____________________ Employee Questionnaire

Interviewer: for cases in construction, agriculture, or uncertain:

Workers' Compensation. Workers in the construction industry or in agriculture are not covered by the federal OSHA lead Standard. However, workers injured or made ill by exposures to lead on the job may be entitled to worker's compensation benefits. California's workers' compensation program pays medical bills for job-related injuries and illnesses. In addition, people who have disabilities from job-related injuries or illnesses may be entitled to income replacement benefits. Steps to obtain these benefits must be taken within specified time periods. If you are in the construction industry or agriculture and if you wish to seek benefits, you should contact an attorney specializing in worker's compensation, or the local Information and Assistance Office at the State Worker's Compensation Appeals Board. The telephone number at the office nearest you is: (xxx) xxx-xxxx.

OSHA Complaint. Under federal/state regulations, workers have a legal right to file a confidential complaint to OSHA regarding workplace conditions.

2. Do you want the address or phone number of the nearest OSHA office to find out more about filing a complaint? ___Yes (1) ___No (2)

Also, at your request, health professionals such as myself, a union representative or other authorized representative can refer a complaint without mentioning your name.

3. Do you want me to make a referral to OSHA for you? ___Yes (1) ___No (2)

4. If you are in a union, do you object to our contacting your union representative without mentioning your name? ___Yes (1) ___No (2)

5. Interviewer: Is there anything about your work or health that you think is important, but we haven't asked about?

____

____

____

"Thank you for your participation. We will be sending you some information packets. If you have any questions, you may contact us at Occupational Health Surveillance and Evaluation Program Lead Registry (xxx) xxx-xxxx."

6. Time (finished) __ __:__ __ (Hr Min) AM/PM (circle)

Patient No. ___________________ Employer Questionnaire

EMPLOYER QUESTIONNAIRE

CALIFORNIA LEAD REGISTRY (Adults)

Priority Cases, > 60 (μg/dl)

Interviewer: Hello, my name is ________________________. |__|__|__|
first last ID

I am with the Occupational Health Surveillance and Evaluation Program, California Department of Health Services—the State health department. Since January 1987, California medical laboratories have been required to report the results of blood tests for lead in California residents, whenever the test is higher than 25. We recently received a notice that one or more persons you employ had a reportable blood lead level.

Under Section 429.11 of the State of California Health and Safety Code, our program has the authority to question employers privately and review records collected pursuant to OSHA standards and regulations and other related matters. We are not an enforcement or regulatory agency, but we can offer useful advice and educational materials to assist you.

Our program would like to assist your effort to provide as safe and healthy work environment as possible. I would like to ask you a few questions about your occupational health and safety program and employee exposure to lead, if any.

1. Would you agree to a 10-minute interview now? ___Yes ___No
   1 2

   If NO to Question 1,

Interviewer: If you want information later or wish to contact us, ask for Dr. ____________, Occupational Health Surveillance and Evaluation Program Lead Registry, Berkeley, CA. Tel. (xxx) xxx-xxxx.

Also, for advice on your legal obligations under OSHA for medical monitoring and industrial hygiene measures you can contact:

DOSH Consultation Services
525 Golden Gate Ave.
San Francisco, CA 94101

2. Today's date: __ __/__ __/__ __ Time: __ __:__ __ AM/PM (circle)
   Dy Mo Yr Hr Min

I. Employer Demographics

1. What industry are you engaged in? ________________________________

2. What year did you start operations at ____________? 19 __ __
   street

3. How many workers does this company employ at the ___________ facility? __ __ __ __
   street

Patient No. ___________________ Employer Questionnaire

4. How many workers do you employ in _________ __ __ __ __
(department/building where the index case was employed)?

5. Do the following processes or activities take place at the company? And, if so, how many workers are employed at each operation?

___ 1 Storage battery manufacturing

___ 2 Lead smelting

___ 3 Radiator repair

___ 4 Painting with lead based paints

___ 5 Casting lead, bronze, brass,

___ 6 Ferrous or nonferrous foundry operations

___ 7 Plating with lead-containing materials

___ 8 Gasoline Station

___ 9 Sanding, cutting or welding surfaces that might be painted with leaded paints

___ 10 Cutting or welding sheets, pipes, or constructions made of lead containing metals

___ 11 Manufacture of leaded paints, inks, dyes, glazes or pigments

___ 12 Auto body repair

___ 13 Manufacture of ceramic items

___ 14 Other:_____________________

II. Environmental Monitoring

1. Who would be the best person to contact for information about environmental monitoring programs for lead at this company?

Contact Person First Name |__|__|__|__|__|__|__|__|__|__| M.I. |__|

Last Name |__|__|__|__|__|__|__|__|__|__|__|__|__|__|__|__|__|__|__|__|

Position |__|__|__|__|__|__|__|__|__|__|__|__|__|__|__|__|

Street|__|__|__|__|__|__|__|__|__|__|__|__|__|__|__|__|__|__|__|__|

City |__|__|__|__|__|__|__|__|__|__|__|__|__|__|__|__|

State |__|__| Zip |__|__|__|__|__|

Telephone (__|__|__) |__|__|__| -|__|__|__|__|

2. What kinds of ventilation are used to remove lead fumes or dusts?

Patient No. ____________________ Employer Questionnaire

___none ___hood ___other local exhaust
1 2 3
___ventilation ___other:________________________________
4 system with fans 5

____

3. Has the amount of lead in the air ever been measured at this company? ___Yes ___No
1 2

If NO, "Your establishment may be covered by the OSHA lead standard. If so, you are required to conduct an initial air sampling for lead, and based on those results you may have to implement an industrial hygiene program, including air monitoring, engineering controls, a respirator program for employees, and a medical surveillance program. Private employers may contact, free of charge, DIR Consultation Services at (xxx) xxx-xxxx for technical information about your obligations as an employer under the OSHA standard." Skip to Section III.

4. What year did you start monitoring air for lead? 19 __ __

5. What month and year did you last monitor air for lead? __ __/__ __
Mo Yr

6. Have you ever been told that the lead in the air was above the PEL or action level? ___Yes ___No
1 2

III. Medical Monitoring

1. Does this company have a medical program that routinely measures the levels of lead in the blood of workers who are exposed to lead? ___Yes ___No
1 2

IF NO, "Under the OSHA lead standard, employers are required to establish a medical monitoring program for each worker with exposure to lead above an action level. The medical monitoring program is to be run by the employer's medical supervisor, who, under the OSHA regulation, is required, at a minimum, to provide the following for each eligible employee:

a. an annual physical examination
b. blood tests for lead every 2 months with elevated blood lead levels
c. a repeat blood test within 2 weeks for any blood lead exceeding 40 μg/dl, and then monthly tests until the blood lead is below 40.
d. a recommendation to the employer to remove an employee from lead exposure when any single blood lead test exceeds 60 μg/dl."

If NO, skip to Question 4.

2. What month and year did you last monitor blood leads? __ __/__ __
Mo Yr

3. Have workers ever been medically removed for elevated blood lead? ___Yes ___No
1 2

Patient No. ___________________ Employer Questionnaire

Who is the medical supervisor of this program?

Dr. First Name: |__|__|__|__|__|__|__|__|__|__|__| M.I. |__|

Last Name: |__|__|__|__|__|__|__|__|__|__|__|__|__|__|__|__|__|__|__|__|__|

Position |__|__|__|__|__|__|__|__|__|__|__|__|__|__|__|__|

Street|__|__|__|__|__|__|__|__|__|__|__|__|__|__|__|__|__|__|__|__|

City |__|__|__|__|__|__|__|__|__|__|__|__|__|__|__|__|

State |__|__| Zip |__|__|__|__|__|

Telephone (__|__|__) |__|__|__| -|__|__|__|__|

4. Interviewer: We will be sending you information about the health effects of lead, and employer's obligations under the OSHA lead standard. If you want additional information or wish to contact us, ask for Dr. ______________, Occupational Health Surveillance and Evaluation Program Lead Registry, Berkeley, CA 94704. Tel. (xxx) xxx-xxxx.

Also, for advice on your legal obligations under OSHA for medical monitoring and industrial hygiene measures you can contact:

DOSH Consultation Services
525 Golden Gate Ave.
San Francisco, CA 94101
(xxx) xxx-xxxx

We would like to thank you for your participation.

5. Time (finished) __ __:__ __ AM/PM (circle)
Hr Min

Patient No. ___________________ Physician Questionnaire

PHYSICIAN QUESTIONNAIRE CALIFORNIA LEAD REGISTRY (Adults)
Priority Cases, > 60 (μg/dl)

Interviewer: Hello, my name is _________________________. |__|__|__|
first name last name ID

I am with the Occupational Health Surveillance and Evaluation Program, California Department of Health Services —- the State health department. Since January 1987, California medical laboratories have been required to report the results of blood tests for lead in California residents, whenever the test is higher than 25. We recently received a notice that:

__________________ employed by ____________________________________
Patient name Employer name, Street, City
was reported to have a blood lead level of _______ from a sample taken on ______________ .
date

Our program would like to assist your effort to diagnose and manage lead-related health problems in patients. I would like to ask you a few questions about medical surveillance of lead-exposed workers. We are primarily interested in the extent of potential lead exposure among household contacts and coworkers of persons under your care. We are not an enforcement or regulatory agency, but we can provide technical assistance, if you request. This interview is confidential. Information that is being collected for statistical purposes will not identify you, employers, or patients by name.

1. Would you agree to a 5-minute interview now? ___Yes ___No
1 2

If NO to Question 1,

Interviewer: If you want information later or wish to contact us, ask for Dr. _______________, Occupational Health Surveillance and Evaluation Program Lead Registry, Berkeley, CA 94704. Tel. (xxx) xxx-xxxx.

Also, if you supervise an employer's medical monitoring progam for lead exposures, you can contact the following agencies for advice on your obligations under OSHA for medical monitoring and industrial hygiene measures:

DIR Consultation Services
525 Golden Gate Ave.
San Francisco, CA 94101

(xxx) xxx-xxxx.

Hazard Evaluation System and
Information Service (HESIS)
Berkeley, CA 94704

(xxx) xxx-xxxx

2. Today's date: __ __/__ __/__ __ Time: __ __:__ __ AM/PM (circle)
Dy Mo Yr Hr Min

3. Are you the supervisor for ___________ (employer's) ___Yes ___No
medical program? 1 2

If NO, do you know who is ________ (employer's) medical supervisor?

Patient No. ___________________ Physician Questionnaire

Dr. |__|__|__|__|__|__|__|__|__|__| |__|
First name MI

|__|__|__|__|__|__|__|__|__|__|__|__|__|__|__|__|__|__|__|__|
Last name

Organization |__|__|__|__|__|__|__|__|__|__|__|__|__|__|__|__|

Street|__|__|__|__|__|__|__|__|__|__|__|__|__|__|__|__|__|__|__|__|

City |__|__|__|__|__|__|__|__|__|__|__|__|__|__|__|__|

State |__|__| Zip |__|__|__|__|__|

Telephone (__|__|__) |__|__|__| -|__|__|__|__|

4. Why did you request the blood lead test to be done?

___ Company screening 1 ___Symptomatic patient 2 ___Other:______________ 3

5. How many other workers, if any, employed by _____________(employer) at ____________ (street), __________(city) have you treated for lead-related health problems in the past 12 months? ___ ___

6. Have you made a recommendation to the employer to remove this individual from exposure to lead? ___Yes 1 ___No 2

Interviewer: If NO, "Most clinical authorities recognize that blood levels exceeding 80 μg/dl are immediately injurious, and recommend removal from the source of exposure as part of treatment. Also, under the OSHA lead standard, workers are required to be medically removed from their job when their blood lead levels exceed 50 μg/dl."

7. Have you made a recommendation to the patient's family concerning possible take-home exposures to lead? ___Yes 1 ___No 2

8. Do you know if any of the patient's family also has an elevated blood lead level? ___Yes 1 ___No 2

"Lead on work clothing taken home may cause household contamination. If take-home exposures are a potential concern we recommend that family members be considered for medical follow-up, too."

9. Are you familiar with the procedures for medical monitoring of workers under the OSHA lead standard? ___Yes 1 ___No 2

IF NO, "Under the OSHA lead standard, employers are required to establish a medical monitoring program for each worker with exposure to lead above an action level. The medical monitoring program is to be run by

Patient No. ___________________ Physician Questionnaire

the employer's medical supervisor, who, under the OSHA regulation, is required, at a minimum, to provide the following for each eligible employee:

a. an annual physical examination
b. blood tests for lead every 2 months.
c. a repeat blood test within 2 weeks for any blood lead exceeding 40 μg/dl, and then monthly tests until the blood lead is below 40
d. a recommendation to the employer to remove an employee from lead exposure when any single blood lead test exceeds 60 μg/dl

10. Are you familiar with the reporting program called "Doctor's First Report of Work-Related Illness", which is run by the California Department of Industrial Relations? ___Yes (1) ___No (2)

11. Have you filed a Doctor's First Report for _______ (Employee)? ___Yes (1) ___No (2)

IF NO, "Under the Doctor's First Report program, physicians are legally required to file a form for each case of suspected or proven work-related illness to the California Department of Industrial Relations, or the employer's worker compensation insurance carrier."

Interviewer: We will be sending you some information regarding medical guidelines for lead-exposed workers. If you want additional information or wish to contact us, ask for Dr. ______________, Occupational Health Surveillance and Evaluation Program Lead Registry, Berkeley, CA 94704. Tel. (xxx) xxx-xxxx.

Also, for advice on your obligations under OSHA for medical monitoring and industrial hygiene you can contact:

DOSH Consultation Services
525 Golden Gate Ave., 3rd Floor
San Francisco, CA 94101
(xxx) xxx-xxxx

Hazard Evaluation System and
Information Service (HESIS)
Berkeley, CA
(xxx) xxx-xxxx

* * * Thank you for your participation * * *

12. Time (finished): __ __ (Hr) : __ __ (Min) AM/PM (circle)

Appendix H

Field Investigation: Evaluation of Selected Jobs for Risk Factors for Carpal Tunnel Syndrome and Other Cumulative Trauma Disorders, Food Manufacturing Workers, Santa Clara County

BARBARA A. SILVERSTEIN, DAVID P. REMPEL, AND NEIL A. MAIZLISH

INTRODUCTION

The California Occupational Health Program (COHP) of the California Department of Health Services is working with the National Institute for Occupational Safety and Health (NIOSH) to develop a model program for reporting occupational diseases and investigate ways to prevent them. This program is called Sentinel Event Notification System for Occupational Risks (SENSOR). The model is based on a network of community-based, primary care physicians, and other health care providers who report suspected cases of occupational illness to COHP. COHP then follows up these reports to confirm cases, identify work-related risk factors, and to make recommendations for preventive actions at worksites. Reported work-related risk factors for carpal tunnel syndrome (CTS) include:

1. highly repetitive motions (cycle time less than 30 seconds or repeated series of motions occurring within a work cycle more than 50% of the cycle time)
2. high hand force (10-pound load on the tendons of the wrist). This load may be achieved by holding a 10-pound object. It may also be achieved by holding a much lighter object:
   - in a pinch grip
   - with a flexed or hyperextended wrist
   - with a low coefficient of friction (slippery)
   - that is producing segmental vibration
   - with poor fitting gloves
   - in a cold environment
3. localized external pressure or contact stress on the soft tissues of the wrist and base of the palm

When high force and high repetitiveness are combined in the same job, the risk of CTS has been reported to increase about 4 times as much as when just one of these factors is present, and 16 times as much as when neither of these factors is present.[1]

This site visit was requested by SENSOR to identify work-related risk factors for CTS on jobs where three index cases and symptomatic coworkers worked and were reported to SENSOR. Management and local union representatives accompanied the SENSOR staff to three different work areas where employees may have experienced CTS symptoms.

BACKGROUND

There are approximately 205 hourly and 23 salaried employees at this facility that manufactures two different types of food products. The breakfast food product requires a three-shift operation with relatively constant production and employs 7 machine operators and 10 inspector helpers per shift. The dessert product manufacturing is a two-shift operation, which is somewhat seasonal with the busiest season from May through December. In the lighter season, layoffs last from 1 to 6 months. Although employment figures vary, at the time of our visit, there were approximately 23 machine operators and 46 helper/inspectors in the production area and 8 machine operators and 18 helper/inspectors in the packaging area. Other areas of the plant were not visited. During the busy season, 45–55 hours of work per week are common. The mean plant seniority was reported to be around 5 years although there were a number of workers with more than 25 years seniority. High turnover usually occurs in the first 3 months of employment in this plant. Efforts are made to hire new employees before the busy season starts to facilitate training with a senior worker for about a week for inspection and helper jobs. The plant is currently working with outside consultants to improve their job training program.

According to the Industrial Relations Manager, there has been a health and safety committee in the past but it was not particularly active. They intend to reinstitute the committee and have employee involvement on it. Monthly safety meetings (5–15 minutes) are held with crews on each line to discuss safety rules. Hearing protection is required throughout the plant. The overall plantwide lost time incidence rate was running 15.1 per 200,000 hours. Rates for musculoskeletal disorders in general and carpal tunnel syndrome in particular, were not immediately available. In addition to six workers' compensation cases of carpal tunnel syndrome among inspectors, back and shoulder disorders were viewed as a problem among helpers. The plant has recently changed medical providers and plans to have the providers tour the plant. Additionally, California Division of Workers' Compensation Form RB-90s are being completed by supervisors on all jobs. This information, which includes basic job requirements, will be given to the providers and the Industrial Relations Manager, so that restrictions can be more precisely determined.

METHODS

A brief risk factor checklist was used to facilitate recording observations of the selected jobs. After preliminary discussions with the production manager, steward, and employees, the work was observed and workstation layout measurements obtained (relevant heights and reach distances). Final product weights were ascertained from packages and production rates were obtained from the production manager. Checklists were completed based on observing work activities of several workers for approximately 20–30 minutes per job.

FINDINGS

JOB 1: Breakfast Food Production Inspectors

Production has increased 66% in the last 2 years by increasing the number of cooking irons on the wheel. There has not been a 66% increase in inspectors to handle the increase in production. There are three different inspector jobs in the breakfast food area and workers rotate every hour between these jobs: (*1*) wheel inspector, (*2*) prefreezer inspector, (*3*) stacking inspector. The product is automatically poured into small forming cookers on a large wheel (160 cookers per wheel). The cooker top is automatically opened, and the product is removed by vacuum belt. Occasionally the product sticks to the cooker. The wheel inspector uses an ice pick type tool in the right hand, a cotton gloved left hand, or both to gently remove the product from the cooker top (48 inches high and 24 inch reach) or bottom without damaging the product. Damaged product is tossed aside and undamaged product slides in a chute to the conveyor belt. This picking tends to occur about 40–50 times per minute.

The product moves from one of three wheels by conveyor belt to the fast freeze area. Just prior to entering the freezing unit, two prefreezer inspectors visually inspect the products as they move 6 across a 39-inch wide by 37-inch high conveyor belt at a rate of 822 per minute. This job requires the inspector to check color and irregularities and to remove the defective product before freezing. Additionally, the inspector repositions product if it is bunched up.

The product moves from the freezer via three conveyor lines, through automated stacking machines (manual operation until 5–6 years ago) on their way to being plastic wrapped. Two stacker inspectors wearing cotton gloves, visually inspect and manually reposition some of the 205 stacks of frozen product (4 per stack per minute). The metal rim of the conveyor is approximately 41.5 inches high and the belt is 15 inches wide. The product continues on the conveyor belt (separated in the middle by a metal guard) to the packaging area. Another stacker inspector is positioned before the wrapper machine to move the product from one side of the belt to the other if a backup starts to take place. All of these jobs were performed standing stationary on rubber mats.

Risk Factors for Carpal Tunnel Syndrome and Other Cumulative Trauma Disorders

Risk factors observed in these jobs included:

1. Very high repetitiveness due to line speed. Although handling was not required for each product as it went by on the conveyor or wheel, inspectors' hands were in continual motion to be ready to remove defective products or reposition them. The delicacy required to reposition product and prevent damage, increases the load on the entire upper limb in order to have maximum control of finger motion. This increases localized fatigue. Rotation between the inspector jobs probably does little to reduce the repetitive load on the hands because in all of these jobs, the fingers are in constant motion.
2. Localized contact stresses against the palmar side of the wrist and forearm, particularly in the prefreezer and stacker inspection jobs, caused by the

hard metal edges of the conveyor guard when the inspector supported the arm on the edge to stabilize the position.

3. Awkward postures were required in several jobs. The wheel inspector used an ice pick type tool to remove the product from the top of the cooker, a 24-inch horizontal reach at approximately 46 inches from the floor. This is above shoulder height for the smallest 5% of the female work force. The horizontal reach distance is greater than the shoulder-grip distance for 50% of the female work force. Because this is a repetitive task, excessive stress is being placed on the shoulder. Using the in-line pick to carefully remove the product requires a severely bent wrist to flick the product off and into the chute or disposal bin. The gloved left hand lightly pinches the product and also is bent when discarding damaged product.

Conveyor heights on the other inspector jobs were similar but the reach distance was not as great (approximately 15–18 inches). Discarding damaged product required wrist flexion by the prefreezer inspector whereas repositioning of the warm delicate product required light pinching with cotton-gloved hands. The prewrapper inspector used repetitive wrist flexion and light pinching when transferring stacks of product from one side of the conveyor to the other over a 4-inch high by 1/4-inch thick metal divider.

Recommendations

1. Increase rest allowances or the number of inspectors to reduce the repetitiveness of these jobs. Rotation between them is probably good to reduce some of the visual demands of these jobs but it is not a particularly useful strategy for reducing repetitiveness because all of these inspector jobs require rapid hand–wrist activity, particularly of the flexor tendons. Job enlargement may also decrease the repetitiveness by increasing the number of different tasks the inspector does (such as cleaning, some machine adjustments, etc.).
2. Use light-weight but sturdy platforms for shorter workers to reduce shoulder flexion. Providing adjustability in platform height would accommodate most workers.
3. Use a T-bar handle or ball-shaped handle with a hook at the end of a longer pick to reduce reach distance, ulnar deviation, and the need for wrist flexion when removing product in the wheel inspector job.
4. Cover the conveyor guards with compressible material where inspectors are working to reduce contact stresses when the inspectors use the guards to rest and stabilize their arms and wrists. Another alternative would be to flange the edges to provide a wider surface area for resting the arms.
5. Provide sit–stand stools to reduce the static loading and postural fatigue associated with standing stationary for long periods of time.

Operators on the automatic wrapping machines were observed loading 35-pound plastic wrap rolls (16-inch long by 10.5-inch diameter) onto shafts located 66 inches from floor level. This is above the shoulder height of 95% of the male work force. Although they do this infrequently, once every 1.75 hours, there is a risk for both back and shoulder strain. This risk could be reduced by using a mechanical lever to lower and raise the shaft for loading.

The cartoning machine operator was observed loading large stacks of prescored small cartons into the machine from boxes (131 boxes per day, 49,320 cartons). The operator uses an extended pinch grip to grasp as many cartons as possible at one time. This method requires high pinch force. Operator training should include placing smaller quantities of cartons at any one time. Training should also include ways to get to the other side of the machine without climbing over a moving conveyor.

JOB 2: Dessert Food Production Inspectors

There are four lines in this department. Although there have been no major process changes over the last 9 years, production has been increasing in the last 5 years. Plans are under way to automate the material flow process between production through freezing and into packaging. In the meantime, some of the product is transferred via 16-tray metal racks with sharp edged lips. The bottom row is 10 inches from the floor. Approximately five trays are below knee height and five trays are at or above shoulder height. The product ranges from 26 to 47 oz., depending on size. The inspector visually inspects the product as it passes on the conveyor belt (at 42 products per minute). The inspector adds or removes components as necessary and discards damaged product. One inspector forms or manually presses the top of the product. Other inspectors tear down the product if it doesn't meet specifications and puts the components into separate bins. The endline inspector places two products at a time on the racks for transport to the freezer. It is anticipated that this racking will be eliminated with the automated system. However, even with the automated system, some racking will be required as a buffer for system overflow. Most of the conveyor lines are about 38 inches high. In some areas, metal platforms are provided for the inspectors. Inspectors rotate on these lines.

Carpal Tunnel Syndrome Risk Factors

Risk factors observed on these inspector jobs include:

1. Repetitiveness. The product is manually manipulated by an inspector approximately 20,000 times per 8-hour shift. Some inspectors work up to 14–16 hours a day during the busy season.
2. Contact stress on the backs and sides of the fingers during racking due to the thin metal lip on the edge of the trays.
3. Awkward postures during rack loading and off-loading. This is particularly a problem when the full racks are being loaded or off-loaded because wrist extension or flexion is required for lower and higher trays, as is shoulder flexion for higher trays and back flexion for low trays. The racking operation requires the inspector to use either a pinch grip with ulnar deviation to hold the edge of the product (pinching a 2–3-pound part requires as much force as gripping an 8–12 pound part), or full supination of the forearm with wrist flexion–extension to hold the product in the palm of the hand. The endline inspector must continually twist to the side to load the racks. This twisting increases the risk of low back pain. This inspector is also exposed to cold from the nearby freezer. The inspectors racking as part of a buffer for the line are required to flex their backs as they lean over the conveyor to load or unload product to the belt.

Recommendations

1. Use only the middle trays in the loading and off-loading operations to reduce awkward shoulder and back postures. For those racks used in buffering the overflow or underflow of products, (stationary), consider using spring-loaded tray devices (with adequate spacing to prevent crushing the product) to reduce awkward postures.
2. Increase rest allowances or increase the number of inspectors to reduce the repetitiveness of these jobs. Rotation between inspectors is probably good to reduce some of the visual demands of these jobs but it is not a particularly useful strategy for reducing repetitiveness because all of these inspector jobs require rapid hand–wrist activity, particularly of the flexor tendons. Job enlargement may also decrease the repetitiveness by increasing the number of different tasks the inspector does (such as cleaning, some machine adjustments, etc.).
3. Pad the edges of the metal rack trays to reduce contact stresses against the backs and sides of the fingers as well as the wrists.
4. Provide sit–stand stools to reduce postural fatigue due to stationary standing.

JOB 3: Dessert Food Packaging Inspectors

Helpers push the product racks from the freezer to the packaging conveyor belts. Inspectors, wearing cotton gloves, remove two frozen products at a time from the racks to the conveyor belt for packaging at a rate of 40–42 per minute per inspector. These inspectors rotate with an indexer inspector who repositions product just before it goes into cartoning and packing. For one line, the product is transported from the freezer via conveyor rather than by tray racks. Although this appears to be a superior method that is planned for both lines, it does not eliminate all racking. After boxing the product, a helper loads the boxes (6 products/box) onto a pallet for storing and shipping.

Carpal Tunnel Syndrome Risk Factors

Risk factors observed in these jobs include:

1. Highly repetitive use of the hands and wrists to off-load product (more than 20,000 per 8-hour shift). Even when the product was automatically transferred to the packing line, the buffering (for over or underloading the line) required racking and unracking 24–50 products per minute.
2. Contact stress against the wrists, and backs and sides of the fingers due to the sharp metal lip on the cold trays.
3. Forceful finger pinches when removing the frozen product from and to the trays on the rack.
4. Cold exposure to the hands and wrists due to handling frozen product and coming in contact with the cold trays.
5. Awkward postures including wrist flexion and extension with a pinch grip while loading and offloading the product from the trays. For inspectors doing the manual transfer, severe back flexion and shoulder flexion are required when handling product from the top five and bottom five trays.

Recommendations

1. Increase rest allowances or increase the number of inspectors to reduce the repetitiveness of these jobs. Rotation between inspector jobs is probably good to reduce some of the visual demands of these jobs but it is not a particularly useful strategy for reducing repetitiveness because all of these inspector jobs require rapid hand–wrist activity, particularly of the flexor tendons. Job enlargement may also decrease the repetitiveness by increasing the number of different tasks the inspector does (such as cleaning, some machine adjustments, etc.).
2. Automate the transfer process as planned. Provide spring-loaded tray devices for the buffering of excess or reduced product on the packing line. Consider using slides from the tray to the conveyor belt so the product can be pawed rather than requiring a pinch grip. This would reduce both forceful and awkward postures.
3. Provide swivel sit–stand stools so the inspector can turn in the stool rather than the torso to off-load, and thus relieve postural loading on the spine.
4. Provide a better insulated glove (not necessarily thicker because it would reduce sensory feedback from the fingers and increase force requirements).

In passing, the manual palletizing operation at the end of the packaging line was observed. The helper manually transfers a 9" × 18" × 9" 12-pound box to the pallet every 15 seconds. The pallet holds 10 boxes per 7 rows. The horizontal and vertical locations of extreme lifts may put this job above the action limit for the NIOSH Work Practices Guidelines for Manual Materials Handling.[2] The repetitive severe forward bending is a known risk factor for low back pain.

GENERAL RECOMMENDATIONS

1. Training is an integral component of any program that wants to create change. Supervisory and employee training in work methods, ergonomic awareness, the goals of job modification, etc. are crucial. When new employees enter the area where adjustability has been built in, orientation to the use of equipment and proper adjustment should be integrated into other job training.
2. If new equipment or work methods are to be implemented, employee input into requirements, and testing of the equipment in pilot stages will minimize expense in purchasing unnecessary or uncomfortable equipment, and facilitate implementation.
3. When implementing job or layout modifications, a formalized follow-up process should be instituted to determine whether (*1*) the change reduced the problem and (*2*) the change did not create a new problem. Pre–post discomfort ratings for each body area by employees is one way to accomplish this.[3]
4. In general, inclusion of department and job on daily first aid or medical logs of those with cumulative trauma disorder symptoms can assist the health care providers in identifying problem areas (musculoskeletal as well as other unrelated problems) and follow trends over time to see if any of the programs that are instituted have a positive or negative health effect.
5. A summary of this report, and any action plans or recommendations that are developed by the facility after this report, should be distributed to participating supervisors, and employees and their representatives so they can know what is happening and can contribute to overall plans for change in this area.

CONCLUSIONS

The brief evaluation of inspector jobs in three areas of the plant indicated that there were risk factors present, including highly repetitive hand and wrist motions, awkward postures, contact stresses in all of these jobs and high pinch force in racking activities that can contribute to the development or exacerbation of CTS and other upper extremity disorders. Additionally, stressful back and shoulder postures associated with stooping or reaching were observed. These job specific risk factors are described in the body of this report. Although it may not always be possible to eliminate all risk factors completely, the more of them that are eliminated or reduced, the better the probability of controlling work-related CTS. If nothing is done, CTS will be a continuing and probably increasing problem in this facility. It is commendable that the facility is taking an active role in dealing with these problems by working with the health care provider to characterize job requirements for all jobs. Providers will then have a catalog of job requirements in their offices. This will enhance the medical management component of dealing with these risk factors.

Institution of a local health and safety committee should proceed rapidly, and this committee needs to take an active role in facilitating the recommendations contained in this report. Information obtained from this site visit will be pooled with information from other facilities to form broader conclusions and recommendations. No site specific identifiers will be used in full technical reports.

ACKNOWLEDGMENTS

This report was prepared under a grant from the National Institute for Occupational Safety and Health by the California Occupational Health Program. *Evaluation of Selected Jobs for Risk Factors for Carpal Tunnel Syndrome & Other Cumulative Trauma Disorders, Food Manufacturing Workers, Santa Clara County.* Surveillance Report CDHS(COHP) SR89-002-3. Berkeley: California Department of Health Services, 1989.

REFERENCES

1. Silverstein BA, Fine LJ, Armstrong TJ. Occupational factors and carpal tunnel syndrome. *Am J Ind Med* 1987; 11:343–358.
2. Chaffin DB. Manual material handling and the biomechanical basis for prevention of low-back pain in industry—an overview. *Am Ind Hygiene J* 1987; 48:989–996.
3. Silverstein BA, Armstrong TJ, Longmate A, Woody D. Can in-plant exercise control musculoskeletal symptoms? *J Occup Med* 1988; 30:922–927.

Appendix I

Recommended Medical Screening Protocol for Workers Exposed to Occupational Allergens

KENNETH D. ROSENMAN

There are no legal requirements to perform medical surveillance on individuals exposed to occupational allergens (see Table I.1 for list of common workplace allergens). The Michigan Occupational Safety and Health Administration's (MIOSHA) Respiratory Protection Standard 1910.34 (e) (1) states that the employer shall provide a medical evaluation to determine the employee's ability to use a respirator before the employee is fit tested or required to use the respirator in the workplace.

Annual medical examinations for individuals who are potentially exposed to occupational allergens is good medical practice. It has been well-documented that the longer an individual remains exposed to an occupational allergen that he or she has become sensitized to, the more likely that he or she will have persistent breathing problems even after exposure has ended (see Table I.2 for abstracts of relevant articles from medical literature). The purpose then of an annual medical screening is to identify symptomatic individuals and remove them from exposure so as to reduce the likelihood of causing a chronic disability.

Studies in the medical literature do not support excluding individuals with an allergic disposition (family or personal history) or cigarette smokers identified in a preemployment physical, from working around occupational allergens. The dose that an individual inhales from both usual daily exposure and nonroutine heavy exposures from spills is the best predictor of who will become symptomatic.

Accordingly, medical surveillance is *not* a substitute for good dust and chemical control in the workplace. Controlling exposure is the only effective primary prevention strategy.

PROTOCOL

1. Questionnaire—A standardized questionnaire should be administered during a preemployment physical to obtain a baseline, and on an annual basis. Since the symptoms from occupational allergens can be intermittent particularly when they first begin, the person may have a completely normal physical examination and breathing test and still be having severe attacks of asthma. Key questions that should be included in an annual examination are shown in Table I.3.
2. Physical examination—A physical examination with particular attention to the skin, head, eyes, ears, nose, throat, and lungs should be performed preemployment as a baseline, and on an annual basis.
3. Pulmonary function testing should be done as a baseline and annually. All pulmonary function testing should use equipment and follow the protocol of the American Thoracic Society.[1] The technician administering the test should have completed an accredited training course such as those approved by the National Institute of Occupational Safety and Health.

It is important not only to evaluate the latest pulmonary function test as to whether it is normal or abnormal, but also to observe excessive loss between successive years. Studies on isocyanate exposure have suggested excessive loss (>25–35 ml per year) as a po-

[1] American Thoracic Society. Standardization of Spirometry—1994 Update. American Journal of Respiratory and Critical Care Medicine 1995; 152:1107–1136.

Table I.1 Examples of Agents Capable of Causing Occupational Asthma

Natural Products	
Vegetable gums	Orris root
Flax seed	Flour
Castor bean	Papain
Soybean	Mushroom dust and moldy compost
Natural glues	Wood dusts
Animal danders and other animal antigens	Natural resins
Coffee bean	Animal fat, oil, and products
Insect debris	Fish meal and emulsions
Detergent enzymes	Tobacco dust
Grain dusts and grain products	Pancreatic extracts

Synthetics	
INORGANIC	PHARMACEUTICALS
Platinum, complex salts	Psyllium
Nickel salts	Penicillin
Chromium salts	Ampicillin
Sodium and potasium	Spiramycin
Persulphates	Phenylglycine acid chloride
ORGANIC	Sulphathiasole
Diisocyanates	Bromelin
Toulene	Amprolium hydrochloride
Diphenylmethane	Sulphone choloramides
Hexamethylene	Tetracycline
Anhydrides	MISCELLANEOUS
Phthalic	Formaldehyde
Tetrachlorophthallic	Piperazine
Trimellitic	Organophosphorus insecticides
Amines	Pyrolysis products of polyvinyl chloride
Aminoethyl	Alkylaryl polyether alcohol
Ethanolamine	Tartrazine
Dimethyl ethanolamine	Products of heated adhesives
Ethylene diamine	
Paraphenylenediamine	
Diethylene triamine	
Diethylene tetramine	

tential adverse effect, even in the absence of symptoms of asthma.

Individuals who are suspected to have occupational asthma should have the diagnosis confirmed by pre- and postshift or midshift (depending when the individual becomes symptomatic) pulmonary function testing or measurement of peak flow every 2 hours over a 2-week period with a portable peak flow meter. Sufficient time off work (2 weeks or more) may be necessary to allow recovery and documentation by peak flow measurements.

Individuals with confirmed occupational asthma should, whenever possible, be given the option of transfer to areas of nonexposure. Sensitized individuals may react at extremely low levels of exposure. In order for this transfer option to be a realistic alternative, the individuals should be able to maintain his or her pay rate at the new job.

All individuals should be strongly advised to stop smoking. Some investigations have suggested that smokers given similar levels of exposure will develop occupational asthma in a shorter period than will nonsmokers.

Table I.2 Annotated References

1. Yassi A. Occupational Health Program, University of Manitoba, Winnipeg, Canada. Health and socioeconomic consequences of occupational respiratory allergies: a pilot study using workers' compensation data. *Am J Ind Med* 1988; 14(3):291–298.

Growing evidence suggests that individuals with occupational allergies have long-term health and employment problems. Workers' compensation claims for allergic respiratory disease allowed in Ontario 1975–1981 were reviewed for demographic, risk factor, and exposure data. Diagnoses listed in these 244 claims were reassessed for consistency with criteria for occupational respiratory allergies. Twenty-eight percent of the 154 claimants who met the criteria were granted a permanent disability award from the workers' compensation board (WCB). In response to a questionnaire mailed 2–8 years after claim allowance, 77% of those traced reported improvement, but 59% still required medication and 85% still suffered symptoms. Seventy-six percent of claimants left their employers. Seventy-five percent of those who left did so because of their allergic condition; 95% suffered long-term income loss. The unemployment rate for this cohort was 36%, well above that for the general population. Older workers with longer duration of symptoms and longer duration of exposure prior to the claim had the worst prognoses. The data were consistent with previous studies in suggesting that occupational respiratory allergies may result in serious health and socioeconomic consequences. Exploring the feasibility, acceptability, and potential usefulness of WCB data, it is suggested that this source merits further consideration for both descriptive as well as prognostic studies.

2. Mapp CE, Corona PC, De Marzo N, Fabbri L. Institute of Occupational Medicine, University of Padova, Italy. Persistent asthma due to isocyanates. A follow-up study of subjects with occupational asthma due to toluene diisocyanate (TDI). *Am Rev Resp Dis* 1988 Jun; 137(6):1326–1329.

Thirty-five subjects with occupational asthma due to toluene diisocyanate (TDI) exposure were examined. All the subjects were studied with inhalation challenges with TDI and with methacholine. Toluene diisocyanate asthma was documented by a positive inhalation challenge to low levels of TDI. Airway responsiveness to methacholine was in the range of asthmatic patients at the time of diagnosis. After an average follow-up interval of 10 months, all the subjects were reexamined. Of the 35 subjects examined, 30 subjects (85.7%) left the workplace, and 5 remained in the same job. Twenty-seven subjects (77.1%) continued to have asthmatic attacks requiring medication for relief of symptoms. At follow-up examination, TDI asthma was documented by a positive inhalation challenge to TDI in 27 subjects. Of these 27 TDI reactors, 22 subjects were removed from occupational exposure to TDI. The TDI reactors had persistent respiratory symptoms and airway hyperresponsiveness to methacholine. At follow-up visit, 8 subjects (22.9%) lost sensitization to TDI; 5 subjects (62.5%) in this group also had normal airway responsiveness to methacholine after removal from exposure. Only 1 subject among the TDI nonreactors complained of mild respiratory symptoms. At diagnosis, there were no significant differences between subjects who recovered and those who did not with regard to age, smoking habits, atopy, duration of exposure to isocyanates, duration of symptoms, baseline FEV_1 (% pred), and baseline airway responsiveness to methacholine.

3. Malo JL, Cartier A, Ghezzo H, Lafrance M, McCants M, Lehrer SB. Department of Chest Medicine, Hopital du Sacre-Coeur, Montreal, Canada. Patterns of improvement in spirometry, bronchial hyperresponsiveness, and specific IgE antibody levels after cessation of exposure in occupational asthma caused by snow-crab processing. *Am Rev Resp Dis* 1988 Oct; 138(4):807–812.

Thirty-one workers with occupational asthma caused by snow-crab processing were assessed by a long-term follow-up on three occasions at mean ± SD intervals of 12.8 ± 5.4, 31.4 ± 6.3, and 64.4 ± 6.3 months after leaving work. The diagnosis of work-related asthma was initially confirmed in all of them by specific inhalation challenges at the workplace or by laboratory inhalation of snow-crab boiling water ($N = 24$) or by serial monitoring of airway caliber and bronchial responsiveness to histamine at work and off work ($N = 7$). Total duration of work-related exposure was 12.8 ± 5.6 months (range, 3–21 months), and the duration of symptoms after onset was 6.8 ± 4.2 months (range, 1–18 months). At the time of diagnosis, all 31 subjects required medication for asthma, 11 had a FEV_1 less than or equal to 85% predicted, and all subjects had a PC20 less than or equal to 16 mg/ml. Twelve of 25 serum samples assessed showed high levels of specific immunoglobulin E (IgE) antibodies to crab meat, boiling water, or both. At the time of the first follow-up, there was a reduction in the number of subjects still requiring medication, with a significant reduction in FEV_1, and a PC_{20} less than or equal to 16 mg/mL. However, no further change was observed afterwards. Similarly, the mean FEV_1 and FEV_1/FVC improved significantly from the time of diagnosis to the first follow-up ($p < 0.01$), with a plateau thereafter.

4. Chan-Yeung M. Evaluation of impairment/disability in patients with occupational asthma. *Am Rev Resp Dis* 1987 Apr; 135(4):950–951.

Contrary to popular belief, patients with documented occupational asthma do not necessarily recover completely after removal from exposure. Several follow-up studies (1–7) of patients with occupational asthma because of a variety of agents show that the majority of patients continue to have persistent asthma of varying severity months or years after the cessation of exposure (Table I.1). The persistence of symptoms is accompanied by the presence of nonspecific bronchial hyperresponsiveness as documented by methacholine or histamine inhalation test (2–7). As these patients did not have asthma before they entered the industry and had documented specific reaction to the sensitizing agents, it is fair to assume that their persistent asthma is the result of occupational exposure.

Table I-3 Questions to Be Included in an Annual Medical Exam for Workers Exposed to Occupational Allergens

RECENT MEDICAL HISTORY

1. Do you consider yourself to be in good health?

   ❑ Yes (1) ❑ No (2)

   If no, state reason: ____________________

CHEST COLDS AND CHEST ILLNESSES

2. If you get a cold, does it usually go to your chest? (Usually means more than 1/2 the time).

   ❑ Yes (1) ❑ No (2) ❑ Do no get colds (3)

3. During the past year, have you had any chest illnesses that have kept you off work, indoors at home, or in bed?

   ❑ Yes (1) ❑ No (2)

   If YES to 3:

   A. Did you produce phlegm or mucus with any of these chest illnesses?

      ❑ Yes (1) ❑ No (2) ❑ Did not have chest illness (3)

   B. In the past year, how many such illnesses with phlegm or mucus did you have that lasted a week or more? Number of illnesses ______

MEDICAL HISTORY

4. In the past year have you had:

			If yes, describe
Asthma	❑ Yes (1)	❑ No (2)	____________
Bronchitis	❑ Yes (1)	❑ No (2)	____________
Hay fever	❑ Yes (1)	❑ No (2)	____________
Other allergies	❑ Yes (1)	❑ No (2)	____________
Pneumonia	❑ Yes (1)	❑ No (2)	____________
Tuberculosis	❑ Yes (1)	❑ No (2)	____________
Chest surgery	❑ Yes (1)	❑ No (2)	____________
Other lung problems	❑ Yes (1)	❑ No (2)	____________

WHEEZING

5. Does your chest ever sound wheezy or whistling:

A. When you have a cold?	❑ Yes (1)	❑ No (2)
B. Occasionally apart from colds?	❑ Yes (1)	❑ No (2)
C. Most days or night?	❑ Yes (1)	❑ No (2)

   IF YES to A, B, or C:

   1. For how many years has this been present? Number of years ___________

6. Have you ever had an attack of wheezing that has made you feel short of breath?

❑ Yes (1) ❑ No (2)

IF YES to 6:

A. How old were you when you had your first such attack? Age in years _____

B. Have you had 2 or more such episodes?

❑ Yes (1) ❑ No (2)

C. Have you required medicine or treatment for these attacks?

❑ Yes (1) ❑ No (2)

D. Is there a chemical substance or job at work that you think causes these attacks?

❑ Yes (1) ❑ No (2)

If yes, describe: ______________________________________

7. Do you bring up phlegm or mucus most days of the week (4 out of 7) for a period of 3 months straight (count phlegm or mucus with first smoke or on first going out-of-doors, don't count phlegm or mucus from your nose).

❑ Yes (1) ❑ No (2)

IF YES to 7:

A. How many years have you brought up phlegm or mucus? Number of years _____

CIGARETTE SMOKING

8. Do you smoke cigarettes? ❑ Yes (1) ❑ No (2)

IF YES to 8:

A. How many packs of cigarettes do you smoke each day? Number of packs: _____

Index